Clinical Psychiatry: Placebo and Nocebo Effects

Clinical Psychiatry: Placebo and Nocebo Effects

Editor: Rosio Allan

AMERICAN
MEDICAL PUBLISHERS
www.americanmedicalpublishers.com

AMERICAN
MEDICAL PUBLISHERS
www.americanmedicalpublishers.com

Cataloging-in-Publication Data

Clinical psychiatry : placebo and nocebo effects / edited by Rosio Allan.
p. cm.
Includes bibliographical references and index.
ISBN 979-8-88740-007-5
1. Clinical psychology. 2. Psychiatry. 3. Placebos (Medicine). 4. Nocebos (Medicine).
5. Medicine and psychology. I. Allan, Rosio.
RC467 .C55 2023
616.89--dc23

American Medical Publishers,
41 Flatbush Avenue,
1st Floor, New York,
NY 11217, USA

ISBN 979-8-88740-007-5 (Hardback)

Contents

Preface

Every book is a source of knowledge and this one is no exception. The idea that led to the conceptualization of this book was the fact that the world is advancing rapidly; which makes it crucial to document the progress in every field. I am aware that a lot of data is already available, yet, there is a lot more to learn. Hence, I accepted the responsibility of editing this book and contributing my knowledge to the community.

A placebo is anything that looks like a real medical treatment but is not, in reality. Placebos are medical substances that improve the health status of the person due to the patient's belief that the substance is indeed effective. The opposite of the placebo effect is the nocebo effect. A nocebo is a medical substance with no medical effects that worsens the health status of the person due to the patient's negative beliefs and expectations. In psychiatry, the placebo effect plays a significant role in the majority of mental disorders, including depression, anxiety, addictions, and schizophrenia. A few prominent symptoms of nocebo effect are nausea, itching, bloating and sleeping issues. This book is a compilation of the works of various international experts carrying out research with respect to placebos and nocebo, and their significance in clinical psychiatry. It is a vital tool for all researching or studying placebo and nocebo effects.

While editing this book, I had multiple visions for it. Then I finally narrowed down to make every chapter a sole standing text explaining a particular topic, so that they can be used independently. However, the umbrella subject sinews them into a common theme. This makes the book a unique platform of knowledge.

I would like to give the major credit of this book to the experts from every corner of the world, who took the time to share their expertise with us. Also, I owe the completion of this book to the never-ending support of my family, who supported me throughout the project.

Editor

1

Effects of Placebo Interventions on Subjective and Objective Markers of Appetite

Verena Hoffmann [1], Marina Lanz [1], Jennifer Mackert [1], Timo Müller [2,3], Matthias Tschöp [2,3] and Karin Meissner [1,4]**

[1] Institute of Medical Psychology, Faculty of Medicine, LMU Munich, Munich, Germany, [2] Helmholtz Diabetes Center, Helmholtz Zentrum München, German Research Center for Environmental Health (GmbH), Munich, Germany, [3] German Center for Diabetes Research (DZD), Garching bei München, Germany, [4] Division of Health Promotion, Coburg University of Applied Sciences, Coburg, Germany

Correspondence:
Verena Hoffmann
verena.hoffmann@med.lmu.de
Karin Meissner
karin.meissner@med.lmu.de

Objective: Patients' expectations about the benefit of an intervention are important determinants of the placebo effect. Little is known about the extent to which expectations influence outcomes of treatments in the field of appetite regulation. This study aimed to investigate the effects of treatment-related expectations on subjective and objective markers of appetite.

Methods: 90 healthy participants of normal weight were randomly allocated to either an appetite-enhancing placebo group, a satiety-enhancing placebo group, or a control group. All participants received a placebo capsule along with group-specific verbal suggestions to either be appetite-promoting, or satiety-enhancing, or to have no effect on appetite. Before and during the 2 h following randomization, participants were repeatedly asked to rate feelings of hunger and satiety on visual analog scales (VAS), and blood samples were taken repeatedly to assess plasma ghrelin levels as a physiological marker of hunger.

Results: In comparison to the control group, the satiety-enhancing placebo intervention significantly reduced appetite and increased satiety. The appetite-enhancing placebo intervention did not alter subjective levels of hunger, but increased plasma ghrelin levels in females.

Conclusions: Results provide the first experimental evidence that appetite-regulating placebo interventions can elicit a psychobiological response. Expectations are important factors to consider when evaluating the effects of interventions in the field of appetite regulation.

Keywords: placebo effect, expectation, appetite, satiety, ghrelin

INTRODUCTION

Obesity is a dramatically increasing problem in our society. Treatment approaches for obesity include psychological, pharmacological, and surgical interventions (1–3). To what extent placebo effects, i.e. positive treatment expectations, contribute to the success of obesity treatments is unclear. A recent systematic review of placebo-controlled surgery trials revealed that patients receiving sham bariatric surgery showed on average 71% of the weight loss reported by the patients in the active surgery groups (4). These data suggest a strong inhibitory effect of placebo interventions on appetite.

Eating behavior is closely linked to mental sets. For example, Higgs (5) reported that participants consumed less in a test session when they were reminded of a recent meal. Furthermore, Provencher et al. (6) showed that participants ate less when the meal was perceived as healthy. Crum and colleagues went one step further and evaluated the impact of expectations on plasma levels of the gut hormone ghrelin, a physiological marker of appetite (7). In a within-subjects design, healthy volunteers on two occasions were made believe to receive either a "high-caloric, indulgent milk shake" or a "low-caloric, sensitive milk shake." In truth, both milk shakes were of identical contents. Results showed a different ghrelin response to these milk shakes: In comparison to the "sensible" shake, the ghrelin increase was larger when expecting the "indulgent" milk shake, followed by a sharper decline of ghrelin levels 30 min after drinking the shake. These findings indicate a strong impact of nutrition-specific expectations on appetite and satiety, as evidenced by altered plasma ghrelin levels before and after a test meal. Additionally, differences in eating behavior are linked to gender. Several studies have shown that females tend to eat healthier than men [i.e., avoiding high-fat food and eating more fruit and fiber; (8, 9)]. This has been linked to more concerns of women about their body weight as compared to men (10). Also, it has been reported, that females eat more sweets when perceiving stress than men (11).

In this study, we investigated whether treatment-related expectations can affect appetite, satiety and plasma ghrelin levels. In a between-subjects design, normal-weight participants received a placebo capsule together with the information that its content would either increase appetite, or increase satiety, or would leave appetite and satiety unaffected. We hypothesized that the appetite-enhancing placebo intervention would decrease satiety and increase appetite and plasma ghrelin levels, while the satiety-enhancing placebo intervention would have the opposite effects, both in comparison to a no treatment control group.

MATERIALS AND METHODS

Participants

The study was conducted at the Institute of Medical Psychology at the LMU Munich, Germany. Healthy participants aged 18–36 years were recruited via flyers and a university mailing list. All participants had to be of normal weight (Body Mass Index (BMI) 18–25 kg/m^2). Exclusion criteria included report of pregnancy, breastfeeding, regular use of medication (except hormonal contraceptives and anti-allergic drugs), acute or chronic disease, smoking, surgery in the last 4 weeks before the experiment, elevated fasting blood glucose levels (>100 mg/dl), and elevated levels of anxiety and/or depression scores [>7 in at least one subscale of the Hospital Anxiety and Depression Scale (HADS); (12)]. The study protocol was approved by the ethics committee of the Medical Faculty at LMU Munich. Participants provided written informed consent and received 45 Euro compensation.

Experimental Procedure

Ninty participants were randomly allocated to one of three groups: "control," "enhanced appetite" (placebo), or "enhanced satiety" (placebo). To allow for double-blinding, 6 additional participants were randomized to verum treatments (3 enhanced appetite, 3 enhanced satiety; compare (13); **Figure 1**). Groups were stratified by sex due to sex differences in eating behavior (14) and neurobiological mechanisms of placebo effects (15). At recruitment, participants were informed that the experiment investigated how biological and psychological factors contribute to the regulation of hunger and appetite.

Participants underwent a single test session starting at 8 o'clock in the morning. They were asked to abstain from food for 10–12 h prior to the experiment (intake of small amounts of water was allowed). Upon arrival, participants took seat in a comfortable chair, and blood glucose levels were determined from finger blood samples using a BG Star device (Sanofi-Aventis, Hannover, Germany). An indwelling flexible catheter was then placed in the antecubital vein and kept patent with a saline infusion to allow for repeated blood drawing during the experiment. Electrodes to measure the electrocardiogram (ECG) were attached. Participants were then asked to fill in the "Hospital Anxiety and Depression Scale" [HADS; (12)], the 'Three Factor Eating Questionnaire' [TFEQ; (16)] and to rate current levels of hunger and satiety on 100-mm visual analog scales (VAS). Thereafter, the first blood sample to assess ghrelin levels was collected and the ECG measurement was started. Following a 15-min baseline period, the experimenter opened the randomization envelope, performed the verbal expectancy manipulation according to group allocation ("appetite increase," "satiety increase," or "control") and asked the participants to swallow the provided test capsule with 100 ml of mineral water (standardized temperature of 20°C). After resting periods of 30 and 60 min, respectively, participants were asked to rate current levels of hunger and satiety, and the second and third blood sample for ghrelin assessments were collected.

Blinding and Randomization

A person not directly involved in the experiments prepared an opaque, sequentially-numbered randomization envelope for each participant according to a computer-generated randomization list. The envelopes contained information on the type of intervention ("appetite-stimulating," "satiety-enhancing," or "control") as well as a test capsule. Neither the experimenter nor the participants were informed whether the capsule in the hunger-enhancing and satiety-enhancing conditions was a placebo or contained an active ingredient (double-blinded design).

Capsules

Identical white and opaque vegetarian capsules were used for all interventions. The placebo capsules were filled with lactose (Heirler Cenovis GmbH, Radolfzell, Germany). For the satiety-increasing active intervention, capsules were filled with an alginate complex (lyophilized sodium-alginate complex, added with aluminum- and calciumchoride; CM3 Alginat Kapseln, Easyway GmbH, Monheim, Germany). Alginate reduces hunger

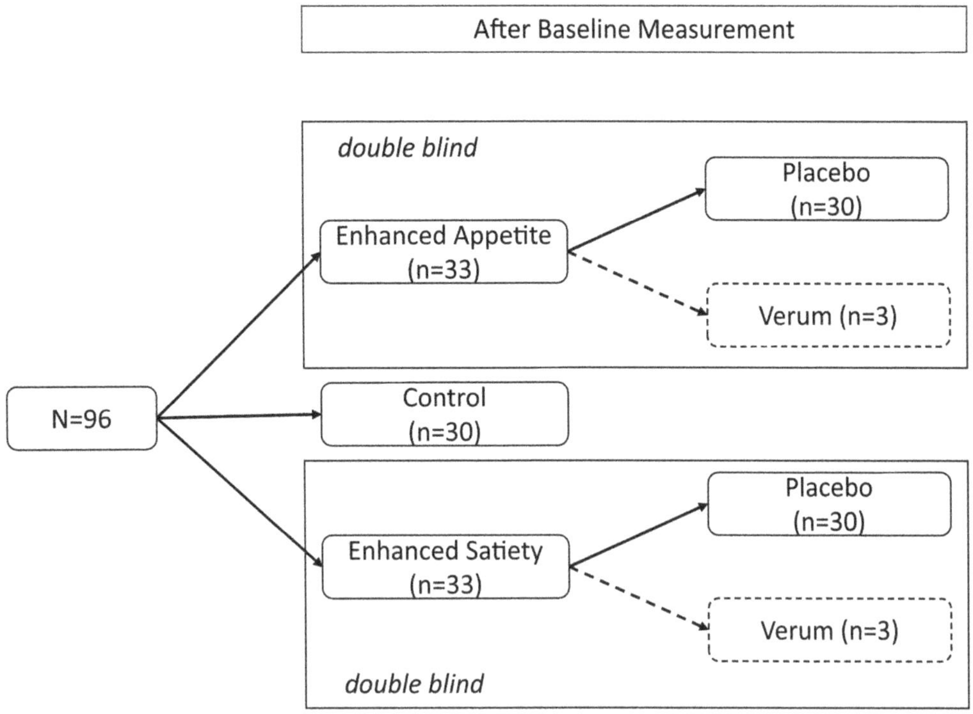

FIGURE 1 | Study design. This randomized, double-blind, controlled trial was conducted in a between-subject design. After the baseline measurement, participants were randomly allocated to one of five groups ("control," "placebo enhanced appetite," "placebo enhanced satiety," "verum enhanced appetite," and "verum enhanced satiety"). The verum groups served only for double-blinding and were not evaluated further.

and increases satiety feelings, which is partly due to its volume-increasing content (17). For the appetite-stimulating active intervention, one tablet of "Appetit-Anreger" with extracts of bitter herbs (Zirkulin Naturheilmittel GmbH, Bremen) was placed in the study capsules. Dietary supplements containing bitters are traditionally used to increase appetite and to support digestion (18).

Expectancy Manipulation

Standardized expectancy manipulations were performed by two female experimenters in white coats (one undergraduate, one graduate student). After opening the randomization envelopes, participants in the appetite-stimulating groups were told to receive either a placebo capsule or a capsule filled with bitters, and that bitters are known to increase secretion of digestive fluids in the stomach and thus are expected to increase appetite within 20–30 min after intake of the capsule. Participants in the satiety-enhancing groups were told to receive either a placebo capsule or a capsule containing alginate, and that alginate is known to increase its volume in the stomach and thus is expected to enhance satiety within 20–30 min after intake of the capsule. They were told to receive either a verum or a placebo intervention (randomization ratio was not disclosed). Participants in the control group received a placebo capsule together with the information that its ingredients would have no effect on gastric activity and appetite.

Measurements

Hunger and Satiety Ratings

Perceived hunger ("How hungry do you feel?") was rated using a 100-mm visual analog scale from "0" ("not at all hungry") to "100" ("extremely hungry"). Perceived satiety ("How full do you feel?") were assessed by means of a 100-mm visual analog rating scale, ranging from 0 ("not at all full") to 100 ("extremely full").

Plasma Ghrelin

To assess the concentration of ghrelin in plasma, blood samples were collected in commercially available EDTA tubes (2.7 ml), complemented with 54 μl 4 mM 4-(2-aminoethyl)benzenesulfonyl fluoride hydrochloride (AEBSF) (19). Blood samples were immediately stored on ice and centrifuged within 30 min for 10 min at 3,000 g and 4°C. Two samples of 500 μl plasma were transferred to Eppendorf tubes and complemented with 100 μl 1 mM HCl. Samples were gently mixed and stored at −70°C until final analysis. Analysis of plasma ghrelin content was performed with the Ghrelin (total) Assay Kit (Catalogue number: EZGRT-89K) from Merck Millipore, Darmstadt, Germany according to protocol.

Electrocardiogram

The electrocardiogram was recorded to evaluate changes in heart rate. A transient increase of heart rate has been described as part of the cephalic phase response when food is anticipated (20). The electrocardiogram signal was measured continuously during the experiment using three disposable Ag/AgCl electrodes, which were positioned in an Einthoven Lead I configuration and connected to the BIOPAC amplifier module ECG100C of a BIOPAC MP 150 device (BIOPAC Systems Inc., Goleta, CA, USA). Data was acquired using AcqKnowledge 3.7.2 software and a sampling rate of 500 Hz. Intervals between successive R peaks (cardiac periods) were extracted from the electrocardiogram signal using the peak-detection function implemented in AcqKnowledge 3.7.2. Heart periods were examined and screened for artifacts based on the procedure developed by Proges and Byrne (21). Average heart rate was calculated for the last five artifact-free minutes of the baseline period and the two post-intervention periods (i.e., minutes 25–30 and minutes 55–60 after randomization).

Questionnaires

The Hospital Anxiety and Depression scale [HADS; (12)] was used to screen for anxiety and/or depression. The Three Factor Eating Questionnaire [TFEQ; (16)] with its three subscales "cognitive restraint of eating," "disinhibition," and "hunger" was used to test for possible differences in eating behavior between groups at baseline.

Female participants were asked for the normal length of their menstrual cycle, the beginning of the last menstruation, and whether they took hormonal contraceptives. Time point of ovulation was estimated by subtracting 14 days from the length of the menstrual cycle (22).

Statistical Analyses

Assuming an effect size partial eta-squared of 0.1, the study was planned to have a power of 90% to detect a significant interaction effect between "group" and "time point" in a mixed ANOVA for changes of hunger, satiety and ghrelin from before to after the intervention (with a type 1 error of 5%) (calculated by GPower Version 3.1.7). However, we later decided to use ANCOVAs to adjust for the slight group differences at baseline. Statistical analyses were performed using SPSS (version 23.0). Hunger ratings, satiety ratings and plasma ghrelin levels were each subjected to 3-way analyses of covariance (ANCOVA), with two levels of "time" (30 min and 60 min after randomization), three levels of "group" (appetite, satiety, control) and two levels of "sex" (male, female). In each model, baseline levels (15 min before randomization) were included as covariates. Bonferroni corrections were applied, where appropriate. A p-value ≤ 0.05 (2-sided) was considered statistically significant.

RESULTS

Participants

One Hundred thirteen participants were assessed for eligibility and 17 were excluded (three did not meet inclusion criteria, 12 declined to participate, one did not show up and one had elevated fasting blood glucose levels). Thirty participants each were assigned to the appetite group, the satiety group, and the control group. All participants completed the experiment.

Study groups were comparable with respect to demographic variables, eating behavior as well as anxiety and depression scores (**Table 1**). Participants had a mean age of 26.6 years (3.2 SD; range: 18–36 years) and a mean BMI of 21.9 kg/m^2 (1.8 SD; range: 18.6–25 kg/m^2). Fourteen women were in the preovulatory phase and two women in the postovulatory phase of the menstrual cycle, while 29 women were using hormonal contraceptives.

Hunger Ratings

The 3-way ANCOVA for post-intervention hunger ratings, controlled for baseline levels, revealed a significant 3-way interaction between "group," "time," and "sex" [$F_{group\times time\times sex(2,83)} = 4.0$, $p = 0.023$]. However, *post hoc* 2-way ANCOVAs performed separately for each sex showed no significant interaction effect between "group" and "time" [women, $F_{group\times time(2,41)} = 3.1$, $p = 0.058$; men, $F_{group\times time(2,41)} = 0.6$, $p = 0.571$). Furthermore, the 3-way ANCOVA showed a significant main effect of "group" [F_{group} (2, 83) $= 6.7$, $p = 0.002$]. Bonferroni-corrected *post hoc* tests indicated significantly lower hunger ratings in the satiety group compared to the control group ($p = 0.033$) and to the appetite group ($p = 0.002$) (**Figure 2**, **Table 2**).

TABLE 1 | Group characteristics at baseline.

Variable	Appetite group (n = 30) mean (SD)	Satiety group (n = 30) mean (SD)	Control group (n = 30) mean (SD)	F (df)	p-value
Age (years)	23.6 (3)	23.4 (2.9)	24 (3.7)	0.243 (2.87)	0.785
Body Mass Index (kg m^2)	21.8 (2)	21.7 (1.7)	22.2 (1.7)	0.632 (2.87)	0.534
Blood Glucose (mg/dl)	93.8 (8.1)	95.3 (9.9)	95.5 (6.6)	0.337 (2.84)	0.715
Hunger ratings (VAS)	4.6 (3.2)	6.3 (2.3)	5.7 (2.6)	2.867 (2.87)	0.062
Satiety ratings (VAS)	3.0 (2.2)	2.6 (2.4)	2.6 (1.9)	1.931 (2.87)	0.151
Ghrelin levels (pg/ml)	495.2 (217.3)	463.2 (180.5)	464 (212.4)	0.215 (2.87)	0.807
HOSPITAL ANXIETY AND DEPRESSION SCALE (HADS)					
Anxiety	3 (2.4)	2.8 (1.9)	3.4 (1.6)	0.560 (2.87)	0.573
Depression	1.4 (1. 5)	1.6 (1.8)	1.9 (2.1)	0.652 (2.87)	0.523
THREE FACTOR EATING QUESTIONNAIRE (TFEQ)					
Cognitive Restraint of Eating	10.6 (2)	10.9 (2.2)	10.1 (2.0)	0.317 (2.87)	0.317
Disinhibition	7.7 (2)	8.3 (2.1)	8.1 (2.2)	0.624 (2.87)	0.538
Hunger	6.3 (2.2)	6.8 (2)	7 (1.9)	0.957 (2.87)	0.388

SD, Standard Deviation.

Satiety Ratings

The 3-way ANCOVA for post-intervention satiety ratings, controlled for baseline levels, revealed a significant main effect of "group" [$F_{(2,83)} = 11.1$, $p < 0.001$]. Bonferroni-corrected *post hoc* tests indicated significantly higher satiety ratings in the satiety group than in the control group ($p < 0.001$) and in the appetite group ($p < 0.001$) (**Figure 3**, **Table 2**). The 3-way interaction between "group," "time," and "sex" was not significant [$F_{\text{group×time×sex}(2,83)} = 2.5, p = 0.102$].

Ghrelin Levels

The 3-way ANCOVA for post-intervention plasma ghrelin levels, controlled for baseline levels, revealed a significant 2-way interaction between "group" and "sex" [$F_{(2,71)} = 3.4, p = 0.040$]. Separate ANCOVAs for male and female participants indicated a significant main effect of "group" in women [$F_{(2,37)} = 4.4$, $p = 0.019$] but not in men [$F_{(2,33)} = 1.5, p = 0.235$]. Bonferroni-corrected *post hoc* tests indicated that the interaction in women was due to higher post-intervention ghrelin levels in the appetite group compared to the control group ($p = 0.019$; **Figure 4**, **Table 2**). Neither the main effect of "group" [$F_{\text{group}(2,71)} = 0.9$, $p = 0.401$) nor the 3-way interaction between "group," "time," and "sex" [$F_{\text{group×time×sex}(2,71)} = 2.7, p = 0.075$] was significant.

Heart Rate

The 3-way ANCOVA for post-intervention heart rate, controlled for baseline levels, revealed no significant main or interaction effects [$F_{\text{group}(2,82)} = 0.1$, $p = 0.922$; $F_{\text{group×time}(2,82)} = 0.2$, $p = 0.812$; $F_{\text{group×time×sex}(2,82)} = 1.1, p = 0.342$; **Table 2**].

Treatment Guesses

Thirteen participants (72.2%) in the satiety group, but only five participants (27.8%) in the appetite group guessed to having received the active agent. The difference between groups was significant ($\chi^2 = 0.1, p = 0.024$).

DISCUSSION

This is the first study designed to evaluate the effects of treatment-related expectations on appetite, satiety, and associated plasma ghrelin levels. Our randomized-controlled double-blinded experiment revealed that the satiety-enhancing placebo intervention successfully altered subjective feelings of appetite and satiety in the suggested direction. Furthermore, the appetite-enhancing placebo intervention increased ghrelin levels in women.

A recent meta-analysis of sham-controlled surgery trials suggested that bariatric surgery for obesity is associated with a large placebo effect on weight loss, equaling 71% of the effect of active bariatric surgery (4). Our finding that the satiety-enhancing placebo intervention indeed increased satiety provides the first experimental evidence that treatment-related expectations contribute to the success of satiety-enhancing medical interventions.

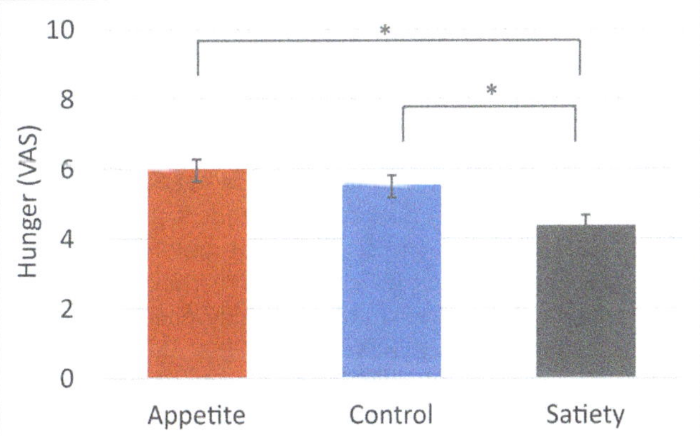

FIGURE 2 | Hunger ratings. Baseline-corrected hunger ratings following the three placebo interventions (estimated means ± SEM). VAS = visual analogue scale. *$p < 0.05$.

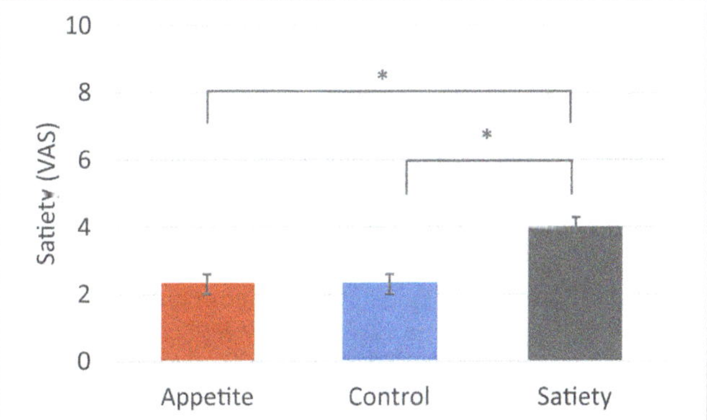

FIGURE 3 | Satiety ratings. Baseline-corrected satiety ratings following the three placebo interventions (estimated means ± SEM). VAS = visual analogue scale. *$p < 0.05$.

TABLE 2 | Post-intervention values (baseline-adjusted) of hunger ratings, satiety ratings, plasma ghrelin levels, and heart rate.

	Appetite group		Satiety group		Control group	
	Males ($n = 15$) Mean (SE)	Females ($n = 15$) Mean (SE)	Males ($n = 15$) Mean (SE)	Females ($n = 15$) Mean (SE)	Males ($n = 15$) Mean (SE)	Females ($n = 15$) Mean (SE)
Hunger ratings (VAS; cm)	6.3 (0.4)	5.5 (0.5)	3.8 (0.4)	5.0 (0.5)	5.8 (0.4)	5.2 (0.5)
Satiety ratings (VAS; cm)	2.5 (0.4)	2.1 (0.4)	4.0 (0.4)	3.9 (0.4)	2.3 (0.4)	2.3 (0.4)
Plasma ghrelin levels (pg/ml)	453.5 (20.2)	535.5 (20.1)	455.6 (20.8)	478.9 (21.0)	504.1 (24.2)	452.8 (20.1)
Heart rate (1/min)	63.2 (1 7)	63.3 (1.7)	65.7 (1.7)	62.2 (1.7)	62.8 (1.7)	64.6 (1.7)

SE, Standard Error; VAS, Visual Analogue Scale.

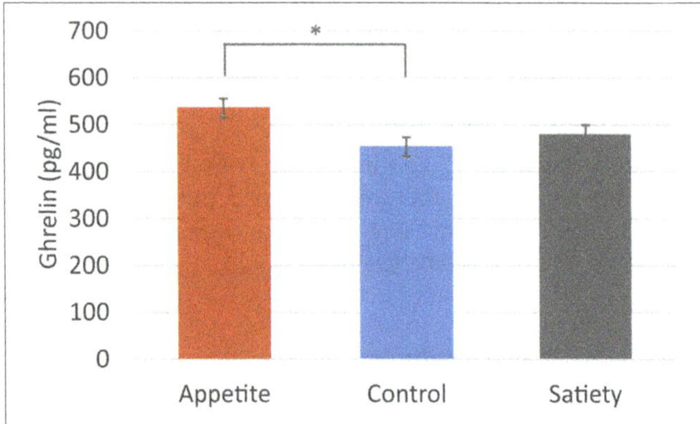

FIGURE 4 | Ghrelin levels in women. Baseline-corrected plasma ghrelin levels (pg/ml) in women following the three placebo interventions (estimated means ± SEM). *$p < 0.05$.

The retrospective evaluation of treatment guesses suggests that the appetite-enhancing placebo intervention was less credible to the participants than the satiety-enhancing placebo intervention. This could explain why the appetite-enhancing placebo intervention did not alter subjective feelings of appetite and satiety. However, the guess of having received placebo does not necessarily mean that the participant did not believe in the effectiveness of the intervention. Recent studies indicate that also open-label placebo administration can lead to positive beliefs and symptom improvement (23–25). Supporting this explanation, we observed an increase in ghrelin levels following the appetite-enhancing placebo intervention in women, suggesting the occurrence of a placebo effect on a physiological level. Ghrelin is secreted by the stomach, with levels peaking just before a meal and declining after feeding. In addition, ghrelin serves as an interoceptive signal for food-seeking behavior (26, 27). A previous study in a predominantly female cohort (65% women) found that plasma ghrelin levels increased when participants anticipated the intake of an "indulgent" milk-shake as compared to a "low-calorie" milk-shake, even though hunger ratings did not change (7). This may indicate that ghrelin is a highly sensitive measure to capture a psychologically mediated increase in appetite that occurs even before behavioral effects are measureable. With regard to the observed sex difference, it is important to note that stronger physiological placebo responses in women have also been reported in studies of placebo analgesia (15, 28). In addition, there is ample evidence that the physiology of appetite differs between sexes (29, 30). For example, women showed higher brain activation in the fusiform gyrus while viewing high-caloric pictures in the hungry state (31). Furthermore, brain activation to calorie-rich foods within the dorsolateral, ventrolateral, and ventromedial prefrontal cortices, the middle/posterior cingulate, and the insula were larger in women than in men (32), regions that play a role in self-reflection (33). Interestingly, sex differences in eating behavior are mediated, among other factors, by the gut hormone ghrelin (14), both in terms of secretion of this hormone and of ghrelin sensitivity (34, 35). Thus, the sex-specific ghrelin response in our experiment is in line with previous studies showing a stronger physiological response to placebo interventions as well as to appetite-enhancing food stimuli in women.

Our results provide first evidence that a placebo intervention to enhance appetite may enhance ghrelin secretion in women even before behavioral effects are measureable. In contrast, we found a strong effect of the satiety-enhancing intervention on ratings of hunger and satiety, notably without changes in circulating levels of total ghrelin. These data collectively suggest that ghrelin secretion is most likely unrelated to the placebo effect on satiety. It could be argued that food ingestion is a prerequisite for the postprandial fall in circulating ghrelin. However, as demonstrated in healthy human volunteers, postprandial suppression of ghrelin secretion did not differ between subjects receiving a mixed meal or who have been sham fed to allow smelling, chewing and tasting but not swallowing of food (26, 36). An anorexigenic hormone such as leptin or peptide YY (37) may still be better suited to capture the hormonal correlates of the placebo effect on satiety.

Several limitations of our results need to be mentioned. First, the short observational period in our experiment does not allow any conclusion on whether placebo effects on hunger and satiety can last longer than a few hours. Second, we performed our experiment in a normal-weight sample. Further studies are needed to clarify whether the findings of our experiment can be replicated in obese and anorectic patients. Third, our study was designed to investigate placebo effects on hunger and satiety induced by verbal suggestions. Learning mechanisms, such as behavioral conditioning and reinforcement learning, are known to affect eating behavior (38) as well as placebo effects (39), and their involvement in placebo effects on appetite-regulation should be evaluated in follow-up studies.

In conclusion, the results of the present study indicate a powerful inhibition of appetite in response to a satiety-enhancing placebo intervention and first evidence for an increase of ghrelin levels in women in response to an appetite-enhancing placebo intervention. Results thus provide the first experimental evidence that expectations are important factors to consider when evaluating the effects of medical interventions in the field of appetite regulation. Further studies with additional physiological outcome parameters are needed to better understand the psychobiological processes triggered by appetite-modulating placebo interventions.

AUTHOR CONTRIBUTIONS

VH and KM designed the experiments. VH, ML and JM performed the experiments. VH and KM analyzed the data. VH, TM, MT, and KM interpreted the data. VH drafted the first version of the manuscript. All authors critically reviewed the manuscript.

ACKNOWLEDGMENTS

KM received support by the Theophrastus Foundation, Germany, the Schweizer-Arau Foundation, Germany, and KM and MT by the Deutsche Forschungsgemeinschaft (ME 3675/1-1).

REFERENCES

1. Wadden TA, Butryn ML, Hong PS, Tsai AG. Behavioral treatment of obesity in patients encountered in primary care settings: a systematic review. *JAMA* (2014) 312:1779–91. doi: 10.1001/jama.2014.14173
2. Yanovski SZ, Yanovski JA. Long-term drug treatment for obesity: a systematic and clinical review. *JAMA* (2014) 311:74–86. doi: 10.1001/jama.2013.281361
3. Ells LJ, Mead E, Atkinson G, Corpeleijn E, Roberts K, Viner R, et al. Surgery for the treatment of obesity in children and adolescents. *Cochrane Database Syst Rev*. (2015) 6:CD011740. doi: 10.1002/14651858.CD011740
4. Jonas WB, Crawford C, Colloca L, Kaptchuk TJ, Moseley B, Miller FG, et al. To what extent are surgery and invasive procedures effective beyond a placebo response? A systematic review with meta-analysis of randomised, sham controlled trials. *BMJ Open* (2015) 5:e009655. doi: 10.1136/bmjopen-2015-009655
5. Higgs S. Memory for recent eating and its influence on subsequent food intake. *Appetite* (2002) 39:159–66. doi: 10.1006/appe.2002.0500
6. Provencher V, Polivy J, Herman CP. Perceived healthiness of food. If it's healthy, you can eat more! *Appetite* (2009) 52:340–4. doi: 10.1016/j.appet.2008.11.005
7. Crum AJ, Corbin WR, Brownell KD, Salovey P. Mind over milkshakes: mindsets, not just nutrients, determine ghrelin response. *Health Psychol*. (2011) 30:424–9; discussion 430–21. doi: 10.1037/a0023467
8. Wardle J, Haase AM, Steptoe A, Nillapun M, Jonwutiwes K, Bellisie F. Gender differences in food choice: the contribution of health beliefs and dieting. *Ann Behav Med*. (2004) 27:107–16. doi: 10.1207/s15324796abm2702_5
9. Westenhoefer J. "Age and gender dependent profile of food choice," in *Diet diversification and Health Promotion* (Basel: Karger Publishers) (2005). pp. 44–51.
10. Pliner P, Chaiken S, Flett GL. Gender differences in concern with body weight and physical appearance over the life span. *Person Soc Psychol Bull*. (1990) 16:263–73.
11. Grogan SC, Bell R, Conner MJA. Eating sweet snacks: gender differences in attitudes and behaviour. *Appetite* (1997) 28:19–31.
12. Zigmond AS, Snaith RP. The hospital anxiety and depression scale. *Acta Psychiatr Scand* (1983) 67:361–70.
13. Benedetti F, Pollo A, Lopiano L, Lanotte M, Vighetti S, Rainero I. Conscious expectation and unconscious conditioning in analgesic, motor, and hormonal placebo/nocebo responses. *J Neurosci* (2003) 23:4315–23. doi: 10.1523/JNEUROSCI.23-10-04315.2003
14. Asarian L, Geary N. Sex differences in the physiology of eating. *Am J Physiol Regul Integr Comp Physiol*. (2013) 305:R1215–67. doi: 10.1152/ajpregu.00446.2012
15. Colloca L, Pine DS, Ernst M, Miller FG, Grillon C. Vasopressin boosts placebo analgesic effects in women: a randomized trial. *Biol Psychiatry* (2016) 79:794–802. doi: 10.1016/j.biopsych.2015.07.019
16. Stunkard AJ, Messick S. The three-factor eating questionnaire to measure dietary restraint, disinhibition and hunger. *J Psychosom Res*. (1985) 29:71–83.
17. Georg MG, Kristensen M, Belza A, Knudsen JC, Astrup A. Acute effect of alginate-based preload on satiety feelings, energy intake, and gastric emptying rate in healthy subjects. *Obesity* (2012) 20:1851–8. doi: 10.1038/oby.2011.232
18. Länger R, Schiller H. *Gesundheit aus der Naturapotheke: Richtiger Umgang mit pflanzlichen Arzneimitteln*. Heidelberg: Springer-Verlag (2011).
19. Liu J, Prudom CE, Nass R, Pezzoli SS, Oliveri MC, Johnson ML, et al. Novel ghrelin assays provide evidence for independent regulation of ghrelin acylation and secretion in healthy young men. *J Clin Endocrinol Metab*. (2008) 93:1980–7. doi: 10.1210/jc.2007-2235
20. Mattes RD. Physiologic responses to sensory stimulation by food: nutritional implications. *J Am Diet Assoc*. (1997) 97:406–13. doi: 10.1016/S0002-8223(97)00101-6
21. Porges SW, Byrne EA. Research methods for measurement of heart rate and respiration. *Biol Psychol*. (1992) 34:93–130.
22. Fehring RJ, Schneider M, Raviele K. Variability in the phases of the menstrual cycle. *J Obstet Gynecol Neonatal Nurs*. (2006) 35:376–84. doi: 10.1111/j.1552-6909.2006.00051.x
23. Kaptchuk TJ, Friedlander E, Kelley JM, Sanchez MN, Kokkotou E, Singer JP, et al. Placebos without deception: a randomized controlled trial in irritable bowel syndrome. *PLoS ONE* (2010) 5:e15591. doi: 10.1371/journal.pone.0015591
24. Hoenemeyer TW, Kaptchuk TJ, Mehta TS, Fontaine KR. Open-label placebo treatment for cancer-related fatigue: a randomized-controlled clinical trial. *Sci Rep*. (2018) 8:2784. doi: 10.1038/s41598-018-20993-y
25. Schaefer M, Sahin T, Berstecher BJPO. Why do open-label placebos work? A randomized controlled trial of an open-label placebo induction with and without extended information about the placebo effect in allergic rhinitis. *PLoS ONE* (2018) 13:e0192758. doi: 10.1371/journal.pone.0192758
26. Müller TD, Nogueiras R, Andermann ML, Andrews ZB, Anker S, Argente J, et al. Ghrelin. *Mol Metab*. (2015) 4:437–60. doi: 10.1016/j.molmet.2015.03.005
27. Heisler LK, Lam DD. An appetite for life: brain regulation of hunger and satiety. *Curr Opin Pharmacol*. (2017) 37:100–6. doi: 10.1016/j.coph.2017.09.002
28. Theysohn N, Schmid J, Icenhour A, Mewes C, Forsting M, Gizewski E, et al. Are there sex differences in placebo analgesia during visceral pain processing? A fMRI study in healthy subjects. *Neurogastroenterol Motil*. (2014) 26:1743–53. doi: 10.1111/nmo.12454
29. Davy SR, Benes BA, Driskell JA. Sex differences in dieting trends, eating habits, and nutrition beliefs of a group of midwestern college students. *J Am Diet Assoc*. (2006) 106:1673–7. doi: 10.1016/j.jada.2006.07.017
30. Marino M, Masella R, Bulzomi P, Campesi I, MalorniW, Franconi, FJM. Nutrition and human health from a sex–gender perspective. *Mol Aspects Med*. (2011) 32:1–70. doi: 10.1016/j.mam.2011.02.001
31. Frank S, Laharnar N, Kullmann S, Veit R, Canova C, Hegner YL, et al. Processing of food pictures: influence of hunger, gender and calorie content. *Brain Res*. (2010) 1350:159–66. doi: 10.1016/j.brainres.2010.04.030
32. Killgore WD, Yurgelun-Todd DA. Sex differences in cerebral responses to images of high versus low-calorie food. *Neuroreport* (2010) 21:354–8. doi: 10.1097/WNR.0b013e32833774f7
33. Moran JM, Heatherton TF, Kelley WM. Modulation of cortical midline structures by implicit and explicit self-relevance evaluation. *Soc Neurosci*. (2009) 4:197–211. doi: 10.1080/17470910802250519
34. Sakata I, Tanaka T, Yamazaki M, Tanizaki T, Zheng Z, Sakai T. Gastric estrogen directly induces ghrelin expression and production in the rat stomach. *J Endocrinol*. (2006) 190:749–57. doi: 10.1677/joe.1.06808
35. Clegg DJ, Brown LM, Zigman JM, Kemp CJ, Strader AD, Benoit SC, et al. Estradiol-dependent decrease in the orexigenic potency of ghrelin in female rats. *Diabetes* (2007) 56:1051–8. doi: 10.2337/db06-0015
36. Arosio M, Ronchi CL, Beck-Peccoz P, Gebbia C, Giavoli C, Cappiello V, et al. Effects of modified sham feeding on ghrelin levels in healthy human subjects. *J Clin Endocrinol Metab*. (2004) 89:5101–4. doi: 10.1210/jc.2003-032222
37. Chan J, Stoyneva V, Kelesidis T, Raciti P, Mantzoros C. Peptide YY levels are decreased by fasting and elevated following caloric intake but are not regulated by leptin. *Diabetologia* (2006) 49:169–73. doi: 10.1007/s00125-005-0041-2
38. Jansen A. A learning model of binge eating: cue reactivity and cue exposure. *Behav Res Ther*. (1998) 36:257–72.
39. Colloca L, Benedetti F. Placebo and nocebo effects: unfolding the complex interplay between distinct phenotypes and physiological mechanisms. *Psychol Conscious Theory Res Pract*. (2016) 3:162. doi: 10.1037/cns0000054

2

How Placebo Needles Differ from Placebo Pills?

Younbyoung Chae [1], Ye-Seul Lee [1,2] and Paul Enck [3]*

[1] Acupuncture and Meridian Science Research Center, College of Korean Medicine, Kyung Hee University, Seoul, South Korea, [2] Department of Anatomy and Meridians, College of Korean Medicine, Gachon University, Seongnam, South Korea, [3] Department of Internal Medicine, Psychosomatic Medicine and Psychotherapy, University of Tübingen, Tübingen, Germany

***Correspondence:**
Younbyoung Chae
ybchae@khu.ac.kr*

Because acupuncture treatment is defined by the process of needles penetrating the body, placebo needles were originally developed with non-penetrating mechanisms. However, whether placebo needles are valid controls in acupuncture research is subject of an ongoing debate. The present review provides an overview of the characteristics of placebo needles and how they differ from placebo pills in two aspects: (1) physiological response and (2) blinding efficacy. We argue that placebo needles elicit physiological responses similar to real acupuncture and therefore provide similar clinical efficacy. We also demonstrate that this efficacy is further supported by ineffective blinding (even in acupuncture-naïve patients) which may lead to opposite guesses that will further enhances efficacy, as compared to no-treatment, e.g., with waiting list controls. Additionally, the manner in which placebo needles can exhibit therapeutic effects relative to placebo pills include enhanced touch sensations, direct stimulation of the somatosensory system and activation of multiple brain systems. We finally discuss alternative control strategies for the placebo effects in acupuncture therapy.

Keywords: acupuncture, blinding, control, placebo, physiology

INTRODUCTION

Acupuncture is a therapeutic intervention performed by "inserting one or more needles into specific sites on the body surface for therapeutic purposes" (1). Placebo needles were developed and validated to evaluate the efficacy of acupuncture treatment in randomized controlled clinical trials (RCTs) (2, 3). Due to the indistinguishably inert nature of placebo controls compared with active treatments, placebo-controlled studies enable determination of the therapeutic effects of target treatments from unspecific treatment effects, such as medical context and consequent expectation. Similarly, placebo needles must be indistinguishable from real acupuncture needles and not produce any physiological therapeutic effects. To achieve this, non-penetrating needles with a similar appearance to real acupuncture needles, which retract telescopically into the needle handle when pressed on the skin, were developed because they provide patients with the visual illusion that their skin is being penetrated, much like a stage dagger in theater performances.

Non-penetrating needles have been commonly used as placebo controls for acupuncture research over several decades (4), and are often seen as standard when investigating the mechanisms underlying the acupuncture effects (5). Interestingly, several studies have shown that the effectiveness of placebo acupuncture needles is similar to that of real acupuncture needles. A systematic review of clinical trials revealed only a small difference between real and placebo needles in terms of pain relief, whereas a moderate difference was found between placebo treatment and no treatment at all, e.g., during a waiting period (6). RCTs have shown that real and placebo acupuncture treatments are equally effective and that both are superior to "treatments as usual" (TAU) for chronic pain (7, 8). Taken together, these findings imply that acupuncture treatment is equally effective as placebo acupuncture and therefore, that acupuncture treatment effects are placebo effects (9). However, the adequacy of the controls being used in these studies remains to be determined (10). Many discussions of whether placebo needles are appropriate controls for acupuncture research have followed the development of these needles (11), and there has been some criticism from a physiological perspective that placebo needles may not be proper controls for acupuncture studies (12). In fact, placebo needles are neither fully indistinguishable from regular needles nor physiologically inert (13, 14). Similarly, a recent meta-analysis suggested that neither the Streitberger device nor the Park Sham device is adequate inert controls for clinical studies (15).

This issue pertains not only to acupuncture needles, but also to other treatment devices that involve physical contact with the patient, such as injections, transcutaneous electrical nerve stimulation, manual therapy, and surgical interventions. Placebo devices, including placebo injections and placebo acupuncture needles, exhibit stronger effects than do oral placebo pills (16). Similarly, a meta-analysis showed that subcutaneous placebo administrations produce greater effects than do oral placebos for the acute treatment of migraine (17). A more recent meta-analysis of the effects of placebo interventions across all clinical conditions showed that physical placebo interventions, including acupuncture, have greater effects than do pill controls (18); sham acupuncture has been shown to have even greater effects than other physical placebos (19). A clinical trial revealed that placebo needles have greater effects than placebo pills on self-reported pain and severity of symptoms in patients with persistent arm pain (20). Expectations on the potential benefit induced in the recipient, influenced by the magnitude of the invasiveness of the intervention, leads to therapeutic effects following a placebo treatment (21). The greater effect of placebo devices compared with placebo pills may be due to the additional physical contact or the tactile component of the intervention, which is minimally present with the use of pharmaceutical pills. Therefore, the contextual effects associated with the preparation of acupuncture treatment devices are multisensory and have a broader impact on the patient. The tactile context of treatment devices such as during acupuncture is essential for the establishment of therapeutic effects (22). In contrast to the use of oral placebo pills, this context has two components: physiological action and ineffective blinding, which initially takes effect once the treatment is applied, and which, therefore, is different from the gradual unblinding due to experiences of adverse events during the drug applications.

Thus, the purpose of the present article was to review the two components of placebo devices, physiological action and effective blinding, and to discuss how these features result in stronger placebo effects relative to oral pills.

PHYSIOLOGICAL ACTIONS OF PLACEBO NEEDLES

The "Specific" Effect of Placebo Needles Due to Tactile Stimulation

Pharmaceutical research involving a placebo requires a verum preparation with a specific drug and a placebo preparation without that drug, with the difference in the effects of these two preparations indicating the effectiveness of the target drug. The aims of this type of study design are to exclude any other possible factor that might influence the general effects of medical treatment, such as natural history, regression to the mean, and/or methodological biases, and to test the "true" therapeutic effects of the novel compound (23). Additionally, the non-specific effects of the treatment can be observed by comparing the response with placebo to a no-treatment control condition, e.g., a waiting list; these effects are caused by the treatment preparation itself within a medical context, i.e., the attention the patient receives. The context provided by the medical setting may be referred to as the "specific" effect of the placebo (24). In fact, placebo effects are regarded as brain–body responses to contextual information that promote health and well-being (24).

In the case of placebo needles, tactile stimulation is an additional component that is associated with the treatment context of acupuncture, which is absent in a pharmaceutical context. Due to this component, the expected difference in effect between placebo needle treatment and waiting list groups includes a tactile context that has been overlooked in previous studies. The tactile context provided by the placebo needles, much like the medical context under which a pill is given, cannot be physiologically inert, and this stimulation can even exert similar therapeutic actions by enhancing touch sensations in the body (25). Furthermore, the touch of the placebo needles experienced by the patient initiates a multisensory process and thereby activates bodily self-awareness. Overall, tactile stimulation provides a broader range of contexts that contribute to the effect and improve the healing process relative to other placebo interventions (26). The effect of the tactile component on the patient can be categorized accordingly into sensory-discriminative and affective-social aspects. These aspects of the tactile component play important roles in the therapeutic effect of acupuncture treatment in clinical practice (22), which is examined in the context of placebo needles in the following sections.

The Sensory-Discriminative Aspect of the Touch Component of Placebo Needles

Several studies have examined in depth the sensory-discriminative aspect of acupuncture needles. The process of needle insertion and the types of needle manipulation (27) activate diverse touch perception processes and stimulate mechanically sensitive pain fibers (28). This tactile stimulation process produces what is known as the *de qi* sensation (a combination of various sensations that include heaviness, numbness, soreness, and distention), which is fundamental for the therapeutic outcome of acupuncture treatment (29, 30).

Placebo needles were first validated as a sufficient control in acupuncture studies under the assumption that a lesser degree of *de qi* sensation would be evoked, thereby leading to less effective clinical outcomes (2, 3). In the initial validation studies of placebo needles, participants were not able to distinguish the placebo needles from real needles, but they experienced a greater degree of *de qi* sensation with real needles than with placebo needles (2, 3, 31) (**Figure 1**).

On the other hand, a recent validation study of the Streitberger needle conducted with a large population showed no significant difference in *de qi* sensation between patients treated with real and placebo needles, even though the placebo needle does not penetrate the skin (32). Additionally, a study investigating Park Sham devices revealed that the *de qi* sensation induced by real and placebo needles is not distinguishable (33). *De qi* sensation, a composite of unique sensations produced during acupuncture, has been considered to be one of the essential components for clinical efficacy (22). Considering the lack of a significant difference between treatments administered with real and placebo needles, we can assume that the placebo needle exerts an action that is similar to those exerted during real acupuncture.

The somatosensory system is activated directly by placebo needles, which exert various physiological actions in the body that are similar to those exerted by real acupuncture needles. Real and placebo needles produce enhanced skin conductance responses and decrease the heart rate, suggesting that placebo needles are not physiologically inert in terms of autonomic response patterns (14). Furthermore, these autonomic responses to placebo needles might be derived from the patient's orienting responses, or bodily self-awareness (34). A functional magnetic resonance imaging study demonstrated that tactile stimulation, which mimics acupuncture stimulation, not only induces activation in sensorimotor processing regions and deactivation in default-mode network regions, but also modulates higher cognitive areas in the brain (35). Additionally, a meta-analysis of brain imaging studies showed that placebo needles produce weaker, but similar, patterns of brain activation compared with real acupuncture (36). When the placebo needle touches the skin and evokes activity in cutaneous afferent nerves, it seems to act in the brain and result in a limbic touch response (37).

In the pharmaceutical trials, active pills have "true" therapeutic effects of the novel compound in the capsules while placebo pills use the same types of capsules without active components. Placebo pills, of course, can induce tactile sensation on the tongue, but it is not likely that such tactile sensation can be related with the therapeutic effects in the trials. On the other hand, placebo needles can induce tactile sensations around the acupoints that is similar to real acupuncture needles; these tactile sensations themselves could produce physiological actions through the body in the acupuncture trials.

The Affective-Social Aspect of the Touch Component of Placebo Needles

The process of treatment with placebo needles involves a component of touch between the patient and the practitioner. This affective-social aspect, involving slow gentle touch stimulation, activates unmyelinated C tactile fibers (CT afferents) and induces feelings of calm and well-being (38, 39). Prior to

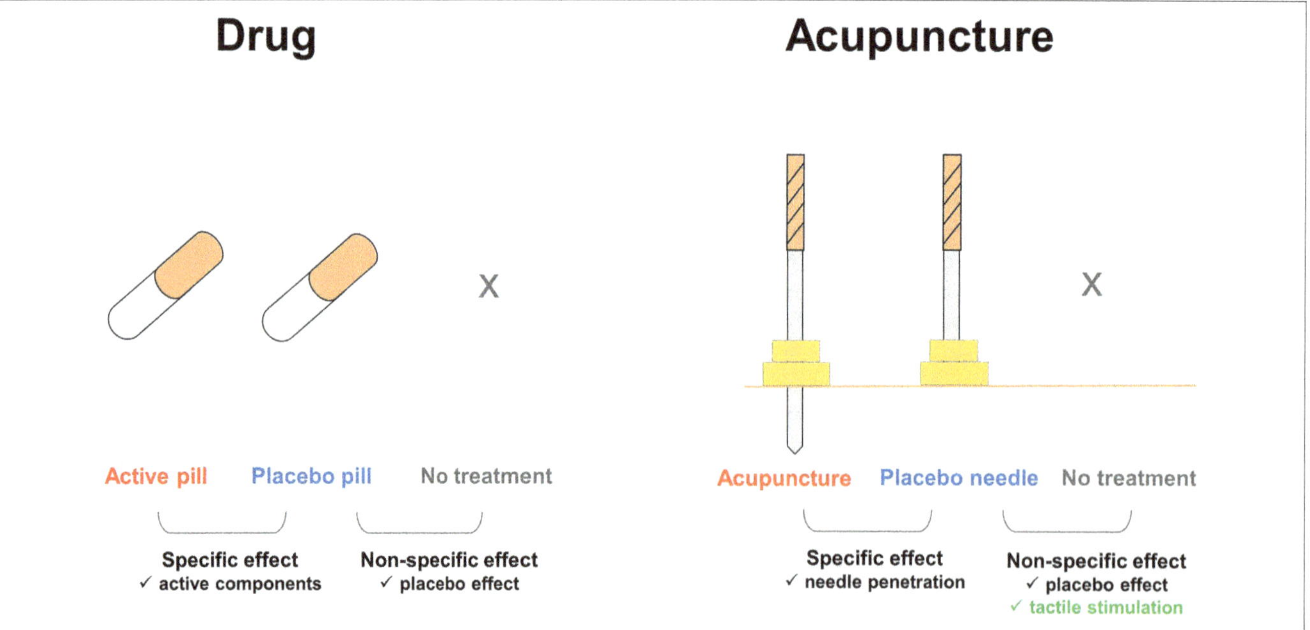

FIGURE 1 | Additional components involved in the effects of placebo needles. In pharmaceutical trials, the nonspecific effects of treatments can be ruled out by comparing the placebo pill group with an untreated group, e.g., on a waiting list. In acupuncture trials, tactile stimulation is an additional factor that affects the placebo needle and untreated groups. Enhanced touch sensations, which are distinct during acupuncture treatment, but absent with placebo pills, remain substantial during placebo needle administration. Thus, placebo needles not only play a role as a cue for treatment expectations, but also evoke the somatosensory system and directly activate multiple brain systems.

inserting and stimulating the needle, the practitioner touches the patient to assess the skin tissue and identify the region to which the needle will be applied. This process of gently touching the patient's skin activates CT afferents and alleviates unpleasantness. Furthermore, this type of pleasant touch reestablishes the patient's sense of self-esteem and well-being by inducing a limbic touch response (39). A clinical study (40) supports the role of affective-social touch in treatments with acupuncture and placebo needles because the enhanced patient–doctor relationship produced greater improvements in patients with irritable bowel syndrome. Additionally, the entirety of the procedure, including warmth, empathy, and the communication of positive expectations, might influence clinical outcomes (40).

Gentle touch, which is always a component of acupuncture treatment, plays a crucial role in the overall outcome of the medical treatment. Gentle touch by a nurse before a surgical operation decreases subjective and objective levels of stress in the patient (41). Furthermore, gentle touch plays a direct moderating role in the physiological responses of the patient such that it lowers blood pressure, enhances transient sympathetic reflexes, and increases pain thresholds (42). The affective-social components of gentle touch also enhance the patient–doctor relationship, even when patients are treated with placebo needles (40). Although the gentle touch component prior to the application of real or placebo needles is not considered to be part of the active component of placebo treatment, it is nevertheless part of the placebo preparation in a clinical acupuncture trial. Thus, compared with the effects observed in a waiting list group or a group receiving another placebo intervention, this component generates a stronger doctor–patient relationship and enhances the placebo effect.

Although the placebo needle acts as a control due to its non-penetrating qualities, the tactile component is not completely removed; thus, its application in acupuncture trials may additionally produce crucial effects such as directly evoking the somatosensory system, strengthening the doctor–patient relationship, and enhancing the patient's general condition. The biophysical effects of placebo needles influence the patient's expectations and contextualization, which likely also play roles in his or her cognitive perception during the treatment process regarding the alleviation of symptoms.

BLINDING OF PLACEBO NEEDLE APPLICATIONS

The Blinding Components of Placebo Needles

Placebo needles were developed based on a visual illusion that induces the belief that one's skin has been penetrated (2, 3). The tip of the placebo needle is blunt and retracts into the needle's handle; thus, a placebo needle has a shape similar to that of a real needle, but is dissimilar in that it does not penetrate the skin. Because the placebo needle induces the sensation of pricking and appears to penetrate the skin, the patient is more likely to classify placebo needle treatment as active relative to placebo pills. Placebo pills are indistinguishable in appearance from the active drug, but the patient must be convinced that they are receiving real treatment. The chance of determining whether a pill is a placebo or an active treatment is theoretically equal in pharmaceutical trials due to the indistinguishable appearance, smell, and taste of placebo pill compared to active drugs; in contrast, the chance of determining whether a needle is placebo or real is not completely equal, since the patient receiving the treatment while looking at and feeling the needle would be inclined to believe that the placebo treatment is active. Consequently, the probability of a patient determining placebo and real needle would be even more biased, if they have prior experience of acupuncture needling and have felt its therapeutic effects.

Blinding is another important issue that can minimize bias or the potential effect of context on the outcomes of RCTs (43). The blinding index (BI) was developed to assess the success of blinding in clinical trials (44) and is interpreted as a "correct guess beyond chance." For example, a BI of 1 indicates that all guesses are correct, a BI of -1 indicates that all guesses are incorrect, and a BI of 0 indicates that the probabilities of correct and incorrect guesses are equal (45). When classifying the blinding results of trials, BI values > 0.2 are considered to indicate failed blinding because more participants guessed correctly, BI values < 0.2 and > -0.2 are considered to be random guesses, and BI values < -0.2 are also considered to indicate failed blinding because more participants guessed incorrectly (45). An assessment of blinding in trials involving pharmacological interventions for psychiatric disorders yielded average BI values of 0.18 and 0 in the active treatment and placebo control groups, respectively (46). This finding implies that blinding was established successfully, which is an ideal result from a scientific perspective.

In contrast, people more often respond to placebo needles because they are more likely to believe that they are receiving active treatment, which is also known as an opposite guess (15, 46). Although a recent systematic review of the use of placebo needles for acupuncture in clinical trials with limited reporting of the credibility of blinding showed that participant blinding was successful in most cases (15), participants were less likely than chance levels to believe that the needles were real, rather than placebos. When a BI calculation was applied to this review, the average BI values were 0.55 and -0.33 for the real and placebo needle groups, respectively (15), indicating unsuccessful blinding. Additionally, based on the classification rules for blinding scenarios, 86% of studies have involved unblinded participants in the real acupuncture group (BI > 0.2) and participants making opposite guesses in the placebo group (BI< -0.2) (15).

A recent acupuncture study showed that 61 and 68% of patients administered real and placebo treatments, respectively, perceived treatment type correctly, which implies that blinding was unsuccessful (47). One possible reason for this unsuccessful blinding is the experience of the *de qi* sensation, which could contribute to the correct identification of the treatment (47), even though placebo needling sessions produce substantial levels of this sensation. Another possible explanation is that smaller insertion and pullout forces are used during placebo needling

(13). Differences in biomedical forces may be a crucial reason for the association of different somatosensory processes with the use of real and placebo needles (7) (**Figure 2A**).

Greater Expectations During Placebo Needling Produced Greater Placebo Effects

According to systematic reviews of the BI in clinical trials, pharmacological placebo pills have an approximately 50% chance of being perceived as active, whereas this assumption is not necessarily true for placebo needles (15, 46). While in the aforementioned studies the adverse events of drug trials indicate the risk of unblinding, the BI index seem to have been uncompromised, possibly due to the occurrence time and the frequency of such events.

The discussed BI patterns are often thought to indicate adequate blinding, but a greater probability of believing that a placebo is real might be due to wishful thinking rather the well-known psychological preference toward real or better treatment (48). The greater probability of opposite guesses in placebo needle groups may be related to greater expectations regarding symptom alleviation. Placebo effects, or any improvement in the symptoms or physiological condition of an individual receiving a placebo treatment (23), are based largely on the expectation of receiving actual treatment, cued and contextual conditioning, and/or observational and social learning (49). Thus, patients may have higher levels of expectation during placebo needling than when receiving placebo pills, which could contribute to treatment efficacy (50). In this manner, placebo responses may be more frequent in placebo needles than in placebo pills because patients are more likely

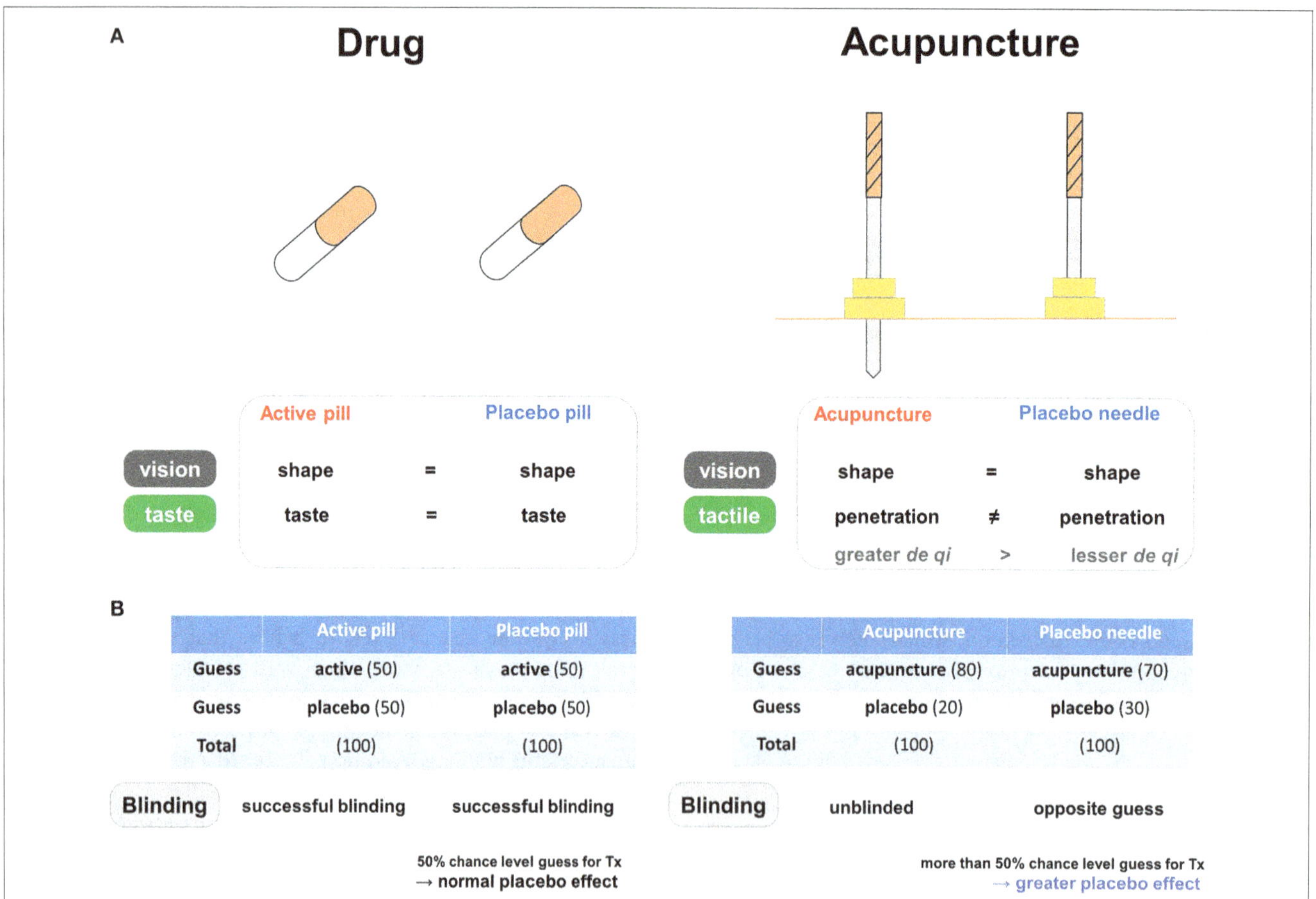

FIGURE 2 | The blinding components of placebo needles. **(A)** Differences in blinding characteristics between placebo needles and placebo pills. In pharmaceutical trials, the similar shapes and tastes of the active and placebo pills prevent patients from correctly guessing whether they are in the treatment group. In acupuncture trials, placebo needles are similar to real acupuncture devices in terms of shape, but not in terms of penetration when applied to the skin. **(B)** Both active and placebo pills have a 50% chance level of being perceived as active in the pharmaceutical trials, whereas both real and placebo acupuncture causes a tendency to believe that they are receiving active treatment in the acupuncture trials. Differences in blinding scenarios for placebo needles and placebo pills. In pharmaceutical trials, successful blinding in the treatment and placebo groups results in patients making random guesses about whether they are receiving active or placebo pills. Acupuncture trials involve different blinding scenarios: "unblinded participants" in the real acupuncture group and participants making "opposite guesses" in the placebo needle group. Due to this unique pattern of blinding, individuals more often respond to placebo needles because they are more likely to believe they are receiving active treatment (i.e., opposite guess).

to perceive the use of placebo needles as active treatment (**Figure 2B**).

ALTERNATIVE CONTROL STRATEGIES

When blinding becomes difficult (as with sham acupuncture needles) or even impossible (such as with psychotherapy), alternative control strategies are required to separate specific therapy effects from unspecific (e.g., contextual) effects as well as from spontaneous remission and response biases (23). Ineffective or impossible blinding also precludes conventional cross-over designs where each patient serves as his/her own control, thereby reducing the data variance and allowing trials with far less patients than with a parallel-group design. However, cross-over designs carry another risk: that of carry-over effects from one phase to the next. If the carry-over effect is based on Pavlovian conditioning of responses (51), even longer wash-out phases cannot prevent it to occur.

A number of design alternatives have been discussed which all exhibit both specific advantages and pitfalls.

No Treatment Controls (NTC)

To separate "spontaneous variation" from "placebo responses", a "no-treatment" control group appears necessary that determines how much of the unspecific effects can be attributed to spontaneous variation and recovery. Since this is rarely done, the exact size of the contribution of spontaneous variation to the placebo response is known only for minor and benign clinical conditions and may account here for approximately 50% of the placebo effect (52). In experimental settings, "no treatment controls" may also serve to control for habituation and sensitization effects that may occur with repetitive stimulation, e.g. in pain and placebo analgesia experiments.

NTC are limited by ethical rules when patients with a severe clinical condition require treatment and cannot be offered trial participation that would assign them to a NTC group, as set by the Declaration of Helsinki of the World Medical Association (53).

Waiting List Control (WLC), Treatment as Usual (TAU)

Assigning patients to a "no treatment" group may be ethically problematic, e.g., in case of severe diseases, or when for other reasons the patients require treatment; in such cases WLC and TAU are control strategies for non-drug testing when an inert "placebo" is not available, e.g., in psychotherapy, physical/manual therapy, surgery, and "instrumental" therapies (TENS, transcranial magnetic or direct current stimulation, laser or light therapy), including acupuncture (see above). While some of these therapies have "sham therapy techniques" that can serve as placebo controls, e.g., in acupuncture, others must rely on WLC and TAU as their only control condition.

However, WLC and TAU face significant limitations: while patients expect to receive effective therapy, they are randomized to routine treatment most of them have had in the past (TAU), or (in case of WLC) have to wait for the treatment they were recruited for, resulting in disappointment and potentially nocebo effects (21). This affects only recruitment and compliance, and biases patient populations in such studies.

To avoid WLC and TAU and the associated disadvantages, studies in acute and chronic pain are often conducted comparing a novel drug with another drug already available rather than with placebos (54, 55).

Comparative Effectiveness Research (CER)

One approach to circumvent the placebo dilemma in RCT (for ethical as well as for methodological reasons) has recently been favored by drug approval authorities, by boards of medical societies, and by ethics committees, namely to avoid utilization of placebos in clinical trials. Comparative effectiveness research (CER) compares novel treatments to already approved therapies: to the best of our knowledge, this has never been done for acupuncture therapy, e.g., in chronic pain conditions.

However, as has been shown in a number of meta-analyses in depression, schizophrenia. and other diseases, comparing a new therapy to a comparator increases the response solely driven by the higher likelihood of patients to receive active treatments (100%) as compared to placebo-controlled trials (56). In such trials therefore, the placebo response is high but cannot be controlled anymore. Of specific interest is the fact that CER studies need to test for "non-inferiority" of the novel drug, resulting in higher patient numbers (57).

Cohort Multiple Randomized Controlled Trial (CMRCT) Design

The "cohort multiple randomized controlled trial" (CMRCT) (58)—formerly also known as the Zelen design (59)—splits the "no treatment" control arm of a drug trial (done for the purpose of mere observation of the natural course of the disease) from the drug trial itself, by recruiting a large cohort of patients for an "observational study" in which patients are followed under their TAU condition.

The observational cohort then serves as the basis for the recruitment of a subsample for the treatment study, either placebo-controlled or CER: patients are randomly approached, but can be selected based on a number of factors accounting for statistical representativeness.

A number of limitations apply, however: "the observational cohort needs to be monitored over time (a cross-sectional sample analysis would not be sufficient to account for changes occurring over time), and it needs to be representative for complete patient cohort affected by the diseases, both in terms of disease features (e.g., symptom severity) as well as disease management (diagnosis, TAU). Once such a cohort it established it may be used for more than one RCT" (21).

DISCUSSION AND CONCLUSION

Similar to other placebo types, placebo needles play an important contextual role in treatment expectations; however, they also directly evoke the somatosensory system and activate multiple brain systems. Placebo preparations are applied in studies to blind participants, and they enable the calculation of chance levels for patients' guesses about whether interventions are therapeutic or inert. However, the probability of making an opposite guess is greater for placebo needles than for placebo pills, which is often explained by patients' greater expectations. Because patients are more likely to perceive placebos as active treatment in placebo needle trials, placebo responses may be observed more frequently to placebo needles than to placebo pills.

The tactile components of acupuncture needle use are crucial factors during treatment preparation and could not be fully controlled for as placebo needles were being developed. The distinctive touch sensations experienced during acupuncture treatment are substantial, even during the administration of placebo needles. Due to the physical contact necessary when applying placebo needles, the validity of these needles as controls has been in question from the perspectives of physiological inertness and blinding. These factors may result in placebo needles exerting stronger placebo effects than do other types of placebo preparation that do not include tactile components. Thus, the development of a technique to control for the tactile components of acupuncture interventions while participants are consciously receiving treatment is an important consideration. The studies reviewed here demonstrated that the *de qi* sensation cannot be completely accounted for when using placebo needles without controlling for the tactile components, which suggests some level of clinical efficacy. Placebo needle administrations may inadvertently, albeit less robustly, activate the somatosensory system and induce regulatory mechanisms that are also triggered by acupuncture needling. Furthermore, placebo needles, or what we have considered to be control needles for experimental studies, may be a form of acupuncture treatment that is low dose or that provides weak stimulation.

In clinical trials, the placebo control should be indistinguishable from the active treatment (i.e., blinding success) and yet physiologically inert (less *deqi* sensation in this case). In the case of acupuncture, however, it is difficult to meet these two criteria simultaneously (60). Most importantly, our argument on the inadequacy of placebo needles as controls in acupuncture trials should not inhibit further acupuncture trials with randomized, controlled designs. Placebo needles indeed are more likely to induce placebo responses than placebo pills, which is largely due to the tactile component that cannot be separated from the components of the real acupuncture needles. In other words, conversely, our arguments imply that acupuncture needles contain a substantial level of placebo effect, which was not completely ruled out by controlling the penetration. It is also important to note that waiting lists do produce unspecific effects on their own (61). Furthermore, recent studies in acupuncture have employed study designs such as pragmatic trials, which compare acupuncture treatment with waiting lists and usual care (62–64), while other innovative control strategies still await validation with acupuncture. In the meantime, the discussion on the effect of the tactile components of placebo needles in its effectiveness as placebos, as well as effective blinding, needs to be continued.

Taken together, the placebo needles do have different characteristics from placebo pills in clinical trials. Our exploration does not imply that acupuncture may be more effective than placebo, but suggests that we have to consider these unique characteristics of placebo needles before we draw premature conclusions that acupuncture itself is just a placebo.

AUTHOR CONTRIBUTIONS

Conceived and designed the paper: YC and PE. Wrote the first draft of the paper: YC Y-SL, and PE. Revised the paper and approved the final version: YC, Y-SL, and PE.

ACKNOWLEDGMENTS

This research was supported by Basic Science Research Program through the National Research Foundation of Korea (NRF) funded by the Ministry of Education, Science and Technology (2014K2A3A1000166 & 2015R1D1A1A01058033 & 2015M3A9E3052338).

REFERENCES

1. Liu T. Acupuncture: what underlies needle administration? *Evid Based Complement Alternat Med.* (2009) **6**:185–93. doi: 10.1093/ecam/nen002
2. Streitberger K, Kleinhenz J. Introducing a placebo needle into acupuncture research. *Lancet* (1998) **352**:364–5. doi: 10.1016/S0140-6736(97)10471-8
3. Park J, White A, Stevinson C, Ernst E, James M. Validating a new non-penetrating sham acupuncture device: two randomised controlled trials. *Acupunct Med.* (2002) **20**:168–74. doi: 10.1136/aim.20.4.168
4. Dincer F, Linde K. Sham interventions in randomized clinical trials of acupuncture–a review. *Complement Ther Med.* (2003) **11**:235–42. doi: 10.1016/S0965-2299(03)00124-9
5. Hu B, Bai F, Xiong L, Wang Q. The endocannabinoid system, a novel and key participant in acupuncture's multiple beneficial effects. *Neurosci Biobehav Rev.* (2017) **77**:340–57. doi: 10.1016/j.neubiorev.2017.04.006
6. Madsen MV, Gotzsche PC, Hrobjartsson A. Acupuncture treatment for pain: systematic review of randomised clinical trials with acupuncture, placebo acupuncture, and no acupuncture groups. *BMJ* (2009) **338**:a3115. doi: 10.1136/bmj.a3115
7. Schneider A, Enck P, Streitberger K, Weiland C, Bagheri S, Witte S, et al. Acupuncture treatment in irritable bowel syndrome. *Gut* (2006) **55**:649–54. doi: 10.1136/gut.2005.074518
8. Cherkin DC, Sherman KJ, Avins AL, Erro JH, Ichikawa L, Barlow WE, et al. A randomized trial comparing acupuncture, simulated acupuncture, and usual care for chronic low back pain. *Arch Intern Med.* (2009) **169**:858–66. doi: 10.1001/archinternmed.2009.65
9. Solomon S. Acupuncture for Headache. It's Still All Placebo. *Headache* (2017) **57**:143–46. doi: 10.1111/head.12975
10. Enck P, Klosterhalfen S, Zipfel S. Acupuncture, psyche and the placebo response. *Auton Neurosci.* (2010) **157**:68–73. doi: 10.1016/j.autneu.2010.03.005
11. Langevin HM, Hammerschlag R, Lao L, Napadow V, Schnyer RN, Sherman KJ. Controversies in acupuncture research: selection of controls and outcome measures in acupuncture clinical trials. *J Altern Complement Med.* (2006) **12**:943–53. doi: 10.1089/acm.2006.12.943
12. Lundeberg T, Lund I, Naslund J, Thomas M. The Emperors sham - wrong assumption that sham needling is sham. *Acupunct Med.* (2008) **26**:239–42. doi: 10.1136/aim.26.4.239
13. Chae Y, Um SI, Yi SH, Lee H, Chang DS, Yin CS, et al. Comparison of biomechanical properties between acupuncture and non-penetrating

sham needle. *Complement Ther Med.* (2011) **19**(Suppl. 1), S8–12. doi: 10.1016/j.ctim.2010.09.002
14. Kang OS, Chang DS, Lee MH, Lee H, Park HJ, Chae Y. Autonomic and subjective responses to real and sham acupuncture stimulation. *Auton Neurosci.* (2011) **159**:127–30. doi: 10.1016/j.autneu.2010.07.027
15. Zhang CS, Tan HY, Zhang GS, Zhang AL, Xue CC, Xie YM. Placebo devices as effective control methods in acupuncture clinical trials: a systematic review. *PLoS ONE* (2015) **10**:e0140825. doi: 10.1371/journal.pone.0140825
16. Kaptchuk TJ, Goldman P, Stone DA, Stason WB. Do medical devices have enhanced placebo effects? *J Clin Epidemiol.* (2000) **53**:786–92. doi: 10.1016/S0895-4356(00)00206-7
17. De Craen AJ, Tijssen JG, De Gans J, Kleijnen J. Placebo effect in the acute treatment of migraine: subcutaneous placebos are better than oral placebos. *J Neurol.* (2000) **247**:183–8. doi: 10.1007/s004150050560
18. Hrobjartsson A, Gotzsche PC. (2010). Placebo interventions for all clinical conditions. *Cochrane Database Syst Rev.* **20**:CD003974. doi: 10.1002/14651858.CD003974.pub3
19. Linde K, Niemann K, Meissner K. Are sham acupuncture interventions more effective than (other) placebos? A re-analysis of data from the Cochrane review on placebo effects. *Forsch Komplementmed.* (2010) **17**:259–64. doi: 10.1159/000320374
20. Kaptchuk TJ, Stason WB, Davis RB, Legedza AR, Schnyer RN, Kerr CE, et al. Sham device v inert pill: randomised controlled trial of two placebo treatments. *BMJ* (2006) **332**:391–7. doi: 10.1136/bmj.38726.603310.55
21. Weimer K, Enck P. Traditional and innovative experimental and clinical trial designs and their advantages and pitfalls. In: Barrett JE, Flockerzi V, Frohman MA, Geppetti P, Hofmann FB, Michel MC, Page CP, Rosenthal W, Wang K, editors. *Handbook of Experimental Pharmacology*. Berlin: Springer (2014). p. 237–72.
22. Chae Y, Olausson H. The role of touch in acupuncture treatment. *Acupunct Med.* (2017) **35**:148–52. doi: 10.1136/acupmed-2016-011178
23. Enck P, Bingel U, Schedlowski M, Rief W. The placebo response in medicine: minimize, maximize or personalize? *Nat Rev Drug Discov.* (2013) **12**:191–204. doi: 10.1038/nrd3923
24. Wager TD, Atlas LY. The neuroscience of placebo effects: connecting context, learning and health. *Nat Rev Neurosci.* (2015) **16**:403–18. doi: 10.1038/nrn3976
25. Kerr CE, Shaw JR, Conboy LA, Kelley JM, Jacobson E, Kaptchuk TJ. Placebo acupuncture as a form of ritual touch healing: a neurophenomenological model. *Conscious Cogn.* (2011) **20**:784–91. doi: 10.1016/j.concog.2010.12.009
26. Lee YS, Chae Y. Powerful effects of placebo needles. *Acupunct Med.* (2018) doi: 10.1136/acupmed-2017-011516
27. Seo Y, Lee IS, Jung WM, Ryu HS, Lim J, Ryu YH, et al. Motion patterns in acupuncture needle manipulation. *Acupunct Med.* (2014) **32**:394–9. doi: 10.1136/acupmed-2014-010585
28. Zhao ZQ. Neural mechanism underlying acupuncture analgesia. *Prog Neurobiol.* (2008) **85**:355–75. doi: 10.1016/j.pneurobio.2008.05.004
29. Kong J, Fufa DT, Gerber AJ, Rosman IS, Vangel MG, Gracely RH, et al. Psychophysical outcomes from a randomized pilot study of manual, electro, and sham acupuncture treatment on experimentally induced thermal pain. *J Pain* (2005) **6**:55–64. doi: 10.1016/j.jpain.2004.10.005
30. Choi YJ, Lee JE, Moon WK, Cho SH. Does the effect of acupuncture depend on needling sensation and manipulation? *Complement Ther Med.* (2013) **21**:207–14. doi: 10.1016/j.ctim.2012.12.009
31. White P, Lewith G, Hopwood V, Prescott P. The placebo needle, is it a valid and convincing placebo for use in acupuncture trials? A randomised, single-blind, cross-over pilot trial. *Pain* (2003) **106**:401–9. doi: 10.1016/j.pain.2003.08.013
32. Xie CC, Wen XY, Jiang L, Xie MJ, Fu WB. Validity of the "streitberger" needle in a chinese population with acupuncture: a randomized, single-blinded, and crossover pilot study. *Evid Based Complement Alternat Med.* (2013) **2013**:251603. doi: 10.1155/2013/251603
33. Liang ZH, Xie CC, Li ZP, Zhu XP, Lu AP, Fu WB. Deqi sensation in placebo acupuncture: a crossover study on chinese medicine students. *Evid Based Complement Alternat Med.* (2013) **2013**:620671. doi: 10.1155/2013/620671
34. Napadow V, Lee J, Kim J, Cina S, Maeda Y, Barbieri R, et al. Brain correlates of phasic autonomic response to acupuncture stimulation: an event-related fMRI study. *Hum Brain Mapp.* (2013) **34**:2592–606. doi: 10.1002/hbm.22091
35. Napadow V, Dhond RP, Kim J, Lacount L, Vangel M, Harris RE, et al. Brain encoding of acupuncture sensation–coupling on-line rating with fMRI. *Neuroimage* (2009) **47**:1055–65. doi: 10.1016/j.neuroimage.2009.05.079
36. Chae Y, Chang DS, Lee SH, Jung WM, Lee IS, Jackson S, et al. Inserting needles into the body: a meta-analysis of brain activity associated with acupuncture needle stimulation. *J Pain* (2013) **14**:215–22. doi: 10.1016/j.jpain.2012.11.011
37. Lund I, Naslund J, Lundeberg T. Minimal acupuncture is not a valid placebo control in randomised controlled trials of acupuncture: a physiologist's perspective. *Chin Med.* (2009) **4**:1. doi: 10.1186/1749-8546-4-1
38. Campbell A. Role of C tactile fibres in touch and emotion–clinical and research relevance to acupuncture. *Acupunct Med.* (2006) **24**:169–71. doi: 10.1136/aim.24.4.169
39. Lund I, Lundeberg T. Are minimal, superficial or sham acupuncture procedures acceptable as inert placebo controls? *Acupunct Med.* (2006) **24**:13–15. doi: 10.1136/aim.24.1.13
40. Kaptchuk TJ, Kelley JM, Conboy LA, Davis RB, Kerr CE, Jacobson EE, et al. Components of placebo effect: randomised controlled trial in patients with irritable bowel syndrome. *BMJ* (2008) **336**:999–1003. doi: 10.1136/bmj.39524.439618.25
41. Whitcher SJ, Fisher JD. Multidimensional reaction to therapeutic touch in a hospital setting. *J Pers Soc Psychol.* (1979) **37**:87. doi: 10.1037/0022-3514.37.1.87
42. Mcglone F, Wessberg J, Olausson H. Discriminative and affective touch: sensing and feeling. *Neuron* (2014) **82**:737–55. doi: 10.1016/j.neuron.2014.05.001
43. Wood L, Egger M, Gluud LL, Schulz KF, Juni P, Altman DG, et al. Empirical evidence of bias in treatment effect estimates in controlled trials with different interventions and outcomes: meta-epidemiological study. *BMJ* (2008) **336**:601–5. doi: 10.1136/bmj.39465.451748.AD
44. Baethge C, Assall OP, Baldessarini RJ. Systematic review of blinding assessment in randomized controlled trials in schizophrenia and affective disorders 2000-2010. *Psychother Psychosom.* (2013) **82**:152–60. doi: 10.1159/000346144
45. Bang H, Ni L, Davis CE. Assessment of blinding in clinical trials. *Control Clin Trials* (2004) **25**:143–56. doi: 10.1016/j.cct.2003.10.016
46. Freed B, Assall OP, Panagiotakis G, Bang H, Park JJ, Moroz A, et al. Assessing blinding in trials of psychiatric disorders: a meta-analysis based on blinding index. *Psychiatry Res.* (2014) **219**:241–7. doi: 10.1016/j.psychres.2014.05.023
47. Vase L, Baram S, Takakura N, Takayama M, Yajima H, Kawase A, et al. Can acupuncture treatment be double-blinded? An evaluation of double-blind acupuncture treatment of postoperative pain. *PLoS ONE* (2015) **10**:e0119612. doi: 10.1371/journal.pone.0119612
48. Bang H. Random guess and wishful thinking are the best blinding scenarios. *Contemp Clin Trials Commun.* (2016) **3**:117–21. doi: 10.1016/j.conctc.2016.05.003
49. Colloca L, Miller FG. How placebo responses are formed: a learning perspective. *Philos Trans R Soc Lond B Biol Sci.* (2011) **366**:1859–69. doi: 10.1098/rstb.2010.0398
50. Colloca L, Lopiano L, Lanotte M, Benedetti F. Overt versus covert treatment for pain, anxiety, and Parkinson's disease. *Lancet Neurol.* (2004) **3**:679–84. doi: 10.1016/S1474-4422(04)00908-1
51. Suchman AL, Ader R. Classic conditioning and placebo effects in crossover studies. *Clin Pharmacol Ther.* (1992) **52**:372–7. doi: 10.1038/clpt.1992.157
52. Krogsboll LT, Hrobjartsson A, Gotzsche PC. Spontaneous improvement in randomised clinical trials: meta-analysis of three-armed trials comparing no treatment, placebo and active intervention. *BMC Med Res Methodol.* (2009) **9**:1. doi: 10.1186/1471-2288-9-1
53. World Medical Association. World Medical Association Declaration of Helsinki: ethical principles for medical research involving human subjects. *JAMA* (2013) **310**:2191–4. doi: 10.1001/jama.2013.281053
54. Saarto T, Wiffen PJ. Antidepressants for neuropathic pain. *Cochrane Database Syst Rev.* (2007) **20**:CD005454. doi: 10.1002/14651858.CD005454.pub2
55. Quilici S, Chancellor J, Lothgren M, Simon D, Said G, Le TK, et al. Meta-analysis of duloxetine vs. pregabalin and gabapentin in the treatment of diabetic peripheral neuropathic pain. *BMC Neurol* (2009) **9**:6. doi: 10.1186/1471-2377-9-6

56. Weimer K, Colloca L, Enck P. Placebo effects in psychiatry: mediators and moderators. *Lancet Psychiatry* (2015) **2**:246–57. doi: 10.1016/S2215-0366(14)00092-3
57. Leon AC. Evolution of psychopharmacology trial design and analysis: six decades in the making. *J Clin Psychiatry* (2011) **72**:331–40. doi: 10.4088/JCP.10r06669
58. Relton C, Torgerson D, O'cathain A, Nicholl J. Rethinking pragmatic randomised controlled trials: introducing the "cohort multiple randomised controlled trial" design. *BMJ* (2010) **340**:c1066. doi: 10.1136/bmj.c1066
59. Zelen M. A new design for randomized clinical trials. *N Engl J Med.* (1979) **300**:1242–5. doi: 10.1056/NEJM197905313002203
60. Chae Y. The dilemma of placebo needles in acupuncture research. *Acupunct Med.* (2017) **35**:382–3. doi: 10.1136/acupmed-2017-011394
61. Gold SM, Enck P, Hasselmann H, Friede T, Hegerl U, Mohr DC, et al. Control conditions for randomised trials of behavioural interventions in psychiatry: a decision framework. *Lancet Psychiatry* (2017) **4**:725–32. doi: 10.1016/S2215-0366(17)30153-0
62. Witt CM, Jena S, Selim D, Brinkhaus B, Reinhold T, Wruck K, et al. Pragmatic randomized trial evaluating the clinical and economic effectiveness of acupuncture for chronic low back pain. *Am J Epidemiol.* (2006) **164**:487–96. doi: 10.1093/aje/kwj224
63. Macpherson H, Tilbrook H, Bland JM, Bloor K, Brabyn S, Cox H, et al. Acupuncture for irritable bowel syndrome: primary care based pragmatic randomised controlled trial. *BMC Gastroenterol* (2012) **12**:150. doi: 10.1186/1471-230X-12-150
64. Chung VC, Ho RS, Liu S, Chong MK, Leung AW, Yip BH, et al. Electroacupuncture and splinting versus splinting alone to treat carpal tunnel syndrome: a randomized controlled trial. *CMAJ* (2016) **188**:867–75. doi: 10.1503/cmaj.151003

3

Mental Training for Better Achievement: Effects of Verbal Suggestions and Evaluation (of Effectiveness) on Cognitive Performance

Kristina Fuhr and Dustin Werle*

Clinical Psychology and Psychotherapy, Department of Psychology, University of Tuebingen, Tuebingen, Germany

***Correspondence:**
Kristina Fuhr
kristina.fuhr@uni-tuebingen.de

Objective: There is only some literature regarding the influence of verbal suggestions on cognitive performance in healthy volunteers. For example, the performance in a knowledge test was enhanced when participants were told that they had subliminally received the correct answer. However, enhancing cognitive performance only via verbal suggestions without prior conditioning phases has not yet been examined. The goal of our study was therefore to investigate the effects of a mental training based on verbal suggestions compared to a control training on cognitive performance in a student population using a balanced-placebo-design.

Methods: In total, 103 participants were randomly assigned either to listening to a 20 min audio-taped mental training or to a 20 min philosophy lecture (control training) via headphones. Participants were individually tested before and after the training concerning their cognitive performance. Information about the type of training were varied in both intervontion conditions ("You are part of our experimental condition and you will receive an effective mental training" or "You are part of our control group and you will receive the control condition"). At the end of the assessment, participants were asked what kind of training they believed they had received and how effective they would rate the received training.

Results: Overall, the cognitive performance improved in all participants, $F_{(1, 99)} = 490.01, p < 0.001$. Contrary to our hypotheses, we found no interaction of the type of training and type of instruction on the cognitive performance. Participants who rated the received training as being effective at the end of the experiment (regardless if it was the mental or the control training), have before experienced a greater improvement in their cognitive performance [$F_{(2,100)} = 7.26, p = 0.001$] and showed higher scores in the ability to absorb [$F_{(2, 99)} = 3.75, p = 0.027$].

Conclusion: The subjects' own experiences in the task might have influenced the rating of the training rather than the actual training or the information they receive regarding the type of training. This finding underlines the relevance of enhancing the subjective beliefs and self-efficacy in situations where cognitive attention processes are important and of individually tailoring mental trainings.

Keywords: placebo, mental training, cognitive performance, verbal suggestions, effectiveness rating

INTRODUCTION

The influence of expectations and suggestions on the placebo response was shown in different experimental studies concerning psychological aspects like for example pain [e.g., (1)]. In the context of pain, the given verbal instructions did not only influence the subjective analgesic effect but also reduced the amount of requests for opioid doses (1). However, verbal suggestions alone (without any preconditioning) could only influence pain tolerance in healthy subjects and motor performance in Parkinson's patients, but not for example hormonal secretion (2). Little is known about placebo effects on cognitive performance. For example, cognitive processes like attention could be improved after suggesting participants they had consumed caffeine similar to the improvement after they really consumed caffeine [e.g., (3)]. Comparable results were found when college students believed that they had received a "neuro-enhancing" stimulant. The cognitive performance improved in some scales and the participants also evaluated their subjective results as better (4). However, the placebo effect concerning the cognitive processes was only investigated when providing the participants with some kind of substance or placebo. Therefore, it would be interesting if similar to the results that were found in pain, cognitive processes might also be influenced by evoking specific expectations just via receiving verbal suggestions, i.e., verbal instructions but also via psychological interventions. Automatic visual perception and cognitive processes, as they are for example assumed for the Stroop effect, can be influenced and even controlled just by receiving verbal suggestions during a hypnotic experience. This effect was most pronounced in highly suggestible individuals (5, 6). For example, the interference in the Stroop effect, when the ink color and the word color are incongruent, could be eliminated when suggesting subjects to view word stimuli as neutral and meaningless (5). Furthermore, the performance of counting visual stimuli was reduced when suggesting participants after a hypnotic induction that a wooden board would cover the screen (6). In one study, the performance in the Flanker task, for example, was only influenced by posthypnotic suggestions in highly suggestible participants compared to (the same) non-hypnotic suggestions in an alert state (7). Thus, the advantage of using verbal suggestions after a hypnotic induction or with highly suggestible participants instead of only verbal instructions is that hypnotic suggestions were able to even demonstrate control over some cognitive processes, as described before (5, 6). However, there is only some literature regarding the enhancement of cognitive performance only via verbal suggestions. For example, the performance in a knowledge test was enhanced when participants believed that they had subliminally received the correct answer (placebo condition) compared to those who were told that they subliminally only received a flash [control condition, (8)]. Even the results in an intelligence test could be enhanced when positive expectations were evolved only via the way participants were recruited (9). Another study found that it was more the subjective evaluation of the own performance that was influenced by expectations rather than the objective performance [as for example reaction times or success rates, see (10)]. However, in previous studies, expectancy effects on placebo were usually paired with some previous test phase in which participants already underwent a specific conditioning paradigm and therefore could already build according expectations regarding the relevant test phase (10).

Taken together, previous results imply that some suggestions can block cognitive processes that were assumed to be automatic and not directly influenceable. However, the magnitude of the placebo effect on enhancing cognitive performance only based on verbal suggestions without previous experience has not yet been examined.

Concerning placebo effects in psychotherapy, as in well-established treatments like for example cognitive behavioral therapy, it is impossible to conduct double-blind trials and challenging to develop "placebo" control groups that are not distinguishable from the specific treatment that is to be tested (11). However, it was demonstrated that psychological placebo interventions show equivalent effects as specific psychotherapies if they were structurally equally designed (12). That's why some researchers emphasize the relevance/superiority of the "common factors" in psychotherapy over the specific therapeutic ingredients (13, 14). Investigating mechanisms of change and differentiating specific and non-specific/common therapeutic "ingredients" is more or less impossible since every specific ingredient is transmitted also via words, verbal suggestions, and other therapeutic rituals (15). Studies are lacking that directly manipulate some of the non-specified factors as for example expectations (16). Using hypnotic verbal suggestions could be one possibility to use some kind of psychological intervention that is not based on specific treatment strategies but directly addresses the non-specific factors like expectations (17) and hypnosis can thus be used as a "non-deceptive placebo" (18).

The goal of our study was therefore to investigate the effects of a mental training based on hypnotic verbal suggestions compared to a control training consisting of a philosophy lecture on the cognitive performance in a student population using a "balanced-placebo-design" (19). We paired the trainings with evoking different expectations in the participants concerning the "efficacy" of the mental training. We expected the strongest effects on cognitive performance when participants received both the mental training and the suggestion of this training as being "effective" compared to the conditions in which they received incongruent information (received mental training and were told "ineffective" or received control training and were told "effective") or the control training paired with the information of being "ineffective."

MATERIALS AND METHODS

Study Design

The study used a mixed 2 × 2 × 2 design with the within-factor time and the between-factors intervention and information, see **Figure 1**. As dependent variable, we assessed the cognitive performance in a specific attention/concentration task (see Assessments). With the within-factor time, cognitive performance was measured before and after the intervention. The factor intervention consisted of the mental training vs.

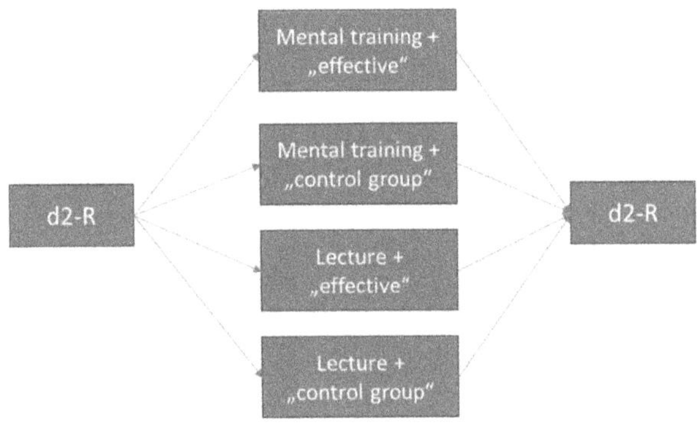

FIGURE 1 | Study design and procedure.

the control training. Concerning the factor information, half of the participants of each intervention condition was told to receive an effective training ("You are part of our experimental group and you will receive an effective mental training") vs. the other half was told that they are part of the control group ("You are part of our control group and you will receive the control condition"). With pairing the factors intervention and information, a balanced-placebo-design was established. Subjects were randomly assigned to one of the four experimental conditions. We chose random numbers between one to four that were equally distributed to do so (source: https://rechneronline.de/zufallszahlen/).

The study protocol was approved by the local Ethics Committee for Psychological Research of the Faculty of Science at the University of Tuebingen (Az 2016/1123/26). All subjects gave written informed consent in accordance with the Declaration of Helsinki.

Participants

The a priori sample size was defined at 100 participants.

Participants for the current study were recruited at the University of Tuebingen via announcements in social media (e.g., facebook groups of psychology students and of the students who were interested in study participation) and in cafeterias and libraries. Inclusion criteria were (1) being at the age of 18 to 50 years old, (2) no uncorrected ametropia, (3) normal hearing, and (4) providing written informed consent to participate in the study. Participants were alerted to the fact that they might be incompletely informed about some part of the study ["authorized deception," see (20)]. After study completion, every participant was completely debriefed in case of prior deception. The "misinformation" of participants was necessary in these experimental conditions where the type of intervention and the type of information were not congruent (mental training and told that "being part of the control group"; control training and told that "being part of the experimental group and receiving an effective training"). The goal of the incomplete information was to evoke specific expectations in participants concerning the effectiveness of the following intervention. The so-called "authorized deception" is a possibility in experimental placebo studies to overcome an important ethical dilemma. On one hand, the deception of participants is necessary to demonstrate the effect of expectancy on outcome. On the other hand, the ethical norms request the participant's free choice of taking part in a study only after every aspect of the study was fully displayed (21). It was shown that the use of "authorized deception" does not affect the placebo effect and therefore is a very useful tool (20).

In total, 103 participants were investigated in the present study. Eighty-three of the subjects (80.6%) were female, all of them being students, about 50% were studying psychology ($n = 43$, 41.7%) or cognitive science ($n = 10$, 9.7%) in the first or second year. The mean age was 23.35 years ($SD = 4.18$).

Interventions

In both conditions, participants individually listened to a 20 min audio-take via headphones. The mental training consisted of different indirect hypnotic verbal suggestions for enhancing the cognitive performance: reminding participants of their own experience when learning some new procedures, creating the image of an archer, giving metaphors with the goal to concentrate and focus on relevant aspects of a task whereas irrelevant aspects can be ignored. Participants were thus not directly but indirectly told to focus more on the cognitive performance task. The control training consisted of a part of a lecture in philosophy about the humans' free will. Listening to the lecture should not evoke an enhancement of the cognitive performance in the subjects. The "control training" was parallelized in the length to the mental training.

Assessments

The cognitive performance of participants was individually tested with the d2R (22) before and after receiving the intervention. The d2R measures attention and concentration performance within 5 min. Participants have to cancel out every "d" with two dashes in between distractors across several rows within a specific time limit. We used the measure of concentration performance of the d2R as overall measure for the participants' attention ability.

Depressive symptoms within the last 14 days were assessed with the Beck Depression Inventory II at baseline [BDI II, (23)].

The participants' ability to absorb in thoughts and imaginings was assessed with the Tellegen Absorption Scale with 34 items at baseline [TAS, (24)].

The BDI-II and the TAS were included as covariates in the data analysis.

At baseline, we also asked participants via questionnaire about some sociodemographic variables.

At the end of the assessment, participants were asked to rate (1) the effectiveness of the training and (2) what type of training the believed they received.

Study Procedure

The investigators of the study followed a specific protocol with standardized instructions when interacting with the participants. Investigators were not blinded to the intervention and the information condition of the participants. After oral and written informed consent, participants received the BDI-II, the TAS, and a sociodemographic questionnaire. At baseline, the d2R was administered the first time. Afterwards, information about the type of training was varied according the participant's experimental condition ("You are part of our experimental condition and you will receive an effective mental training" or "You are part of our control group and you will receive the control condition"). Afterwards, participants received either the mental training or the philosophy lecture via headphones for 20 min. After listening to the audios, the participants were again tested with the d2R. After the task, they were asked to answer the previously described questions about the training they have received before. At the end of the assessment, all participants were debriefed following again a standardized protocol. The assessment took 1 h in total per participant. Subjects received either monetary compensation or got hourly credit for participating in the study.

Statistical Analysis

We computed a three-way analysis of variance, with the between-subjects factors intervention (mental training vs. control training) and information ("effective training" vs. "part of the control group"), and the within-subjects factor time (before and after the training). The dependent variable was cognitive performance measured before and after receiving the training. For baseline correction, we conducted an analysis of covariance with the factors intervention and information, as well as cognitive performance at baseline as covariate. Cognitive performance after the training was used as dependent variable.

RESULTS

The four study groups were comparable at baseline regarding age, $F_{(3, 99)} = 0.21$, $p = 0.890$, sex, $X^2_{(3)} = 3.79$, $p = 0.285$, the TAS, $F_{(3, 99)} = 0.56$, $p = 0.644$, and the BDI-II, $F_{(3, 99)} = 0.41$, $p = 0.748$.

There were differences in the four groups in the cognitive performance at baseline, almost reaching significance, $F_{(3, 99)} = 2.61$, $p = 0.056$, see also the following analyses.

The cognitive performance significantly improved in all participants, $F_{(1,99)} = 490.01$, $p < 0.001$. Means and standard deviations are displayed in **Table 1**. We found no effect of the type of intervention, $F_{(1, 99)} = 0.11$, $p = 0.747$, and no interaction between the factors intervention and time, $F_{(1, 99)} = 0.06$, $p = 0.802$. Further, we found no interaction between information and time, $F_{(1, 99)} = 0.71$, $p = 0.402$, and between information and intervention, $F_{(1, 99)} = 0.85$, $p = 0.358$. However, we found a significant interaction between all three factors, $F_{(1, 99)} = 4.08$, $p = 0.046$ and a significant effect of type of information, $F_{(1, 99)} = 4.79$, $p = 0.031$. This was due to significant differences in the cognitive performance at baseline regarding the type of information, $F_{(1, 101)} = 5.72$, $p = 0.018$. The participants that were later told to be in the control group were actually faster than those who were later instructed to receive an effective mental training ("effective mental training": $M = 166.4$, $SD = 34.8$ vs. "control group": $M = 183.1$, $SD = 36.1$).

When controlling for baseline differences in cognitive performance, there was an interaction between type of training and type of instruction, almost reaching significance, $t_{(98)} = -12.77$, $p = 0.063$. The cognitive performance in groups with congruent information and training did not improve as much, as in groups with incongruent information (improvement "congruent": $M = 33.89$, $SD = 20.11$ vs. improvement "incongruent": $M = 40.55$, $SD = 12.38$).

The covariate depressive symptoms, assessed with the BDI-II, was not related to the cognitive performance, $F_{(1, 96)} = 0.13$, $p = 0.723$, nor was the ability to absorb, as measured with the TAS, $F_{(1, 96)} = 0.46$, $p = 0.500$.

When we compared the cognitive performance of the participants regarding their effectiveness rating at the end of the intervention, a significant interaction between time and the rating of the training was found. We observed an improvement of the cognitive performance, when the participants afterwards rated the training as neutral or effective at the end of the assessment, compared to those who rated the training as ineffective, $F_{(2, 100)} = 7.26$, $p = 0.001$, see also **Table 2**. The improvement in cognitive performance was, however, independent of the fact if participants correctly identified the training condition or not, $F_{(1, 101)} = 1.75$, $p = 0.189$.

The actual training they received had no significant effect on the evaluation of the effectiveness, $X^2_{(2)} = 5.50$, $p = 0.064$, see **Table 3**. The effectiveness rating at the end of the intervention was rather significantly associated with their own belief, what type of training they received, $X^2_{(2)} = 10.67$, $p = 0.005$, see **Table 4**.

These participants who rated the training as neutral or effective, showed higher scores in absorption (TAS) at baseline compared to those who rated the training as ineffective, $F_{(2, 99)} = 3.75$, $p = 0.027$ (ineffective: $M = 42.0$, $SD = 19.6$; neutral: $M = 46.4$, $SD = 18.3$; effective: $M = 56.1$, $SD = 25.4$; *post hoc* Bonferroni: effective vs. ineffective: $p = 0.038$). No differences were found regarding age, depressive symptoms, and sex.

TABLE 1 | Cognitive performance before and after the intervention in all four experimental conditions.

Intervention	Information	d2-R KL pre *M (SD)*	d2-R KL post *M (SD)*
Mental training	"Effective mental training" (*n* = 29)	169.8 (32.8)	205.3 (36.1)
	"Control group" (*n* = 24)	176.7 (32.4)	216.3 (36.5)
Lecture (Control training)	"Effective mental training" (*n* = 25)	162.6 (37.3)	204.1 (39.0)
	"Control group" (*n* = 25)	189.3 (39.0)	221.2 (40.5)
	total (*n* = 103)	174.4 (36.2)	211.4 (38.1)

M, mean; SD, standard deviation; n, sample size.

TABLE 2 | Cognitive performance before and after the intervention regarding effectiveness ratings.

	d2-R KL pre *M (SD)*	d2-R KL post *M (SD)*
Training was ineffective (*n* = 24)	179.71 (36.45)	205.75 (34.18)
Training was neutral (*n* = 29)	171.90 (32.55)	212.59 (38.65)
Training was effective (*n* = 50)	173.26 (38.56)	213.50 (40.02)

M, mean; SD, standard deviation; n, sample size.

TABLE 3 | Effectiveness rating in the two actual intervention conditions.

	Mental training: *n*	Lecture: *n*
Training was ineffective ($n = 24$)	8	16
Training was neutral ($n = 29$)	14	15
Training was effective ($n = 50$)	31	19

n, sample size, $X^2_{(2)} = 5.50$, $p = 0.064$.

TABLE 4 | Effectiveness rating in the two assumed intervention conditions.

	Mental training assumed: *n*	Lecture assumed: *n*
Training was ineffective ($n = 24$)	8	16
Training was neutral ($n = 29$)	8	21
Training was effective ($n = 50$)	31	19

n, sample size, $X^2_{(2)} = 10.67$, $p = 0.005$.

DISCUSSION

Contrary to our hypothesis, that a mental training, which is only based on verbal suggestions, or the information about the effectiveness of the training could enhance cognitive performance, there was no effect of the training and the information about the training on their actual performance. Overall, we found that the cognitive performance of all participants improved. This result might be due to practicing or an effect of repeated measures [see also (22)]. However, the participant's own rating about the effectiveness of the training was significantly influenced by the cognitive performance change irrespective of the actual type of intervention or information they received. Our results suggest that it was either the perception of their own performance improvement that influenced their rating about the effectiveness at the end of the assessment. The effectiveness rating, however, was independent of the actual training they received and also of the fact if they correctly identified the training condition. Thus, another interpretation of the results could be that the subjective evaluation influenced the participant's performance in the second trial. Unfortunately, we did not assess expectations regarding the mental training and its influence on cognitive performance before the assessment.

Mental practice is known to enhance performance in general, because it involves training of specific behaviors, especially in cognitive tasks (25). Another study found that mental practicing - imagining a specific motor activity—could enhance the outcome in that specific motor task (26). This finding could be interpreted as a top-down mechanism that somehow activated the brain regions that are also associated with the concrete task and thus enhance performance. Similarly, if a mental training is able to activate areas that are associated with cognitive performance, the performance itself can be improved. However, the mental practice should be regularly trained for maintaining effects (25). In our study, participants received only one session of mental training. Furthermore, several cognitive abilities are needed for assessing attention performance in a specific task like the d2R that was used in our study, for example performance speed, accuracy, inhibition of distractors etc. (22). It might be possible that our mental training was not able to activate the specific abilities that were necessary for the attention task that we measured. Our training, which consisted of suggestions that might indirectly influence their performance, did not include any mental practice of the specific attention task. However, some higher order cognitions, as for example self-efficacy (27) or other meta-cognitive aspects like self-regulation or motivation (28), could have been more important for the cognitive outcome that we measured. Especially in student samples, perceived self-efficacy can influence the cognitive performance (29). The finding of another study, that verbal suggestions could enhance creativity, was explained by the idea that it was driven by intrinsic motivation and the belief in the own competence of the participant (30). If we transfer that explanation to our results, we could hypothesize that the participant's own motivation and belief in their performance had the biggest effect on their actual performance regardless of the information given by the investigator or the suggestions that were used in the mental training. Their own evaluation of the effectiveness of the training was consequently not based on external information but on their own intrinsic standards. The participants' motivation to improve or their perceived self-efficacy therefore influenced their performance the most. Our results are also in line with previous findings that it was rather the subjective evaluation than the objective performance that was influenced by verbal suggestions [see (7)]. The (almost significant) result that the cognitive performance improved more when subjects were given information about the type of training that was not congruent to the actual training they received, is extremely interesting within the previously discussed explanation. We interpret that result in the way that the participants' motivation to improve was even triggered more when receiving incongruent information.

We found that participants who rated the training as effective had higher hypnotic suggestibility than those who rated the training as ineffective. The effectiveness rating, however, was significantly influenced by the intervention they perceived they have received rather than the actual intervention condition that they received. This potential placebo effect implies that highly suggestible subjects might base their expectations on the owns appraisal instead of external information. We argue that the effect of enhancing cognitive performance was more pronounced in a subgroup of participants with high intrinsic motivation, high self-efficacy, and high suggestible ability. Similarly, patients with high suggestibility suffering from depression showed greater responses to suggestions and expectations regarding the effects and side effects they perceived together with taking an antidepressant medication (31). The ability to absorb in images, also known as hypnotic suggestibility [see (24)], might therefore mediate the effect of expectations on outcome [see also (31)]. However, the ability to absorb in our study had no impact on the cognitive performance itself but on the participants' own evaluation of the effectiveness of the treatment. This underlines the importance of tailoring interventions to some of the participants' characteristics or needs. Personalized medicine, also used in the psychiatric context, is based on that idea of optimizing the fit between patient characteristics and treatment choice and therefore enhancing treatment outcome and benefit [e.g., (32)]. Furthermore, interventions that are based on hypnotic verbal suggestions should have the goal of increasing the self-efficacy and the belief in the own competence (33). This idea can be underlined by the findings regarding the influence of non-specific/common factors on the outcome of psychotherapy (34).

Placebo effects on cognitive performances were found when participants suffer from mild cognitive or attentional deficits as for example in some nicotine-smokers that were deprived before (35). Some patients with Major Depression also suffer from a cognitive impairment [see (36)], and attention or concentration problems are also included in the list of typical symptoms and criteria of depression. Mental trainings and other psychological interventions for enhancing cognitive performance might even be more effective for these patients compared to healthy academically high performers like university students. This is in line with a study that found that older adults might also profit in their cognitive performance after receiving some kind of cognitive training (37). Future studies should evaluate the effects of a mental training that focuses on cognitive enhancement especially in patients with Major Depression. Within this context, the influence of placebo effects on the cognitive performance should also be investigated.

LIMITATIONS

There are several factors that limit the generalizability of the current study.

One limitation of the current study is that we did not conduct any pilot study to figure out if the mental training that we conceptualized was effective or not. We also did not obtain any feedback about the quality of the mental training from the participants. However, we have to note, that it was not our goal to evaluate the mental training. In contrast, we were more interested in differentiating the effects of direct suggestions and information that were given by the investigators compared to creating some images (within the mental training) that might indirectly influence the participants' performance. However, the mental training should have been evaluated in different samples regarding its effectiveness on enhancing cognitive performance. For this purpose, a full deceptive placebo design could be used. In summary, our mental training was not specifically effective for the cognitive performance in the student sample.

Second, our study sample was not representative. We measured a very young and highly educated student sample. Comparing the means of the present sample with the norms of the d2R, it was obvious that even at baseline the student sample showed an extremely high concentration performance [norms of the d2R at the age of 20–39: $M = 158.6$, $SD = 29.4$, see (22); current sample: $M = 174.38$, $SD = 36.24$]. This might be based on motivation differences regarding the assessment or some previous experience in the task [see also (22)].

We found differences in the cognitive performance of participants at baseline regarding the factor type of information. The differences were found at baseline where the instruction were not yet given to the subject. Thus, we might have created an investigator's effect. Even if the participants were randomly assigned to the experimental condition, the investigator was not blind regarding the intervention and information condition that the subjects received when interacting with him or her. Especially when the investigator knew the fact that the participant will be later told to receive the control condition, it might have been that he or she behaved in a different way when interacting with the participant that may have influenced and increased their performance. We wanted to avoid any influence of the investigator on the subject by using a standardized protocol for instructing the subjects. But maybe they were already influencing the subjects' performance unconsciously or via indirect communication. In sum, a potential investigators' allegiance effect may have confounded the results [see also (38)]. Future studies should either avoid investigator effects by blinding the investigator who is interacting with the participants regarding the type of training they receive. Another possibility could also be to directly manipulate and vary of some aspects of the contact with the participants. For example, placebo effects were enhanced when a practitioner contact was longer and focused more on the nature and history of symptom assessment compared to a relationship with only limited contact (39) and a warm empathic contact with a clinician could even result in subjective and objective ratings of improvement of cold duration and severity (40).

CONCLUSIONS

The participants' own evaluation of the effectiveness of the training was most probably driven by their own performance in the first and second trial of the task or by their own motivation to perform. The own experiences and ratings were subsequently more important for their cognitive performance than the efficacy of a specific training or information about the training they receive. This finding underlines the relevance of enhancing the self-efficacy in situations where cognitive attention processes are important and of individually tailoring psychological trainings or interventions accordingly. The relevance of mental trainings for people with psychological disorders with a mild cognitive impairment as for example in patients with mild to moderate Major Depression Episodes should be investigated in future studies. Within this context, especially the participant's belief in the efficacy of a specific treatment should enhance their actual treatment response. The ability to absorb in images, also known as hypnotic suggestibility [see (24)], might mediate the effect of expectations on outcome and should be investigated in future psychotherapy studies.

AUTHOR CONTRIBUTIONS

Both authors contributed to the conception and design of the study. KF wrote the first draft of the manuscript. KF and DW conducted the statistical analysis. Both authors approved the submitted version.

FUNDING

The study was funded by the University Program for the Promotion of Junior Researchers at the Eberhard Karls Universität of Tübingen, awarded to KF, between July 2016 to December 2017. We acknowledge support from Deutsche Forschungsgemeinschaft and Open Access Publishing Fund of University of Tuebingen.

ACKNOWLEDGMENTS

We want to thank our investigators Neele Alberts, Lia Heubner, Isabell Kunze, and Tina Lorenz for helping with the data acquisition.

REFERENCES

1. Pollo A, Amanzio M, Arslanian A, Casadio C, Maggi G, Benedetti F. Response expectancies in placebo analgesia and their clinical relevance. *Pain* (2001) 93:77–84. doi: 10.1016/S0304-3959(01)00296-2
2. Benedetti F, Pollo A, Lopiano L, Lanotte M, Vighetti S, Rainero I. Conscious expectation and unconscious conditioning in analgesic, motor, and hormonal placebo/nocebo responses. *J. Neurosci.* (2003) 23:4315–23. doi: 10.1523/JNEUROSCI.23-10-04315.2003
3. Dawkins L, Shahzad FZ, Ahmed SS, Edmonds CJ. Expectation of having consumed caffeine can improve performance and mood. *Appetite* (2011) 57:597–600. doi: 10.1016/j.appet.2011.07.011
4. Cropsey KL, Schiavon S, Hendricks PS, Froelich M, Lentowicz I, Fargason R. Mixed-amphetamine salts expectancies among college students: is stimulant induced cognitive enhancement a placebo effect? *Drug Alcohol Depend.* (2017) 178(Suppl. C):302–9. doi: 10.1016/j.drugalcdep.2017.05.024
5. Lifshitz M, Bonn NA, Fischer A, Kashem IF, Raz A. Using suggestion to modulate automatic processes: From Stroop to McGurk and beyond. *Cortex* (2013) 49:463–73. doi: 10.1016/j.cortex.2012.08.007
6. Schmidt B, Hecht H, Naumann E, Miltner WHR. The Power of mind: blocking visual perception by hypnosis. *Sci. Rep.* (2017) 7:4889. doi: 10.1038/s41598-017-05195-2
7. Iani C, Ricci F, Gherri E, Rubichi S. Hypnotic suggestion modulates cognitive conflict: the case of the flanker compatibility effect. *Psychol. Sci.* (2006) 17:721–7. doi: 10.1111/j.1467-9280.2006.01772.x
8. Weger UW, Loughnan S. Mobilizing unused resources: using the placebo concept to enhance cognitive performance. *Q. J. Exp. Psychol.* (2013) 66:23–8. doi: 10.1080/17470218.2012.751117
9. Foroughi CK, Monfort SS, Paczynski M, McKnight PE, Greenwood PM. Placebo effects in cognitive training. *Proc Natl Acad Sci USA.* (2016) 113:7470–4. doi: 10.1073/pnas.1601243113
10. Schwarz KA, Büchel C. Cognition and the placebo effect–dissociating subjective perception and actual performance. *PloS One* (2015) 10:e0130492. doi: 10.1371/journal.pone.0130492
11. Wampold BE, Minami T, Tierney SC, Baskin TW, Bhati KS. The placebo is powerful: estimating placebo effects in medicine and psychotherapy from randomized clinical trials. *J Clin Psychol.* (2005) 61:835–54. doi: 10.1002/jclp.20129
12. Baskin TW, Tierney SC, Minami T, Wampold BE. Establishing specificity in psychotherapy: a meta-analysis of structural equivalence of placebo controls. *J Consult Clin Psychol.* (2003) 71:973–9. doi: 10.1037/0022-006X.71.6.973
13. Asay TP, Lambert MJ. The empirical case for the common factors in therapy: quantitative findings. In: Hubble MA, Duncan BL, Miller SD, editors. *The Heart and Soul of Change: What Works in Therapy* (1999). p. 23–55. doi: 10.1037/11132-001
14. Messer SB, Wampold BE. Let's face facts: common factors are more potent than specific therapy ingredients. *Clin Psychol.* (2002) 9:21–5. doi: 10.1093/clipsy.9.1.21
15. Butler SF, Strupp HH. Specific and nonspecific factors in psychotherapy: a problematic paradigm for psychotherapy research. *Psychotherapy* (1986) 23:30–40. doi: 10.1037/h0085590
16. Greenberg RP, Constantino MJ, Bruce, N. Are patient expectations still relevant for psychotherapy process and outcome? *Clin Psychol Rev.* (2006) 26:657–78. doi: 10.1016/j.cpr.2005.03.002
17. Erickson MH. The interpersonal hypnotic technique for symptom correction and pain control. *Am J Clin Hypnosis* (1966) 8:198–209. doi: 10.1080/00029157.1966.10402492
18. Kirsch I. Clinical hypnosis as a nondeceptive placebo: empirically derived techniques. *Am J Clin Hypnosis* (1994) 37:95–106. doi: 10.1080/00029157.1994.10403122
19. Enck P, Klosterhalfen S, Zipfel S. Novel study designs to investigate the placebo response. *BMC Med Res Methodol.* (2011) 11:1–8. doi: 10.1186/1471-2288-11-90
20. Martin AL, Katz J. Inclusion of authorized deception in the informed consent process does not affect the magnitude of the placebo effect for experimentally induced pain. *Pain* (2010) 149:208–15. doi: 10.1016/j.pain.2009.12.004
21. Miller FG, Wendler D, Swartzman LC. Deception in research on the placebo effect. *PLoS Med* (2005) 2: e262. doi: 10.1371/journal.pmed.0020262
22. Brickenkamp R, Schmidt-Atzert L, Liepmann D. *Test d2-Revision: Aufmerksamkeits-und Konzentrationstest.* Göttingen: Hogrefe (2010).
23. Beck AT, Steer RA, Brown GK. *Manual for the Beck Depression Inventory-II.* San Antonio, TX: Psychological Corporation (1996).
24. Tellegen A, Atkinson G. Openness to absorbing and self-altering experiences ("absorption"), a trait related to hypnotic susceptibility. *J Abnorm Psychol.* (1974) 83:268–77. doi: 10.1037/h0036681
25. Driskell JE, Copper C, Moran A. Does mental practice enhance performance? *J Appl Psychol.* (1994) 79:481–92. doi: 10.1037/0021-9010.79.4.481
26. Papadelis C, Kourtidou-Papadeli C, Bamidis P, Albani M. Effects of imagery training on cognitive performance and use of physiological measures as an assessment tool of mental effort. *Brain Cogn.* (2007) 64:71–85. doi: 10.1016/j.bandc.2007.01.001
27. Bandura A. Perceived self-efficacy in cognitive development and functioning. *Educ Psychol.* (2010) 28:117–148. doi: 10.1207/s15326985ep2802_3
28. Pintrich PR, De Groot EV. Motivational and self-regulated learning components of classroom academic performance. *J Educ Psychol.* (1990) 82:33–40. doi: 10.1037/0022-0663.82.1.33
29. Bouffard-Bouchard T. Influence of self-efficacy on performance in a cognitive task. *J Soc Psychol.* (2010) 130:3:353–63. doi: 10.1080/00224545.1990.9924591
30. Rozenkrantz L, Mayo AE, Ilan T, Hart Y, Noy L, Alon U. Placebo can enhance creativity. *PloS ONE* (2017) 12:e0182466. doi: 10.1371/journal.pone.0182466
31. Nitzan U, Chalamish Y, Krieger I, Erez HB, Braw Y, Lichtenberg P. Suggestibility as a predictor of response to antidepressants: a preliminary prospective trial. *J Affect Dis.* (2015) 185:8–11. doi: 10.1016/j.jad.2015.06.028
32. Cuijpers P, Reynolds CF, Donker T, Li J, Andersson G, Beekman A. Personalized treatment of adult depression: medication, psychotherapy, or both? A systematic review. *Depress Anxiety* (2012) 29:855–64. doi: 10.1002/da.21985
33. Doering BK, Glombiewski JA, Rief W. Expectation-focused psychotherapy to improve clinical outcomes. *Int Rev Neurobiol.* (2018) 138:257–70. doi: 10.1016/bs.irn.2018.02.004
34. Ilardi SS, Craighead WE. The role of nonspecific factors in cognitive-behavior therapy for depression. *Clin Psychol* (1994) 1:138–55. doi: 10.1111/j.1468-2850.1994.tb00016.x

35. Hammersley JJ, Gilbert DG, Rzetelny A, Rabinovich NE. Moderation of nicotine effects on covert orienting of attention tasks by poor placebo performance and cue validity. *Pharmacol Biochem Behav.* (2016) 149:9–16. doi: 10.1016/j.pbb.2016.07.006
36. Reppermund S, Ising M, Lucae S, Zihl J. Cognitive impairment in unipolar depression is persistent and non-specific: further evidence for the final common pathway disorder hypothesis. *Psychol Med.* (2009) 39:603–14. doi: 10.1017/S003329170800411X
37. Ball K, Berch DB, Helmers KF, Jobe JB, Leveck MD, Marsiske M, et al. Effects of cognitive training interventions with older adultsa randomized controlled trial. *JAMA* (2002) 288:2271–81. doi: 10.1001/jama.288.18.2271
38. Berman JS, Reich CM. Investigator allegiance and the evaluation of psychotherapy outcome research. *Eur J Psychother Counsel.* (2010) 12:11–21. doi: 10.1080/13642531003637775
39. Kaptchuk TJ, Kelley JM, Conboy LA, Davis RB, Kerr CE, Jacobson EE, et al. Components of placebo effect: randomised controlled trial in patients with irritable bowel syndrome. *BMJ* (2008) 336:999–1003. doi: 10.1136/bmj.39524.439618.25
40. Rakel DP, Hoeft TJ, Barrett BP, Chewning BA, Craig BM, Niu M. Practitioner empathy and the duration of the common cold. *Fam Med.* (2009) 41:494–501.

4

The Influence of Expectancy Level and Personal Characteristics on Placebo Effects: Psychological Underpinnings

Lili Zhou[1,2], *Hua Wei*[3], *Huijuan Zhang*[1,2], *Xiaoyun Li*[3], *Cunju Bo*[4], *Li Wan*[4*], *Xuejing Lu*[1,2*] *and Li Hu*[1,2,3,4]

[1] CAS Key Laboratory of Mental Health, Institute of Psychology, Chinese Academy of Sciences, Beijing, China, [2] Department of Psychology, University of Chinese Academy of Sciences, Beijing, China, [3] Key Laboratory of Cognition and Personality, Ministry of Education, Faculty of Psychology, Southwest University, Chongqing, China, [4] Department of Pain Management, The State Key Clinical Specialty in Pain Medicine, The Second Affiliated Hospital of Guangzhou Medical University, Guangzhou, China

***Correspondence:**
Xuejing Lu
luxj@psych.ac.cn
Li Wan
wanli5000cn@163.com

Placebo effects benefit a wide range of clinical practice, which can be profoundly influenced by expectancy level and personal characteristics. However, research on the issue of whether these factors independently or interdependently affect the placebo effects is still in its infancy. Here, we adopted a 3-day between-subject placebo analgesia paradigm (2-day conditioning and 1-day test) to investigate the influence of expectancy levels (i.e., No, Low, and High) and personal characteristics (i.e., gender, dispositional optimism, and anxiety state) on placebo effects in 120 healthy participants (60 females). Our results showed that the reduction of pain intensity in the test phase was influenced by the interaction between expectancy and gender, as mainly reflected by greater reductions of pain intensity in females at Low expectancy level than females at No/High expectancy levels, and greater reductions of pain intensity in males than in females at High expectancy level. Additionally, the reduction of pain unpleasantness was not only modulated by the interaction between expectancy and gender, but also by the interaction between expectancy and dispositional optimism, as well as the interaction between expectancy and anxiety state. Specifically, participants who were more optimistic in Low expectancy group, or those who were less anxious in High expectancy group showed greater reductions of pain unpleasantness. To sum up, we emphasized on regulating the expectancy level individually based on the assessment of personal characteristics to maximize placebo effects in clinical conditions.

Keywords: expectancy, placebo analgesia, gender, dispositional optimism, anxiety state

INTRODUCTION

Placebo commonly refers to an inert substance or a medicinally inactive treatment that can generate clinically-useful effects. A person who receives a placebo treatment usually experiences actual improvements in his/her physical condition, which is well-known as the *placebo effect*. The placebo effect can be beneficial in a wide range of clinical situations, such as modulating the therapeutic effects of deep brain stimulation on Parkinson's disease, generating antidepressant responses in depression, and reducing unpleasantness in patients with anxiety (1, 2). It can also enhance the effectiveness of physical interventions (3–5) and provide an alternative approach to avoid side effects of drug treatments (6, 7).

Although placebo effect is a complex phenomenon that can be affected by multiple factors (e.g., memory, motivation, anxiety, learning, patient-provider interaction, and previous treatment experience) (1, 8–10), response expectancy has been recognized as one of the main psychological mechanisms underlying this effect (11). Response expectancy has been defined as the expectancy to the occurrence of non-volitional responses (i.e., responses experienced as occurring automatically without volitional efforts, including fear, sadness, sexual arousal, pain, etc.) to situational cues (12). According to *Response Expectancy Theory*, such response expectancy could affect the probability that an individual would engage in a particular behavior (e.g., increased/decreased pain responses), as non-volitional responses have positive and negative reinforcement values (12). Consistent with this theory, accumulating evidence has shown that the placebo effect (e.g., placebo analgesia) could be altered by changing individual expectancy (3, 7, 13–19).

In general, response expectancy is composed of two distinct aspects: (1) the expected magnitude of a change (i.e., expectancy level), and (2) the subjective probability that the change will occur (i.e., individual belief) (12). With regards to the first aspect of response expectancy, a greater placebo effect is usually associated with a higher level of positive expectancy (4, 5, 20–23). However, these observations are not guaranteed under some circumstances. For example, in laboratory settings, even individual expectation of placebo effects has been successfully acquired during the classical conditioning phase, unrealistically high expectancy that does not match with one's present experience would weaken individual belief in the placebo treatment during the test phase (24).

In terms of the second aspect of response expectancy, previous studies have demonstrated that individual belief in the current experience has a critical influence on response expectancy through learning mechanisms (21, 24). Such a belief is easily affected by personal characteristics, thus contributing to the differentiation of individual expectancy (25, 26), and subsequently leading to individual variability in response to placebos (27, 28). For instance, gender has been verified as a factor contributing to the variability of placebo effects—some studies suggested that males reported greater pain reductions after placebo treatments compared to females (29–31), whereas other studies described a better respondence to placebos in females than in males (29, 32–34). Additionally, the influence of other personal characteristics on placebo responses has been frequently reported in the literature. For example, dispositional optimism, referred to a generalized positive outcome expectancy for the future (35), is inextricably linked to proneness of increased placebo effects (36, 37). Comparatively, individuals with low anxiety level are more likely to respond to a placebo treatment (36).

However, research on the issue of whether expectancy level and personal characteristics independently or interdependently affect the placebo effects is still in its infancy. Here, we adopted a between-subject placebo analgesia paradigm to test the influence of expectancy levels (i.e., No, Low, and High) and personal characteristics (i.e., gender, dispositional optimism, and anxiety state) on placebo effects.

MATERIALS AND METHODS

Participants

A total of 120 healthy, right-handed participants (60 females) were recruited from the local community. None of them reported a history of illness or concurrent medication. Participants were informed that they were attending a study aimed to test the effect of lidocaine (a local anesthetic that could be topically applied on the skin) on alleviating pain, and they were asked not to consume products containing caffeine, alcohol, or nicotine at least 12 h before the experiment. All the participants gave their written informed consents and were told their rights to discontinue participation at any time during the study. Each participant was randomly assigned to one of the three experimental groups divided by the manipulated expectancy levels (i.e., No, Low, and High) during the Conditioning phase (as described below), with 40 participants (20 females) in each group. After the whole experiment, all participants were fully debriefed.

Experimental Materials

Pain Stimuli

The electrical pain stimuli were delivered using a constant-current stimulator (model DS7A; Digitimer, UK) with three stainless steel concentric bipolar needle electrodes (38, 39). Pain stimuli were intraepidermal electrical pulses delivered to the inner side of the left forearm through the electrodes (located according to an equilateral triangle shape), which have been proved to preferentially activate the Aδ nociceptive fibers in the superficial skin layers (40, 41). Each electrode consisted of a needle cathode (length = 0.1 mm, diameter = 0.2 mm) surrounded by a cylindrical anode (diameter = 1.4 mm). Each stimulus consisted of 100 rapidly succeeding constant-current, square-wave pulses at 50 Hz (0.5-ms duration for each pulse).

Dispositional Optimism

The Chinese version of the Life Orientation Test-Revised (LOT-R) was adopted to assess participants' dispositional optimism, as its reliability has been well-established (Cronbach alpha of positive subscale = 0.73, $N = 479$; Cronbach alpha of negative subscale = 0.82, $N = 479$) (42). In the current sample, the reliability of the scale was satisfactory (Cronbach alpha = 0.66, $N = 120$).

Anxiety State

The state subscale of Chinese version of State-Trait Anxiety Inventory (STAI-S) was adopted to assess participants' anxiety state. The reliability of the Chinese version of STAI-S (Cronbach alpha = 0.90, $N = 2{,}150$) (43) has been well-established. Notably, the reliability of the subscale in the current sample was satisfactory (STAI-S: Cronbach alpha = 0.89, $N = 120$).

Experimental Procedure

A randomized, single-blinded between-subject experimental paradigm of placebo analgesia was adopted in the present study (7). Participants were firstly familiarized with the electrical stimulation prior to the formal experiment. The stimulus intensities were adjusted individually using the method of limits, to identify the thresholds for each participant that would elicit a low sensation (~2 rating), moderate sensation (~4 rating), and high sensation (~6 rating) on an 11-point self-report Numeric Rating Scale (NRS, 0 = no sensation, 10 = unbearable pain). Specifically, the stimuli at ~2 rating elicited a non-painful sensation, whereas the stimuli at ~4 and ~6 ratings elicited a painful pinprick sensation. Once these stimulus intensities were determined, a randomized sequence of pain stimuli with different intensities was delivered to participants until they were able to reliably distinguish the intensities of these stimuli. Notably, these determined stimuli with varied intensities were used during the conditioning procedure (see Conditioning Phase section) to ensure a successful manipulation of expectancy level during the experiment.

The experiment consisted of two phases in three consecutive days: *Conditioning phase* (Day 1 and Day 2) and *Test phase* (Day 3). On each day, participants underwent three sessions: (1) a pre-treatment session, (2) a treatment session, and (3) a post-treatment session (see **Figure 1**). To rule out possible confounding effects related to the gender of experimenter (44, 45), half of participants in each group with an equal number of males ($n = 20$) and females ($n = 20$) were instructed by a female experimenter, while the rest were guided by a male experimenter. Both female and male experimenter wore white coats and had received systematic training of procedure prior to the formal experiment.

Conditioning Phase

The Conditioning phase started with a pre-treatment session consisting of 20 trials. Each trial started with a 1 s white fixation centered on the screen with a black background. After a 5 s waiting, an electrical stimulus at ~6 ratings (0.80 ± 0.29 mA) lasting for 2 s was delivered to the left forearm of the participant. Being waiting for another 5 s, participants were required to verbally rate the perceived intensity (0 = no sensation, 10 = unbearable pain) and unpleasantness (0 = not unpleasant, 10 = extremely unpleasant) of pain evoked by the electrical stimulus (with 8 s per each rating, 16 s in total). The inter-trial interval varied between 8 and 12 s. The stimulus intensity in the pre-treatment session was identical across groups and the whole session lasted for ~16 min.

In the treatment session, a non-active skin cream was applied on the palmar side of the participant's left forearm. Being waiting for 5 min, participants were instructed to remove the cream and have a 10 min rest. Meanwhile, in order to strength expectancy level, participants were given one of the following verbal interventions, depending on treatment assignment:

(1) participants in No expectancy group were told that "*the skin cream is ineffective to relieve or eliminate pain*";
(2) participants in Low expectancy group were told that "*the skin cream can reduce but not eliminate pain*";
(3) participants in High expectancy group were told that "*the skin cream can completely eliminate pain.*"

The treatment session lasted for ~15 min.

The Conditioning phase ended with a post-treatment session consisting of 40 trials. The procedure was identical to the pre-treatment session, except that different intensities of electrical stimuli were set for different groups: inducing a painful sensation at ~6 rating (0.69 ± 0.16 mA) for No expectancy group, at ~4 rating (0.47 ± 0.17 mA) for Low expectancy group, and a non-painful sensation at ~2 rating (0.28 ± 0.08 mA) for High expectancy group. Such changes of stimulus intensity for different groups were intended to strengthen the power of verbal intervention to response expectancy, which has been frequently applied in previous placebo-related studies (46–48). The post-treatment session lasted for ~37 min.

Test Phase

The Test phase also consisted of a pre-treatment session, a treatment session, and a post-treatment session. The procedure of this phase was identical to the *Conditioning phase*, except that the intensity of electrical stimuli applied in the post-treatment session was identical for all participants across groups, i.e., inducing a painful pinprick sensation at ~6 rating (0.78 ± 0.26 mA). Participants were first required to complete the psychological questionnaires upon arriving to the laboratory on the Test day. To make sure that the expectancy manipulation was successful, participants in the Low and High Expectancy groups were required to verbally rate the strength of expectancy to drug efficacy on an 11-point NRS (0 = without any expectancy, 10 = full expectancy) at the end of the test. The average ratings of expectancy to drug efficacy were significantly different between groups (Low: 6.90 ± 1.31, High: 8.39 ± 0.80, $t = -6.11$, $P < 0.001$), indicating a successful expectancy manipulation. For participants in No expectancy group, the expectancy to drug efficacy was not assessed to avoid extra response bias to the expectancy manipulation.

Statistical Analysis

To assess the magnitude of placebo effects, we calculated the changes of subjective pain intensity and unpleasantness by subtracting the ratings in the post-treatment session from those in the pre-treatment session in Test phase (49). To demonstrate the influence of personal characteristics on the modulation of expectancy level on placebo effects, we performed a statistical analysis using a "split into three subgroups" strategy (13-14-13 split). Specifically, we sorted the LOT-R scores in ascending order and split the data into low (13 participants), middle (14 participants), and high LOT-R subgroups (13 participants) for each experimental condition. Following, we performed three-way analyses of variance (ANOVAs) on the indicators

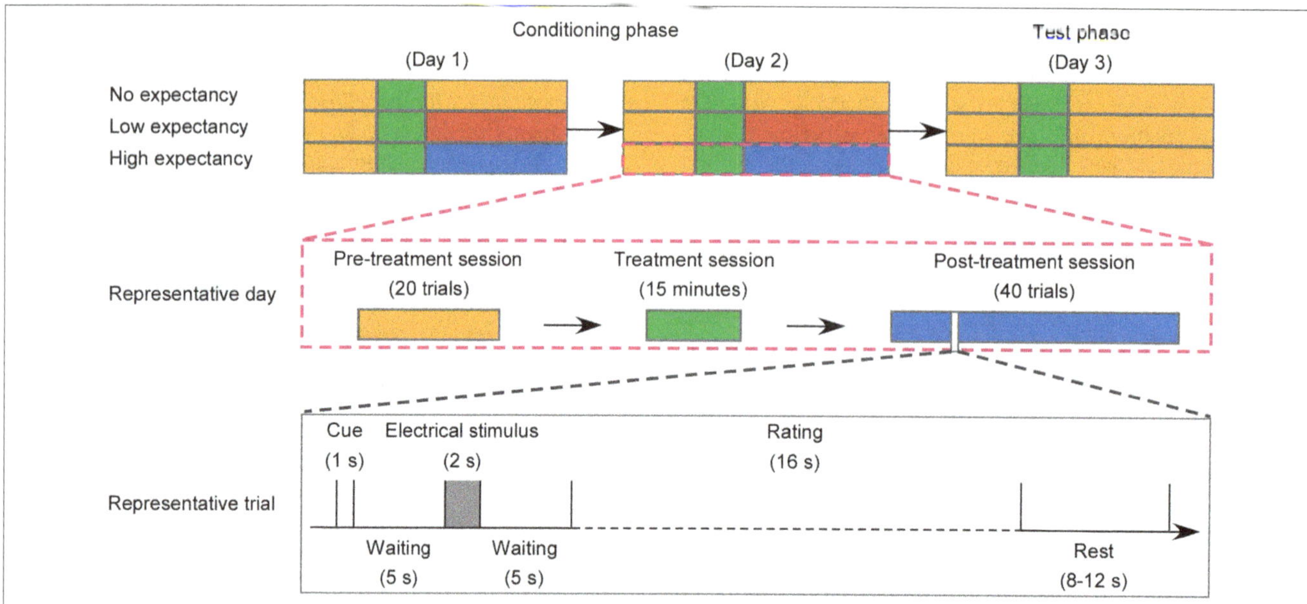

FIGURE 1 | Flowchart of the experimental design. **(Top)** For each experimental group (No, Low, and High expectancy), the experiment consisted of two phases: Conditioning phase (Day 1 and Day 2) and Test phase (Day 3), and each day consisted of three sessions: a pre-treatment session, a treatment session, and a post-treatment session. Sessions, in which the electrical stimuli elicit a low sensation at ~2 rating, moderate sensation at ~4 rating, and high sensation at ~6 rating on the 11-point Numerical Rating Scale, are marked in blue, red, and orange, respectively. Treatment sessions are marked in green. **(Middle)** The experimental procedure in a representative day contained a 20-trial pre-treatment session, a 15 min treatment session, and a 40-trial post-treatment session, which are marked in orange, green, and blue, respectively. **(Bottom)** A representative trial of the pre-treatment session or the post-treatment session was starting with a 1-s cue, followed by a 5 s waiting, a 2 s electrical stimulus, another 5 s waiting, and a 16 s rating of the perception of pain intensity, unpleasantness, anxiety level, and satisfaction of drug officacy (post-treatment session in Low and High expectancy groups). The trial was ended with a rest of 8–12 s.

of placebo effects, with "expectancy level" (No, Low, and High), "dispositional optimism (LOT-R)" (low and high), and "gender" (female and male) as between-subject factors. Likewise, scores of anxiety state (STAI-S) were sorted and analyzed using the same statistical strategy. The statistical *P*-values were adjusted with Greenhouse-Geisser correction to avoid violation of the sphericity assumption, when necessary. *Post hoc* pairwise comparisons were performed with Bonferroni adjustments, when the main effects or interactions reach statistical significance. The effect size and statistical power in the present sample were estimated by partial eta-squared and 1-β, respectively. For partial eta-squared (η_p^2), an effect size of 0.0099 is deemed as a "small" effect, around 0.0588 as a "medium" effect, and 0.1379 to infinity as a "large" effect (50). For 1- β, 0.8 is the commonly acceptable statistical power. To detect the effectiveness of sample size used in the current study, we performed a prior computation on the required sample size using G*power (an online free software for power analysis, available at http://www.gpower.hhu.de/en.html) by setting statistical power at 0.8 with large effect size ($\eta_p^2 = 0.1379$). The result showed a minimal sample size of 64 in total to detect the main effects and interactions between independent variables, which indicated that our sample size ($N = 120$) was enough to detect these effects. All statistical analyses were carried out in SPSS 22.0 statistical analysis package (SPSS Inc., New York, USA). Statistical threshold was set at 0.05.

RESULTS

Participant Characteristics

Participant characteristics for each experimental group are summarized in **Table 1**. The age was not significantly associated with "expectancy level" (No, Low, and High) and "gender" (female and male) [$F_{(2,114)} = 2.84$, $P = 0.06$, $\eta_p^2 = 0.05$]. This result, together with the counterbalanced experimental design for gender, indicated that all the participants across groups were age- and gender-matched, thus avoiding possible bias when assessing placebo effects.

Influence of Expectancy Level, Dispositional Optimism, and Gender on Placebo Effects

Significant main effects of "expectancy level" [$F_{(2,72)} = 7.06$, $P = 0.002$, ${\eta_p}^2 = 0.172$] and "dispositional optimism (LOT-R)" [$F_{(1, 72)} = 5.18$, $P = 0.026$, ${\eta_p}^2 = 0.071$] were observed, while no significant main effect of "gender" [$F_{(1, 114)} = 0.04$, $P = 0.848$, ${\eta_p}^2 = 0.001$] was showed in the reduction of pain intensity (see **Table 2**). *Post hoc* comparisons on "expectancy level" showed that participants in Low expectancy group elicited a greater reduction of pain intensity than both No ($P < 0.001$) and High ($P = 0.055$) expectancy groups, while the latter two had no significant difference ($P = 0.29$). Neither the interaction between "expectancy level" and "dispositional

TABLE 1 | Characteristics of participants in each experimental group (data are expressed as mean ± standard deviation, M ± SD).

Group	Gender	*N*	Age
No expectancy	F	20	20.20 ± 1.15
	M	20	21.30 ± 1.38
Low expectancy	F	20	20.95 ± 1.28
	M	20	21.55 ± 1.73
High expectancy	F	20	21.40 ± 1.39
	M	20	21.00 ± 1.59

F, Female; M, Male.

TABLE 2 | The changes of pain intensity from pre-treatment to post-treatment sessions in all experimental groups (data are expressed as M ± SD).

Personal characteristics		Response expectancy		
		No	Low	High
Gender	F	−0.04 ± 1.14	1.70 ± 1.27	−0.004 ± 1.35
	M	0.41 ± 0.99	1.09 ± 0.87	1.37 ± 1.77
LOT-R	Low	0.58 ± 1.21	1.78 ± 1.44	0.59 ± 1.83
	High	−0.10 ± 0.68	0.93 ± 0.68	0.31 ± 0.85
STAI-S	Low	−0.22 ± 1.16	0.94 ± 0.69	1.21 ± 1.83
	High	0.39 ± 1.31	1.54 ± 1.38	0.75 ± 1.89

F, Female; M, Male; LOT-R, Life Orientation Test-Revised; STAI-S, State subscale of State-Trait Anxiety Inventory. Changes of pain intensity were obtained by subtracting the ratings in post-treatment sessions from those in pre-treatment sessions.

TABLE 3 | The changes of pain unpleasantness from pre-treatment to post-treatment sessions in all experimental groups (data are expressed as M ± SD).

Personal characteristics		Response expectancy		
		No	Low	High
Gender	F	−0.03 ± 0.71	0.36 ± 0.66	−0.34 ± 0.78
	M	0.02 ± 0.54	−0.04 ± 0.66	0.32 ± 0.92
LOT-R	Low	0.32 ± 0.52	−0.07 ± 0.56	−0.08 ± 0.84
	High	−0.09 ± 0.50	0.40 ± 0.58	−0.03 ± 0.64
STAI-S	Low	−0.25 ± 0.56	0.07 ± 0.72	0.47 ± 1.11
	High	0.35 ± 0.71	0.21 ± 0.81	−0.13 ± 0.86

F, Female; M, Male; LOT-R, Life Orientation Test-Revised; STAI-S, State subscale of State-Trait Anxiety Inventory. Changes of pain unpleasantness were obtained by subtracting the ratings in post-treatment sessions from those in pre-treatment sessions.

optimism (LOT-R)" [$F_{(1, 72)} = 0.79$, $P = 0.460$, $\eta_p^2 = 0.023$] (**Figure 3**, left panel), nor the interaction between "dispositional optimism (LOT-R)" and "gender" [$F_{(2,72)} = 0.20$, $P = 0.655$, $\eta_p^2 = 0.003$] (see **Figure 2**, left panel) was significant. However, the interaction between "expectancy level" and "gender" [$F_{(2,114)} = 4.29$, $P = 0.018$, $\eta_p^2 = 0.112$] was significant. *Post-hoc* comparison on this interaction revealed that (1) female participants in the Low expectancy group reported a greater reduction of pain intensity due to placebo treatment than females in No ($P < 0.001$) and High ($P = 0.001$) expectancy groups; (2) for participants in High expectancy group, males reported a greater reduction of pain intensity due to placebo treatment than females ($P = 0.01$).

In contrast, main effects of "expectancy level" [$F_{(2,72)} = 1.00$, $P = 0.374$, $\eta_p^2 = 0.029$], "dispositional optimism (LOT-R)" [$F_{(1, 72)} = 0.05$, $P = 0.832$, $\eta_p^2 = 0.001$], and "gender" [$F_{(1, 72)} = 0.03$, $P = 0.874$, $\eta_p^2 < 0.001$] were not significant on the reduction of pain unpleasantness (see **Table 3**). Except of non-significant interaction between "dispositional optimism (LOT-R)" and "gender" [$F_{(2,72)} = 0.78$, $P = 0.379$, $\eta_p^2 = 0.011$], both the interaction between "expectancy level" and "dispositional optimism (LOT-R)" [$F_{(2,72)} = 3.26$, $P = 0.044$, $\eta_p^2 = 0.084$] (**Figure 3**, right panel), and the interaction between "expectancy level" and "gender" [$F_{(2,72)} = 3.38$, $P = 0.040$, $\eta_p^2 = 0.091$] (**Figure 2**, right panel) were statistically significant. *Post-hoc* comparison on the interaction between "expectancy level" and "dispositional optimism (LOT-R)" showed that (1) for participants with high LOT-R scores, those in Low expectancy group experienced a greater reduction of unpleasantness due to placebo treatment than those in No expectancy group ($P = 0.046$); (2) for Low expectancy group, participants with high LOT-R scores had a tendency to report a greater reduction of unpleasantness than those with low LOT-R scores ($P = 0.056$; see **Table 3**). Similar to the results of pain intensity, *post-hoc* pairwise comparisons showed that (1) female participants in the Low expectancy group reported a greater reduction of unpleasantness due to placebo treatment than those in High expectancy group ($P = 0.039$); (2) for participants in High expectancy group, males tended to report a greater reduction of unpleasantness due to placebo treatment than females ($P = 0.073$).

Influence of Expectancy Level, Anxiety State, and Gender on Placebo Effects

For the reduction of pain intensity, there was a significant main effect of "expectancy level" [$F_{(2, 72)} = 4.14$, $P = 0.02$, $\eta_p^2 = 0.026$]. *Post-hoc* comparisons showed that participants in Low expectancy group reported a greater reduction of pain intensity than those in No expectancy group ($P = 0.007$). No significant main effect of "gender" [$F_{(1, 72)} = 3.07$, $P = 0.082$, $\eta_p^2 = 0.09$] or "anxiety state (STAI-S)" [$F_{(1, 72)} = 1.21$, $P = 0.26$, $\eta_p^2 = 0.02$] was found. No significant interaction between "expectancy level" and "anxiety state (STAI-S)" [$F_{(2, 72)} = 1.68$, $P = 0.19$, $\eta_p^2 = 0.05$] (see **Figure 4**, left panel), or between "anxiety state" and "gender" [$F_{(2, 72)} = 1.27$, $P = 0.26$, $\eta_p^2 = 0.02$] was observed. However, the interaction between "expectancy level" and "gender" was significant [$F_{(2, 72)} = 4.04$, $P = 0.02$, $\eta_p^2 = 0.11$]. *Post-hoc* comparison on this interaction revealed the same pattern as the results reported in the previous section ("Influence of expectancy level, dispositional optimism, and gender on placebo effects").

With regard to the reduction of unpleasantness, no main effect of "expectancy level" [$F_{(2,72)} = 0.12$, $P = 0.891$, $\eta_p^2 = 0.003$], "anxiety state (STAI-S)" [$F_{(1, 72)} = 0.07$, $P = 0.796$, $\eta_p^2 = 0.001$], or "gender" [$F_{(1, 72)} = 1.28$, $P = 0.263$, $\eta_p^2 = 0.018$] was observed. The interaction between "expectancy level" and "anxiety state (STAI-S)" [$F_{(2, 72)} = 4.05$, $P = 0.022$, $\eta_p^2 = 0.106$] (**Figure 4**, right panel), and the interaction between "expectancy level" and "gender" [$F_{(2, 72)} = 4.49$, $P = 0.015$, $\eta_p^2 = 0.117$] (**Figure 2**,

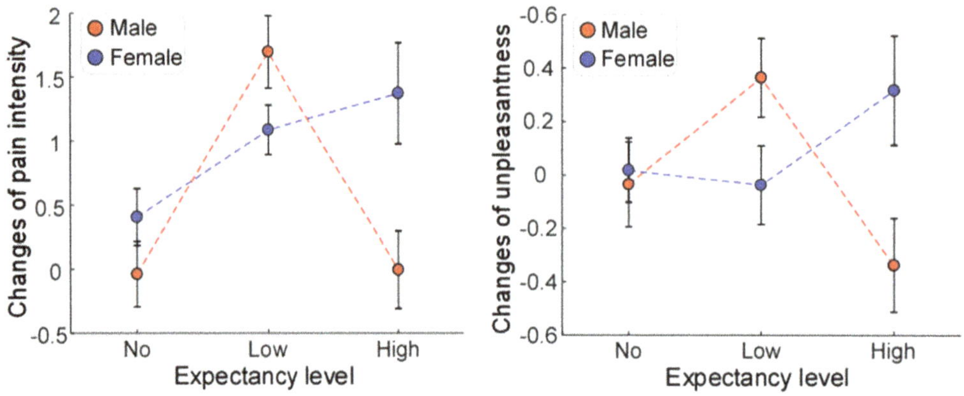

FIGURE 2 | The influences of expectancy level and gender on placebo effects. Significant main effect of expectancy level was only observed for changes of pain intensity **(Left)**. Significant interactions of expectancy level and gender were observed for changes of pain intensity **(Left)** and unpleasantness **(Right)**. Error bars indicate standard error, and data from female and male participants are marked in blue and red, respectively.

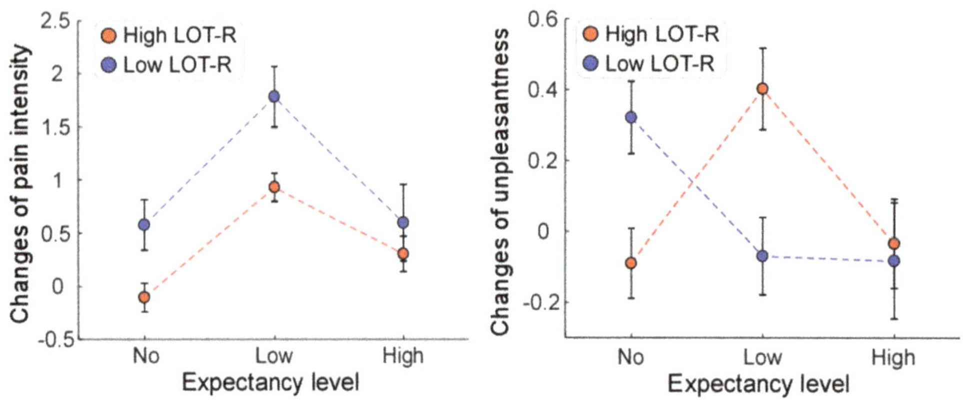

FIGURE 3 | The influences of expectancy level and dispositional optimism (LOT-R) on placebo effects. Significant main effect of expectancy level was only observed for changes of pain intensity **(Left)**. Significant interaction of expectancy level and dispositional optimism (LOT-R) was observed for changes of unpleasantness **(Right)**, but not for changes of pain intensity **(Left)**. Error bars indicate standard error, and data from participants with low and high scores of Life Orientation Test-Revised (Low LOT-R and High LOT-R) are marked in blue and red, respectively.

right panel) were significant. *Post-hoc* pairwise comparisons on the interaction between "expectancy level" and "anxiety state (STAI-S)" showed that for participants with low STAI-S scores, those in High expectancy group felt less pain unpleasantness due to the placebo treatment than those in No expectancy group ($P = 0.027$). *Post-hoc* comparison on interaction between "expectancy level" and "gender" revealed the same pattern as the results reported in the previous section ("Influence of expectancy level, dispositional optimism, and gender on placebo effects"). No significant interaction was observed between "anxiety state (STAI-S)" and "gender" [$F_{(2, 72)} = 2.39$, $P = 0.127$, $\eta_p{}^2 = 0.034$].

DISCUSSION

In the present study, we demonstrated that placebo effects were not only influenced by expectancy level or personal characteristics alone, but also depended on their interactions. Specifically, we observed that the reductions of pain intensity and pain unpleasantness in the Test phase were influenced by the interaction between expectancy level and gender, as mainly reflected by greater reductions of pain intensity and pain unpleasantness in females at Low expectancy level than females at No/High expectancy levels, and greater reductions of pain intensity and pain unpleasantness in males than in females at High expectancy level. Additionally, the reduction of pain unpleasantness was modulated by the interaction between expectancy level and dispositional optimism, as well as the interaction between expectancy level and anxiety state. Participants who were more optimistic in Low expectancy group, or those who were less anxious in High expectancy group showed greater reductions of pain unpleasantness.

Firstly, placebo effects, defined as the reduction of pain intensity or unpleasantness, depended on the interaction between expectancy level and gender. We found female participants elicited maximal placebo effects in Low rather than No and High expectancy groups, which is in line with the previous

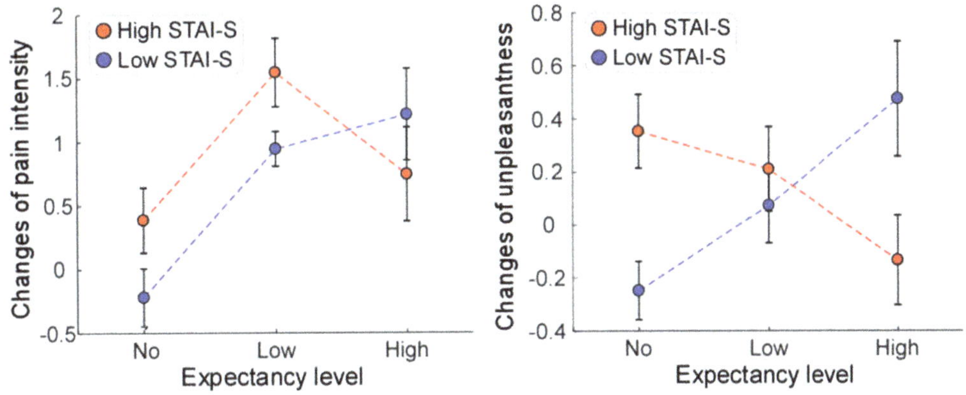

FIGURE 4 | The influences of expectancy level and anxiety state (STAI-S) on placebo effects. Significant main effect of expectancy level was only observed for changes of pain intensity **(Left)**. Significant interaction of expectancy level and anxiety state (STAI-S) was observed for changes of unpleasantness **(Right)**, but not for changes of pain intensity **(Left)**. Error bars indicate standard error, and data from participants with low and high scores of State subscale of State-Trait Anxiety Inventory (Low STAI-S and High STAI-S) are marked in blue and red, respectively.

study showing that placebo effects, as quantified by systolic blood pressure, alertness, and tension, were stronger at the moderate expectancy level than at the extremely low and high expectancy levels (24). In other words, a realistically reasonable expectancy, rather than the unrealistic expectancy level, is more likely to enhance individual belief of the treatment, which is essential to maximize placebo effects (21, 24, 51). However, when compared with female participants, males exhibited a different pattern: in High expectancy group, they reported a greater reduction of pain intensity/unpleasantness due to placebo treatment. These findings suggested that a placebo response to an expectancy manipulation can vary tremendously by gender. However, we failed to observe the main effect of gender in placebo responses, which is inconsistent with a few previous studies (33, 34, 52). Admittedly, the issue of gender discrepancy in placebo responses is still controversial, and further investigation on this issue is highly needed. Please note that gender-specific placebo effects would have tremendous implications for medical research and clinical conditions, such as pain and neurological disorders, in which placebo responses are commonly considered relevant (53, 54).

Secondly, we provided evidence showing that placebo effects, defined as the reduction of pain unpleasantness, were influenced by the interaction between expectancy level and other personal characteristics, such as dispositional optimism and anxiety state. Previous evidence proved that individuals with high scores of dispositional optimism or low scores of anxiety state were more likely to respond to placebo treatment (36, 37). This is in line with our results demonstrating that optimists (those with high LOT-R scores) or participants with low STAI-S scores showed greater placebo responses after treatments. Obviously, being more optimistic or less anxious has a positive influence on the experience to a placebo treatment, as these individuals have a tendency to hold positive expectation (55). In particular, the present results might help explain the consistent correlation between dispositional optimism and positive medical outcomes (56–58). It is suggested that the different respondence between optimists and pessimists (those with low LOT-R scores) to placebo-related expectations may contribute to placebo response discrepancy. Noted that such an effect of dispositional optimism on placebo effects was confirmed in our study, but only observed in Low expectancy group, suggesting that a realistically reasonable, but not an overly-positive expectancy could optimize the influence of dispositional optimism on the placebo response. In other words, since optimists cannot be frequently driven by negative expectancy as forcefully as pessimists can, they might experience fewer negative events. Further, may it be the optimists, not the pessimists, who could be most likely to respond to a placebo-related expectancy for positive outcomes. The above speculation is consistent with a study on persuasion, in which optimists were more likely than pessimists to be persuaded by positively structural arguments (59). Therefore, an individual with high dispositional optimism might not only be less susceptible to negative expectancy, but also be more possible than those with lower dispositional optimism to benefit from positive expectancy, particularly at realistically optimized expectancy level. This is also prompted that patients with high dispositional optimism should be informed more frequently about a certain treatment with realistically positive expectancy to strengthen their responses in medical care. Future studies are needed to explore this issue under clinical conditions.

Importantly, in line with previous studies demonstrating that people's belief can be influenced by personal characteristics, such as optimism, neuroticism, and extraversion (25, 26, 60), our observation provides further evidence suggesting that the placebo effect can be jointly affected by the expectancy level and personal characteristics, which is fitted well with the Response Expectancy Theory (24, 51). Notably, there are tremendous differences in personal characteristics between healthy population and patients. For example, depressive, persistent social phobic, neurotic, fearful, and obsessive-compulsive personality characteristics are very common in pain sufferers compared to healthy population, whereas patients undergoing injectable aesthetic treatments scored significantly higher on extraversion, agreeableness, openness to experience, and neuroticism (61–63). Thus, the next important step is to replicate the main findings of the present study in clinical conditions. To note, a growing body of neurobiological researches on placebo effects indicated the influence of cognitive progressing on the modulation of pain perception (64, 65), which implied that an integrated model combining cognitive factors with psychological factors is warranted to comprehensively explore the placebo mechanisms.

LIMITATIONS

There are two limitations in the present study. First, although we assigned both male and female experimenters randomly to the participants, we did not control the potential influence of experimenters' gender well-enough, which still could have increased error variance. Selecting either a male or a female experimenter might be more suitable for further investigations. Second, we examined the effect of the interaction between expectancy level and personal characteristics on placebo effects within a non-clinical population, and it calls for clinical studies to replicate the main findings of the present study.

CONCLUSION

Considering that placebo effects have been recognized as effective psychobiological events attributing to the improvement of the overall therapeutic outcomes, we believe that our findings not only advance our understanding of the psychological underpinnings of placebo effects, but also suggest a constructive way (regulating the expectation level individually based on the assessment of personal characteristics) to maximize placebo effects in various clinical applications.

AUTHOR CONTRIBUTIONS

HW, LW, XJL, and LH conceived and designed the experiments. HW and HZ performed the experiments. LZ, XJL, and LH analyzed the data. LZ, HW, XYL, CB, LW, XJL, and LH wrote the paper. All authors approved the final manuscript and agreed to be accountable for all aspects of the work.

FUNDING

This work was supported by the National Natural Science Foundation of China (No. 31671141, 31701000, 31822025), the Informatization Special Project of Chinese Academy of Sciences (No. XXH13506-306), and the Scientific Foundation project of Institute of Psychology, Chinese Academy of Sciences (No. Y6CX281007, Y6CX021008, KLMH2018ZG02). The funders had no role in study design, data collection, data analysis, decision to publish, or preparation of the manuscript.

REFERENCES

1. Benedetti F. Mechanisms of placebo and placebo-related effects across diseases and treatments. *Annu Rev Pharmacol Toxicol.* (2008) 48:33–60. doi: 10.1146/annurev.pharmtox.48.113006.094711
2. Finniss DG, Kaptchuk TJ, Miller F, Benedetti F. Biological, clinical, and ethical advances of placebo effects. *Lancet* (2010) 375:686–95. doi: 10.1016/S0140-6736(09)61706-2
3. Bingel U, Wanigasekera V, Wiech K, Ni Mhuircheartaigh R, Lee MC, Ploner M., et al. The effect of treatment expectation on drug efficacy: imaging the analgesic benefit of the opioid remifentanil. *Sci Transl Med.* (2011) 3:70ra14. doi: 10.1126/scitranslmed.3001244
4. Colloca L, Lopiano L, Lanotte M, Benedetti F. Overt versus covert treatment for pain, anxiety, and Parkinson's disease. *Lancet Neurol.* (2004) 3:679–84. doi: 10.1016/s1474-4422(04)00908-1
5. Pollo A, Amanzio M, Arslanian A, Casadio C, Maggi G, Benedetti F. Response expectancies in placebo analgesia and their clinical relevance. *Pain* (2001) 93:77–84. doi: 10.1016/S0304-3959(01)00296-2
6. Benedetti F, Amanzio M, Vighetti S, Asteggiano G. The biochemical and neuroendocrine bases of the hyperalgesic nocebo effect. *J Neurosci.* (2006) 26:12014–22. doi: 10.1523/jneurosci.2947-06.2006
7. Benedetti F, Pollo A, Lopiano L, Lanotte M, Vighetti S, Rainero I. Conscious expectation and unconscious conditioning in analgesic, motor, and hormonal placebo/nocebo responses. *J Neurosci.* (2003) 23:4315–23. doi: 10.1523/JNEUROSCI.23-10-04315.2003
8. Price DD, Finniss DG, Benedetti F. A comprehensive review of the placebo effect: recent advances and current thought. *Annu Rev Psychol.* (2008) 59:565–90. doi: 10.1146/annurev.psych.59.113006.095941
9. Kessner S, Forkmann K, Ritter C, Wiech K, Ploner M, Bingel U. The effect of treatment history on therapeutic outcome: psychological and neurobiological underpinnings. *PLoS ONE* (2014) 9:e109014. doi: 10.1371/journal.pone.0109014
10. Kessner S, Wiech K, Forkmann K, Ploner M, Bingel U. The effect of treatment history on therapeutic outcome: an experimental approach. *JAMA Intern Med.* (2013) 173:1468–9. doi: 10.1001/jamainternmed.2013.6705
11. Milling LS, Reardon JM, Carosella, G.M. Mediation and moderation of psychological pain treatments: response expectancies and hypnotic suggestibility. *J Consult Clin Psychol.* (2006) 74:253–62. doi: 10.1037/0022-006x.74.2.253
12. Kirsch I. Response expectancy as a determinant of experience and behavior. *Am Psychol.* (1985) 40:1189. doi: 10.1037/0003-066X.40.11.1189
13. Kirsch I. Response expectancy and the response to antidepressant medication. *EBioMedicine* (2017) 25:13. doi: 10.1016/j.ebiom.2017.09.038
14. Koyama T, McHaffie JG, Laurienti PJ, Coghill RC. The subjective experience of pain: where expectations become reality. *Proc Natl Acad Sci USA.* (2005) 102:12950–5. doi: 10.1073/pnas.0408576102
15. Kirsch IE. *How Expectancies Shape Experience.* Washington, DC: American Psychological Association (1999).
16. Kong J, Gollub RL, Rosman IS, Webb JM, Vangel MG, Kirsch I., et al. Brain activity associated with expectancy-enhanced placebo analgesia as measured by functional magnetic resonance imaging. *J Neurosci.* (2006) 26:381–8. doi: 10.1523/jneurosci.3556-05.2006
17. Montgomery GH, Kirsch I. Classical conditioning and the placebo effect. *Pain* (1997) 72:107–13.

18. Wager TD, Rilling JK, Smith EE, Sokolik A, Casey KL, Davidson RJ., et al. Placebo-induced changes in FMRI in the anticipation and experience of pain. *Science* (2004) 303:1162–7. doi: 10.1126/science.1093065
19. Zubieta JK, Bueller JA, Jackson LR, Scott DJ, Xu Y, Koeppe RA., et al. Placebo effects mediated by endogenous opioid activity on μ-opioid receptors. *J Neurosci.* (2005) 25:7754–62.
20. De Pascalis V, Chiaradia C, Carotenuto E. The contribution of suggestibility and expectation to placebo analgesia phenomenon in an experimental setting. *Pain* (2002) 96:393–402. doi: 10.1016/S0304-3959(01)00485-7
21. Enck P, Bingel U, Schedlowski M, Rief W. The placebo response in medicine: minimize, maximize or personalize? *Nat Rev Drug Discov.* (2013) 12:191–204. doi: 10.1038/nrd3923
22. Price DD, Milling LS, Kirsch I, Duff A, Montgomery GH, Nicholls SS. An analysis of factors that contribute to the magnitude of placebo analgesia in an experimental paradigm. *Pain* (1999) 83:147–56. doi: 10.1016/S0304-3959(99)00081-0
23. Wei H, Zhou L, Zhang H, Chen J, Lu X, Hu L. The influence of expectation on nondeceptive placebo and nocebo effects. *Pain Res Manag.* (2018) 2018:8459429. doi: 10.1155/2018/8459429
24. Kirsch I, Weixel LJ. Double-blind versus deceptive administration of a placebo. *Behav Neurosci.* (1988) 102:319–23.
25. Evans AM, Revelle W. Survey and behavioral measurements of interpersonal trust. *J Res Pers.* (2008) 42:1585–93.
26. Warren ME. *Democracy and Trust.* Cambridge: Cambridge University Press (1999).
27. Colagiuri B, Schenk LA, Kessler MD, Dorsey SG, Colloca L. The placebo effect: from concepts to genes. *Neuroscience* (2015) 307:171–90. doi: 10.1016/j.neuroscience.2015.08.017
28. Colloca L, Grillon C. Understanding placebo and nocebo responses for pain management. *Curr Pain Headache Rep.* (2014) 18:419. doi: 10.1007/s11916-014-0419-2
29. Saxon L, Hiltunen AJ, Hjemdahl P, Borg S. Gender-related differences in response to placebo in benzodiazepine withdrawal: a single-blind pilot study. *Psychopharmacology* (2001) 153:231–7. doi: 10.1007/s002130000574
30. Aslaksen PM, Bystad M, Vambheim SM, Flaten MA. Gender differences in placebo analgesia: event-related potentials and emotional modulation. *Psychosom Med.* (2011) 73:193–9. doi: 10.1097/PSY.0b013e3182080d73
31. Butcher BE, Carmody JJ. Sex differences in analgesic response to ibuprofen are influenced by expectancy: a randomized, crossover, balanced placebo-designed study. *Eur J Pain* (2012) 16:1005–13. doi: 10.1002/j.1532-2149.2011.00104.x
32. Pud D, Yarnitsky D, Sprecher E, Rogowski Z, Adler R, Eisenberg E. Can personality traits and gender predict the response to morphine? An experimental cold pain study. *Eur J Pain* (2006) 10:103. doi: 10.1016/j.ejpain.2005.01.010
33. Gear RW, Miaskowski C, Gordon NC, Paul SM, Heller PH, Levine JD. The kappa opioid nalbuphine produces gender-and dose-dependent analgesia and antianalgesia in patients with postoperative pain. *Pain* (1999) 83:339–45. doi: 10.1016/S0304-3959(99)00119-0
34. Olofsen E, Romberg R, Bijl H, Mooren R, Engbers F, Kest B., et al. Alfentanil and placebo analgesiano sex differences detected in models of experimental pain. *Anesthesiol J Am Soc Anesthesiol.* (2005) 103:130–9. doi: 10.1097/00000542-200507000-00020
35. Brissette I, Scheier MF, Carver CS. The role of optimism in social network development, coping, and psychological adjustment during a life transition. *J Personal Soc Psychol.* (2002) 82:102. doi: 10.1037//0022-3514.82.1.102
36. Morton DL, Watson A, El-Deredy W, Jones AK. Reproducibility of placebo analgesia: effect of dispositional optimism. *Pain* (2009) 146:194–8. doi: 10.1016/j.pain.2009.07.026
37. Geers AL, Wellman JA, Fowler SL, Helfer SG, France CR. Dispositional optimism predicts placebo analgesia. *J Pain* (2010) 11:1165–71. doi: 10.1016/j.jpain.2010.02.014
38. Hu L, Zhao C, Li H, Valentini E. Mismatch responses evoked by nociceptive stimuli. *Psychophysiology* (2013) 50:158–73. doi: 10.1111/psyp.12000
39. Zhao C, Valentini E, Hu L. Functional features of crossmodal mismatch responses. *Exp Brain Res.* (2015) 233:617–29. doi: 10.1007/s00221-014-4141-4
40. Inui K, Tran TD, Hoshiyama M, Kakigi R. Preferential stimulation of Adelta fibers by intra-epidermal needle electrode in humans. *Pain* (2002) 96:247–52. doi: 10.1016/S0304-3959(01)00453-5
41. Kakigi R, Inui K, Tamura Y. Electrophysiological studies on human pain perception. *Clin Neurophysiol.* (2005) 116:743–63. doi: 10.1016/j.clinph.2004.11.016
42. Li CH. Validation of the Chinese version of the life orientation test with a robust weighted least squares approach. *Psychol Assess.* (2012) 24:770–6. doi: 10.1037/a0026612
43. Shek DT. Reliability and factorial structure of the Chinese version of the State-Trait Anxiety Inventory. *J Psychopathol Behav Assess.* (1988) 10:303–17.
44. Aslaksen PM, Myrbakk IN, Høifødt RS, Flaten MA. The effect of experimenter gender on autonomic and subjective responses to pain stimuli. *Pain* (2007) 129:260–8. doi: 10.1016/j.pain.2006.10.011
45. Kállai I, Barke A, Voss U. The effects of experimenter characteristics on pain reports in women and men. *Pain* (2004) 112:142–7. doi: 10.1016/j.pain.2004.08.008
46. Colloca L, Benedetti F. How prior experience shapes placebo analgesia. *Pain* (2006) 124:126–33. doi: 10.1016/j.pain.2006.04.005
47. Jensen K, Kirsch I, Odmalm S, Kaptchuk TJ, Ingvar M. Classical conditioning of analgesic and hyperalgesic pain responses without conscious awareness. *Proc Natl Acad Sci USA.* (2015) 112:7863–7. doi: 10.1073/pnas.1504567112
48. Jensen KB, Kaptchuk TJ, Kirsch I, Raicek J, Lindstrom KM, Berna C., et al. Nonconscious activation of placebo and nocebo pain responses. *Proc Natl Acad Sci USA.* (2012) 109:15959–64. doi: 10.1073/pnas.1202056109
49. Kong J, Gollub RL, Polich G, Kirsch I, Laviolette P, Vangel M., et al. A functional magnetic resonance imaging study on the neural mechanisms of hyperalgesic nocebo effect. *J Neurosci.* (2008) 28:13354–62. doi: 10.1523/jneurosci.2944-08.2008
50. Cohen J. *Statistical Power Analysis for the Social Sciences.* Hillsdale, NJ: Lawrence Erlbaum Associates (1988).
51. Kirsch I. *Changing Expectations: A Key to Effective Psychotherapy.* Pacific Grove, CA: Thomson Brooks/Cole Publishing Co (1990).
52. Averbuch M, Katzper M. Gender and the placebo analgesic effect in acute pain. *Clin Pharmacol Ther.* (2001) 70:287–91. doi: 10.1067/mcp.2001.118366
53. Castelnuovo G, Giusti EM, Manzoni GM, Saviola D, Gabrielli S, Lacerenza M., et al. What is the role of the placebo effect for pain relief in neurorehabilitation? Clinical implications from the italian consensus conference on pain in neurorehabilitation. *Front Neurol.* (2018) 9:310. doi: 10.3389/fneur.2018.00310
54. Skyt I, Moslemi K, Baastrup C, Grosen K, Svensson P, Jensen TS, et al. Does conditioned pain modulation predict the magnitude of placebo effects in patients with neuropathic pain? *Eur J Pain* (2018) 22:784–92. doi: 10.1002/ejp.1164
55. Hodo DW. Personality characteristics of patients with pain. *Am J Psychiatry* (2002) 159:336.
56. Williams NL. Optimism and pessimism: implications for theory, research, and practice. *J Cogn Psychother.* (2003) 17:200. doi: 10.1891/088983903780906174
57. Geers AL, Helfer SG, Kosbab K, Weiland PE, Landry SJ. Reconsidering the role of personality in placebo effects: dispositional optimism, situational expectations, and the placebo response. *J Psychosom Res.* (2005) 58:121–7. doi: 10.1016/j.jpsychores.2004.08.011
58. Scheier MF, Carver CS. Effects of optimism on psychological and physical well-being: theoretical overview and empirical update. *Cogn Ther Res.* (1992) 16:201–28.
59. Geers AL, Handley IM, McLarney AR. Discerning the role of optimism in persuasion: the valence-enhancement hypothesis. *J Personal Soc Psychol.* (2003) 85:554. doi: 10.1037/0022-3514.85.3.554
60. Hiraishi K, Yamagata S, Shikishima C, Ando J. Maintenance of genetic variation in personality through control of mental mechanisms: a test of trust, extraversion, and agreeableness. *Evol Hum Behav.* (2008) 29:79–85. doi: 10.1016/j.evolhumbehav.2007.07.004

61. Naylor B, Boag S, Gustin SM. New evidence for a pain personality? A critical review of the last 120 years of pain and personality. *Scand J Pain* (2017) 17:58–67. doi: 10.1016/j.sjpain.2017.07.011
62. Scharschmidt D, Mirastschijski U, Preiss S, Brähler E, Fischer T, Borkenhagen A. Body image, personality traits, and quality of life in Botulinum Toxin A, and dermal filler patients. *Aesthetic Plast Surg.* (2018) 42:1119–25. doi: 10.1007/s00266-018-1165-3
63. Taiminen T, Kuusalo L, Lehtinen L, Forssell H, Hagelberg N, Tenovuo O, et al. Psychiatric (axis I) and personality (axis II) disorders in patients with burning mouth syndrome or atypical facial pain. *Scand J Pain* (2011) 2:155–60. doi: 10.1016/j.sjpain.2011.06.004
64. Wiech K. Deconstructing the sensation of pain: the influence of cognitive processes on pain perception. *Science* (2016) 354:584–7. doi: 10.1126/science.aaf8934
65. Zhang H, Zhou L, Wei H, Lu X, Hu L. The sustained influence of prior experience induced by social observation on placebo and nocebo responses. *J Pain Res.* (2017) 10:2769. doi: 10.2147/JPR.S147970

5

Mechanisms of Perceived Treatment Assignment and Subsequent Expectancy Effects in a Double Blind Placebo Controlled RCT of Major Depression

Johannes A. C. Laferton [1,2,3†], Sagar Vijapura [4†], Lee Baer [4‡], Alisabet J. Clain [4], Abigail Cooper [4§], George Papakostas [4], Lawrence H. Price [5], Linda L. Carpenter [5], Audrey R. Tyrka [5], Maurizio Fava [4] and David Mischoulon [4]*

[1] Department of Psychiatry, Brigham and Women's Hospital, Harvard Medical School, Harvard University, Boston, MA, United States, [2] Department of Clinical Psychology and Psychotherapy, Friedrich-Alexander-Universität Erlangen-Nürnberg, Erlangen, Germany, [3] Department of Clinical Psychology and Psychotherapy, Psychologische Hochschule Berlin, Berlin, Germany, [4] Depression Clinical and Research Program, Department of Psychiatry, Massachusetts General Hospital, Harvard Medical School, Boston, MA, United States, [5] Mood Disorders Research Program, Laboratory for Clinical and Translational Neuroscience, Butler Hospital, Department of Psychiatry and Human Behavior, Alpert Medical School, Brown University, Providence, RI, United States

***Correspondence:**
David Mischoulon
dmischoulon@mgh.harvard.edu

† These authors have contributed equally to this work and share first authorship

‡ Deceased

§ Abigail Cooper, Fairleigh Dickinson University, Teaneck, NJ, United States

Objective: It has been suggested that patients' perception of treatment assignment might serve to bias results of double blind randomized controlled trials (RCT). Most previous evidence on the effects of patients' perceptions and the mechanisms influencing these perceptions relies on cross-sectional associations. This re-analysis of a double blind, placebo controlled RCT of pharmacological treatment of major depression set out to gather longitudinal evidence on the mechanism and effects of patients' perceived treatment assignment in the pharmacological treatment of major depression.

Methods: One-hundred eighty-nine outpatients with DSM-IV diagnosed major depression were randomized to SAMe 1,600–3,200 mg/d, escitalopram 10–20 mg/days, or placebo for 12 weeks. Data on depressive symptoms (17-item Hamilton Depression Scale; HDRS-17), adverse events and patients' perceived treatment assignment was collected at baseline, week 6, and week 12. The re-analysis focused on $N = 166$ (out of the originally included 189 participants) with available data on perceived treatment assignment.

Results: As in the parent trial, depressive symptoms (HDRS-17) significantly decreased over the course of 12 weeks and there was no difference between placebo, SAMe or escitalopram. A significant number of patients changed their perceptions about treatment assignment throughout the trial, especially between baseline and week 6. Improvement in depressive symptoms, but not adverse events significantly predicted perceived treatment assignment at week 6. In turn, perceived treatment assignment at week 6, but not actual treatment, predicted further improvement in depressive symptoms at week 12.

Conclusions: The current results provide longitudinal evidence that patients' perception of treatment assignment systematically change despite a double blind procedure and in turn might trigger expectancy effects with the potential to bias the validity of an RCT.

Parent study grant number: R01 AT001638
Parent study ClinicalTrials. gov Identifier: NCT00101452

Keywords: major depressive disorder, SAMe, escitalopram, placebo, perceived treatment assignment, un-blinding, double blind randomized controlled trial, bias

INTRODUCTION

The belief that one is taking a medication can lead to improvement in numerous health conditions regardless of the presence or absence of a pharmacologic agent (1, 2). This expectation effect is specifically pronounced in the pharmacological treatment of depression (3, 4). Double blind randomized controlled trials (RCTs) assume that these expectations are equally balanced across treatment arms. Yet, the effectiveness of blinding in RCTs is rarely assessed or reported, and there are suggestions in the literature that patients are frequently un-blinded (5–7). If patients do learn which treatment arm they are in, expectancy effects due to perceived treatment assignment are no longer controlled for. This introduces a considerable amount of bias, as meta-epidemiological studies typically find un-blinded studies to exaggerate effect size by more than 30% compared to blinded studies (8–10). Moreover, it is important to note that not only an actual un-blinding, but any between-groups imbalance of the perceived treatment assignment can bias the results of a trial (11, 12).

Possible mechanisms that may influence perceived treatment assignment include the physical characteristics of the medication and the placebo, medication side effects, or beneficial effects on the health condition (13). Regarding the former, taste, color, shape, size, route and process of administration (13) might lead to un-blinding, if they differ between drug and placebo. Moreover, medication side effects could inadvertently serve to influence perception of treatment assignment (14, 15). Studies have shown that side effects are associated with patients and independent evaluators guessing treatment assignment (15, 16). The experience of side effects could then increase the treatment effect by enhancing the patient's expectation of benefit. This possibility is supported by both experimental and clinical evidence. Thus, for example, in an experimental pain task (17), participants receiving a placebo that produces side effects (so called, "active placebo") achieved higher pain thresholds than those who received a non-active placebo. Clinical trials on the pharmacological treatment of pain or depression using active placebos as a control condition have found smaller differences between active medication and the placebo arm compared to similar trials using non-active placebos (18–21). It should be noted that in order for physical characteristics or side effects to influence perceived treatment assignment, the participant needs at least a certain amount of knowledge about these characteristics of the drug. Finally, improvement of symptoms may also indicate participants' perception of treatment assignment. Previous studies among various health conditions have shown an association between clinical improvement and patient perceptions regarding treatment assignment (22–27). However, a major limitation of most of those analyses is that perceived treatment assignment was elicited either before or after treatment, making it impossible to investigate mechanisms of un-blinding and its prospective impact on treatment outcome. If assessed at the beginning of a trial, it cannot be concluded whether mechanisms such as side effects or health improvement have had an influence on the perception of treatment assignment. In contrast, assessment at the end of a study does not indicate whether more side effects or greater improvement in health were due to the perceived treatment assignment, or whether the perception of treatment assignment was due to experienced side effects or improvement in health. Experimental evidence suggests that experienced improvement influences perceived treatment assignment, which in turn influences treatment outcome (28). Whether this is true for clinical trials remains unclear so far. Moreover, when using a single time point assessment, one cannot determine whether participants change their perception of treatment assignment throughout a trial.

To better understand (1) whether the perception of the treatment assignment changes over the course of a study, (2) and whether these changes are influenced by side effects or health improvement, and (3) whether the perceived treatment assignment is prospectively related to the treatment effects, a re-analysis of a three-armed, double blind RCT on the treatment of major depression was conducted. The parent trial (29) examined the effects of escitalopram or S-adenosyl-L-methionine (SAMe) vs. placebo in patients with major depression and assessed perceived treatment assignment at several points throughout the trial. Moreover, in the parent study, no significant differences in improvement in the 17-item Hamilton Depression Rating Scale (HDRS-17) total score or response rates were found between the three treatment arms, making it particularly interesting to investigate expectancy effects due to possible bias in perceived treatment.

MATERIALS AND METHODS

Study Design and Procedure

This study is a secondary analysis of a two center, three-arm, double blind RCT (29) on the treatment of major depression with escitalopram or SAMe vs. placebo (clinical trials.gov: NCT00101452) conducted at two academic psychiatry centers in the U.S. Detailed methods for the parent trial have been described elsewhere (29). The study was approved by both local Institutional Review Boards.

Participants

One-hundred eighty-nine outpatients, 18–80 years old, who met criteria for current major depressive episode according to Structured Clinical Interview for DSM-IV (30) plus screening and baseline scores of ≥25 on the Inventory of Depressive Symptomatology-Clinician-Rated (31), were recruited from April 2005 to December 2009 through clinician referral and general advertisement (e.g., "Have you lost interest in things you used to enjoy, had appetite or sleep changes? Are you interested in natural remedies? Participate in a research study of a naturally occurring supplement called SAMe in treating Major Depressive Disorder") in local newspapers, radio, and television. A ≥ 6 week use of SAMe or escitalopram during the concurrent episode as well as severe medical or other primary psychiatric disorder were exclusion criteria [for detailed description of exclusion criteria see (29)].

Procedure

After written informed consent participants were randomized in a 1:1:1 manner (stratified by center) for 12 weeks of double-blind treatment with SAMe (1,600 mg/d), escitalopram (10 mg/d), or placebo. A double-dummy design was used to maintain the blind, since SAMe tablets differed in appearance from escitalopram tablets. Participants were made aware of their odds of receiving any particular one of the three possible treatments. At week 6, for non-responders (<50% HAM-D reduction) escitalopram dose could be increased to 20 mg/d and SAMe to 3,200 mg/d for weeks 7–12. Participants who experienced intolerable side effects at the higher dose were allowed to decrease their dose to the previous level.

Assessment

Assessment relevant for the reanalysis took place during baseline, visit 4 (week 6) and visit 7 (week 12; end of active treatment). Antidepressant efficacy was assessed with the Hamilton 17-item Depression Rating Scale [HDRS-17; (32)]. Side effects were assessed using the Systematic Assessment for Treatment Emergent Events-Systematic Inquiry [SAFTEE (33)]. Side effects documented on the SAFTEE were categorized by severity as 0 (none), 1 (mild), 2 (moderate), and 3 (severe). Scores were calculated based on the number of adverse events reported by each subject that were treatment-emergent, which we defined as any SAFTEE side effect for which severity increased by 1 or more levels from baseline. Besides an overall side effect score, sub-category scores for gastrointestinal and sexual functioning side effects were calculated based on known pharmacologic profiles of the active treatments and side effect patterns reported in the parent study (29). In order to assess perception of treatment assignment patients were asked to guess whether they believed to have received SAMe, escitalopram or placebo.

Data Analysis

This re-analysis focused on the acute treatment phase only (baseline-12 weeks) including $N = 166$ participants from the intent-to-treat sample, with at least one post-baseline visit and available data on perceived treatment assignment. Patients with missing data on perceived treatment assignment did not differ from those included in the analysis with regard to HRDS-17 scores and side effects at the respective time points.

Frequency distribution, means and standard deviations were assessed for each variable. Non-normally distributed variables were $\log_{10}$-transformed in order to satisfy the statistical assumptions of parametric tests. Baseline differences were tested with analysis of variance (ANOVA) for parametric data, and χ^2-tests for categorical data. Change in clinical variables was analyzed with mixed ANOVAs with treatment assignment as the between-participant factor and time as the within-participants factor. Significant main or interaction effects were analyzed by Bonferroni corrected *post-hoc* tests. Differences in perceived treatment assignment distributions were analyzed using χ^2-tests. To assess whether clinical improvement or side effects were prospectively associated with perceived treatment assignment, logistic regression analyses were performed using clinical improvement and side effects as predictors, actual treatment assignment (dummy coded with placebo as the reference condition) and previous perceived treatment assignment (active treatment vs. placebo) as covariates, and whether participants perceived themselves to be on active medication [placebo = 0; active treatment (SAMe or escitalopram) = 1] at the successive time point as the dependent variable. To assess whether perceived active treatment affected subsequent clinical improvement, linear multiple regression analysis were performed with perceived treatment [placebo = 0; active treatment (SAMe or escitalopram) = 1] as predictor, actual treatment assignment (dummy coded with placebo as the reference condition) and pre HDRS-17 score as covariates, and successive HDRS-17 score as dependent variable. To test for treatment arm specific effects of perceived treatment, the interaction term between actual treatment assignment and perceived treatment assignment was added to the multiple regression analysis and additional Bonferroni corrected *post-hoc* tests were carried out for each treatment arm individually. For all analyses, two-tailed significance was set at $p < 0.05$. All calculations were performed with SPSS Version 23 (Chicago, Illinois).

RESULTS

Trial Characteristics

Demographic and baseline clinical characteristics for each treatment group are reported in **Table 1**. No significant differences were observed between the treatment groups.

Changes in Depressive Symptoms and Side Effects Over Time

Depressive symptoms significantly declined over time (see **Table 1**). However, there was no significant between-group difference or group × time interaction. For both total side effect score and gastrointestinal side effects (see **Table 1**), there was

TABLE 1 | Demographic and clinical characteristics throughout trial.

	Placebo (n = 52)	SAMe (n = 59)	Escitalopram (n = 55)	Baseline differences
Age years *M (SD)*	43.68 (16.51)	45.04 (14.16)	46.12 (13.47)	$F_{(2, 163)} = 0.39, p = 0.674$
Sex *f (%)* female	27 (51.9)	32 (54.2)	27 (49.1)	$\chi^2(2) = 0.30; p = 0.682$
Race *f (%)* Caucasian (*MD* = 15)	43 (84.3)	41 (82.0)	40 (80.0)	$\chi^2(2) = 0.32; p = 0.852$
Education *f (%)* college (*MD* = 8)	37 (72.5)	39 (70.9)	37 (71.2)	$\chi^2(2) = 0.04; p = 0.980$
Currently married/living with someone	14 (28.0)	10 (18.2)	15 (18.2)	$\chi^2(2) = 2.02; p = 0.364$
Employment *f (%)* working	13 (25.0)	28 (47.5)	20 (36.4)	$\chi^2(2) = 1.49; p = 0.473$
Dose increase at week 6 *f (%; MD* = 39)	29 (67.4)	20 (47.6)	27 (64.3)	$\chi^2(2) = 3.99; p = 0.136$
DEPRESSIVE SYMPTOMS (HAMD)				
Baseline *M (SD)*	19.44 (4.03)	19.12 (4.81)	19.71 (4.84)	Main effect time: $F_{(2, 93)} = 79.58, p < 0.001$
Week 6 *M (SD; MD* = 38)	13.42 (5.69)	11.09 (7.22)	13.22 (6.99)	Main effect group: $F_{(2, 94)} = 0.79, p = 0.454$
Week 12 *M (SD; MD* = 69)	12.00 (6.96)	11.12 (6.74)	10.78 (6.58)	Interaction group × time: $F_{(4, 94)} = 1.34, p = 0.257$
SIDE EFFECTS (SAFTEE)				
Overall				
Week 6 *M (SD; MD* = 40)	4.41 (4.48)	3.84 (3.56)	5.40 (4.42)	Main effect time: $F_{(1, 93)} = 0.16, p = 0.690$
Week 12 *M (SD; MD* = 70)	4.16 (3.62)	4.28 (4.15)	4.82 (4.29)	Main effect group: $F_{(2, 93)} = 1.51, p = 0.227$
				Interaction group × time: $F_{(2, 93)} = 0.19, p = 0.191$
Gastrointestinal				
Week 6 *M (SD; MD* = 40)	0.29 (0.51)	0.58 (0.91)	0.55 (0.86)	Main effect time: $F_{(1, 93)} = 0.22, p = 0.644$
Week 12 *M (SD; MD* = 70)	0.35 (0.61)	0.83 (1.23)	0.48 (0.74)	Main effect group: $F_{(2, 93)} = 2.03, p = 0.137$
				Interaction group × time: $F_{(2, 93)} = 0.90, p = 0.409$
Sexual Function				
Week 6 *M (SD; MD* = 40)	0.17 (0.54)	0.19 (0.59)	0.54 (0.89)	Main effect time: $F_{(1, 93)} = 0.09$,
Week 12 *M (SD; MD* = 70)	0.23 (0.56)	0.18 (0.58)	0.72 (0.96)	Main effect group: $F_{(2, 93)} = 7.01$,
				Interaction group × time: $F_{(2, 93)} = 0.04, p = 0.964$.

MD, Missing Data.

no significant change from week 6 to week 12, between-group difference, or group × time interaction. For sexual functioning side effects (see **Table 1**), there was no significant change from week 6 to week 12, or group × time interaction, but the between-group difference was significant. Bonferroni-corrected *post-hoc* tests revealed that sexual functioning side effects were significantly higher with escitalopram compared to SAMe ($p = 0.002$) and to placebo ($p = 0.009$), but not different between SAMe and placebo ($p = 0.714$).

Changes in Perceived Treatment Assignment Distributions Over Time

Participants' perceptions of treatment assignment throughout the study can be seen in **Figure 1**. At baseline (before application of treatment), participants in the SAMe group ($\chi^2 = 14.00$, $df = 2$, $p = 0.001$), the escitalopram group ($\chi^2 = 18.88$, $df = 2$, $p < 0.001$) and the placebo group ($\chi^2 = 11.41$, $df = 2$, $p = 0.003$) were expecting to receive SAMe significantly more often than would be expected, based on an equal assignment probability (1/3). At week 6, only participants in the escitalopram arm perceived themselves to be on SAMe more often than by chance ($\chi^2 = 6.37$, $df = 2$, $p = 0.041$). Participants' perceived treatment assignment in the SAMe ($\chi^2 = 2.00$, $df = 2$, $p = 0.368$) and placebo groups ($\chi^2 = 2.53$, $df = 2$, $p = 0.282$) did not significantly differ from that expected in an equal treatment distribution.

At week 12, participants' perceived treatment assignment did not significantly differ from an equal distribution in the SAMe arm ($\chi^2 = 4.36$, $df = 2$, $p = 0.113$), the escitalopram arm ($\chi^2 = 1.92$, $df = 2$, $p = 0.283$) or the placebo arm ($\chi^2 = 0.54$, $df = 2$, $p = 0.764$). There was no association between participants' baseline perceived treatment assignment and drop out by week 6 ($\chi^2 = 0.04$, $df = 2$, $p = 0.982$) and week 6 perceived treatment assignment and drop out by week 12 ($\chi^2 = 1.90$, $df = 2$, $p = 0.387$).

Overall, almost twice as many patients changed their perceived treatment assignment between baseline and week 6 (48.9%), compared to between week 6 and week 12 (26.0%; see **Table 2** for detailed within-person change patterns). Between baseline and week 6 patients in the placebo group changed their perceived treatment assignment more often (60%) than patients in the SAMe and the escitalopram group (42.4%; 48.6%). Between week 6 and week 12 patients in the SAMe group changed their perception of treatment assignment more frequently (38.8%) than in the escitalopram and the placebo group (both: 20.8%).

Factors Associated With Perceived Treatment Assignment

Prospective associations of clinical improvement and side effects with whether participants perceived to be on an active medication (SAMe or escitalopram) or placebo are reported in **Table 3**. At week 6, participants were significantly more likely to perceive that they were receiving active medication if they experienced clinical improvement. Among participants who experienced a reduction in HDRS-17 score of 13 or greater, all perceived that they were

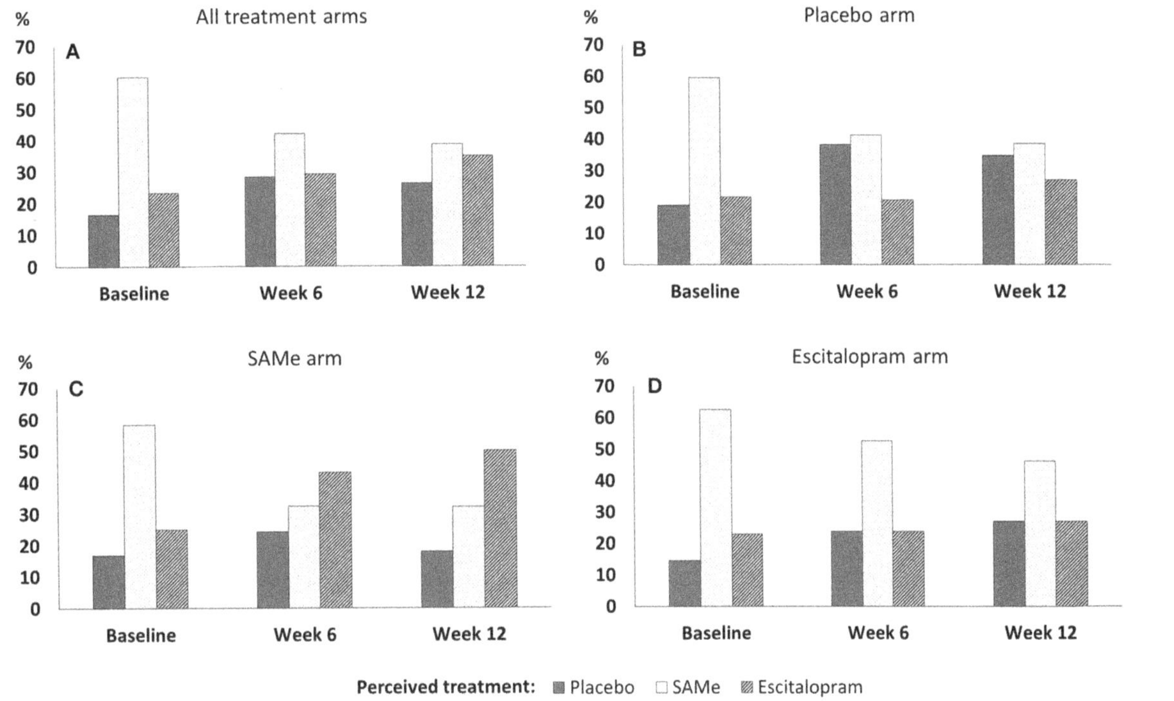

FIGURE 1 | Perceived treatment assignment throughout the trial in **(A)** all treatment arms, **(B)** the placebo arm, **(C)** the SAMe arm, and **(D)** the escitalopram arm.

assigned to an active medication group. There was no threshold below which participants would certainly perceive themselves to be on placebo. Side effects and actual treatment assignment were not associated with participants' perception that they were receiving an active medication at week 6. Clinical improvement between week 6 and week 12, side effects, and actual treatment assignment, were not associated with participants' perceived treatment assignment at week 12.

Prospective Associations of Perceived Treatment Assignment and Subsequent Improvement

Prospective associations of participants' perceived treatment assignment (active vs. placebo) and actual treatment assignment on clinical improvement are shown in **Table 4**. Controlling for baseline HDRS-17, neither actual nor perceived treatment assignment predicted HDRS-17 scores at week 6. However, controlling for week 6 HDRS-17, patients' perceived treatment assignment at week 6, but not actual treatment assignment predicted week 12 HDRS-17 scores. Participants perceiving they were taking active medication at week 6 showed significantly higher improvement in depressive symptoms at week 12 than participants believing they were taking placebo. *Post-hoc* analysis revealed no significant interaction between actual treatment assignment and week 6 perceived treatment predicting HDRS-17 improvement at week 12 [$R^2 = 0.02$, $F_{(2,76)} = 1.28$, $p = 0.284$]. However, Bonferroni corrected *post-hoc* sub group analyses of the effect of perceived treatment at week 6 on treatment outcome at week 12 within each treatment group individually (**Table 5**) indicated that the effect of perceived treatment assignment was significant in the escitalopram treatment arm but not in the placebo and SAMe treatment arm (**Figure 2**).

DISCUSSION

This re-analysis of a three arm, two-center, double blind RCT of SAMe or escitalopram vs. placebo for the treatment of major depression shows that a significant number of patients did change their perception of treatment assignment throughout the trial, corroborating previous analyses on longitudinal changes of perceived treatment assignment in clinical trials (11, 23). The large majority of change in perceived treatment assignment happened throughout the first 6 weeks of treatment and was significantly predicted by the preceding improvement in depressive symptomatology. Side effects did not seem to have influenced perceived treatment assignment. Although side effects are frequently mentioned as a potential mechanism informing perceived treatment assignment, this result is consistent with another re-analysis of an RCT containing two active treatments for opioid dependency. Oviedo-Joekes et al. (34) found that desired drug effects (drug related highs) but not overall side effects were associated with perceived treatment allocation. Possibly, in trials with more than one active treatment, side effects might not be a pivotal mechanism influencing perceived treatment assignment, since it may be more difficult to guess between two active treatments based simply on side effects. Moreover, patients randomized to placebo in the current re-analysis did not differ from the active treatment groups in terms

TABLE 2 | Changes in perceived treatment assignment from baseline to week 6 and week 6 to week 12 by actual treatment group.

	Change baseline to week 6 f (%)	Change week 6 to week 12 f (%)
Active medication = PBO	*n* = 25	*n* = 24
no change	10 (40.0)	19 (79.2)
SAMe to ESC	4 (16.0)	1 (4.2)
SAMe to PBO	5 (20.0)	1 (4.2)
ESC to SAMe	2 (8.0)	0 (0.0)
ESC to PBO	2 (8.0)	0 (0.0)
PBO to SAMe	1 (4.0)	2 (8.3)
PBO to ESC	1 (4.0)	1 (4.2)
Active medication = SAMe	*n* = 32	*n* = 25
no change	19 (57.6)	16 (61.5)
SAMe to ESC	6 (18.2)	4 (15.4)
SAMe to PBO	2 (6.1)	1 (3.8)
ESC to SAMe	1 (3.0)	2 (7.7)
ESC to PBO	1 (3.0)	1 (3.8)
PBO to SAMe	2 (6.1)	2 (7.7)
PBO to ESC	2 (6.1)	0 (0.0)
Active medication = ESC	*n* = 35	*n* = 24
no change	18 (51.4)	19 (79.2)
SAMe to ESC	4 (11.4)	2 (8.3)
SAMe to PBO	6 (17.7)	0 (0.0)
ESCto SAMe	4 (11.4)	1 (4.2)
ESC to PBO	0 (0.0)	1 (4.2)
PBO to SAMe	2 (5.7)	1 (4.2)
PBO to ESC	1 (2.9)	0 (0.0)

PBO, placebo; SAMe, S-adenosyl-L-methionine; ESC, escitalopram.

of side-effects indicating a nocebo effect (35, 36). Hence, variance in side effects might not have been heterogeneous enough to be associated with perceived treatment. While a majority of patients expected to receive SAMe before treatment began, there was no imbalance of perceived group allocation in favor of actual group allocation during the active treatment phase. This indicates that patients overall were successfully blinded regarding their specific treatment allocation until the end the treatment phase.

However, patients believing to be on active medication at week 6 showed significantly higher improvement in depressive symptoms at week 12 than patients believing to be on placebo, indicating expectancy effects due to perceived treatment assignment. The expectancy effect did not seem to be influenced by selective drop out, given the lack of association between perceived treatment and subsequent attrition. It remains unclear whether the expectancy effect was of the same or different magnitude among all treatment arms. *Post-hoc* analysis suggests that this effect might have been more pronounced in the escitalopram treatment arm. However, the omnibus test for an interaction between perceived and actual treatment was not significant. Therefore, this suggestion remains speculative for the trial at hand and should encourage better powered re-analyses to further explore this issue.

Notwithstanding, while most previous studies—due to their cross-sectional analysis—were unable to differentiate whether the perception of receiving active medication enhanced the treatment response via expectancy effects, or whether the improvement at the end of these trials influenced the final perception of treatment assignment, this re-analysis indicates that both might be true successively. The suggested pathway of expectancy effects due to perceived treatment assignment found in experimental research (28)–improvement influences perceived treatment, which in turn influences treatment outcome-appears to be validated within this re-analysis of a clinical trial.

In view of the above, this re-analysis now longitudinally confirms expectancy effects in double blind RCTs, and further ads to research highlighting important limitations for the interpretation of effects found in double blind placebo controlled RCTs. In clinical practice, patients do not have reason to doubt that they are receiving active medication. In placebo controlled RCTs, however, this doubt is justified and potentially induces decreased expectancy, which results in an underestimation of the effectiveness of a drug compared to routine clinical practice (37, 38). More generally, double blind RCTs evaluate the specific treatment effect of a pharmacologic verum by comparing it to the response generated by the unspecific treatment effect in the placebo group. If the verum group's treatment response exceeds that in the placebo group, the drug is considered to have drug specific effects. However, such a judgment is only justifiable under the assumption that the treatment response in the verum group consists of the equivalent unspecific effects observed in the placebo group plus the specific effects of the verum ("additive model"). Such an additive model of drug and placebo effects, however, has frequently been questioned theoretically and empirically (39–41). In fact evidence from clinical trials and both behavioral and neuro-physiological experiments suggest that drug specific and unspecific effects can interact (38, 39) and hence might not be equal between a verum and a placebo arm. Therefore, drug specific effects can be both over and underestimated in double blind RCTs. Although results regarding differential expectancy effects with the treatment arms are inconclusive in the current re-analysis, based on the results of this RCT, it cannot be said with absolute certainty that neither SAMe nor escitalopram do have or do not have drug specific efficacy. There is the possibility that specific characteristics of the SAMe or esctitalopram arm induced expectancy effects, which would have led to an overestimation of drug specific effects. On the other hand, RCTs with more than one active treatment arm have been found to show enhanced expectancy effects since the uncertainty of receiving active treatment is lower (38). As a result, this might have led to ceiling effects masking the drug specific expectancy. To circumvent these pitfalls, new study designs to better evaluate the effects of pharmacological treatment have been proposed; these include the balanced placebo design, the balanced cross over design, balanced open-hidden design or delayed response design [see (39, 40) for more details]. However, until such innovations for testing

TABLE 3 | Improvement and adverse effects predicting patients' perception to be on active medication (SAMe or escitalopram) or placebo at week 6 and week 12 using logistic regression analysis.

	B (SE)	*p*	*OR (95%–CI)*
PERCEIVED TREATMENT ASSIGNMENT AT WEEK 6 (n = 92)			
Improvement (Baseline – week 6; HDRS-17)	0.21 (0.06)	0.001	1.23 (1.09; 1.39)
Side Effects Week 6 (SAFTEE)			
Overall	−0.06 (1.15)	0.957	0.94 (0.09; 8.92)
Gastrointestinal	1.26 (1.95)	0.519	3.52 (0.07; 161.09)
Sexual function	−2.42 (1.72)	0.160	0.09 (0.01; 2.59)
Drug Assignment			
SAMe (vs. placebo)	0.84 (0.75)	0.266	2.31 (0.53; 10.10)
Escitalopram (vs. placebo)	1.00 (0.72)	0.165	2.73 (0.66; 11.25)
Baseline Perceived Treatment Assignment			
Active medication (vs. placebo)	1.41 (0.73)	0.054	4.10 (0.98; 17.23)
Constant	1.44 (1.11)	0.193	0.236
R^2 = 0.28 (Cox & Snell) 0.42 (Nagelkerke) $\chi^2_{(7)} = 30.66$, $p < 0.001$			
PERCEIVED TREATMENT ASSIGNMENT AT WEEK 12 (n = 71)			
Improvement (week 6–week 12; HDRS-17)	−0.03 (0.06)	0.653	0.97 (0.86; 1.10)
Side Effects Week 12 (SAFTEE)			
Overall	−1.35 (1.63)	0.408	0.26 (0.01; 6.36)
Gastrointestinal	1.88 (2.23)	0.400	7.12 (0.09; 515.08)
Sexual function	−1.18 (2.36)	0.617	0.37 (0.00; 31.27)
Drug Assignment			
SAMe (vs. placebo)	0.00 (0.95)	0.998	1.00 (0.16; 6.41)
Escitalopram (vs. placebo)	−0.02 (0.95)	0.980	0.98 (0.15; 6.29)
Week 6 Perceived Treatment Assignment			
Active medication (vs. placebo)	3.25 (0.75)	<0.001	25.89 (5.91; 113.31)
Constant	−0.03 (1.12)	0.975	0.966
R^2 = 0.36 (Cox & Snell) 0.52 (Nagelkerke) $\chi^2(7) = 31.32$, $p < 0.001$			

The predictors drug assignment and perceived treatment assignment were dummy coded with placebo as reference condition.

TABLE 4 | Longitudinal associations of patients' perceived treatment assignment and actual drug assignment with subsequent improvement in depression (HDRS-17).

	ß	*B [CI]*	*SE (B)*	*t*	*p*
WEEK 6 HDRS-17 (n = 104)					
Baseline HDRS-17	0.28	0.41 [0.14; 0.69]	0.14	2.97	0.004
Drug Assignment					
SAMe (vs. placebo)	−0.21	−2.92 [−6.03; 0.19]	1.57	1.86	0.065
Escitalopram (vs. placebo)	−0.03	−0.39 [−3.54; 2.67]	1.57	0.25	0.802
Week 6 perceived treatment assignment = active (vs. placebo)	−0.07	−1.32 [−4.69; 2.05]	1.69	0.78	0.440
R^2= 0.11, $F_{4, 99} = 3.71$, $p = 0.007$					
WEEK 12 HDRS-17 (n = 83)					
Week 6 HDRS-17	0.47	0.47 [0.26; 0.68]	0.11	4.40	<0.001
Drug Assignment					
SAMe (vs. placebo)	0.09	1.21 [−1.77; 4.19]	1.49	0.81	0.420
Escitalopram (vs. placebo)	−0.06	−0.82 [−3.88; 2.27]	1.54	0.51	0.605
Week 6 perceived treatment assignment = active (vs. placebo)	−0.22	−3.10 [−6.12; −0.09]	1.51	2.05	0.044
R^2= 0.13, $F_{(4, 78)} = 10.41$, $p < 0.001$					

The predictors drug assignment and perceived treatment assignment were dummy coded with placebo as reference condition.

pharmacological interventions become more established, double blind RCTs should at least assess and test for expectancy effects in a systematic manner.

Concerning the assessment of expectancy effects, the results of this re-analysis suggest that the current practice of measuring perceived treatment assignment only once—either at the

TABLE 5 | Longitudinal associations of patients' perceived treatment assignment with subsequent improvement in depression (HDRS-17) at week 12 individually by treatment group.

	ß	*B [CI]*	*SE (B)*	*t*	*p*
ACTUAL TREATMENT = PLACEBO (*n* = 26)					
Week 6 HDRS-17	0.09	0.15 [−0.42; 0.65]	0.26	0.45	0.999
Week 6 perceived treatment assignment = active (vs. placebo)	−0.27	−3.80 [−9.89; 2.93]	2.95	1.29	0.630
R^2= 0.10, $F_{(2, 23)}$ = 1.32, p = 0.286					
ACTUAL TREATMENT = SAMe (*n* = 30)					
Week 6 HDRS-17	0.65	0.60 [0.28; 0.92]	0.16	3.89	0.003
Week 6 perceived treatment assignment = active (vs. placebo)	0.00	−0.00 [−5.39; 5.93]	2.63	0.00	0.999
R^2= 0.42, $F_{(1, 28)}$ = 9.80, p = 0.001					
ACTUAL TREATMENT = ESCITALOPRAM (*n* = 27)					
Week 6 HDRS-17	0.58	0.59 [0.32; 0.87]	0.13	4.42	<0.010
Week 6 perceived treatment assignment = active (vs. placebo)	−0.37	−5.18 [−9.03; −1.33]	1.87	2.78	0.030
R^2= 0.73, $F_{(2, 24)}$ = 32.46, p < 0.001					

Perceived treatment assignment was dummy coded with placebo as reference condition. p-values have been adjusted for multiple testing using Bonferroni correction.

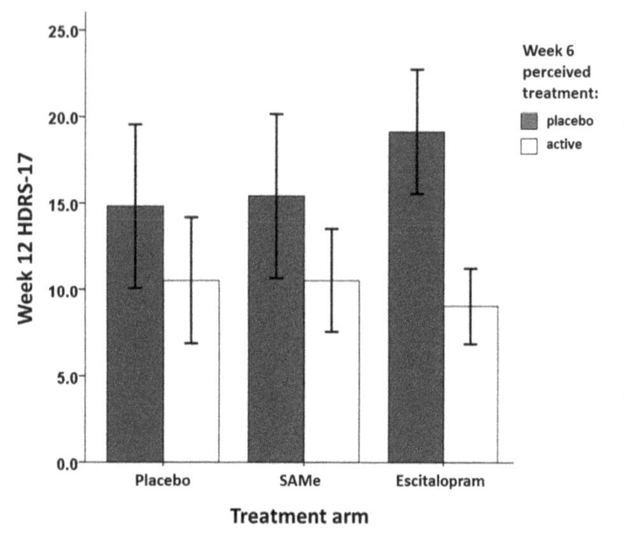

FIGURE 2 | Mean week 12 treatment outcome by week 6 perceived treatment and actual treatment assignment.

beginning or at the end of a trial—is questionable. The disadvantages of end of trial assessment of perceived treatment assignment have already been mentioned above. However, some previous studies used baseline or early assessment of perceived treatment allocation for their analysis of blinding or expectancy effects. Yet, in this re-analysis the perception of treatment assignment at the start of the trial did not at all reflect the perception of treatment assignment throughout the trial, making it a very unreliable measure to operationalize un-blinding or expectancy effects. Future trials should use repeated assessment of patients' perceived treatment assignment to determine un-blinding and evaluate expectancy effects. In addition, it would be even more advisable to assess patients' outcome expectations throughout a trial. First, a patient who believes to be on a specific active medication but does not believe the medication to be effective will most likely not have any expectancy effects (37), a case that would not be differentiated by only assessing perceived treatment assignment. Secondly, expectations can be assessed on parametric (or at least ordinal) scales, giving the advantage of statistical power over the assessment of perceived treatment assignment assessed as nominal data. For further details on the assessment of patients' expectations in medical treatment see (42).

While not the focus of this re-analysis, one additional finding is of interest: a large majority of patients before the start of treatment expected to receive SAMe, despite being informed about the equal assignment probability. A similar pattern in favor of the "new" treatment has been observed in other trials before (11, 34). This might shed interest on the role of drug trial advertisement. For the trial of this re-analysis, advertisements emphasized the treatment of depression with SAMe, because it was thought that this would attract more participants interested in taking a natural product; this could have influenced patients' expectations. While the current re-analysis did not find any indication that these expectations influenced treatment effects, one might see some indication of advertisement or novelty effect (14) in the newest net-work meta-analysis on anti-depressants (43). Cipriani et al. did find that the same anti-depressant had a positive pooled effect size in trials when evaluated as a new agent, and negative effect sizes when evaluated as the "old" comparator agent. Hence, in trials with two or more active comparators it might be worthwhile to investigate whether framing such as "new" vs. "old" toward participants is an additional source of bias. If such a "novelty effect" existed, this would pose further evidence against an additive model.

Some limitations have to be considered when interpreting the results presented. First, the external validity is limited by the fact that the re-analysis was based on a three arm RCT with SAMe and escitalopram as the active treatments. As discussed above expectancy effects are considered to be higher in a study with two active treatments. Generalization to clinical practice is limited since patients usually have no doubt about receiving active medication. However, patients in clinical practice are likely to have expectations regarding the efficacy of the medication or expectations about side effects (42), which might also serve to influence treatment effects. Additionally, both active treatments are reasonably well tolerated. Therefore, it remains unclear, whether results would be different among active treatment with stronger side effect profiles (e.g., tricyclic antidepressants). Moreover, it remains unclear whether comparing a "classical" anti-depressant with a natural supplement anti-depressant might have different mechanisms of perceived treatment than in other trials. Related to that, it is unclear whether trial advertisement attracted individuals with specific interest in natural remedies, who might for example have more negative expectations about "classical" anti-depressants. Further, although there was no difference in participants providing perceived treatment data regarding depressive symptoms and side effects, nor an association with drop-out, one can not completely rule out whether missing guess data might be a source of bias.

In conclusion, this re-analysis showed that patients' perceptions about treatment assignment do change throughout a trial, that these perceptions appeared to be influenced by preceding improvement in depressive symptoms, and that perceptions about treatment assignment predicted further improvement. Building on previous cross-sectional and experimental evidence the current results further highlight issues with the interpretation of effects found in double blind RCTs. Future RCTs should apply multiple assessment of perceived treatment assignment and/or expectations throughout the trial. This would permit testing for possible expectation effects that might bias the comparison for specific efficacy, and provide the opportunity to further explore mechanisms of bias in double blind RCTs. Moreover, new study designs for testing pharmacological interventions should be considered, to get a more concise estimate of the specific effects of a pharmacological treatment.

ETHICS STATEMENT

This study was carried out in accordance with the recommendations of the U.S. Food and Drug Administration (FDA) guidelines with written informed consent from all subjects. All subjects gave written informed consent in accordance with the Declaration of Helsinki. The protocol was approved by the Institutional Review Boards of the Massachusetts General Hospital in Boston, MA and the Butler Hospital in Providence, RI.

AUTHOR CONTRIBUTIONS

JL, SV, and DM designed the re-analysis, conducted data analysis, and wrote the current manuscript. DM, LP, LC, AT, and MF designed and conducted the original randomized controlled trial this re-analysis is based on. LB and AJC assisted with the statistical analysis. GP and AC assisted with the writing of the manuscript.

FUNDING

The original study was supported by the NIH and the National Center for Complementary and Alternative Medicine (NCCAM), R01 grant R01AT001638. SAMe tosylate and matching placebo were supplied by Pharmavite LLC, CA, United States. JL was supported by a fellowship within the Postdoc-Program of the German Academic Exchange Service (DAAD).

REFERENCES

1. Enck P, Bingel U, Schedlowski M, Rief W. The placebo response in medicine: minimize, maximize or personalize? *Nat Rev Drug Discov.* (2013)12:191–204. doi: 10.1038/nrd3923
2. Benedetti F. Mechanisms of placebo and placebo-related effects across diseases and treatments. *Annu Rev Pharmacol Toxicol.* (2008) 48:33–60. doi: 10.1146/annurev.pharmtox.48.113006.094711
3. Kirsch I, Moore TJ, Scoboria A, Nicholls SS. The emperor's new drugs: an analysis of antidepressant medication data submitted to the u.s. food and drug administration. *Prev Treat.* (2002) 5:23. doi: 10.1037/1522-3736.5.1.523a
4. Kirsch I, Deacon BJ, Huedo-Medina TB, Scoboria A, Moore TJ, Johnson BT. Initial severity and antidepressant benefits: a meta-analysis of data submitted to the food and drug administration. *PLoS Med.* (2008) 5:0260–8. doi: 10.1371/journal.pmed.0050045
5. Baethge C, Assall OP, Baldessarini RJ. Systematic review of blinding assessment in randomized controlled trials in schizophrenia and affective disorders 2000-2010. *Psychother Psychosom.* (2013) 82:152–60. doi: 10.1159/000346144
6. Hróbjartsson A, Forfang E, Haahr MT, Als-Nielsen B, Brorson S. Blinded trials taken to the test: an analysis of randomized clinical trials that report tests for the success of blinding. *Int J Epidemiol.* (2007) 36:654–63. doi: 10.1093/ije/dym020
7. Bello S, Moustgaard H, Hróbjartsson A. Unreported formal assessment of unblinding occurred in 4 of 10 randomized clinical trials, unreported loss of blinding in 1 of 10 trials. *J Clin Epidemiol.* (2017) 81:42–50. doi: 10.1016/j.jclinepi.2016.08.002
8. Wood L, Egger M, Gluud LL, Schulz KF, Jüni P, Altman DG, et al. Empirical evidence of bias in treatment effect estimates in controlled trials with different interventions and outcomes: meta-epidemiological study. *BMJ* (2008) 336:601–5. doi: 10.1136/bmj.39465.451748.AD
9. Hróbjartsson A, Emanuelsson F, Thomsen ASS, Hilden J, Brorson S. Bias due to lack of patient blinding in clinical trials. a systematic review of trials randomizing patients to blind and nonblind sub-studies. *Int J Epidemiol.* (2014) 43:1272–83. doi: 10.1093/ije/dyu115
10. Hróbjartsson A, Sofia A, Thomsen S. Observer bias in randomised clinical trials with binary outcomes: systematic review of trials with

both blinded and non-blinded outcome assessors. *BMJ* (2012) 1119:1–11. doi: 10.1136/bmj.e1119
11. Rees JR, Wade TJ, Levy DA, Colford JM, Hilton JF. Changes in beliefs identify unblinding in randomized controlled trials: a method to meet CONSORT guidelines. *Contemp Clin Trials.* (2005) 26:25–37. doi: 10.1016/j.cct.2004.11.020
12. Mathieu E, Herbert RD, McGeechan K, Herbert JJ, Barratt AL. A theoretical analysis showed that blinding cannot eliminate potential for bias associated with beliefs about allocation in randomized clinical trials. *J Clin Epidemiol.* (2014) 67:667–71. doi: 10.1016/j.jclinepi.2014.02.001
13. Desbiens NA. In randomized controlled trials, should subjects in both placebo and drug groups be expected to guess that they are taking drug 50% of the time? *Med Hypotheses* (2002) 59:227–32. doi: 10.1016/S0306-9877(02)00205-0
14. Schulz KF, Grimes DA. Blinding in randomised trials: hiding who got what. *Lancet* (2002) 359:696–700. doi: 10.1016/S0140-6736(02)07816-9
15. Turner JA, Jensen MP, Warms CA, Cardenas DD. Blinding effectiveness and association of pretreatment expectations with pain improvement in a double-blind randomized controlled trial. *Pain.* (2002) 99:91–9. doi: 10.1016/S0304-3959(02)00060-X
16. White K, Kando J, Pharm D, Park T, Waternaux C, Brown WA. Side effects and the "Blindability" of clinical drug trials. *Am J Psychiatry* (1992) 149:1730–1.
17. Rief W, Glombiewski JA. The hidden effects of blinded, placebo-controlled randomized trials: An experimental investigation. *Pain* (2012) 153:2473–7. doi: 10.1016/j.pain.2012.09.007
18. Gilron I, Tu D, Holden RR. Sensory and affective pain descriptors respond differentially to pharmacological interventions in neuropathic conditions. *Clin J Pain* (2013) 29:124–31. doi: 10.1097/AJP.0b013e31824ce65c
19. Kinney MAO, Mantilla CB, Carns PE, Passe MA, Brown MJ, Hooten WM, et al. Preoperative gabapentin for acute post-thoracotomy analgesia: a randomized, double-blinded, active placebo-controlled study. *Pain Pract.* (2012) 12:175–83. doi: 10.1111/j.1533-2500.2011.00480.x
20. Simmonds MK, Rashiq S, Sobolev IA, Dick BD, Gray DP, Stewart BJ, et al. The effect of single-dose propofol injection on pain and quality of life in chronic daily headache: a randomized, double-blind, controlled trial. *Anesth Analg.* (2009) 109:1972–80. doi: 10.1213/ANE.0b013e3181be3f86
21. Moncrieff J, Wessely S, Hardy R. Active placebos versus antidepressants for depression. *Cochrane Database Syst Rev.* (2004):CD003012. doi: 10.1002/14651858.CD003012.pub2
22. Dar R, Barrett SP. The effects of beliefs regarding drug assignment in experimental and field studies of nicotine delivery devices: a review. *J Psychopharmacol.* (2014) 28:1071–9. doi: 10.1177/0269881114548295
23. Correa JB, Heckman BW, Marquinez NS, Drobes DJ, Unrod M, Roetzheim RG, et al. Perceived medication assignment during a placebo-controlled laboratory study of varenicline: temporal associations of treatment expectancies with smoking-related outcomes. *Psychopharmacology* (2014) 231:2559–66. doi: 10.1007/s00213-013-3420-2
24. Colagiuri B, Morley K, Boakes R, Haber P. Expectancy in double-blind placebo-controlled trials: An example from alcohol dependence. *Psychother Psychosom.* (2009) 78:167–71. doi: 10.1159/000206871
25. Thomas JL, Guo H, Lynam IM, Powell JN, Okuyemi KS, Bronars CA, et al. The impact of perceived treatment assignment on smoking cessation outcomes among African-American smokers. *J Gen Intern Med.* (2008) 23:1361–6. doi: 10.1007/s11606-008-0656-3
26. McRae C, Cherin E, Yamazaki TG, Diem G, Vo AH, Russell D, et al. Effects of perceived treatment on quality of life and medical outcomes in a double-blind placebo surgery trial. *Arch Gen Psychiatry* (2004) 61:412–20. doi: 10.1001/archpsyc.61.4.412
27. Chen JA, Papakostas GI, Youn SJ, Baer L, Clain AJ, Fava M, et al. Association between patient beliefs regarding assigned treatment and clinical response: reanalysis of data from the Hypericum Depression Trial Study Group. *J Clin Psychiatry* (2011) 72:1669–76. doi: 10.4088/JCP.10m06453
28. Colagiuri B, Boakes R. Perceived treatment, feedback, and placebo effects in double-blind RCTs: an experimental analysis. *Psychopharmacology* (2010) 208:433–41. doi: 10.1007/s00213-009-1743-9
29. Mischoulon D, Price LH, Carpenter LL, Tyrka AR, Papakostas GI, Baer L, et al. A double-blind, randomized, placebo-controlled clinical trial of S-adenosyl-L -methionine (SAMe) vs. escitalopram in major depressive disorder. *J Clin Psychiatry* (2014) 75:370–6. doi: 10.4088/JCP.13m08591
30. First MB, Spitzer RL, Gibbon M, Williams JB. *Structured Clinical Interview For DSM-IV Axis I Disorders: Clinician Version (SCID-CV).* Washington, DC: American Psychiatric Press (1997).
31. Rush AJ, Gullion CM, Basco MR, Jarrett RB, Trivedi MH. The inventory of depressive symptomatology (IDS): psychometric properties. *Psychol Med.* (1996) 26:477–86. doi: 10.1017/S0033291700035558
32. Hamilton M. A rating scale for depression. *J Neurol Neurosurg Psychiatry* (1960) 23:56–62. doi: 10.1136/jnnp.23.1.56
33. Levine J, Schooler NR. SAFTEE: a technique for the systematic assessment of side effects in clinical trials. *Psychopharmacol Bull.* (1986) 22:343–81.
34. Oviedo-Joekes E, Marchand K, Palis H, Guh D, Brissette S, Lock K, et al. Predictors of treatment allocation guesses in a randomized controlled trial testing double-blind injectable hydromorphone and diacetylmorphine for severe opioid use disorder. *Addict Res Theory* (2017) 25:263–72. doi: 10.1080/16066359.2016.1263729
35. Barsky AJ, Saintfort R, Rogers MP, Borus JF. Nonspecific medication side effects and the nocebo phenomenon. *JAMA* (2002) 287:622–7. doi: 10.1001/jama.287.5.622
36. Colloca L, Finniss D. Nocebo effects, patient-clinician communication, and therapeutic outcomes. *JAMA* (2012) 307:567–8. doi: 10.1001/jama.2012.115
37. Colagiuri B. Participant expectancies in double-blind randomized placebo-controlled trials: potential limitations to trial validity. *Clin Trials.* (2010) 7:246–55. doi: 10.1177/1740774510367916
38. Enck P, Klosterhalfen S, Weimer K, Horing B, Zipfel S. The placebo response in clinical trials: more questions than answers. *Philos Trans R Soc B Biol Sci.* (2011) 366:1889–95. doi: 10.1098/rstb.2010.0384
39. Kube T, Rief W. Are placebo and drug-specific effects additive? questioning basic assumptions of double-blinded randomized clinical trials and presenting novel study designs. *Drug Discov Today* (2017) 22:729–35. doi: 10.1016/j.drudis.2016.11.022
40. Enck P, Klosterhalfen S, Zipfel S. Novel study designs to investigate the placebo response. *BMC Med Res Methodol.* (2011) 11:90. doi: 10.1186/1471-2288-11-90
41. Kirsch I. Are drug and placebo effects in depression additive? *Biol Psychiatry* (2000) 47:733–5. doi: 10.1016/S0006-3223(00)00832-5
42. Laferton JAC, Kube T, Salzmann S, Auer CJ, Shedden-Mora MC. Patients' expectations regarding medical treatment: a critical review of concepts and their assessment. *Front Psychol.* (2017) 8:233. doi: 10.3389/fpsyg.2017.00233
43. Cipriani A, Furukawa TA, Salanti G, Chaimani A, Atkinson LZ, Ogawa Y, et al. Comparative efficacy and acceptability of 21 antidepressant drugs for the acute treatment of adults with major depressive disorder: a systematic review and network meta-analysis. *Lancet* (2018) 1–10. doi: 10.1016/S0140-6736(17)32802-7

6

Influencing Side-Effects to Medicinal Treatments: A Systematic Review of Brief Psychological Interventions

Rebecca K. Webster[1,2]* *and G. James Rubin*[1,2]

[1] *Department of Psychological Medicine, Institute of Psychiatry, Psychology & Neuroscience, King's College London, London, United Kingdom,* [2] *The National Institute for Health Research Health Protection Research Unit in Emergency Preparedness and Response, King's College London, London, United Kingdom*

Correspondence:
Rebecca K. Webster
Rebecca.webster@kcl.ac.uk

Background: Nocebo effects contribute to a large proportion of the non-specific side-effects attributed to medications and are mainly generated through negative expectations. Previous reviews show that interventions designed to change participants' expectations have a small effect on pain experience. They are also effective in reducing side-effects caused by exposure to sham medications. To date, there has been no review of the influence of such interventions on symptoms attributed to real medicinal treatments.

Objective: To review studies using a randomized controlled design testing the effect of brief psychological interventions compared to usual practice on the side-effect experience to medicinal treatments in healthy volunteers and patients.

Methods: We searched Web of Science, Scopus, Medline, PsycINFO, PsycARTICLES, and Cochrane CENTRAL using search terms for randomized controlled trials along with "nocebo," "placebo effect," "medication," "side-effects," and associated terms. Studies were eligible if they studied a human population, used an active medicine, delivered a brief psychological intervention intended to influence side-effect reporting compared to usual care or no intervention, and used a randomized controlled design. Because of the heterogeneity of the literature we used a narrative synthesis and assessed evidence quality using the GRADE approach.

Results: Our database search and supplementary search of the reference sections of included studies retrieved 50,140 citations. After screening, full text review and manual reference searches, 27 studies were included. The quality of the studies and evidence was judged to be low. The strongest and most consistent effect came from omitting side-effect information, although surprisingly de-emphasizing side-effects did not affect side-effect reporting. Other techniques, including priming, distraction, and altering the perception of branding, produced mixed results.

Conclusion: Brief psychological interventions can influence side-effect reporting to active medications. Research is currently investigating new ways to de-emphasize side-effects whilst still upholding informed consent, but larger confirmatory trials with suitable control groups are needed. The literature in this area would be improved by more detailed reporting of studies.

Keywords: review, side-effects, medicine, nocebo effect, interventions, side-effect information

INTRODUCTION

Nocebo effects, sometimes dubbed the placebo effect's "evil twin," are the experience of noxious symptoms in response to an inert exposure (1). Nocebo effects can also refer to negative clinical outcomes which are not attributable to the actual pharmacological or physiotherapeutic action of an intervention (2). It is estimated that between 38 and 100% of side-effects reported to drugs taken for a large range of medical conditions are related to the treatment context, rather than the active ingredients of the medication itself (3).

These nocebo-related side-effects are important, as they can affect a patient's well-being (4) and influence their decision as to whether to adhere to their treatment regimen (5, 6). For example adverse media coverage surrounding the safety of statins and their reported side-effects has resulted in around 2,00,000 patients who are no longer taking their statins as directed leading to a predicted increase of 2,000 cardiovascular events in the next decade (7). This is despite the fact that most of these side-effects are probably nocebo-related (8). Perhaps unsurprisingly, side-effects can also result in substantial additional health care costs in terms of additional primary care and hospital visits and also the cost of wasted medication due to non-adherence (9).

Of the multiple factors that may contribute to the development of nocebo effects, expectations of symptoms appear to be the main contributor. These can be generated through verbal and written suggestions about what symptoms to expect, be implied by the apparent dose of a drug, and be learnt through classical conditioning and social observation (10). Studies have used these psychological mechanisms as a means to alter peoples' experience of experimentally induced pain (11), as well as pain following acute medical procedures, such as injections (12) and surgery (13). These effects have been studied in multiple reviews, showing that brief psychological interventions designed to change expectation of pain following treatment have a small but reliable effect on relieving patients' pain compared to usual care (14–16).

However, to our knowledge, there has been no review of whether such interventions can alter patient experience ofside-effects to medicinal treatments. Although evidence demonstrates that such interventions can be effective in altering side-effects reported following exposure to inert substances (10), it is also important to assess if these effects can be transferred to clinical practice. We therefore set out to review studies using a randomized controlled design testing the effect of brief psychological interventions compared to usual practice on the side-effect experience to medicinal treatments in healthy volunteers and patients. To answer the question: can brief psychological interventions influence the side-effect experience to medications?

METHODS

Our reporting of this systematic review adheres to the standards for the Preferred Reporting Items for Systematic reviews and Meta-Analyses (17). The protocol for this review was prospectively registered on PROSPERO (CRD42018091903).

Identification of Studies

We searched the following electronic databases with a predefined search strategy: Web of Science, Scopus, OvidSp (Medline, PsycINFO, and PsycARTICLES) and Cochrane CENTRAL. We included Web of Science and Scopus for their coverage of the sciences and social sciences. OvidSp was chosen for its coverage of journals chiefly in the area of health sciences, and also for its inclusion of the databases PsycINFO and PsycARTICLES. Cochrane CENTRAL was included due to its coverage of randomized controlled trials and because it includes records which are derived from other sources to the ones already chosen.

In preliminary work we tested a variety of search strategies in an effort to balance specificity and sensitivity. Our final search strategy used the recommended search terms to identify randomized controlled trials (18) along with the terms and associated words for "nocebo," "placebo effect," "medication," and "side-effects." We used separate search strategies for each of the databases as these needed to be modified due to differences in MeSH terms, boolean operators and wildcards. A copy the search strategy we used for Medline can be seen in the **Supplementary Material**.

Review Process

The search was initially carried out on 22nd March 2018 and updated on 22nd June 2018 following the identification of a relevant study published between this time. The initial electronic searches were combined using EndNote and duplicates were identified and deleted. The titles and abstracts of citations were then screened for potential relevance. If relevance was not clear from the abstract, the study was taken forward to the full text review. All full text versions of papers that were potentially relevant were then screened in relation to the inclusion criteria. Papers that met the inclusion criteria had their reference sections manually searched for other studies that could be included.

Selection Criteria

Studies were eligible for inclusion in this review if they met the criteria below.

Population

Human population (healthy volunteers, patients and children were allowed).

Exposure

Active medicinal treatment (i.e., contains a pharmacological agent), associated with side-effects.

Intervention

A brief, psychological intervention delivered in one session and that could be feasibly introduced within a single doctor-patient consultation or treatment appointment. By psychological we mean an intervention that targets certain psychological processes, such as cognitive expectations, attention or learning. Interventions requiring biological or chemical stimuli were excluded because these are not purely psychological. As we wanted to identify interventions that could be easily incorporated into clinical practice, in-depth psychological interventions, such as cognitive behavior therapy, mindfulness, relaxation training or guided imagery, or that consisted of intensive educational packages were excluded as these typically are not delivered in one session and often take place over the course of a treatment.

Comparator

Usual care. We excluded studies with control conditions involving a different type of intervention.

Outcome

We included studies with an outcome of side-effects measured via self-report or inferred through objective measures. We followed the NICE (19) definition of a side-effect as "An effect of a drug (or treatment or intervention) that is additional to the main intended effect. It could be good, bad or neutral, depending on the circumstances." For some studies, e.g., those concerning infant experience to vaccinations, side-effects were measured within minutes of the procedure. We excluded these on the bases that the "side-effects" were presumably related to the insertion of the needle rather than the effects of the vaccine itself.

Study Design

Used an experimental design in which participants were randomized or quasi randomized to receive the intervention or the control condition.

Other Criteria

Published in the English language.

Data Extraction

We extracted data from the final set of studies using a data extraction table developed for this systematic review. Data extracted included the study design and methodology, main demographics of participants, description of intervention and control conditions, side-effect measures, statistical approach and results. We also extracted details about the mode of the intervention, its content and duration.

Quality Assessment

We assessed the quality of all eligible studies using the Cochrane Collaboration's Risk of Bias tool for randomized controlled trials (20).

Data Synthesis and Analysis

Due to the heterogeneity in the interventions that we included and the way that side-effects were measured, scored and analyzed, we used a narrative synthesis to analyse the results. There is no general consensus on the best way to carry out a narrative synthesis for systematic reviews (21). As such we decided to use a weight of evidence approach by identifying the quality of evidence for each type of intervention reviewed. To do this we used the GRADE approach (22) which is a transparent framework used to grade the quality of evidence included in systematic reviews and the strength of recommendations.

RESULTS

Search Results

The database search retrieved 50,133 citations and searching the reference lists of included studies retrieved another 7, giving a total of 50,140. After removing duplicates 40,346 citations remained. After screening titles and abstracts, we reviewed the full text of 63 articles relating to 66 studies. Of these, 39 studies were excluded for not meeting the inclusion criteria, resulting in a total of 26 articles reporting on 27 studies. One article (23) reported results on two separate studies and is referred to in the text and tables as Study 1 or Study 2 where necessary. The number of studies at each stage of the search strategy and the reasons for exclusion are shown in **Figure 1**.

Study Characteristics

See **Table 1** for a full summary of the characteristics of the included studies. The 27 studies included in the review reported on a total of 3,459 participants. There was a range of patient groups and treatments under investigation. The most common of these were patients with cancer receiving chemotherapy (26, 31, 39, 41–44, 46), and patients with depression prescribed anti-depressants (29, 32, 35–37). All studies used a between participants RCT design apart from Cildag et al. (24), Myers and Calvert (36), Redd et al. (39), and Schagen et al. (42) which used a quasi-randomized approach, and Faasse et al. (28) who used a within-subjects RCT design. Some studies used a factorial design in their RCT involving different experimental conditions or baseline variables entered as independent factors (23, 31, 39, 41–43). In these cases, we have reported the main effects of the relevant intervention under investigation.

There were a variety of interventions used by included studies. We looked for common themes and content of the various interventions and were able to group the studies into five different types, these were: priming, distraction, branding, omitting side-effects, and de-emphasizing side-effects, plus a miscellaneous group.

The majority of studies used an un-validated questionnaire specifically designed for their study to measure side-effects, and measures were generally completed within days/weeks following treatment initiation.

Quality Assessment

The quality of included studies was poor (see **Figures 2**, **3**). The main problem was a lack of clear reporting within the papers. Over half of the studies neglected to mention how they carried out randomization, and four were at high risk for using a quasi-randomized approach. Because of the unclear reporting of random sequence generation, the risk for allocation concealment bias followed a similar pattern, and six studies were at high risk because their randomization approach allowed research staff to foresee subsequent allocations. For blinding of participants and personnel, studies often failed to state whether the experimenters were blind to the manipulation that accompanied the active treatment, leaving the risk of bias unclear. Only seven studies used adequate blinding procedures, with one not using blinding at all. Nineteen studies used side-effect measures which were completed by participants, as such blinding of the outcome assessment was judged unlikely to influence these results. For the remaining eight studies it was unclear if participants filled in the measures themselves or if they were administered by a blind/non-blind member of the study team. For 16 studies, drop outs were not addressed, or if they were, the paper typically failed

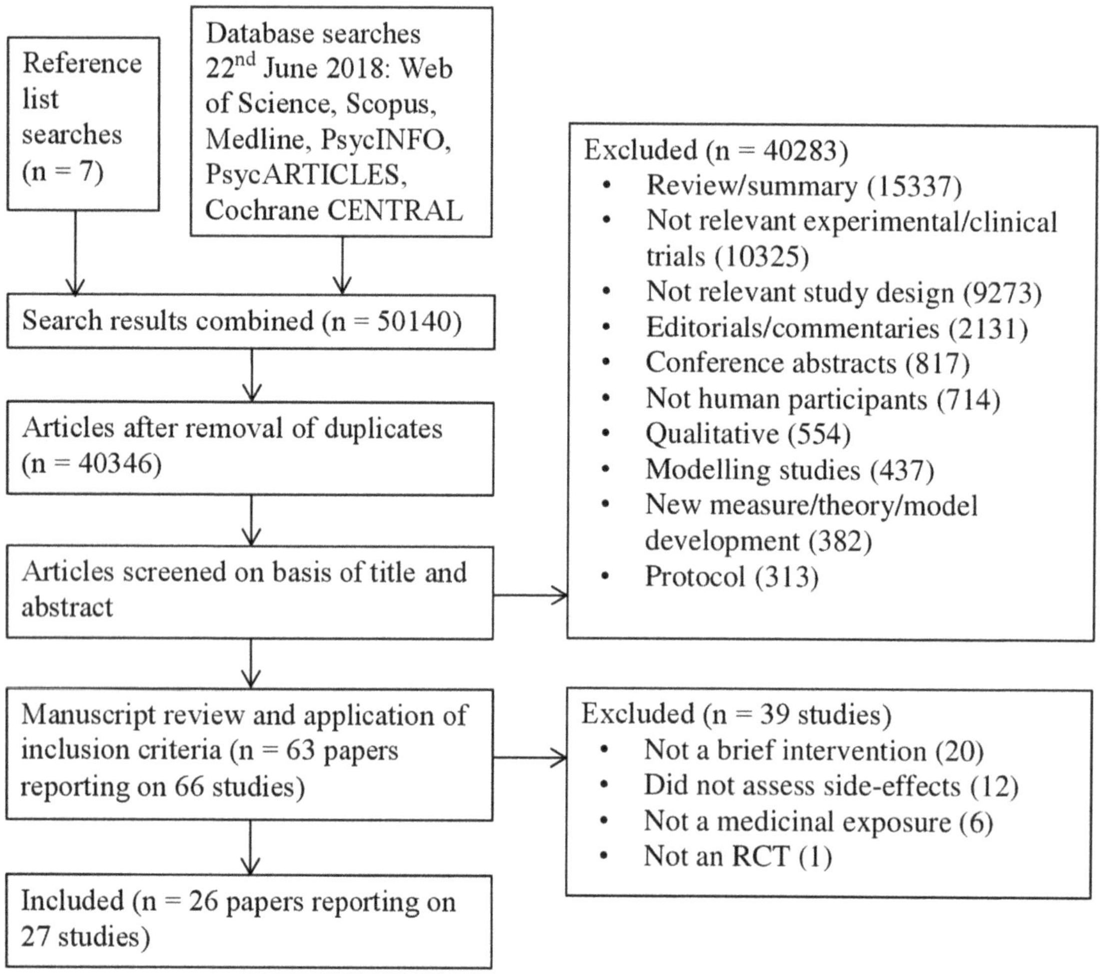

FIGURE 1 | Flow diagram of the selection process of studies including the number of events and reasons for exclusion.

to explain how this affected the results, leaving the risk of bias unclear; the remaining 11 studies provided adequate information and reasoning behind drop outs. Only two studies had lodged a protocol in a publicly accessible registry before the start of recruitment, leaving us unable to assess the risk for selective reporting for the remaining studies, apart from one in which there was a change in the prespecified primary analysis suggesting there was a high risk of bias.

Quality of the Evidence

The quality of evidence regarding priming, distraction, omitting side-effect information and de-emphasizing side effects, and doctor characteristic intervention(s) was very low. This is because most of the information came from studies at low or unclear risk of bias, in which plausible bias could alter the results. There was also some evidence of inconsistency and imprecision in the results due to opposite findings, wide confidence intervals and some small studies which may not have been adequately powered. Due to the broad nature of this systematic review, there is no evidence of indirectness, as all included studies helped to answer the question. It is plausible however, there may have been some publication bias due to the preponderance of smaller studies.

The quality of evidence regarding the branding intervention studies was low. This was graded similarly due to the reasons discussed for the above interventions, however the inconsistency in the results could perhaps be explained by differences in the interventions, and we judged that the small studies were probably due to this literature representing an early evidence base, rather than publication bias.

Finally, the quality of evidence for the deception intervention was moderate. There was some imprecision evident and the sample size was small, however the study was judged to have a low overall risk of bias, and there was no evidence of indirectness. As only one study was included, inconsistency and publication bias could not be determined.

Effect of Interventions on Side-Effect Reporting

Priming

Four studies looked at the effect of priming on side-effect reporting following chemotherapy with mixed results (see

TABLE 1 | Summary table of included studies.

References (intervention type)	Design	Sample (N, M age, %Male)	Treatment	Experimental group (n)	Control group (n)	Side-effect measure (main outcome)	Timing of measure
Cildag et al. (24) (Distraction)	Quasi RCT	Patients undergoing drug provocation test (112, 41.8, 32.1)	Various drug provocation tests	Kept busy filling questionnaires, arranging files and doing archiving (63)	Did not perform any tasks (49)	? (yes)	During provocation test
Cocco (25) (Omitting)	RCT	Patients with arterial hypertension (114, 57.7, 100)	Metroprolol	1. Metroprolol given under a code number with no information about active substance. Informed of all possible side-effects apart from erectile dysfunction (38) 2. Informed taking metroprolol and about all possible side-effects apart from erectile dysfunction (38)	Informed taking metroprolol and erectile dysfunction might occur (38)	IIEF (yes)	At the end of the 60-day trial
Colagiuri et al. (26) (Priming)	RCT	Patients undergoing chemotherapy (91, 60.5, 42.9)	Chemotherapy	Assessed expectancies for nausea, fatigue, sadness, and loss of appetite before first infusion (46)	No assessment of expectancies (45)	SSQ and EORTC QLQ-C30 (yes)	After first chemotherapy cycle
Colgan et al. (27) (Branding)	RCT	People with frequent headaches (69, 21, 21.7)	Branded and generic ibuprofen	Video interviewing health specialists and providing accurate information addressing misperceptions of generic medicines (34)	Video interviewing a neurologist about the different types of headaches and their global epidemiology (35)	Modified GASE (no)	An hour after taking ibuprofen for a headache
Faasse et al. (28) (Branding)	RCCT	Students with frequent headache (81, 20.8, 17)	Ibuprofen	Ibuprofen labeled with the brand name "nurofen" (81)	Ibuprofen labeled "generic ibuprofen" (81)	SSQ (yes)	An hour after taking ibuprofen for a headache
Faria et al. (29) (Misc)	RCT	Patients with seasonal affective disorder (46, 31.8, 60.9)	Escitalopram	Deceptively told they would receive the active placebo, likely to induce side-effects similar to escitalopram but out of which no symptom-improvement could be expected (22)	Correctly informed about the SSRI treatment and the expected improvement (24)	? (no)	?
Flam et al. (30) (Omitting)	RCT	Patients undergoing a myelogram (30, ?,43.3)	Myelogram	1. No tape-recorded message (10) 2. Tape-recorded message about the techniques performed during a myelogram (10)	Tape-recorded message about the sensations to expect during a myelogram (10)	Interview (no)	The day following the myelogram
Jacobs et al. (31) (Priming)	RCT	Patients with breast cancer (175, 49.4, 0)	Chemotherapy	1. Informed about the possibility of cognitive problems after chemotherapy (56) 2. Same information plus reassurance that there are still patients who score well on memory tests (59)	Received a one sentence neutral introduction without reference to chemotherapy or cognitive difficulties (60)	Cognitive failure questionnaire (yes)	After study introduction
John et al. (32) (Omitting)	RCT	Patients with depression (39, 34.0, 38)	Antidepressants	Asked about their symptoms, their prescription was explained to them and they were encouraged to take their medicines as advised (22)	Face-to-face, 10-min education session about depression, treatment, efficacy and adverse effects of the prescribed drug, and plan of management (17)	KAE questionnaire (no)	Six weeks after prescription
Lauder et al. (33) (De-emphasizing)	RCT	Patients undergoing hysterectomy (195, 43.4, 0)	Anesthesia	Informed of the use of two perioperative antiemetics to reduce the incidence of emetic symptoms to anesthesia after operation (95)	Informed that this was a study of post-operative well-being with no information about emetic symptoms (100)	Recorded by nursing staff (yes)	Immediately, 4, 8, and 24 h after surgery (combined)

(Continued)

TABLE 1 | Continued

References (intervention type)	Design	Sample (N, M age, %Male)	Treatment	Experimental group (n)	Control group (n)	Side-effect measure (main outcome)	Timing of measure
Mondaini et al. (34) (Omitting)	RCT	Patients with benign prostatic hyperplasia (107, 60.5, 100)	Finasteride	Finasteride concealed as an "X compound of proven efficacy for the treatment of BPH" (52)	Finasteride concealed as an "X compound of proven efficacy for the treatment of BPH. It may cause erectile dysfunction, decrease libido, problems of ejaculation but it is uncommon" (55)	Male sexual function-4, and SSQ (yes)	12 months after prescription
Mukherjee and Sahay (23) Study 1 (Omitting)	RCT 2 × 2	Business graduates (117, ?, ?)	Skin cream	No information given. Price was manipulated at two levels: 1. low (?) 2. high (?)	Read a news item about skin creams and their potential side-effects. Price was manipulated at two levels: 1. low (?) 2. high (?)	SSQ (yes)	?
Mukherjee and Sahay (23) Study 2 (Omitting)	RCT 2 × 3	Business students (149, ?, ?)	Skin Cream	Presented with an excerpt devoid of any negative aspects. Price was manipulated at three levels 1. low (?) 2. high (?) 3. discounted (?)	Read a news item about skin creams and their potential side-effects. Price was manipulated at three levels 1. low (?) 2. high (?) 3. discounted (?)	SSQ (yes)	?
Myers and Calvert (35) (Omitting)	RCT	Patients with depression (93, 40.4, 39.8)	Amitriptyline	Told only that the drug was being given to cure their depression (46)	Told the drug was being given to cure their depression and listed a series of side-effect they might experience (47)	SSQ (yes)	Two weeks after initial dose
Myers and Calvert (36) (Omitting)	RCT	Patients with depression (89, 38.9, 33.7)	Dothiepin	Told only that the drug was being given to cure their depression (43)	Told the drug was being given to cure their depression and listed a series of side-effect they might experience (46)	SSQ (yes)	Two weeks after initial dose
Myers and Calvert (37) (Omitting)	RCT	Patients with depression (120, 43.3, 25.8)	Dothiepin	1. Told only that the drug was being given to treat their depression and received no written information (40) 2. Verbal and written information about beneficial effects (40)	Verbal and written information about side-effects (40)	SSQ (no)	3 and 6 weeks after prescription
O'Connor et al. (38) (De-emphasizing)	RCT	Patients eligible for flu vaccine (292, 52.5, 6.7)	Influenza vaccine	Described the percentage who remain influenza and side-effect free. Accompanied by flip charts and decision aid poster highlighting the key points (148)	Described the percentage who acquire influenza and vaccine side effects. Accompanied by flip charts and decision aid poster highlighting the key points (144)	SSQ (no)	3 days after vaccination
Redd et al. (39) (Distraction)	Quasi RCT	Pediatric patients undergoing chemotherapy (26, 14.0, 73.2)	Chemotherapy	Played from a choice of video games for 10 min (13)	Permitted access to toys, books, games, and television (13)	Visual analog scale (yes)	10 min later
Rickels et al. (40) (Misc)	RCT	Patients with psychiatric disorders (169, 31.9, 34.3)	Tranquilisers	Study doctor who was a psychiatrist that was drug "enthusastic" (?)	Study doctor who was a psychiatrist that was drug "skeptical" (?)	Recorded by doctor (no)	2 and 4 weeks after prescription (combined)
Roscoe et al. (41) (De-emphasizing)	RCT	Patients with breast cancer (53, 51.5, 0)	Chemotherapy	Handout showing positive interpretation of the data from two acupressure band studies. A 12 min CD involving visualizing pleasant scenes and explaining the efficacy of the acupressure bands (25)	Handout thanked patients for participating in the study, and the CD did not discuss the efficacy of the bands (28)	Diary (yes)	Each day for 5 days following chemotherapy (combined)

(Continued)

TABLE 1 | Continued

References (intervention type)	Design	Sample (N, M age, %Male)	Treatment	Experimental group (n)	Control group (n)	Side-effect measure (main outcome)	Timing of measure
Schagen et al. (42) (Priming)	Quasi RCT 2 × 2 × 2	Patients with breast cancer (261, 53.7, 0)	Chemotherapy	Told that some patients treated with cytotoxic agents experience cognitive problems and the goal of the study was to obtain more insight into the relation between chemotherapy and cognitive problems' (130)	Received a neutral introduction (131)	SSQ (yes)	After study introduction
Schagen et al. (43) (Priming)	RCT 2 × 2	Patients with cancer (236, 48.4, 10.1)	Chemotherapy	Received the introduction that some patients treated with chemotherapy experience cognitive problems (116)	Received a neutral introduction (120)	Cognitive failure questionnaire (yes)	After study introduction
Shelke et al. (44) (De-emphasizing)	RCT	Patients undergoing chemotherapy (322, 57.6, 27)	Chemotherapy	Standard educational materials plus a handout explaining how effective ondansetron, would likely be in controlling nausea and vomiting (159)	Standard educational materials given to new patients (163)	SSQ (no)	Treatment day until four days after (combined)
Silvestri et al. (45) (Omitting)	RCT	Patients with newly diagnosed CVD (96, 52.0, 100)	Atenolol	1. Blinded to drug given (32) 2. Informed on drug given but not on the side-effects (32)	Informed on drug given and its side-effects on erectile function (32)	IIEF (yes)	After 3 months of treatment
Vasterling et al. (46) (Distraction)	RCT	Patients with cancer (60, 51, 35)	Chemotherapy	Played video games during chemotherapy treatment and told this would keep their minds off their treatment, making it less unpleasant and reducing the severity of its side effects (?)	Rested quietly in the treatment room before chemotherapy and told if a patient was relaxed, it would be less unpleasant, and the severity of the side-effects would be reduced (?)	SSQ (no)	After each of the 5 chemotherapy sessions (combined)
Wilhelm et al. (47) (De-emphasizing)	RCT	Healthy males (80, 24.5, 100)	Metoprolol	Informed of side-effects including headache, stomach pain or nausea. Dizziness is also mentioned, but is explained as a sign that the drug is starting to work and means that your body is responding to the beta-blocker particularly well (40)	Informed of side-effects including headache, stomach pain or nausea. Dizziness is also mentioned and explained as a potentially unpleasant, but already known side-effect of the drug (40)	Modified GASE (yes)	?
Wise et al. (48) (Omitting)	RCT	Patients with Asthma (237, 37, 23.8)	Montelukast	The computer presentation showed the same basic education but did not show positive messages about the expected benefits of montelukast and did not contain the television commercial. The capsules were off-white and referred to as montelukast (117)	Viewed a computer presentation for 10–20 min emphasizing the value and potency of the treatment including a television commercial for montelukast. The commercial also described potential side-effects. The capsules were 2-tone blue, and referred to as Singulair (120)	? (no)	After 2 and 4 weeks of treatment (combined)

RCT, randomized controlled trial; RCCT, randomized controlled crossover trial; ?, not reported; CVD, cardiovascular disease; IIEF, international index of erectile dysfunction; SSQ, study specific questionnaire; EORTC QLQ-30, European Organization for Research and Treatment of Cancer Quality of Life Questionnaire; GASE, generic assessment of side effects scale; KAE, knowledge, attitudes, and experiences questionnaire.

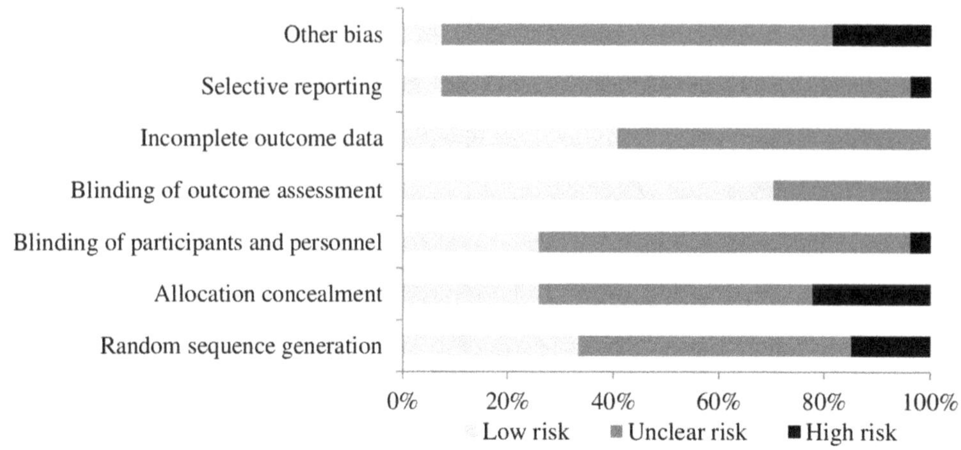

FIGURE 2 | Quality assessment across included studies.

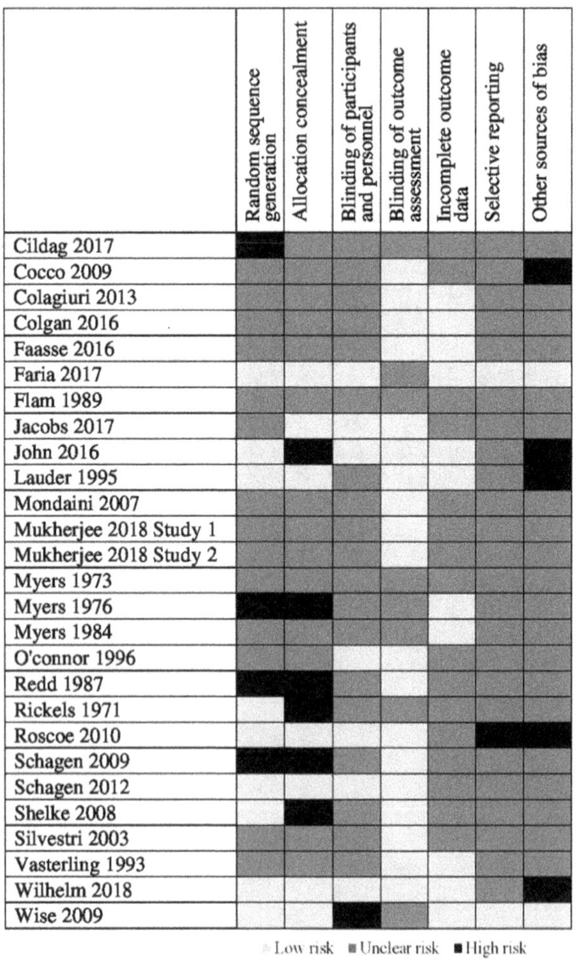

FIGURE 3 | Quality assessment between included studies.

Table 2). Colagiuri et al. (26) found a slight trend for priming patients by assessing their expectancies for side-effects vs. no assessment on subsequent nausea. Jacobs et al. (31) and Schagen et al. (42) found no indication of an effect of priming patients by mentioning that chemotherapy is associated with cognitive problems on retrospectively reported cognitive side-effects. However, Schagen et al. (43) in a similar study did find a small effect of priming leading to increased reporting of previous cognitive side-effects to chemotherapy compared to those in a control group who received no such information.

Distraction

Three studies looked at the effect of distraction on side-effect reporting following chemotherapy and drug provocation tests, showing some evidence that distraction can reduce side-effect reporting (see **Table 3**). Cildag et al. (24) found that keeping patients busy with filling/archiving files significantly reduced the occurrence of adverse reactions compared to a control group, but only by a small amount. Redd et al. (39) found that distracting pediatric cancer patients with video games significantly reduced chemotherapy nausea from baseline, compared to those in the control group. However, for adult cancer patients, Vasterling et al. (46) found that video games were not effective in reducing chemotherapy nausea or vomiting compared to a control group.

Branding

Two studies looked at the effect of branding on side-effect reporting to ibuprofen showing some evidence that branding can affect side-effect reporting (see **Table 4**). Colgan et al. (27) found that a video designed to correct participants' beliefs about generic medicines significantly reduced side effects for both branded and generic ibuprofen compared to those in a control group, showing a large effect. However, Faasse et al. (28) found that simply changing the labeling of ibuprofen from branded to generic did not significantly affect side-effect reporting.

Omitting Side-Effect Information

Eleven studies looked at the effect of omitting side-effect information on side-effect reporting to a range of different treatments, showing that omitting side-effects significantly decreases side-effect reporting (see **Table 5**). Eight studies

TABLE 2 | Priming intervention results.

References	Side-effect outcome and analysis	Results	Effect size (95% CI)	Evidence quality
Colagiuri et al. (26)	Occurrence: Multiple logistic regression	Nausea: Ns, priming group > control group, $p = 0.06$	OR = 3.19 (0.95, 10.69)	
		Fatigue, sadness, loss of appetite: Ns, lowest $p = 0.31$	–	
	Severity: Multiple linear regression	Nausea, fatigue, sadness, loss of appetite: Ns, lowest $p = 0.24$	–	
Jacobs et al. (31)	Frequency: 2 × 2 ANCOVA-group and chemotherapy experience as independent factors	Cognitive problems: Ns for those with chemotherapy experience	–	
Schagen et al. (42)	Severity: 2 × 2 × 2 ANOVA-group, pre-existing knowledge, and chemotherapy experience as independent factors	Cognitive problems: Ns, priming group (M = 2.53, SE = 0.11) < control group (M = 2.68, SE = 0.12) for those with chemotherapy experience, $p = 0.34$	d = −0.11 (−0.36, 0.13)	+ Very Low
		Other complaints: Ns, priming group (M = 3.00, SE = 0.09) > control group (M = 2.95, SE = 0.10) for those with chemotherapy experience, $p = 0.75$	d = 0.05 (−0.20, 0.29)	
Schagen et al. (43)	Severity: 2 × 2 ANOVA-group and chemotherapy experience as independent factors	Cognitive problems: Priming group (M = 21.20, SD = 6.4) > control group (M = 18.98, SD = 6.7) for those with chemotherapy experience, $p = 0.032$	d = 0.34 (0.08, 0.60)	

Ns, non-significant; M, mean; SE, standard error; SD, standard deviation; OR, odds ratio; d, Cohen's d; –, insufficient detail to calculate effect size.

TABLE 3 | Distraction intervention results.

References	Side-effect outcome and analysis	Results	Effect size (95% CI)	Evidence quality
Cildag et al. (24)	Occurrence: Chi square	Adverse reaction: Distraction group (7.9%) < control group (34.7%), $p = 0.0004$	OR = 0.16 (0.05, 0.48)	
Redd et al. (39)	Severity: Repeated measures ANOVA-group as an independent factor and time as a within-groups factor	Nausea: Distraction group (M decrease = −16.92, SD = 8.70), $p < 0.001$. Control group (M decrease = −1.77, SD = 8.96), $p > 0.05$	–	+ Very Low
Vasterling et al. (46)	Frequency: Univariate analysis	Vomiting: Ns	–	
	Severity: Univariate analysis	Nausea: Ns	–	

Ns, non-significant; M, mean; OR, odds ratio; –, insufficient detail to calculate effect size.

found that not informing patients about potential side-effects significantly decreased side-effect reporting to metropolol (25), a myelogram (30), antidepressants (32), finasteride (34), skin cream (23) (study 1 and 2), atenolol (45), and montekulast (48) compared to a control group which received side-effect information, each showing large effect sizes. Similarly Myers and Calvert (36) found a trend for a decrease in side-effect reporting when patients were not informed about the side-effects to the antidepressant dothiepin compared to a control group, and Myers and Calvert (37) found that side-effects significantly decreased to dothiepin when comparing the group that only received beneficial information to groups that received no information and side-effect information. Only one study, Myers and Calvert (35), found no effect of side-effect information on subsequent side-effect reporting.

De-emphasizing Side-Effects

Five studies looked at the effect of de-emphasisng side-effects on side-effect reporting to range of different treatments, showing evidence that this seems to have no effect (see **Table 6**). Three studies found that informing patients of side-effects but in a way that does not make them seem as bad had no effect on side-effect reporting to anesthesia (33), or chemotherapy (41, 44), however this was compared to a control group that did not receive any information about side-effects. O'Connor et al. (38) found that positively framing side-effects to emphasize those that remain side-effect free and comparing to a control group that received standard information about side-effects significantly reduced side-effect reporting to the flu vaccine. Wilhelm et al. (47) found that positively framing side-effects by explaining they are a sign that the drug is working did not significantly reduce side-effects to metoprolol compared to those who received standard information.

Other Interventions

Two other studies investigated interventions which do not fall into the above categories (see **Table 7**). Faria et al. (29) deceptively told seasonal affective disorder patients that they would receive an active placebo which would produce similar side-effects to escitalopram when in fact they received the active drug itself

TABLE 4 | Branding intervention results.

References	Side-effect outcome and analysis	Results	Effect size (95% CI)	Evidence quality
Colgan et al. (27)	Frequency: Linear mixed models	Side-effects across both types of ibuprofen: Generic medicines video group ($M = 1.18$, $SE = 0.40$) < control group ($M = 2.57$, $SE = 0.39$), $p = 0.02$	$d = -0.68$ (-1.17, -0.20)	
		Side-effects within each type of ibuprofen: Generic medicines video group < control group, for both branded, $p = 0.02$, and generic, $p = 0.035$	–	++ Low
Faasse et al. (28)	Severity: Linear mixed models	Side-effects: Ns, branded ($M = 3.41$, $SE = 0.47$) > generic ($M = 2.95$, $SE = 0.46$) ibuprofen, $p = 0.16$.	–	

Ns, non-significant; M, mean; SE, standard error; d, Cohen's d; –, insufficient detail to calculate effect size.

and found this showed a trend in decreasing reported side-effects compared to a control group who were correctly informed. Rickels et al. (40) found no effect of the prescribing psychiatrist being a drug "enthusiast" or drug "skeptical" on reported side-effects to tranquilisers among psychiatric patients.

DISCUSSION

Summary of Main Findings

Although previous literature has looked at altering side-effects generated in response to inert exposures, it is important to test if these interventions also work in the clinical setting and affect side-effects to real medications which may be initiated or exacerbated through a nocebo effect. This can then provide the basis for introducing into clinical practice strategies to reduce these side-effects. Unfortunately, the quality of the studies identified in this review were generally low quality mainly due to the lack of clear reporting, inadequate randomization and allocation procedures, and unpowered effects. Our overriding recommendation, therefore, is that additional, better quality work is needed in this field.

This point notwithstanding, from the results of the included studies, the strongest and most consistent effect in altering side-effects experienced following medical treatments was omitting information about side-effects. Other techniques, such as priming, distraction and altering the perceptions of branding produced mixed results. More tentatively, studies which investigated over the counter medications, common prescription medications, and vaccines seemed to be more susceptible to these interventions than those which studied chemotherapy.

The finding that omitting side-effect information produced the most consistent and strongest effect supports the evidence from the literature on inert exposures (10) which recommends that in order to reduce side-effects induced by nocebo effects we should avoid giving suggestions of side-effects associated with medications to patients. It also echoes what is found in experimental nocebo studies which find that altering information about side-effects alters side-effect experience to infrasound (49), and electrical pain stimuli (50). In addition, this supports previous work showing that interventions designed to change patients' expectations of pain by altering verbal suggestions about the pain to expect after a treatment or procedure can relieve (placebo) or increase (nocebo) patients baseline pain depending on the suggestion (15, 16), highlighting the role that expectations play in both placebo and nocebo effects. Perhaps unsurprisingly no study looked at the effect of omitting information about side-effects to chemotherapy, and therefore we cannot say if the results extend to chemotherapy too. However, as chemotherapy is already well-known for its side-effects, it may be that omitting side-effect information would do little to alter subsequent side-effect reporting in this group.

Not mentioning side-effects to patients in order to reduce these effects is ethically problematic and may not meet the requirements of informed consent, something which has been widely discussed in the literature (51, 52). An alternative approach is to explain the potential side-effects to patients in a way that de-emphasizes them and reduces their apparent likelihood or severity (53). At first look, the results of studies which have used this approach do not appear promising. Most studies have showed no effect of de-emphasizing side-effects on subsequent side-effect experience. However, this might be an artifact relating to the design of these studies, in which the groups that received the de-emphasized side-effect information were compared to a control groups that received no side-effect information at all. Explaining side-effects to patients, albeit in a positive light, is still likely to increase the perceived likelihood of side-effects compared to not describing side-effects. It would be interesting for future studies to test the effects of de-emphasizing side-effects of medication compared to a suitable control group which receives standard side-effect information. In other studies which used an appropriate control group, positive framing of side-effects was shown to be beneficial, a finding that has also been reproduced in healthy adults taking an inert tablet (54). There is also scope for further investigations about framing the side-effects of medication as a sign that the drug is working. This was investigated in a pilot study that, although not powered to find an effect, nonetheless showed a decrease in side-effect measures among participants who believed the medicine to be harmful (47). This idea of de-emphasizing side-effects has shown some promise in the placebo literature on pain, in which positive messages which focus more on the beneficial outcome of treatments rather than the potential side-effects may be more effective in relieving patients pain compared to usual care messages (14).

TABLE 5 | Omitting side-effect information intervention results.

References	Side-effect outcome and analysis	Results	Effect size (95% CI)	Evidence quality
Cocco (25)	Occurrence: Chi square	Erectile dysfunction: No side-effect information group (8%) < drug information group (13%) < control group (32%), $p < 0.01$	–	
Flam et al. (30)	Frequency: Independent t test	Side-effects: Procedural information group (M = 2.1) < control group (M = 4.3), $p < 0.05$	d = −0.94 (−1.86, −0.02)	
		Side-effects: No side-effect information group (M = 1.6) < control group (M = 4.3), $p < 0.05$	d = −1.23 (−2.19, −0.27)	
John et al. (32)	Frequency: Mann Whitney U	Side-effects: No side-effect information group (M = 1.7, SD = 1.9) < control group (M = 3.5, SD = 2.6), $p = 0.044$	d = −0.81 (−1.47, −0.15)	
Mondaini et al. (34)	Occurrence: Mann Whitney U	One or more side-effects: No side-effect information group (15.3%) < control group (43.6%), $p = 0.03$	OR = 0.23 (0.09, 0.59)	
		Erectile dysfunction: No side-effect information group (9.6%) < control group (30.9%), $p = 0.02$	OR = 0.24 (0.08, 0.70)	
		Decreased libido: No side-effect information group (7.7%) < control group (23.6%), $p = 0.04$	OR = 0.27 (0.08, 0.89)	
		Ejaculation disorders: Ns, No side-effect information group (5.7%) < control group (16.3%), $p = 0.06$	OR = 0.31 (0.08, 1.23)	
Mukherjee and Sahay (23) study 1	Severity: Two-way ANCOVA with group and price as independent factors	Skin dryness: No side-effect information group < control group, $p = 0.01$	$\eta p^2 = 0.05$	
		Skin dryness: Ns difference between pricing, $p > 0.70$	–	
		Skin dryness: Interaction between pricing and side-effect information, $p = 0.02$. No side-effect information group (M = 1.85, SD = 1.38) < control group (M = 3.39, SD = 1.98) at low price. Ns between no side-effect information group (M = 2.51, SD = 1.09) and control group (M = 2.72, SD = 1.51) at high price	$\eta p^2 = 0.04$	
Mukherjee and Sahay (23) study 2	Severity: Two-way ANCOVA with group and price as independent factors	Skin dryness: No side-effect information group < control group, $p = 0.01$	$\eta p^2 = 0.04$	+ Very Low
		Skin dryness: Ns difference between pricing, $p = 0.32$	–	
		Skin dryness: Ns interaction between pricing and side-effect information, $p = 0.19$	–	
Myers and Calvert (35)	Occurrence: Chi square	Side-effects: Ns, no side-effect information group (73.9%) < control group (80.9%), $p > 0.05$	OR = 0.67 (0.25, 1.79)	
Myers and Calvert (36)	Occurrence: Chi square	Side-effects: Ns, no side-effect information group (51.2%) < control group (71.7%) $p > 0.05$	OR = 0.41 (0.17, 1.00)	
Myers and Calvert (37)	Occurrence: ?	Side-effects at 3 weeks: Ns, no side-effect information group (67.7%), beneficial information group (48.4%), control group (73.7%), $p > 0.05$	–	
		Side-effects at 6 weeks: Ns, %), no side-effect information group (63.6%), beneficial information group (29.6), control group (57.1%), $p > 0.05$	–	
		Side-effects at 3 weeks: Beneficial information group (48.4%) < combined no side-effect information group and control group (70.5%), $p < 0.05$	OR = 0.39 (0.16, 0.96)	
		Side-effects at 6 weeks: Beneficial information group (29.6%) < combined no side-effect information group and control group (60.0%), $p < 0.05$	OR = 0.28 (0.10, 0.76)	
Silvestri et al. (45)	Occurrence: Chi square	Erectile dysfunction: Blind to drug group (3.1%) < drug information group (15.6%) < control group (31.2%), $p < 0.01$	–	
Wise et al. (48)	Occurrence: Logistic regression	Headaches: No side-effect information group (29%) < control group (37%), $p = 0.02$.	–	
		Lethargy, gastrointestinal distress, fever, rhinitis, cough, "flu," and skin rash: Ns	–	

Ns, non-significant; M, mean, SD, standard deviation; OR, odds ratio; d, Cohen's d; ηp^2, partial eta squared; –, insufficient detail to calculate effect size; ?, not reported.

TABLE 6 | De-emphasizing side-effects intervention results.

References	Side-effect outcome and analysis	Results	Effect size (95% CI)	Evidence quality
Lauder et al. (33)	Occurrence: Chi square	Vomiting: Ns, positive suggestion group (40.4%) < control group (46.9%), $p = 0.363$	OR = 0.77 (0.43, 1.36)	
		Nausea: Ns, positive suggestion group (63.4%) < control group (73.2%), $p = 0.148$	OR = 0.64 (0.34, 1.18)	
	Severity: Mann Whitney U	Nausea: Ns, positive suggestion group (M = 1.45, SD = 1.88) < control group (M = 1.80, SD = 1.89), $p = 0.087$	d = −0.19 (−0.50, 0.13)	
O'Connor et al. (38)	Occurrence: Chi square	Sore arm, weakness, fever: Ns	–	
		Myalgia: Positive frame group < control group, $p = 0.01$	–	
		Chills: Positive frame group < control group, $p = 0.003$	–	
Roscoe et al. (41)	Severity: Two-way ANCOVA with group and baseline expectancy as two independent factors	Average nausea: Ns, positive suggestion group (M = 1.94, SD = 1.07) < control group (M = 1.96, SD = 0.99), $p > 0.05$	d = −0.02 (−0.56, 0.52)	
		Peak nausea: Ns, positive suggestion group (M = 3.56, SD = 2.09) < control group (M = 3.57, SD = 1.88), $p > 0.05$	d = −0.01 (−0.54, 0.53)	+ Very Low
Shelke et al. (44)	Occurrence: Chi square	Nausea: Ns, positive suggestion group (79%) > control group (73%), $p = 0.19$	OR = 1.41 (0.84, 2.37)	
	Severity: Independent t test	Nausea: Ns, positive suggestion group (M = 1.86, SE = 0.76) > control group (M = 1.76, SE = 0.76), $p = 0.34$	d = 0.01 (−0.21, 0.23)	
Wilhelm et al. (47)	Frequency: Independent t test	Specific side-effects: Ns, positive suggestion group (M = 1.38, SD = 1.56) < control group (M = 1.75, SD = 1.77), $p = 0.318$	d = −0.22 (−0.66, 0.22)	
		Nonspecific side-effects: Ns, positive suggestion group (M = 0.68, SD = 1.02) < control group (M = 1.15, SD = 1.93), $p = 0.174$	d = −0.30 (−0.75, 0.14)	
	Severity: Independent t test	Specific side-effects: Ns, positive suggestion group (M = 1.60, SD = 2.00) < control group (M = 1.85, SD = 2.02), $p = 0.580$	d = −0.12 (−0.56, 0.31)	
		Nonspecific side-effects: Ns, positive suggestion group (M = 0.83, SD = 1.60) < control group (M = 1.30, SD = 3.12), $p = 0.396$	d = −0.20 (−0.63, 0.25)	

Ns, non-significant; M, mean; SE, standard error; SD, standard deviation; OR, odds ratio; d, Cohen's d; –, insufficient detail to calculate effect size.

TABLE 7 | Miscellaneous results.

References	Side-effect outcome and analysis	Results	Effect size (95% CI)	Evidence quality
Rickels et al. (40)	Occurrence: ?	Side-effects: Ns	–	+ Very Low
Faria et al. (29)	Frequency: Independent t test	All side-effects: Ns, $p = 0.17$	–	+ + +Moderate
		Drug related side-effects: Ns, covert group (M = 2.22, SD = 1.38) < control group (M = 3.39, SD = 2.62), $p = 0.06$	d = −0.55 (−1.14, 0.04)	

Ns, non-significant; M, mean; SD, standard deviation; d, Cohen's d; –, insufficient detail to calculate effect size; ?, not reported.

Priming patients by informing them about the side-effects to chemotherapy and then asking them to recall side-effects, or by asking about their expectations of chemotherapy side-effects overall showed little impact on side-effect reporting. This may be due to the treatment under investigation. Chemotherapy is a high-profile treatment, and as such it is likely patients are already aware of the side-effects that accompany it, limiting the effect that priming could have. In experimental studies, priming patients using pain-related fear has been shown to increase sensitivity to heat stimuli (55). It may be that priming patients about side-effects to lower profile drugs find more promising effects.

Distraction techniques have been shown to be effective in the field of pain research for example experimental and needle-related pain (56, 57), but in terms of medication side-effects, the evidence base is not as large, limiting conclusions. From the results, it seems that distraction tasks should be relevant to the patients to have the greatest chance of being effective. For example, while video games are suitable for reducing side-effects to chemotherapy in pediatric patients they are less effective in adults (39, 46).

The effect of branding on side-effects shows some effect, something also reflected in the inert literature (58). However given the early evidence base, future studies are needed to test the effects of branding on prescribed drugs, and interventions to alter patients' perceptions of prescribed generic drugs.

Quality of Original Research

It is possible that some of our conclusions may be due to differences in quality between those studies that found an effect and those that did not. We did not observe any clear trend for lower quality studies to report more or fewer significant results than higher quality studies. However, overall the quality of the studies included in this review was limited due to poor reporting of key issues in experimental research, such as randomization, allocation concealment, blinding, and not registering a study protocol prior to initiating recruitment. In addition, the quality of evidence from these studies was low, partially due to these risk of bias issues, but also the fact that the samples sizes of studies were relatively small, adding to evidence of imprecision and indirectness due to the wide confidence intervals, and sometimes contradictory findings.

Quality of This Review

Search strategies for systematic reviews based on nocebo effects are difficult to balance in terms of their specificity and sensitivity (10). In this instance we deliberately opted for a broad search strategy in order to identify as many relevant studies as possible. Due to time constraints, screening, data extraction and quality assessment were done by primarily one author. However, there were regular weekly meetings with both authors to discuss screening, data extraction, quality assessment and writing up of the results, allowing us to resolve any issues as they arose.

Other limitations of the review reflect the way we grouped the results. We aggregated studies based on the type of intervention under investigation. These groupings contained different side-effect outcomes, treatments and participants. It is possible that interactions exist between these variables and the interventions under investigation. Unfortunately, due to the small number of studies investigating each intervention, we did not have enough data to explore this in any depth. However, it does appear that chemotherapy might not be as susceptible to brief psychological interventions compared to prescription and over-the-counter drugs.

Implications and Future Directions

Not mentioning potential side-effects to patients has the most consistent effect in reducing side-effects to medical treatments, especially for over-the-counter and prescription drugs. Whether this meets ethical or regulatory requirements is debatable, however (53, 59). De-emphasizing side-effects through positive framing has potential and could be introduced within doctor-patient consultations and in accompanying patient information leaflets for patients to read at home. Further testing of this method especially in terms of reframing side-effects as signs that the drug is working is needed in an adequately powered trial. In addition, it is important for future studies testing ways of de-emphasizing side-effects to adequately compare them to a control group that receives the standard side-effect information.

Besides framing, it is also important for doctors to consider patients beliefs about generic medicines if prescribing generic drugs or switching patients from a previously branded medication to a generic. Colgan et al. (27) suggest that a simple explanation of how the pharmacological ingredients in generic drugs do not actually differ with branded drugs would be useful. So far, the effects of branding have been studied in over the counter and inert tablets: research with prescribed medication is now needed. In addition, distraction could be beneficial for use if age appropriate tasks are used.

Finally, only one study investigated the effect of doctor characteristics on side-effects. This represents a surprising gap in the literature. Doctor characteristics, such as empathy have been shown to be important in benefitting patients for a range of clinical conditions, especially pain (60). We believe this is an important avenue for future research to investigate in terms of benefitting patients by reducing medication side-effects.

CONCLUSION

This review was restricted by the quality and heterogeneity of the included studies, limiting the conclusions that can be drawn. It does however, provide an indication of which brief psychological interventions are effective in reducing side-effects to active medical treatment. The clearest effect was from omitting information about side-effects to participants before exposure. Although withholding side-effect information would be one way to reduce this, it is ethically and legally problematic. Current work is looking at how we can effectively de-emphasize side-effects while still giving patients the information needed for informed consent, and this shows promise. Potential strategies include positively framing the risk of side-effects, focusing more on the benefits of the drug, and framing side-effects in terms of signs that the drug is working. However further research is needed in larger trials with suitable control groups. There is also a gap for future research to consider doctor characteristics, such as empathy, as a means of reducing patients' experience of side-effects. Finally, better reporting of studies is essential in future, allowing for more concrete determinations of study quality.

AUTHOR CONTRIBUTIONS

RKW and GJR developed the initial research question for the systematic review and the search strategy. RKW carried out the search, screening, data extraction and quality assessment with regular input from GJR. RKW wrote the first draft which was subsequently revised by GJR.

FUNDING

RKW and GJR are affiliated to the National Institute for Health Research Health Protection Research Unit (NIHR HPRU) in Emergency Preparedness and Response at King's College London in partnership with Public Health England (PHE), in collaboration with the University of East Anglia and Newcastle University. The views expressed are those of the authors and not necessarily those of the NHS, the NIHR, the Department of Health or Public Health England.

REFERENCES

1. Kennedy WP. The nocebo reaction. Medicina experimentalis. *Int J Clin Exp Med.* (1961) 95:203–5.
2. Kaptchuk TJ. Powerful placebo: the dark side of the randomised controlled trial. *Lancet* (1998) 351:1722–5. doi: 10.1016/s0140-6736(97)10111-8
3. Mahr A, Golmard C, Pham E, Iordache L, Deville L, Faure P. Types, frequencies, and burden of nonspecific adverse events of drugs: analysis of randomized placebo-controlled clinical trials. *Pharmacoepidemiol. Drug Saf.* (2017) 26:731–41. doi: 10.1002/pds.4169
4. Ammassari A, Murri R, Pezzotti P, Trotta MP, Ravasio L, De Longis P, et al. Self-reported symptoms and medication side effects influence adherence to highly active antiretroviral therapy in persons with HIV infection. *J Acquir Immune Defic Syndr.* (2001) 28:445–9. doi: 10.1097/00042560-200112150-00006
5. Horne R, Chapman SCE, Parham R, Freemantle N, Forbes A, Cooper V. Understanding patients' adherence-related beliefs about medicines prescribed for long-term conditions: a meta-analytic review of the necessity-concerns framework. *PLoS ONE* (2013) 8:e80633. doi: 10.1371/journal.pone.0080633
6. Kardas P, Lewek P, Matyjaszczyk M. Determinants of patient adherence: a review of systematic reviews. *Front Pharmacol.* (2013) 4:91. doi: 10.3389/fphar.2013.00091
7. Horton R. Offline: lessons from the controversy over statins. *Lancet* (2016) 388:1040. doi: 10.1016/S0140-6736(16)31583-5
8. Pedro-Botet J, Rubies-Prat J. Statin-associated muscle symptoms: beware of the nocebo effect. *Lancet* (2017) 389:2445–6. doi: 10.1016/s0140-6736(17)31163-7
9. National Institute For Health and Clinical Excellence. (2009). *Medicines Adherence: Involving Patients in Decisions About Prescribed Medicines and Supporting Adherence.* Available online at: http://www.nice.org.uk/guidance/cg76/resources/guidance-medicines-adherence-pdf
10. Webster RK, Weinman J, Rubin GJ. A systematic review of factors that contribute to nocebo effects. *Health Psychol.* (2016) 35:1334–55. doi: 10.1037/hea0000416
11. Klinger R, Soost S, Flor H, Worm M. Classical conditioning and expectancy in placebo hypoalgesia: a randomized controlled study in patients with atopic dermatitis and persons with healthy skin. *Pain* (2007) 128:31–9. doi: 10.1016/j.pain.2006.08.025
12. Varelmann D, Pancaro C, Cappiello EC, Camann WR. Nocebo-induced hyperalgesia during local anesthetic injection. *Anesth Analg.* (2010) 110:868–70. doi: 10.1213/ANE.0b013e3181cc5727
13. Benedetti F, Maggi G, Lopiano L, Lanotte M, Rainero I, Vighetti S, et al. Open versus hidden medical treatments: the patient's knowledge about a therapy affects the therapy outcome. *Prev. Treat.* (2003) 6:1a. doi: 10.1037/1522-3736.6.1.61a
14. Howick J, Lewith G, Mebius A, Fanshawe TR, Bishop F, van Osch M, et al. Positive messages may reduce patient pain: a meta-analysis. *Eur J Integr Med.* (2017) 11:31–8. doi: 10.1016/j.eujim.2017.03.005
15. Mistiaen P, van Osch M, van Vliet L, Howick J, Bishop FL, Di Blasi Z, et al. The effect of patient-practitioner communication on pain: a systematic review. *Eur J Pain* (2016) 20:675–88. doi: 10.1002/ejp.797
16. Peerdeman KJ, van Laarhoven AIM, Keij SM, Vase L, Rovers MM, Peters ML, et al. Relieving patients' pain with expectation interventions: a meta-analysis. *Pain* (2016) 157:1179–91. doi: 10.1097/j.pain.0000000000000540
17. Moher D, Liberati A, Tetzlaff J, Altman DG. Preferred reporting items for systematic reviews and meta-analyses: the PRISMA statement. *PLoS Med.* (2009) 6:97. doi: 10.1371/journal.pmed.1000097
18. Robinson KA, Dickersin K. Development of a highly sensitive search strategy for the retrieval of reports of controlled trials using PubMed. *Int J Epidemiol.* (2002) 31:150–3. doi: 10.1093/ije/31.1.150
19. NICE. (2018). *Glossary.* Retrieved from: https://www.nice.org.uk/Glossaryletter=S
20. Higgins JPT, Altman DG, Gotzsche PC, Juni P, Moher D, Oxman AD, et al. The Cochrane Collaboration's tool for assessing risk of bias in randomised trials. *BMJ* (2011) 343:d5928. doi: 10.1136/bmj.d5928
21. Popay J, Roberts H, Sowden A, Petticrew M, Arai L, Britten N, et al. *Guidance on the Conduct of Narrative Synthesis in Systematic Reviews: Final Report* (2006). Retrieved from Swindon.
22. Grade Working Group. Grading quality of evidence and strength of recommendations. *BMJ* (2004) 328:1490. doi: 10.1136/bmj.328.7454.1490
23. Mukherjee S, Sahay A. Nocebo effects from negative product information: when information hurts, paying money could heal. *J. Cons. Market.* (2018) 35:32–9. doi: 10.1108/JCM-11-2015-1609
24. Cildag S, Senturk T, Sargin G. The effects of distraction on symptoms during drug provocation test. *Clujul Medical* (2017) 90:18–21. doi: 10.15386/cjmed-688
25. Cocco G. Erectile dysfunction after therapy with metoprolol: the Hawthorne effect. *Cardiology* (2009) 112:174–7. doi: 10.1159/000147951
26. Colagiuri B, Dhillon H, Butow PN, Jansen J, Cox K, Jacquet J. Does assessing patients' expectancies about chemotherapy side effects influence their occurrence? *J Pain Symptom Manage.* (2013) 46:275–81. doi: 10.1016/j.jpainsymman.2012.07.013
27. Colgan SL, Faasse K, Pereira JA, Grey A, Petrie KJ. Changing perceptions and efficacy of generic medicines: an intervention study. *Health Psychol.* (2016) 35:1246–53. doi: 10.1037/hea0000402
28. Faasse K, Martin LR, Grey A, Gamble G, Petrie KJ. Impact of brand or generic labeling on medication effectiveness and side effects. *Health Psychol.* (2016) 35:187–90. doi: 10.1037/hea0000282
29. Faria V, Gingnell M, Hoppe JM, Hjorth O, Alaie I, Frick A, et al. Do you believe it? Verbal suggestions influence the clinical and neural effects of escitalopram in social anxiety disorder: a randomized trial. *EBio Med.* (2017) 24:179–88. doi: 10.1016/j.ebiom.2017.09.031
30. Flam B, Spice-Cherry P, Amsel R. Effects of preparatory information of a myelogram on patients' expectations and anxiety levels. *Patient Educ Couns.* (1989) 14:115–26. doi: 10.1016/0738-3991(89)90047-5
31. Jacobs W, Das E, Schagen SB. Increased cognitive problem reporting after information about chemotherapy-induced cognitive decline: the moderating role of stigma consciousness. *Psychol Health* (2017) 32:78–93. doi: 10.1080/08870446.2016.1244535
32. John AP, Singh NM, Nagarajaiah, Andrade C. Impact of an educational module in antidepressant-naive patients prescribed antidepressants for depression: pilot, proof-of-concept, randomized controlled trial. *Indian J. Psychiatry* (2016) 58:425–31. doi: 10.4103/0019-5545.196710
33. Lauder GR, McQuillan PJ, Pickering RM. Psychological adjunct to perioperative antiemesis. *Br J Anaesth.* (1995) 74:266–70. doi: 10.1093/bja/74.3.266
34. Mondaini N, Gontero P, Giubilei G, Lombardi G, Cai T, Gavazzi A, et al. Finasteride 5 mg and sexual side effects: How many of these are related to a nocebo phenomenon? *J Sex Med.* (2007) 4:1708–12. doi: 10.1111/j.1743-6109.2007.00563.x
35. Myers ED, Calvert EJ. The effect of forewarning on the occurrence of side-effects and discontinuance of medication in patients on amitriptyline. *Br J Psychiatry* (1973) 122:461–4. doi: 10.1192/bjp.122.4.461
36. Myers ED, Calvert EJ. The effect of forewarning on the occurrence of side-effects and discontinuance of medication in patients on dothiepin. *J Int Med Res.* (1976) 4:237–40. doi: 10.1177/030006057600400405
37. Myers ED, Calvert EJ. Information, compliance and side-effects: a study of patients on antidepressant medication. *Br J Clin Pharmacol.* (1984) 17:21–5. doi: 10.1111/j.1365-2125.1984.tb04993.x
38. O'Connor AM, Pennie RA, Dales RE. Framing effects on expectations, decisions, and side effects experienced: the case of influenza immunization. *J Clin Epidemiol.* (1996) 49:1271–6. doi: 10.1016/S0895-4356(96)00177-1
39. Redd WH, Jacobsen PB, Die-Trill M, Dermatis H, McEvoy M, Holland JC. Cognitive/attentional distraction in the control of conditioned nausea in pediatric cancer patients receiving chemotherapy. *J Consult Clin Psychol.* (1987) 55:391–5. doi: 10.1037/0022-006X.55.3.391
40. Rickels K, Lipman RS, Park LC, Covi L, Uhlenhuth EH, Mock JE. Drug, doctor warmth, and clinic setting in the symptomatic response to minor tranquilizers. *Psychopharmacologia* (1971) 20:128–52. doi: 10.1007/BF00404367
41. Roscoe JA, O'Neill M, Jean-Pierre P, Heckler CE, Kaptchuk TJ, Bushunow P, et al. An exploratory study on the effects of an expectancy manipulation

on chemotherapy-related nausea. *J Pain Symptom Manage.* (2010) 40:379–90. doi: 10.1016/j.jpainsymman.2009.12.024

42. Schagen SB, Das E, van Dam FSAM. The influence of priming and pre-existing knowledge of chemotherapy-associated cognitive complaints on the reporting of such complaints in breast cancer patients. *Psychooncology* (2009) 18:674–8. doi: 10.1002/pon.1454
43. Schagen SB, Das E, Vermeulen I. Information about chemotherapy-associated cognitive problems contributes to cognitive problems in cancer patients. *Psychooncology* (2012) 21:1132–5. doi: 10.1002/pon.2011
44. Shelke AR, Roscoe JA, Morrow GR, Colman LK, Banerjee TK, Kirshner JJ. Effect of a nausea expectancy manipulation on chemotherapy-induced nausea: a university of Rochester cancer center community clinical oncology program study. *J Pain Symptom Manage.* (2008) 35:381–7. doi: 10.1016/j.jpainsymman.2007.05.008
45. Silvestri A, Galetta P, Cerquetani E, Marazzi G, Patrizi R, Fini M, et al. Report of erectile dysfunction after therapy with beta-blockers is related to patient knowledge of side effects and is reversed by placebo. *Eur Heart J.* (2003) 24:1928–32. doi: 10.1016/j.ehj.2003.08.016
46. Vasterling J, Jenkins RA, Tope DM, Burish TG. Cognitive distraction and relaxation training for the control of side-effects due to cancer-chemotherapy. *J Behav Med.* (1993) 16:65–80. doi: 10.1007/bf00844755
47. Wilhelm M, Rief W, Doering BK. Decreasing the burden of side effects through positive message framing: an experimental proof-of-concept study. *Int J Behav Med.* (2018) 25:381–9. doi: 10.1007/s12529-018-9726-z
48. Wise RA, Bartlett SJ, Brown ED, Castro M, Cohen R, Holbrook JT, et al. Randomized trial of the effect of drug presentation on asthma outcomes: the American Lung Association Asthma Clinical Research Centers. *J Allergy Clin Immunol.* (2009) 124:436–44, 444e431–8. doi: 10.1016/j.jaci.2009.05.041
49. Crichton F, Dodd G, Schmid G, Gamble G, Cundy T, Petrie KJ. The power of positive and negative expectations to influence reported symptoms and mood during exposure to wind farm sound. *Health Psychol.* (2014) 33:1588–92. doi: 10.1037/hea0000037
50. Laarhoven AI, Vogelaar ML, Wilder-Smith OH, Riel PL, Kerkhof PC, Kraaimaat FW, et al. Induction of nocebo and placebo effects on itch and pain by verbal suggestions. *Pain* (2011) 152:1486–94. doi: 10.1016/j.pain.2011.01.043
51. Colloca L. Tell me the truth and I will not be harmed: informed consents and nocebo effects. *Am J Bioeth.* (2017) 17:46–8. doi: 10.1080/15265161.2017.1314057
52. Wells RE, Kaptchuk TJ. To tell the truth, the whole truth, may do patients harm: the problem of the nocebo effect for informed consent. *Am J Bioeth.* (2012) 12:22–9. doi: 10.1080/15265161.2011.652798
53. Webster RK, Weinman J, Rubin GJ. Explaining all without causing unnecessary harm: is there scope for positively framing medical risk information? *Patient Educ Couns.* (2018). doi: 10.1016/j.pec.2018.09.014. [Epub ahead of print].
54. Webster RK, Weinman J, Rubin GJ. Positively framed risk information in patient information leaflets reduces side effect reporting: a double-blind randomized controlled trial. *Ann Behav Med.* (2018) 52:kax064. doi: 10.1093/abm/kax064
55. Kirwilliam SS, Derbyshire SWG. Increased bias to report heat or pain following emotional priming of pain-related fear. *Pain* (2008) 137:60–5. doi: 10.1016/j.pain.2007.08.012
56. DeMore M, Cohen LL. Distraction for pediatric immunization pain: a critical review. *J Clin Psychol Med Settings* (2005) 12:281–91. doi: 10.1007/s10880-005-7813-1
57. Malloy KM, Milling LS. The effectiveness of virtual reality distraction for pain reduction: a systematic review. *Clin Psychol Rev.* (2010) 30:1011–8. doi: 10.1016/j.cpr.2010.07.001
58. Faasse K, Cundy T, Gamble G, Petrie KJ. The effect of an apparent change to a branded or generic medication on drug effectiveness and side effects. *Psychosom Med.* (2013) 75:90–6. doi: 10.1097/PSY.0b013e3182738826
59. Dyer C. Doctors should not cherry pick what information to give patients, court rules. *Br Med J.* (2015) 350. doi: 10.1136/bmj.h1414
60. Howick J, Moscrop A, Mebius A, Fanshawe TR, Lewith G, Bishop FL, et al. Effects of empathic and positive communication in healthcare consultations: a systematic review and meta-analysis. *J R Soc Med.* (2018) 111:240–52. doi: 10.1177/0141076818769477

7

Psychotherapy and Placebos: Manifesto for Conceptual Clarity

Charlotte R. Blease [1,2*]

[1] Program in Placebo Studies, Beth Israel Deaconess Medical Center, Harvard Medical School, Boston, MA, United States,
[2] School of Psychology, University College Dublin, Dublin, Ireland

Keywords: psychotherapy, placebo, placebo effect, common factors across psychotherapies, philosophical psychology, thomas kuhn, placebo studies, placebo research

***Correspondence:**
Charlotte R. Blease
cblease@bidmc.harvard.edu

For nearly as long as the term has existed "placebo" has been a source of debate and disagreement. Scientists and philosophers have been active contributors to the protracted dialog about how best to define the term leading one prominent health researcher to argue that there appears to be "currently no widely accepted definition of placebo" (1). Meanwhile, new theoretical models aimed at resolving conceptual quagmires—once and for all [e.g., (1, 2)]—often seem to confound rather than crack the problem by inviting further questions (3, 4). If discussion about how to conceive placebo terminology seems to "rage" within the sphere of biomedicine (1) when it comes to the domain of psychotherapy conceptual entanglements appear even more complicated. Here the to-and-fro of debate has spanned the decades though been episodic rather than ongoing [e.g., (5–7)] and lately the debate has re-emerged [see: (8–11)]. Reviewing the recent contributions to this discussion, I argue that are indeed stable definitions for the terms *placebo* and *placebo effect* within the science of placebo studies. Furthermore, I argue that it is justified to use these definitions as a starting point for appraising conceptual disagreement, including the (apparently) contentious translation of these terms to psychotherapy. Exploring two provocative yet divergent claims about the relationship between placebo and psychological treatments (9, 10) I conclude that disagreement arises when researchers employ definitions of placebo that are disengaged from implicit scientific usage.

Discussion about conceptual or definitional matters in science may appear to be esoterica, however definitions are important. How we understand placebo concepts carries subtle but significant methodological significant methodological implications for clinical trials as well as for ethical practice in the delivery of care (4, 12, 13). Therefore, gaining clarity about the argumentation within disputes over concepts is not trivial—rather, it might even be viewed as a major priority for the field of placebo research.

In this *Mini Review* I focus on two of the most prominent recent claims about the relationship between placebo concepts and psychotherapy proposed by leading scholars (9–11). I argue that appearances to the contrary, the resultant conceptual quagmire is avoidable, and suggest how and why definitions of placebo and placebo effects have become muddled within the context of psychotherapy. However, to highlight why disagreement arises it is imperative to identify unambiguous definitions for the terms "placebo" and "placebo effect." Fortunately, in this regard, the insights of philosopher of science Thomas Kuhn are instructive (14).

KUHN'S INSIGHTS

In the mid-Twentieth Century Thomas Kuhn helped to re-orientate philosophy of science by arguing that philosophers should move away from *a priori* formulations about the nature of science and pay closer attention to how scientists in fact reason and evaluate theories (15). One of Kuhn's most important (and least controversial) legacies) is his claim that for empirical progress to arise in a given field of enquiry there must be discernible underlying conceptual stability (15). Following

Kuhn and other post-positivist philosophers I argue that the most effective way to clarify conceptual issues is not to start from the philosophical armchair but to ask: How do established scientists *in fact* use these terms? (14).

If we assume that the field of placebo studies has emerged as an established field of science it is a small step to infer—despite the buzz of debate—that key definitions must be relatively settled in order to support the systematic growth of empirical knowledge. In a recent paper I argued that supposedly contested terminology is relatively settled in scientific placebo research (14).

However, before we address the question about what scientific usage reveals about core definitions, it is important to foreground the discussion by flagging up two important points. To begin, scientific concepts of placebo and placebo effect should be differentiated from those meanings ascribed to the terms in other non-expert domains including among medical practitioners, clinical investigators, patients, and research participants. Here I assume that even individuals who use placebos (e.g., in clinical trials, or as prescribing physicians) may not be experts in about how best to define these terms. Indeed, sociological research has demonstrated that both physicians and patients interpret "placebo" and "placebo effect" in myriad ways [see: (16, 17)]. How these non-experts define this terminology is important but not the present concern of this paper which is to inquire how these terms *ought* to be used.

Next, is a residual and paradoxical question: if there *is* conceptual consensus within the scientific placebo community about placebos and placebo effects why, then, is there so much debate about how to define the terms? I suggest three reasons. First, and perhaps most importantly the term "placebo" has been in use for centuries and is embedded within common lay as well as medical usage, further obstructing the possibility of clear and unambiguous meaning change. Second, even if we agree that scientific research into placebo effects is burgeoning—as a field of enquiry it has emerged only recently (14, 18). Therefore, we might still expect to observe a residual hangover of conceptual disputes regardless of whether such disagreement is substantive. Third, and related, even within scientific contexts, conceptual stability can be typified by implicit understanding rather than articulable, explicit definitions among many scientists who, as Kuhn observed, may be "little better than laymen at characterizing the established bases of their field, its legitimate problems and methods" [(15), p. 44].

Despite these challenges, I argue that we can discern conceptual stability over key definitions within the emergent science of placebo studies (14). I suggest that within the empirical research field, "*placebo effects* are understood to be positive health changes that occur as a result of specific psychobiological mechanisms . . . These psychobiological mechanisms are elicited, in turn, by a range of cues in the context of the practitioner-patient encounter" (14). Placebo effects, therefore, can be broadly understood as a natural kind of psychobiological phenomenon.

The term placebo is more nuanced. When it comes to placebo-randomized controlled trials (RCTs) the placebo allocation should ideally be identical to the verum intervention (the treatment under evaluation) in all respects except for its hypothesized remedial factor(s), and patient allocations should be randomized and double-blinded. The function of placebos in RCTs is to act as controls for the experimental "noise" that arises within clinical trials: this includes: regression to the mean, natural progression of an illness, patient or physician/investigator reporting biases, Hawthorne Effects, *as well as* placebo effects. Placebos in RCTs should therefore be conceived as a moving target: an instrument that is designed to mimic the appearance of a verum intervention (14). This means that the appearance and administration of the placebo control should always be dependent on the treatment under scrutiny rather than simply being reified as a particular kind of thing (e.g., "placebos are sugar pills"). Indeed, it would be less misleading to label placebos in RCTs as "control interventions" (4, 14). Placebo researchers also differentiate between *placebo effects* and *placebo responses* (12): the latter comprise the aggregate responses of receiving a placebo in an RCT—the factors associated with so-called "experimental noise" which, as noted, may or may not include placebo effects.

When it comes to the scientific community's definitions of placebos in clinical contexts, things get trickier. However, one place to glean insight is so-called *open-label placebo* experiments. Here the following script has been provided to patient participants in experimental set ups: "placebo pills are made of an inert substance, like sugar pills...have been shown in clinical studies to produce significant improvement in IBS symptoms through mind-body self-healing processes" [(19); see also: (20)]. In these scenarios, there are two implied definitions of placebo: (i) treatments theorized not to be effective for a condition or symptoms by virtue of their intrinsic properties; and secondly, the added notion that (ii) placebos—as described in (i)—*may be* causally implicated in the elicitation of placebo effects: here it is implied that placebos play a role as causal antecedents of psychobiological pathways which, when combined with other proximal conditions and factors in the context of health care (such as practitioner empathy, warmth, and confidence) cause placebo effect(s) (21). With these delineations in mind, I appraise two recently published, divergent analyses of the relationship between placebos and psychotherapy proposed by prominent scholars.

"ALIGNING PLACEBOS AND PLACEBO EFFECTS WITH PSYCHOTHERAPY IS INCOHERENT"

The first claim owed to Kirsch, Wampold and Kelley is that deployment of this terminology within psychotherapy leads to a form of *reductio ad absurdum* (10). The authors argue: "In the context of medical treatment, placebo effects are relatively easy to define. They are the effects produced by factors other than the physical properties of the treatment" [(10), p. 123]. However, in psychological contexts, the authors contend, "Here is the central problem: The effect of psychotherapy is—by definition of the term *psychotherapy*—produced by something other than the physical properties of the treatment. Therefore, if we adhere to the received implicit definition of *placebo* as it has been used in the context of medicine, the effects of psychotherapy are ispo facto placebo effects and psychotherapy is ipso facto a placebo" [(10), p. 123].

First, Kirsch, Wampold and Kelley claim that we can rely on, "the received implicit definition of how placebo has been used in the context of medicine" [(10), p. 123]. Yet, as argued, implicit and explicit conceptualizations of placebos among *non-experts* are unhelpful precisely because the term has been deployed in myriad inconsistent and sometimes confusing ways [e.g., (17)]. To draw on another example, consider "folk biology" which encompasses among other intuitions, in-built ideas about how to classify species (22): this intuitive classification scheme does not provide a foolproof scientific foundation for how species are (in fact) related to one another. Mixing both classification systems would undermine scientific enquiry. Rather, to avoid conceptual quagmires, definitions of placebo must be anchored to how these terms are standardly, even if implicitly, deployed by experts working in the scientific placebo research community.

Second, the authors suggest that *all non-physical responses* to treatments should be conceived as placebo effects. This is incorrect: just because responses are non-physical—i.e., occurring at a *psychological* level—does not mean they are *de facto* placebo effects. This line of reasoning implies that every non-physical effect of a treatment is a placebo effect. Indeed, the logical extension of this argument is there can be no psychological responses *other than* placebo effects in psychotherapy: yet to suggest that the rich variety of psychological events elicited in psychotherapy simply amount to placebo effects is improbable (23). Correlatively, as scientific research in placebo studies has shown, not all *non-physical* responses to placebos are accurately described as *placebo effects*. We might surmise, in this instance, that Kirsch et al. confuse *placebo responses* with *placebo effects.*

Third, and finally, Kirsch, Wampold and Kelley argue, "[I]n evaluating the efficacy of psychotherapy, the placebo effect cannot and *should not be controlled*" [(10), p. 212]. From the premise that psychological responses *just are* equatable with placebo effects they infer the strong conclusion that it is *unjustified* to undertake placebo-RCTs of psychological treatments. This is unwarranted. From the definition of placebos as control interventions only the weaker claim is supported: *in principle* it is possible to design psychotherapy RCTs but *in practice*, the task is fraught with multiple serious challenges.

Indeed, one such problem is the double-blinding requirement (whereby neither therapist nor participant are aware about whether the individual has been allocated to placebo or the intervention under scrutiny). Another problem, which the authors highlight, is the need to control for so-called "common factors" in the delivery of psychotherapy. Here we must pause to consider what the term *common factors* means and how it should be distinguished from *specific treatment factors* in psychotherapy research.

Specific treatment factors vary according to different psychotherapy modalities and theories. So, for example, specific techniques in cognitive behavioral therapy (CBT) involve identifying hypothesized "cognitive distortions" or "maladaptive thoughts" which, according to CBT theorists and practitioners, are believed to have negative effects on behavior (24, 25). Here the goal of specific treatment techniques is to redress "faulty thinking" by promoting "cognitive restructuring" which, proponents of CBT theorize, will thereby elicit more psychologically constructive thoughts and behaviors (24, 25). Similarly, in psychodynamic psychotherapies and humanistic therapies distinctive kinds of specific techniques are theorized. *Common factors* on the other hand—and as the name suggests—refers to those features of treatment that appear to be shared across different psychological interventions. These include verbal and non-verbal therapist factors (e.g. empathy, positive regard); patient factors (e.g. confidence in the therapist); and factors associated with a strong working alliance between patient and psychotherapist.

To the extent that Kirsch et al. argue that controlling for common factors poses a serious obstacle to placebo-controlled clinical trials in psychotherapy we can agree with them. Nonetheless, conceivably this hindrance may yet be overcome. In the future, technological innovations may render it possible to delivery psychological treatments using avatars in the future: in such a scenario, we might hypothesize that the regulation and control of common factors would become practicable within psychotherapy-RCTs.

"PSYCHOTHERAPY IS A PLACEBO"

Gaab et al. (9) and Trachsel and Gaab (11) present a very different interpretation of the relationship between placebo and psychotherapy. Their proposition is that psychotherapy has an "unwanted proximity" to placebos which poses problems for ethical clinical practice in respect of disclosures to patients about how psychotherapy works [(11), p. 493]. Here I will focus on the claim that psychotherapy is interpretable as a "placebo" and sidestep intricate questions about ethical implications of this conjecture (26). Since these arguments rely on: (a) common factors research into psychotherapy; and (b) Grünbaum's model of placebos (6), it is first necessary to set the scene by providing an overview of each premise.

Common Factors Research

Empirical findings indicate that different versions of psychotherapy, which employ different treatment techniques, appear to be equally successful (23). This is often referred to as the "Dodo Bird Verdict"—the label is derived from the words of the Dodo Bird in Alice in Wonderland: "everybody has won and all must have prizes" [(27), p. 995]. Subsequently, it has been proposed that the Dodo Bird Verdict is explained by the common factors hypothesis—namely, that it is the common factors and not the specific factors that are relevant to outcome (23). While the Dodo Bird Verdict is still somewhat contested (28) a considerable body of research nonetheless suggests that the common factors play a significant role in mediating treatment outcomes (29, 30).

Grünbaum's Model of Placebo

The second key idea underpinning Gaab et al. (9) and Trachsel and Gaab's (11) views about the relationship between psychotherapy and placebos, is Adolph Grünbaum's model of placebos. Grünbaum differentiates between "characteristic" and "incidental" features of interventions which he says must be relativized to—that is, determined by—particular theories about how treatments work [(6), p. 33]. So, characteristic factors of (for example) *amoxicillin* are its particular antibiotic formula in the pill; meanwhile, the incidental factors include its coloration, the bulking agent, and price. Placebos, on this framework, are conceived as interventions that lack any remedial *characteristic* treatment factors for a particular condition. Placebo effects, on the other hand, are conceived as those positive effects that arise from the *incidental* features of a treatment.

Embracing the validity of Grünbaum's model and the common factors hypothesis, Gaab et al. argue that the specific techniques of psychotherapy can be equated with Grünbaum's description of characteristic features of treatments and the common factors interpreted as incidental factors (9, 11). From this perspective, it is concluded that psychotherapy risks being conceived as a placebo.

What should we make of this analysis? A positive feature of Grünbaum's framework is his conceptualization of placebos as a moving classification: placebos are not reified as physical "things" e.g., sugar pills. But when it comes to placebo effects problematic discrepancies arise between Grünbaum's model and scientific research. On Grünbaum's account placebo effects are also conceived as moving targets (rather than as a natural kind): this is because they are conceived as the effects of *incidental treatment factors* associated with a particular treatment theory. Even if we modify and narrow this framework to accommodate the view that placebo effects are the *positive effects of incidental factors* (1) the account is still too liberal from the perspective of scientific placebo studies. This is because other positive psychological effects may conceivably be precipitated by incidental factors (e.g., reporting biases or Hawthorne effects which precipitate positive health behaviors, Pygmalion effects, and/or other psychological processes).

Further problems arise when applying this model to psychotherapy research. If: (a) we accept the validity of the common factors hypothesis; and (b) defend Grünbaum's model of placebos, it might be countered that the common factors cannot be interpreted as "incidental factors." This is because theories within psychotherapy typically regard common factors as integral components of treatment [e.g., (25)]. Thus, the terms *specific* and *common factors* may not be construed as conceptually isomorphic with Grünbaum's *characteristic* and *incidental factors*, respectively. Instead, it would be more accurate to describe different versions of therapy as employing *idiosyncratic* treatment factors alongside common factors but that all of these factors are "characteristic," i.e., considered to be necessary factors for psychotherapy to be successful.

CONCLUSIONS AND RECOMMENDATIONS

In conclusion, conceptual clarity in placebo studies will only be settled when we attend to how placebo terminology is *in fact* used within burgeoning scientific research—rather than how disputants say it used.

In examining the relationship between psychotherapy and placebos we must ask: What is the context of our analysis? Placebos in clinical trials, I have argued, are best characterized as control interventions. As with all control interventions, then, the function of placebos in psychotherapy clinical trials is to mimic the appearance of the verum treatment except for its particular, hypothesized, remedial factor. In practice, designing placebos for psychotherapy clinical trials is hugely challenging; though (as suggested) future technological innovations may eventually help to resolve recalcitrant problems.

In clinical contexts it is incorrect to describe psychotherapy as a placebo. Within the scientific placebo field, researchers implicitly define placebos as, "treatments theorized not to be effective for a condition or symptoms by virtue of their intrinsic properties." While research into basic science of psychotherapy mechanisms is not advanced, it appears that common factors play an important role in mediating change. Moreover, these factors are also theorized by proponents of different psychological treatments to be necessary to outcome.

Finally, placebo effects cannot be equated with "all non-physical responses" of a treatment. The growing science of placebo studies informs us that placebo effect(s) are the remedial outcomes of specific psychobiological mechanisms. Such mechanisms may be elicited by psychotherapy—just as they may be triggered in other treatment modalities.

AUTHOR CONTRIBUTIONS

The author confirms being the sole contributor of this work and approved it for publication.

ACKNOWLEDGMENTS

Thanks are due to the reviewer for very helpful feedback and Prof. Paul Enck for the invitation to contribute to this special issue. I also wish to thank Prof. Ted Kaptchuk for fruitful discussions on the themes of this paper. This article was supported by a Fulbright Scholarship Award and an Irish Research Council/Marie Sklowdowska Curie Global Fellowship (CLNE/2017/226) granted to CB.

REFERENCES

1. Howick J. The relativity of 'placebos': defending a modified version of grünbaum's definition. *Synthese* (2017) 194:1363–96. doi: 10.1007/s11229-015-1001-0
2. Moerman DE, Jonas WB. Deconstructing the placebo effect and finding the meaning response. *Ann Internal Med.* (2002) 136:471–6. doi: 10.7326/0003-4819-136-6-200203190-00011
3. Annoni M, and Blease C. A critical (and cautiously optimistic) appraisal of Moerman's meaning response. *Perspect Biol Med.* (2018) 61:349–52.
4. Turner A. Placebos' and the logic of placebo comparison. *Biol Philos.* (2012) 27:419–32. doi: 10.1007/s10539-011-9289-8
5. Rosenthal D, Frank JD. Psychotherapy and the placebo effect. *Psychol Bull.* (1956) 53:294–302. doi: 10.1037/h0044068
6. Grünbaum A. The placebo concept in medicine and psychiatry. *Psychol Med.* (1986) 16:19–38. doi: 10.1017/S0033291700002506

7. Jopling DA. *Talking Cures and Placebo Effects.* Oxford: Oxford University Press (2008).
8. Blease C, Kirsch I. The placebo effect and psychotherapy: Implications for theory, research, and practice. *Psychol Conscious Theor Res Pract.* (2016) 3:105–107. doi: 10.1037/cns0000094
9. Gaab J, Blease C, Locher C, Gerger H. Go open: A plea for transparency in psychotherapy. *Psychol Conscious Theor Res Pract.* (2016) 3:175–98. doi: 10.1037/cns0000063
10. Kirsch I, Wampold B, Kelley JM. Controlling for the placebo effect in psychotherapy: Noble quest or tilting at windmills? *Psychol Conscious Theor Res Pract.* (2016) 3:121–31. doi: 10.1037/cns0000065
11. Trachsel M, Gaab J. Disclosure of incidental constituents of psychotherapy as a moral obligation for psychiatrists and psychotherapists. *J Med Ethics* (2016) 42:493–5. doi: 10.1136/medethics-2015-102986
12. Evers AWM, Colloca L, Blease C, Annoni M, Atlas LY, Benedetti F, et al. Implications of placebo and nocebo effects for clinical practice: consensus of a group of experts. *Psychother Psychosomat.* (2018) 87:204-10. doi: 10.1159/000490354
13. Weimer K, Colloca L, Enck P. Placebo effects in psychiatry: mediators and moderators. *Lancet Psychiatry* (2015) 2:246–57. doi: 10.1016/S2215-0366(14)00092-3
14. Blease C. Conceptual consensus in placebo studies: Lessons from the philosophy of science. *Perspect Biol Med.* (2018) 61:412–30.
15. Kuhn TS. *The Structure of Scientific Revolutions.* Chicago, IL: University of Chicago Press (1962/1970).
16. Bishop FL, Jacobson EE, Shaw JR, Kaptchuk TJ. Scientific tools, fake treatments, or triggers for psychological healing: how clinical trial participants conceptualise placebos. *Soc Sci Med.* (2012) 74:767–74. doi: 10.1016/j.socscimed.2011.11.020
17. Bishop FL, Howick J, Heneghan C, Stevens S, Hobbs FR, Lewith G. Placebo use in the UK: a qualitative study exploring GPs' views on placebo effects in clinical practice. *Family Pract.* (2014) 31:357–63. doi: 10.1093/fampra/cmu016
18. Enck P, Klosterhalfen S, Weimer K. Unsolved, forgotten, and ignored features of the placebo response in medicine. *Clin Ther.* (2017) 39:458–68. doi: 10.1016/j.clinthera.2016.11.016
19. Kaptchuk TJ, Friedlander E, Kelley JM, Sanchez MN, Kokkotou E, Singer JP. Placebos without deception: a randomized controlled trial in irritable bowel syndrome. *PloS ONE* (2010) 5:e15591. doi: 10.1371/journal.pone.0015591
20. Carvalho C, Caetano JM., Cunha L, Rebouta P, Kaptchuk TJ, and Kirsch, I. Open-label placebo treatment in chronic low back pain: a randomized controlled trial. *Pain* (2016) 157:2766–72. doi: 10.1097/j.pain.0000000000000700
21. Kaptchuk TJ, Kelley JM, Conboy LA, Davis RB, Kerr CE, Jacobson EE, et al. Components of placebo effect: randomised controlled trial in patients with irritable bowel syndrome. *BMJ* (2008) 336:999–1003. doi: 10.1136/bmj.39524.439618.25
22. Atran S. Folk biology and the anthropology of science: cognitive universals and cultural particulars. *Behav Brain Sci.* (1998) 21:547–69. doi: 10.1017/S0140525X98001277
23. Wampold BE, Imel ZE. The *Great Psychotherapy Debate: The Evidence for What Makes Psychotherapy Work.* Routledge (2015).
24. Beck A. *Cognitive Therapy and The Emotional Disorders.* London: Penguin (1976).
25. Beck J. *Cognitive Therapy: Basics and Beyond.* New York, NY: The Guilford Press (1995).
26. Blease C, Trachsel M, Grosse Holtforth M. Paternalism, placebos, and informed consent in psychotherapy: the challenge of ethical disclosure. *Verhaltenstherapie* (2016) 26:22–30. doi: 10.1159/000442928
27. Luborsky L, Singer B, Luborsky L. Comparative studies of psychotherapies: is it true that everyone has won and all must have prizes? *Arch Gen Psychiatry* (1975) 32:995–1008. doi: 10.1001/archpsyc.1975.01760260059004
28. Marcus DK, O'Connell D, Norris AL, Sawaqdeh A. Is the Dodo bird endangered in the 21st century? A meta-analysis of treatment comparison studies Clinical Psychology Review. *Clin Psychol Rev.* (2014) 34:519–30. doi: 10.1016/j.cpr.2014.08.001
29. Lambert MJ, Barley DE. Research summary on the therapeutic relationship and psychotherapy outcome. Expectations and preferences. In: Norcross, JC. editor. *Psychotherapy Relationships that Work: Therapist Contributions and Responsiveness to Patients.* London: Oxford University Press (2002). p. 17–32.
30. Cuijpers P. Are all psychotherapies equally effective in the treatment of adult depression? The lack of statistical power of comparative outcome studies. *Evid Based Mental Health* (2016) 19:39–42. doi: 10.1136/eb-2016-102341

8

When your Doctor "Gets It" and "Gets You": The Critical Role of Competence and Warmth in the Patient–Provider Interaction

Lauren C. Howe[1], Kari A. Leibowitz[2] and Alia J. Crum[2]**

[1] Department of Business Administration, University of Zurich, Zurich, Switzerland, [2] Department of Psychology, Stanford University, Stanford, CA, United States

***Correspondence:**
Lauren C. Howe
Lauren.howe@business.uzh.ch
Alia J. Crum
crum@stanford.edu

Background: Research demonstrates that the placebo effect can influence the effectiveness of medical treatments and accounts for a significant proportion of healing in many conditions. However, providers may differ in the degree to which they consciously or unconsciously leverage the forces that produce placebo effects in clinical practice. Some studies suggest that the manner in which providers interact with patients shapes the magnitude of placebo effects, but this research has yet to distill the *specific* dimensions of patient–provider interactions that are most likely to influence placebo response and the mechanisms through which aspects of patient–provider interactions impact placebo response.

Methods: We offer a simplifying and unifying framework in which interactions that boost placebo response can be dissected into two key dimensions: patients' perceptions of *competence*, or whether a doctor "gets it" (i.e., displays of efficiency, knowledge, and skill), and patients' perceptions of *warmth*, or whether a doctor "gets me" (i.e., displays of personal engagement, connection, and care for the patient).

Results: First, we discuss how this framework builds on past research in psychology on social perception of competence and warmth and in medical literature on models of effective medical care, patient satisfaction, and patient–provider interactions. Then we consider possible mechanisms through which competence and warmth may affect the placebo response in healthcare. Finally, we share original data from patients and providers highlighting how this framework applies to healthcare. Both patient and provider data illustrate actionable ways providers can demonstrate competence and warmth to patients.

Discussion: We conclude with recommendations for how researchers and practitioners alike can more systematically consider the role of provider competence and warmth in patient–provider interactions to deepen our understanding of placebo effects and, ultimately, enable providers to boost placebo effects alongside active medications (i.e., with known medical ingredients) and treatment in clinical care.

Keywords: placebo effects, placebo response, patient-provider interactions, warmth, competence, provider characteristics, provider demeanor

INTRODUCTION

The doctor has been called "a powerful therapeutic agent" (p. 1,067) (1) who can evoke healing in her or his patients even by simply interacting with them. One way providers can help their patients heal, and the focus of this paper, is through eliciting *placebo effects,* or "healing that is produced, activated, or enhanced by the context of the clinical encounter, as distinct from the specific efficacy of treatment interventions" (2). Diverse factors can produce placebo effects, including medical rituals (e.g., taking a pill) and provider behaviors (e.g., communication). For example, providers explicitly stating to patients that a treatment will improve their condition makes it more likely that the treatment will do so (3, 4). Placebo effects bolster the efficacy of both active medications (5–7) and treatments with no active medical properties, ranging from sugar pills (8) to inert creams described as pain relievers (9) to sham acupuncture involving fake needles that never pierce the skin (10).

But not all placebo effects are created equal. A series of studies suggests that how providers interact with their patients shapes the magnitude of placebo effects (10–13). But while these studies acknowledge that patient–provider interactions are critical to placebo response, they do not provide a theoretical framework for the *specific* dimensions of the patient–provider interaction that enhance placebo effects and thus shape a patient's physical health outcomes.

In the current article, we address four key questions, which correspond to the four main sections of the article:

1. What are the key dimensions of patient–provider interactions?
2. In what ways do these dimensions moderate placebo response?
3. What are the mechanisms through which these dimensions moderate placebo response?
4. How can providers leverage these dimensions deliberately in clinical care?

In considering these questions, we delineate a novel framework proposing that interactions that boost placebo response can be dissected into two key dimensions: patients' perceptions of *competence*, or whether a doctor "gets it" (i.e., displays of efficiency, knowledge, and skill) and patients' perceptions of *warmth*, or whether a doctor "gets me" (i.e., displays of personal engagement, connection, and care for the patient). We suggest that competence and warmth work together to influence placebo response and therefore shape effective healthcare.

WHAT ARE THE KEY DIMENSIONS OF PATIENT–PROVIDER INTERACTIONS?

Is there a parsimonious way to represent the many diverse qualities that may be present in patient–provider interactions? We tackle this question in three steps. First, we discuss the psychological literature on social perception, which identifies key dimensions that underlie our impressions of others. Second, we introduce a model of patient–provider interactions that explains how key dimensions from social perception apply in the healthcare context. Third, we illustrate how these key dimensions are evident in the medical literature on patient–provider interactions by reviewing theoretical and empirical work on effective patient–provider interactions.

Competence and Warmth: Two Core Dimensions of Social Perception

Psychologists have long been interested in understanding the dimensions on which people judge others when forming first impressions. In order to successfully navigate one's social world, a person must constantly and rapidly make accurate assessments of other people. Should a stranger be approached or avoided? Is a person a suitable friend or romantic partner? Is an expert worthy of trust? To answer such questions, people need to quickly determine whether another person is likely and able to harm or help them. Although many dimensions for the factors that underlie such social judgments have been proposed, over 50 years of research suggests that they can all be distilled into two key dimensions: warmth and competence (14–20).

One study attempting to identify the underlying dimensions of personality asked participants to describe different people they knew by selecting personality traits from a list of over 60 different traits (21). These researchers then evaluated the degree to which these traits co-occurred in people's descriptions of a particular person. They found the traits that co-occurred frequently could be grouped into those that described intellectual qualities that were either good or bad (i.e., competence—e.g., qualities like determined and industrious *vs.* irresponsible and unintelligent) and social qualities that were good or bad (i.e., warmth—e.g., qualities like sincere and good-natured *vs.* irritable and humorless). These two dimensions were independent and accounted for most of the variance in people's judgments of others.

In other research, participants generated descriptions of events that helped them form strong impressions of other people or themselves (22). Of the over 1,000 descriptions generated by these participants, approximately three-fourths depicted considerations of warmth or competence, as rated by independent judges. In yet another study, a pool of 200 diverse traits were rated on a variety of dimensions, including the degree to which they captured warmth and captured competence (23). These ratings of a trait's warmth and competence predicted all but 3% of the variance in ratings of trait favorability, suggesting that these two ingredients are key to describing positive and negative qualities in person perception.

Together these studies, and dozens of others using a variety of methodologies, suggest that warmth and competence are two key dimensions holding the greatest explanatory power when it comes to positive and negative evaluations of others.[1] Qualities like friendliness, honesty, trustworthiness, good-naturedness, empathy, and kindness (*vs.* coldness, deceit, and unreliability) are all essentially different ways to describe a person's general warmth.

[1] For example, the dimensions of warmth and competence also model people's judgments of the characteristics of social groups. Ratings of warmth and competence distinguished a variety of different social groups on the basis of out-group members' stereotypes about these groups (24). Stereotypes of groups could be categorized into four unique clusters: those rated high on warmth and competence, low on warmth and competence, high on warmth but low on competence, and low on competence but high on warmth.

Qualities like intelligence, power, assertiveness, ambition, efficacy, and skill (*vs.* inefficiency, indecisiveness, passivity, and laziness) are all essentially different ways to describe a person's general competence (15, 20). Though these dimensions have sometimes been called by other names [e.g., agency and communion (25–27); for a review see Ref. (17)] regardless of the nomenclature, there is remarkable consistency among researchers in the qualities that are commonly reflected by these two dimensions.

There is a strong evolutionary argument for the primacy of warmth and competence: the need to rapidly determine whether a person intends to, and is capable of, harming or helping an individual. Essentially, warmth encapsulates answers to the question of "Are this person's intentions toward me positive or negative?" and competence encapsulates answers to the question of "Does this person have the ability to enact those positive or negative intentions?" (14). To promote survival, a person must be able to find an answer to these key questions whenever they encounter someone new.

And indeed, people make these judgments rapidly and non-consciously, any time they evaluate someone new. People judge others as warm or competent based on even brief exposure to another person's behavior (28–30). For example, both adults and children form evaluations of warmth and competence after brief, 100-millisecond exposure to a person's face (31, 32). These two dimensions are readily perceived from a variety of limited non-verbal information, such as tone of voice, body posture, and facial expressions (33–35). Further, ratings of warmth predict liking and ratings of competence predict respect for others (25, 36). Warmth and competence thus seem likely to influence both the quality and outcomes of a variety of important interpersonal interactions, including patient–provider interactions.

In summary, decades of research in social, evolutionary, and cognitive psychology have shown that a multitude of qualities can essentially be distilled into the two core dimensions of competence and warmth, and that these dimensions are fundamental to how people form impressions of others. Next, we apply this competence and warmth framework to healthcare.

Judgments of Competence and Warmth in Healthcare: The Provider "Gets It" and "Gets Me" Framework

Patients' assessments of a provider likely also follow these two key dimensions of social perception, but with a slightly different flavor. We propose a healthcare-specific framework in which patients assess competence by judging whether the provider "gets it" (i.e., demonstrates efficiency, knowledge, and skill) and assess warmth by judging whether the provider "gets me" (i.e., demonstrates personal engagement, connection, and care for the patient; in other words, whether a provider sees a patient as a social being, and not just in terms of their health or illness). See **Table 1** for a summary of these dimensions.

When assessing whether a provider "gets it," a patient may pay attention to cues indicating whether a provider has the necessary qualities to conduct relevant procedures, make an accurate diagnosis, and make the best recommendations for treatment. When assessing whether a provider "gets me," a patient may pay attention to cues indicating whether a provider recognizes and respects that this individual is a person with a life outside of the healthcare context who has their own desires, needs, and values.

There are a multitude of qualities that could bolster patients' perceptions that a provider "gets it," all of which involve a practitioner's perceived expertise and ability to help address a patient's medical concerns. Some qualities might foster perceptions of medical competence in a broader sense, such as whether a provider attended a top-tier medical school, if they seem up-to-date on medical research, or if they speak clearly and confidently. Other qualities might instead focus on perceived competence regarding the patient and their particular situation. For example, does a patient feel like the provider knows their family history, has experience with patients who are similar to them, and can answer their specific questions?

Similarly, patients' perceptions that a provider "gets me" could be cultivated in different ways. Some ways involve very general qualities or actions: whether the provider smiles at and sits near the patient, whether they introduce themselves and use the patient's

TABLE 1 | Judgments of competence and warmth in healthcare: the provider "gets it" and "gets me" framework.

	Competence: "My provider gets it"	Warmth: "My provider gets me"
Definition	Patient perceptions of *competence*, i.e., displays of efficiency, knowledge, and skill	Patient perceptions of *warmth*, i.e., displays of personal engagement, connection, and care for the patient
Key question in assessments of this dimension	Does the provider understand the diagnosis, treatment, and procedures?	Does the provider understand me as a person?
Examples of general qualities	Education, diagnostic ability, general medical and procedural knowledge, confidence, articulateness, clarity of explanations, use of technology	General friendliness and social engagement (e.g., smiling, making eye contact), introducing themselves, being polite to co-workers
Examples of patient-specific qualities	Knowledge of patients' family history, experience with similar patients, answering patients' specific questions and concerns	Knowledge of the patient as a person (i.e., outside of the healthcare context), understanding of patient values, active listening, feeling that the provider respects and does not judge the patient
Qualities bridging warmth and competence	Use of patient-friendly language, individualization of patient explanations and/or care, engagement of patients in their own care and/or decision-making	

We define patient-specific qualities as providers' qualities, such as knowledge of important aspects of a patient's life outside of the healthcare context (warmth) and experience working with similar patients (competence), that reflect knowledge of the specific patient's individual needs, desires, and/or perspectives, as opposed to more general qualities of providers, such as general friendliness (warmth) and general medical knowledge (competence), that do not necessarily require knowledge of the specific patient's individual needs, desires, and/or perspectives.

name, and even whether they are polite to their co-workers at the hospital. These qualities and behaviors, as signals of general positive social engagement, may foster the perception that a provider is likely to regard their patient as a social being worthy of human dignity and respect. Cultivating perceived warmth could also involve qualities that are more patient-specific: listening to a patient and acknowledging their individual perspectives, asking a patient questions about their life outside of the healthcare context to get to know them as a person, appearing to understand the social world of the patient and their values, and respecting the patient. Warmth may also encompass interpersonal skills that bolster perceptions of a provider's engagement with and care for the patient (e.g., active listening) as well as their emotional feelings toward the patient (e.g., empathy).[2]

Competence and Warmth in the Medical Literature

We have proposed that patient–provider interactions can be distilled into two key dimensions: whether a provider appears to "get it" (i.e., competence) and "get me" (i.e., warmth). Here we describe how these dimensions, although not always explicitly categorized as such, represent the foundation of existing theories of effective medical care.

Competence and Warmth in Theoretical Models of Medical Care

Competence and warmth surface as two key dimensions in a variety of theoretical models of effective medical care, as outlined in **Table 2**. Major advances in our understanding of medicine have often involved a shift from considering only a provider's competence as critical to patient care to also incorporating a provider's warmth.

One of the earliest calls to incorporate warmth into models of medical care was the shift from biomedical to biopsychosocial models of medicine (40–42). Biomedical models focused on tasks related to medical competence: rooting out physical causes of illness, using diagnostic tests to determine treatment, and intervening at the level of biology. Biopsychosocial models emphasized the critical role of psychological factors (e.g., personality, mood, coping skills) and social context (e.g., culture, family, socioeconomic status) in health. Biopsychosocial models thus encouraged a greater focus on patients' concerns, comfort, values, and goals—the "getting me" of medicine.

[2] A large literature has explored provider empathy in patient-provider interactions and suggests that it can play an important role (e.g., improving patient health outcomes) (37–39). Empathy is a multifaceted construct that may include several different components, including awareness and sharing of others' affect, caring for others' welfare, and/or imagining what others are feeling (39). The literature on social perception distinguishes between warmth and empathy; empathy is subsumed under the umbrella of warmth as a feature that may indicate it, but other qualities that cannot be directly equated to empathy also comprise warmth (e.g., friendliness, honesty, kindness, and good-naturedness) (15). Simply being friendly or honest does not necessarily communicate empathy but could bolster perceived warmth. Thus, since it encompasses a wider variety of relevant provider characteristics and behaviors, we adopt the more general term *warmth* rather than the more specific term *empathy* in our discussion of provider qualities.

The role of warmth alongside competence is further reflected in the shift from a doctor centered, physician-centered, or disease-centered approach (43, 45, 48) to patient-centered medicine (44, 46, 47). As Levenstein and colleagues (47) suggested, in patient-centered medicine "the task of the physician is twofold, to understand the patient and to understand the disease" (p. 24). Patient-centered medicine suggests that most effective treatments based on exceptional knowledge (the "getting it" of medicine) may prove irrelevant if these treatments do not align with a patient's values and desires, which requires recognizing the patient as a social being and putting effort into "getting me." Similarly, other research distinguishes between disease as objective (i.e., abnormalities of the structure and function of body organs and systems) and illness as subjective, e.g., incorporating how a patient perceives the event and how it affects their life (57).

There are similar parallels in the "voice of the lifeworld" and the "voice of medicine" (49), or as "a question of facts" *versus* "a question of personal values" (50), as described in **Table 2**. Engel captured these dimensions neatly as two different patient considerations: the *need to know and understand* and the *need to feel known and understood* (51). A quote from Engel encapsulates the importance of a provider's warmth as well as competence:

> For the patient, to feel understood by the physician means more than just feeling that the physician understands intellectually, that is, 'comprehends' what the patient is reporting and what may be wrong, critical as these are for the physician's scientific task. Every bit as important is that the physician display understanding about the patient as a person, as a fellow human being, and about what he is experiencing and what the circumstances of his life are. (p. 11)

Later models captured competence and warmth as behaviors that are *cure-oriented versus care-oriented* (52, 53), *instrumental versus affective* (54), and *task-oriented versus socio-emotional* behaviors (55). The tradition of narrative medicine (56) suggested directly that "a scientifically competent medicine alone" (p. 1,897) is not sufficient for effective healthcare. This tradition argues that physicians must complement their scientific ability by listening to patients' stories, engaging with them empathetically, and understanding their individual perspectives. By acknowledging the role of personal connections between providers and patients in healthcare, this tradition, as well as the substantial interest in empathy (58, 59) and the emotional aspects of patient–provider communication (60) in the medical literature in recent years, moved medicine closer still toward recognizing the importance of warmth.

In the medical literature, the past decades have involved a shift from a focus on "getting it" to a focus on also "getting the patient." However, often in these models, warmth and competence have been portrayed as in conflict or competition, or as alternative rather than complementary approaches to care. We propose, and the social perception literature supports, that there need not be a trade-off between warmth and competence, and that these two dimensions often bolster one another.

TABLE 2 | Competence (provider "gets it") and warmth (provider "gets me") in theories of medical care.

Competence/"gets it"	Warmth/"gets me"	References
Biomedical: need to know the illness	**Biopsychosocial:** need to know the person who has the disease	Engel (40); McCormick (41); Smith and Hoppe (42)
Physician-centered medicine: focuses on the doctor's interpretation of the evidence and diminishes the importance of human relationships and the role of the patient	**Patient-centered medicine:** focuses on recognizing patients' individual perspectives and taking them into account in medical care	Bensing (43); Brown et al. (44); Grol et al. (45); King and Hoppe (46); Levenstein et al. (47); Smith and Hoppe (42); Sweeney et al. (48)
Voice of medicine: technical aspects, symptoms, and the etiology and treatment of specific diseases	**Voice of the lifeworld:** viewing problems in patients' personal and sociocultural context	Mishler (49)
A question of facts: whether physicians possess the technical expertise necessary for care	**A question of personal values:** whether a treatment resonates with patients' preferences (e.g., lifestyle, health beliefs, goals)	Eddy (50)
Need to know and understand: a provider's scientific role	**Need to feel known and understood:** a provider's caring role	Engel (51)
Cure-oriented: problem-solving (e.g., asking the patient questions and providing them with information)	**Care-oriented:** reducing patient anxiety (e.g., by using empathy, paraphrasing)	De Valck et al. (52); Van Dulmen and Van Den Brink-Muinen (53)
Instrumental/task-oriented: target diagnosis and treatment	**Affective/socio-emotional oriented:** target rapport and relationship building	Bensing et al. (54); Roter and Larson (55)
Scientific ability/competence	**Patient narratives:** listen to patient stories, engage empathetically, take patients' perspectives	Charon (56)

Competence and Warmth in Medical Research on and Measures of Patient Satisfaction

Next, we review some of the most highly-cited measures of patient satisfaction to illustrate that the competence and warmth framework can distill the provider characteristics present in these measures. As can be seen in **Table 3**, widely-used patient satisfaction scales such as the Press Ganey Survey (61) and the Hospital Consumer Assessment of Healthcare Providers and Systems (HCAHPS) (62) capture both warmth (e.g., is courteous) and competence (e.g., is prompt). While these patient satisfaction scales may have their flaws, they nevertheless implicitly assess both competence and warmth, demonstrating that these dimensions are already considered important to effective healthcare.

Competence and warmth also underlie the constructs captured in some of the most highly cited scales used in medical research (from citations from Google Scholar in November 2018), including the Risser Patient Satisfaction Scale (63) (>490 citations), the Picker Patient Experience Questionnaire (64) (PPE-15, >440 citations), the Medical Interview Satisfaction Scale (65) (MISS, >440 citations, the Consultation Satisfaction Questionnaire (66) (CSQ, >410 citations), and the La Monica-Oberst Patient Satisfaction Scale (67) (LOPSS, > 280 citations), as well as more recently devised scales of patient satisfaction (e.g., the Short Assessment of Patient Satisfaction (SAPS) scale) (60) (see **Table 4** and **Supplemental Table 1**). For example, the items in the LOPSS (67) capture warmth (e.g., is pleasant and gentle) and competence (e.g., is thorough and efficient).

Many critical capabilities of providers highlighted in these measures of patient satisfaction rely on both competence and warmth. For example, the Press Ganey Survey assesses the degree to which a provider made efforts to include the patient in decisions about treatment. To effectively engage a patient in the treatment process, a provider needs the competence to advise a patient on the technical aspects of care and to know what treatment options are suitable. But a provider also needs warmth to gain insight into a patient's perspective and values in order to present relevant

TABLE 3 | Competence and warmth in items from patient satisfaction scales commonly utilized in clinical care evaluations (the Press Ganey Survey and Hospital Consumer Assessment of Healthcare Providers and Systems).

Items associated with competence	Items associated with warmth
Press Ganey Outpatient Medical Practice Survey: seven relevant items, out of 10 items	
Explanations the care provider gave you about your problem or condition	Friendliness/courtesy of the care provider
Information the care provider gave you about medications (if any)	Concern the care provider showed for your questions or worries
Instructions the care provider gave you about follow-up care (if any)	
Items bridging competence and warmth	
Degree to which care provider talked with you using words you could understand	
Care provider's efforts to include you in decisions about your treatment	
Hospital Consumer Assessment of Healthcare Providers and Systems (HCAHPS): seven out of seven items	
Items associated with competence	**Items associated with warmth**
After you pressed the call button, how often did you get help as soon as you wanted it?	How often did (nurses/doctors) treat you with courtesy and respect?
	How often did (nurses/doctors) listen carefully to you?
Items bridging competence and warmth	
How often did (nurses/doctors) explain things in a way you could understand?	

TABLE 4 | Competence and warmth in items from patient satisfaction scales developed for medical research.

La Monica-Oberst Patient Satisfaction Scale (LOPSS): sample of 24 relevant items, out of 41 items	
Items associated with competence	**Items associated with warmth**
Should be more thorough (R)	Is not as friendly as (s)/he should be (R)
Seems disorganized and flustered (R)	Makes me feel like a "case," not an individual (R)
Does not follow through quickly enough (R)	Seems more interested in completing tasks than listening to concerns (R)
Tells me what treatment effects to expect	I can share my feelings when I need to talk.
Seems to know what s/he is talking about	Does things to make me feel more comfortable
Would know what to do in an emergency	Is gentle in caring for me
Appears to be skillful at her/his work	Treats me with respect
Makes helpful suggestions	Appears to enjoy caring for me
Gives complete explanations	Is pleasant to have around
Items bridging competence and warmth	
Neglects to be sure I understand importance of my treatments (R)	
Acts like I cannot understand the medical explanation of my illness (R)	
Fails to consider my opinions and preferences regarding plans for my care (R)	
Helps me to understand my illness	
Gives directions at just the right speed	
Shows me how to follow my treatment program	
Risser Patient Satisfaction Scale: sample of 15 relevant items, out of 25 items	
Items associated with competence	**Items associated with warmth**
Technical-professional area (seven items)	*Trusting relationship area (11 items)*
The nurse really knows what s/he is talking about.	The nurse is understanding in listening to a patient's problems.
The nurse is not precise in doing his/her work. (R)	The nurse should be more friendly than s/he is (R).
The nurse is too slow to do things for me. (R)	I'm tired of the nurse talking down to me. (R)
The nurse is skillful in assisting the doctor with procedures.	The nurse is a person who can understand how I feel.
The nurse is often too disorganized to appear calm. (R)	The nurse is pleasant to be around.
Items bridging competence and warmth	
Educational relationship area (seven items)	
The nurse gives directions at just the right speed.	
I wish the nurse would tell me about the results of my tests more than s/he does. (R)	
It is always easy to understand what the nurse is talking about.	
The nurse explains things in simple language.	
Too often the nurse thinks you can't understand the medical explanation of your illness, so s/he just doesn't bother to explain. (R)	

(R) indicates that the item describes a provider who is lower on warmth or lower on competence. Otherwise, the item is representative of higher warmth or higher competence. Some other items in these scales not captured in this table assessed general satisfaction and/or confidence in providers, which may be shaped by perceptions of both warmth and competence.

options to a patient. They need warmth to judge a patient's knowledge and skills appropriately based on their life experiences and to take that into account when conveying information to them. And, they need warmth to cultivate enough approachability to make a patient feel comfortable engaging in their care. Abilities such as advice-giving may function similarly. Of course, a provider needs the competence to know possible recommendations and to explain them clearly to patients, but a provider also needs the warmth to choose advice that is appropriate for a particular patient and to relate it to the patient to encourage adherence. Competence and warmth combined thus form the foundation of many healthcare skills, as highlighted in **Tables 3** and **4**.

Several scales (i.e., Press Ganey, CSQ, MISS, SAPS) include questions assessing how satisfied patients were with the amount of time that their provider spent with them. Some research shows that provider warmth shapes perceptions of the time spent with a provider during a medical exam (68), and so measures of patient satisfaction with visit length may be linked with perceived provider warmth.

Thus, when attempting to measure the quality of interactions with providers, existing scales tap into the core dimensions of competence and warmth or assess skills that require both of these dimensions. Details on the validity of these scales are reported elsewhere (69–71). Here we focus primarily on the fact that all of these scales capture the core dimensions of competence and warmth, therefore providing further evidence that a combination of these qualities are critical to effective healthcare (in this case, as evidenced by patient satisfaction).

Competence and Warmth in Medical Research on and Measures of Patient–Provider Interactions

Research-based measurements of patient–provider interactions also illuminate the core dimensions of competence and warmth (see **Table 5**). Some widely used methods for analyzing patient–provider interactions include the Roter Interaction Analysis System (55, 72) (RIAS, >700 citations), a coding systems for patient–provider communication, and the coding scheme associated with the Four Habits model (73, 74) (>190 citations).

The RIAS categorizes dialogue into two buckets: 1) task-focused behaviors, involving gathering data to determine care and providing patient education and counseling, and 2) affective behaviors, involving building a relationship and rapport with patients and

TABLE 5 | Warmth and competence in behaviors from the Roter Interaction Analysis System and Four Habits Coding Scheme used to code dialogue between patients and providers.

Roter Interaction Analysis System	
Behaviors associated with competence	**Behaviors associated with warmth**
Providing biomedical information (e.g., about medical condition or therapeutic regimen)	Positive talk (e.g., jokes and laughter, approval, compliments)
Orientation (e.g., providing directions and instructions)	Negative talk (e.g., disagreements, disapproval and criticisms) (R)
Providing information about lifestyle and self-care	Social talk (i.e., non-medical chit-chat)
	Emotional talk (e.g., reassurance, empathy)
Asking questions about medical condition or therapeutic regiment	Asking questions about psychosocial topics
Behaviors bridging competence and warmth	
Partnering and activation (e.g., asking for patient opinions, asking for patient understanding)	
Four Habits Coding Scheme	
Behaviors associated with competence	**Behaviors associated with warmth**
Clinician indicates clear familiarity with patient's history/chart (e.g., mentions recent tests performed).	Patient is greeted in a manner that is personal and warm (e.g., clinician asks patient how s/he likes to be addressed, uses patient's name).
The clinician attempts to elicit the full range of the patient's concerns by generating an agenda early in the visit.	Clinician makes non-medical comments, using these to put the patient at ease.
Clinician fully/clearly explains the rationale behind current, past, or future tests and treatments.	Clinician openly encourages/is receptive to the expression of emotion (e.g., through use of continuers or appropriate pauses).
Clinician fully explores barriers to implementation of treatment plan.	Clinician displays non-verbal behaviors that express great interest, concern, and connection (e.g., eye contact, tone of voice, and body orientation) throughout the visit.
Behaviors bridging competence and warmth	
Clinician shows great interest in exploring the patient's understanding of the problem (e.g., asks the patient what the symptoms mean to him/her).	
Clinician attempts to determine in detail/shows great interest in how the problem is affecting the patient's lifestyle (work, family, daily activities).	
Clinician clearly encourages and invites paint's input into the decision-making process.	

(R) indicates that the measure describes a provider who is lower on warmth or lower on competence. Otherwise, the measure is representative of higher warmth or higher competence.

responding to a patient's emotions. Task-focused behaviors often reflect competence, such as asking questions about a medical condition, discussing the results of tests, and giving instructions about treatment. Affective behaviors reflect warmth, such as emotional expressions toward the patient (e.g., concern, optimism, reassurance), verbal attentiveness (e.g., paraphrasing, empathy), social behaviors (e.g., making personal remarks, joking, laughter), and negative talk (e.g., expressing disapproval or criticism) (75–77). The Four Habits model focuses on developing four key families of skills in providers, namely investing in the beginning of the visit, eliciting patient perspectives, demonstrating empathy, and investing in the end of the visit (73, 74). Many of the skills in the model involve warmth (e.g., create rapport quickly, make at least one empathic statement) and many involve competence (e.g., deliver diagnostic information, provide education). As with the patient satisfaction scales, some measures in these scales build on both competence and warmth (e.g., dispensing advice relevant to a patient's lifestyle, checking patients' understanding, and encouraging patients to talk).

Provider empathy has raised much recent interest, particularly given its association with improved patient health outcomes (78–81). One of the most widely used scales of provider empathy is the 20-item Jefferson Scale of Physician Empathy (80) (>600 citations), which essentially assesses to what degree providers personally endorse the importance of "getting the patient"; for example, items include whether a provider agrees that "Physicians' understanding of their patients' feelings and the feelings of their patients' families is a positive treatment factor" and "It is as important to ask patients about what is happening in their lives as it is to ask about their physical complaints." To some degree, these items assess providers' beliefs about whether warmth is relevant to a provider's competence (e.g., whether it is an important part of diagnosis and treatment). These qualities seem likely to bolster perceptions of a provider's warmth.

Echoing measures of patient satisfaction, other research-based measures that dissect patient provider interactions (e.g., dialogue) into important qualities again capture the core dimensions of competence and warmth.

Competence and Warmth in Experimental Research on Patient–Provider Interactions

Some studies have experimentally compared more standard interactions (e.g., meeting basic standards for clinical care, but limiting the social aspects of the interaction) with "enhanced" interactions that focus more on building rapport and positive engagement with a patient. The qualities in these studies can also be organized into the competence and warmth framework. Some manipulations involve verbal statements that indicate competence or warmth explicitly, and others tap into non-verbal behaviors that signal competence and warmth.

In one study, Rakel and colleagues (82) randomly assigned patients with a common cold to meet with a provider in either a standard visit (e.g., taking medical history, physical exams and diagnosis, limiting touch, eye contact, and visit time) or an enhanced visit involving setting more positive expectations about healing, expressing empathy, empowering and connecting with patients, and educating patients about their illness and treatment to a greater extent (83). The "enhanced interaction" examined in this study reduced the severity and duration of patients' colds, and boosted IL-8 and neutrophil count. Though the researchers largely intended this interaction to bolster perceived provider empathy, many of the behaviors map onto the broader and more comprehensive dimensions of competence and warmth. For example, patients in the enhanced condition received more information about care, including written notes (relevant to competence), and experienced warmth-related non-verbal behaviors (e.g., handshakes, increased eye contact). Some manipulations may have simultaneously conveyed both warmth and competence (e.g., individualizing patient care). **Table 6** illustrates how the qualities can be organized along the competence and warmth dimensions.

Another study experimentally altered patient–provider interaction in hypothetical vignettes in order to assess its relationship to malpractice claims (84), focusing on physician communication behaviors that, in pilot data, surfaced as the most important for enhancing patient–provider rapport. They essentially varied provider competence (e.g., giving information and advice) and warmth (e.g., whether they seemed judgmental and critical *vs.* warm, friendly, and attentive), as well as several components bridging competence and warmth (e.g., engaging the patient, using straightforward language) (see **Table 7**).

Several other studies manipulating patient–provider interactions have focused on training communication skills, as reviewed by Kelley et al. (85). These interventions have often leveraged components that can be understood using the competence and warmth framework. For example, one intervention trained physicians on several skills related to competence (e.g., repeating and summarizing important information; making referrals if needed) and several skills related to warmth (e.g., establishing rapport by introducing themselves and making eye contact; conveying empathy), as well as encouraging physicians to check patient preferences and provide information accordingly (i.e., both competence and warmth) (86, 87). Another intervention involved physicians giving more detailed explanations and making thoughtful pauses (competence) and enhanced active listening and positive non-verbal behavior (warmth), as well as developing skills relevant to competence and warmth (e.g., checking patient understanding and sharing the decision-making process) (88, 89). Yet another involved training a variety of skills that require both competence and warmth, such as assessing what the patient knows about their condition and providing information relevant to the patient's understanding and interests (90, 91).

The methods used in these studies highlight the utility of the competence and warmth framework. In these studies, researchers often work to carefully design studies that experimentally test dozens of different components in the patient–provider interaction. Yet all of these components can be understood, categorized, and synthesized within the framework of competence and warmth. This applies across a wide variety of intervention types, including those focused on empathy, communication skills, shared decision-making, and patient-centered care.

Which is More Important in Patient–Provider Interactions: Competence or Warmth?

The question of whether competence or warmth is more important in social interactions has been discussed somewhat in the social perception literature. Importantly, past research suggests that warmth and competence are not necessarily a trade-off (21, 92). In fact, these dimensions often correlate somewhat positively (i.e., someone who is perceived as warmer also tends to be perceived as more competent) (17, 21).

There is some research suggesting that warmth takes primacy, or is prioritized, in judgments of others (14). When asked to list the traits that are most important in others, people tend to list warmth-related traits rather than competence-related traits, and prefer to learn about warmth-related traits in order to form impressions of others (93). Warmth judgments may also be made more quickly than competence judgments (94). Researchers suggest this pattern may occur because warmth more reliably indicates potential costs and benefits associated with interacting with another person (93, 95). Warmth's primacy makes sense from an evolutionary perspective, as its detection separates foe from friend, potential harm from potential help (15, 94) and must be made most rapidly in order to effectively prepare to fight or flee. The primacy of warmth does not, however, indicate that it is fundamentally more important than competence; both remain essential qualities of social interactions and we propose that the same is true for patients' interactions with providers as well.

There are differences in the role of competence and warmth in patient–provider interactions, as compared to social interactions

TABLE 6 | Experimentally varying warmth and competence in enhanced patient–provider interactions, as reported in Rakel et al. (82) and Barrett et al. (83).

	Competence	Warmth
Verbal cues	• Additional information about how to address illness • Provide written instruction on self-care • Responded to questions	• Active listening • Empathetic statements regarding condition (e.g., it's normal to be worried, colds can sap energy) • Used humor where appropriate
	Bridging competence and warmth • Included personalized comments to tailor care to individual	
		Warmth
Non-verbal cues		• Handshake greeting • Caring facial expressions • Increased eye contact

TABLE 7 | Experimentally varying warmth and competence in enhanced patient–provider interactions in Moore et al. (84).

	Competence	Warmth
Verbal cues	• Gave patient additional information about what to expect • Gave patient additional advice/strategies	• Greeted patient warmly • Apologized for delay • Asked informal questions • Made empathetic statements (e.g., offered condolences) • Was not critical or judgmental of patient
	Bridging competence and warmth • Used easy-to-understand language • Explained medical terms when used • Encouraged patient to ask questions	
	Competence	**Warmth**
Non-verbal cues	• Did not seem in a hurry	• Made eye contact • Listened carefully to patient

more generally, that are worth considering. To illustrate this, consider the definitions in the social perception literature of competence as traits that are "self-profitable" (i.e., that benefit the person who possesses them), and warmth as traits that are "other-profitable" (i.e., that benefit the people around the person who possesses them) (27, 96–98). Such definitions could further justify the primacy of warmth, as they portray judgments of another person's warmth (i.e., "Does this person possess traits that are likely to benefit me?") as the most relevant for self-interest. But in medical care, this distinction cannot be made. A provider's competence is clearly also "other-profitable" for patients, as its presence or absence directly affects a patient's health outcomes. A provider needs to have their patient's interests at heart, but without the ability to enact those positive intentions, even the best intentions are rendered meaningless. Similarly, a provider who has the knowledge to treat a patient but lacks the care or concern to thoughtfully administer this treatment will also not be effective. Accordingly, assessments of positive intentions (warmth) and the ability to enact those positive intentions (competence) are both critical in judgments of providers. Thus, a provider who seems *both* credible and likeable may be the most likely to influence patients' health.

Summary

Perceptions of the degree to which a provider "gets it" (i.e., competence) and "gets me" (i.e., warmth) emerge as two key dimensions in a number of important medical sources including: a) theoretical models of effective medical care, b) measures of patient satisfaction, c) measures of effective patient–provider interactions, and d) empirical research on patient–provider interactions. This suggests that the medical literature has implicitly deemed these two dimensions as pervasive and essential even if researchers did not explicitly use the terms competence and warmth. Likewise, the psychological literature has identified these same dimensions as cornerstones of impression formation more generally.

Thus, the psychological and medical literatures can be connected and simplified by utilizing the framework of competence and warmth. Competence and warmth distill a host of complex provider characteristics that are deemed essential to effective healthcare into two core dimensions. Accordingly, the competence and warmth framework can help practitioners and researchers alike identify which provider qualities are influential in patient–provider interactions and foster greater understanding of how to embody these core qualities to patients.

DO COMPETENCE AND WARMTH MODERATE PLACEBO RESPONSE?

We now turn our attention to examining whether the dimensions of competence and warmth moderate placebo response. To do so, we review four empirical studies which experimentally altered elements of patient–provider interactions to test this question (10–13).

One study deliberately manipulated competence and warmth and three of these studies (10, 12, 13) did so implicitly, although the researchers may not have explicitly set out to do so. **Table 8** illustrates how the interpersonal variables altered in these studies map onto the competence and warmth dimensions. Next, we review each of these studies and their methods in detail.

Czerniak et al. (12): Competence and Warmth Moderate Placebo Pain Relief

Czerniak and colleagues (12) found that warm and competent patient–provider interactions increased healthy volunteers' responses to a placebo cream described as an analgesic ($N = 122$). This ostensible analgesic was applied before patients underwent a cold pressor task (99) in which participants immerse their hand in an ice water bath to induce pain. First, all participants underwent the cold pressor task without the administration of placebo cream to assess baseline pain threshold (defined as the number of seconds before participants indicated that they felt pain from the cold) and pain tolerance (defined as the number of seconds before participants withdrew their hand from the cold). Then, a trained actor posing as a doctor administered a placebo cream (i.e., moisturizer lotion) described as a pain relief cream before participants repeated the cold pressor task. The researchers randomly assigned patients to receive this placebo cream either in the context of a standard interaction designed to mimic a routine doctor's visit, or in the context of an enhanced

TABLE 8 | Competence and warmth as dimensions of patient–provider interaction manipulations that enhanced placebo response.

Verbal cues	**Competence**	**Warmth**
Howe et al. (11)	• Articulate *vs.* filler words • Clear, confident tone *vs.* not	• Introduce self *vs.* not • Call patient by name *vs.* never ask for patient name
Czerniak et al. (12)	• Ask patient to describe pain using metaphors *vs.* don't ask patient to describe pain at all • Emphasize has been studying pain for many years *vs.* not	• Stand to greet patient by name *vs.* remain seated • Shake hand and invite in *vs.* not • Repeat patients' answers to questions *vs.* merely type answer
Kaptchuk et al. (10)	• Ask additional questions about symptoms *vs.* state had reviewed questionnaire • States that have had much experience with treatment *vs.* not	• Warm/friendly manner *vs.* state cannot converse with patients • Use empathetic statements *vs.* not • Actively listen (e.g., repeat patient words) *vs.* not • Words of encouragement *vs.* not
Fuentes et al. (13)	• Ask additional questions about patient symptoms	• Actively listen (e.g., repeat patient words) *vs.* not • Use empathetic statements *vs.* not • Words of encouragement *vs.* not
	Bridging competence and warmth • Ask patient how they normally address pain *vs.* not (Czerniak) • Ask additional questions about patient understanding of condition *vs.* not (Kaptchuk) • Ask additional questions about conditions' impact on life *vs.* not (Kaptchuk) • Ask about patient lifestyle (Fuentes) • Ask about patient understanding of causes of symptoms (Fuentes)	
Non-verbal cues	**Competence**	**Warmth**
Howe et al. (11)	• Make no mistakes *vs.* putting blood pressure cuff on upside down	• Make eye contact *vs.* stare at computer • Sit closer to patient *vs.* maintain physical distance
Czerniak et al. (12)	• Look at cell phone *vs.* not interrupted by cell phone • Examine patient closely *vs.* briefly and more distantly • Hand cream to patient with a large gesture *vs.* not	• Make eye contact *vs.* stare at computer • Patient inspection involves touch *vs.* patient inspection is only visual
Kaptchuk et al. (10)	• 20 seconds of thoughtful silence during procedure *vs.* not	
Fuentes et al. (13)		• Use of physical touch *vs.* not • Increased eye contact • Warm tone of voice
Environmental cues	**Competence**	**Warmth**
Howe et al. (11)	• Nametag indicates higher status (i.e., MD) *vs.* lower status (i.e., student doctor) • Professional attire (e.g., long white coat) *vs.* casual, wrinkled clothes, shorter white coat • Room organized, neat *vs.* disorganized, scattered papers	• Posters with warm images (e.g., red panda) *vs.* no personalized posters
Czerniak et al. (12)	• Carefully select cream from jars *vs.* pull from top drawer of desk	

N = number of participants in the study.

interaction involving characteristics of ritual healing. Both the standard and enhanced interactions lasted approximately 5 minutes or less. Placebo response was measured by pain threshold and pain tolerance relative to baseline.

The researchers drew their inspiration for the "enhanced" interaction from a shaman's healing ritual, incorporating performance behaviors. The authors used a variety of performance-relevant behaviors in the enhanced interactions, including verbal behaviors (i.e., dialogue) that was "personal, attentive to the volunteer, and used imagery in the questions and explanations" (12, p. 4), and deliberate non-verbal behaviors, such as dramatic gestures and movement in the room. The dimensions altered, however, can be organized under the simplifying and unifying framework of provider competence and warmth. Some verbal behaviors (e.g., emphasizing that the provider has many years of experience studying pain, helping patients to use metaphors to describe their pain) and non-verbal behaviors (e.g., examining participants' hands more closely, not being distracted by a cell phone during the interaction) likely increased perceived competence. Several other verbal behaviors (e.g., greeting the participant by name) and non-verbal behaviors (e.g., increasing eye contact, using physical touch) likely increased perceived warmth. Some manipulations may have targeted both competence and warmth. In the enhanced interaction, the provider asked the patient to describe how they normally treat pain, thereby taking the patient's own preferences into account (signaling warmth) and gathering additional information to shape treatment decisions (signaling competence).

Participants who experienced the "enhanced" interaction showed a higher pain tolerance during the cold pressor task compared to participants who experienced the standard interaction. However, the effect of the interaction on pain tolerance was limited to participants who were categorized as "placebo responders" (defined as participants who showed at least a 30% increase in pain tolerance after placebo administration), suggesting that participants who were not susceptible to placebos were also not influenced by the differences in provider interactions.

Kaptchuk et al. (10): Competence and Warmth Moderate Placebo Treatment for IBS

Kaptchuk et al. (10) found that warm and competent patient–provider interactions increased patients' response to sham acupuncture administered over the course of 3 weeks to treat irritable bowel syndrome (IBS) ($N = 262$). Sham acupuncture uses a device that creates the appearance of having pierced the skin without actually doing so, in order to mimic the needles used during acupuncture. Patients were randomly assigned to either receive this sham acupuncture in a short interaction in which providers restricted their engagement with patients, or in an enhanced interaction in which providers engaged in additional conversation with patients and incorporated several verbal and non-verbal behaviors to improve the quality of the interaction. Placebo response was measured through self-reported improvement in IBS symptoms, self-reported adequate relief of IBS symptoms, self-reported symptom severity, and the self-reported degree to which the condition interfered with a patient's quality of life.

The enhanced interaction in this study (10) was designed to be "warm, empathetic, and confident" (p. 2), clearly covering the two dimensions of provider competence and warmth. As documented in **Table 5**, several verbal behaviors (e.g., stating that the provider has had much experience with the treatment) and non-verbal behaviors (e.g., pausing in thoughtful silence for 20 s during the procedure) may have evoked competence, and several verbal behaviors (e.g., making empathetic statements, using active listening and words of encouragement) may have evoked warmth, and some behaviors may have evoked both competence and warmth (e.g., asking additional questions about the patient's understanding of the treatment).

Patients who experienced the "enhanced" interaction reported greater relief and improvement in symptoms over the course of the 6-week study. Thus, the positive effects of placebo acupuncture were augmented by a more supportive interaction with a provider.

Fuentes et al. (13): Competence and Warmth Moderate Placebo Treatment for Chronic Low Back Pain

Fuentes et al. (13) used a similar protocol to Kaptchuk et al. (10) to enhance the interaction between therapists and patients with chronic low back pain who were randomly assigned to either undergo active interferential current therapy (IFC) or sham IFC ($N = 117$).

In one condition, patients experienced a limited interaction in which the provider left after briefly introducing themselves and explaining the treatment. Providers also mentioned that they had been instructed not to converse with participants and minimized discussion accordingly. In the "enhanced interaction" condition, patients experienced an enhanced interaction involving several verbal behaviors that may have enhanced perceived competence (e.g., the provider asked patients additional questions about their symptoms), several that may have enhanced perceived warmth (e.g., active listening, making empathetic statements such as "I can understand how difficult this must be for you"), and several that may have targeted both (e.g., asking patients about their lifestyle and assessing their understanding of their condition). Enhanced interactions also employed several non-verbal behaviors that conveyed warmth, including a warmer tone of voice, increased eye contact, and incorporating physical touch into treatment.

The authors found that the enhanced interaction improved outcomes for both active and placebo treatment. As with Kaptchuk et al. (10), the enhanced interaction also involved providers spending more time with patients (5 min in the limited interaction and about 30 min in the enhanced interaction).

Howe et al. (11): Competence and Warmth Moderate Placebo Treatment for Allergic Reactions

The only study to date which has altered provider warmth and competence *independently* from each other in order to tease apart the dimensions was done by Howe and colleagues (11). In this study, healthy volunteers ($N = 164$) underwent a skin prick test using histamine, which was administered by a trained research assistant who acted as the provider. (Histamine causes a mild allergic reaction in which the skin becomes red, itchy, and a small bump called a "wheal" surfaces.) The provider then applied a placebo cream (moisturizer lotion) to the allergic reaction. This study also separated the qualities of the interaction from the expectations set about the placebo treatment. In the positive expectations condition, they stated that the cream was an antihistamine cream that would reduce the reaction and decrease itching. In the negative expectations condition, they stated that the cream was a histamine agonist that would increase the reaction and increase itching. Placebo/nocebo response was measured by the change in participants' wheal size (in mm) after the placebo cream was applied.

The same provider administered the cream to all participants, but was trained to interact with participants in one of four ways to evoke: 1. High warmth and high competence, 2. High warmth and low competence, 3. Low warmth and high competence, or 4. Low warmth and low competence. Competence was evoked through verbal manipulations (e.g., speaking confidently, minimizing filler words), non-verbal manipulations (e.g., executing all procedures flawlessly), and environmental manipulations (e.g., professional attire, room neat and clean). Warmth was also evoked through verbal manipulations (e.g., the provider introducing themselves and calling the participant by name), non-verbal manipulations (e.g., increased eye contact, sitting closer to participant), and environmental manipulations (e.g., hanging posters with warm images in the exam room). All conditions were the same length of time, thereby controlling for time interacting with the provider. Patients' self-reported ratings of the provider at the end of the exam suggested that perceived competence and warmth were substantially impacted through these simple changes, suggesting that perceptions of providers' warmth and competence are readily malleable.[3]

The researchers found that competence and warmth moderated placebo and nocebo responses. When the provider appeared

[3] Effect sizes for the impact of the experimental alterations of competence and warmth on patient perceptions of providers indicated that the changes in provider behavior designed to evoke competence had a medium size effect on patient perceptions of provider competence, Cohen's $d = 0.47$, and the changes in provider behavior designed to evoke warmth had a large effect on patient perceptions of provider warmth, Cohen's $d = 1.75$.

both competent and warm, participants who heard positive expectations about the cream showed a greater decrease in wheal size than participants who heard negative expectations about the cream. However, when participants had interacted with a provider who was low in warmth and low in competence, their wheal size continued to increase at the same rate regardless of whether or not the provider had set positive or negative expectations about the cream. Mixed conditions (i.e., high warmth/low competence and low warmth/high competence) produced moderate effects on the allergic reaction and were indistinguishable from each other.

This study disentangled precise dimensions of patient–provider relationships and found that warmth and competence shape participants' physiological responses to the expectations that a provider sets about treatment. An additional important take-away from this study is that neither warmth nor competence seemed to matter more than the other; rather, it was only when the two qualities worked together that they effectively created an overall interaction that boosted placebo effects.

Summary

Overall, these studies support the notion that a provider's competence and warmth are key dimensions that moderate placebo response: interactions in which a provider demonstrated both competence and warmth resulted in a greater response to placebo and active treatments. Thus, whether a provider "gets it" and "gets me" can affect the potency of a medical treatment. Accordingly, both of these dimensions constitute an important part of effective healthcare.

WHAT ARE THE MECHANISM THROUGH WHICH COMPETENCE AND WARMTH MODERATE PLACEBO RESPONSE?

The patient–provider relationship is frequently cited as a key mechanism of placebo effects in and of itself (10, 83, 85). As discussed in depth above, the patient–provider relationship assessed in placebo research clearly contains dimensions of both competence and warmth. However, the mechanisms through which a competent and warm patient–provider interaction might boost placebo response are unclear from past literature. We propose that provider competence and warmth increases overall placebo effects by boosting known placebo mechanisms, including a) expectations and b) classical conditioning (i.e., repeated associations between a medical stimulus, such as a pill, and the active drug inside the pill, which could lead to a conditioned response) (4, 100). By augmenting the impact of these known placebo mechanisms, provider warmth and competence then boost overall placebo response.

Competence and Warmth Amplify Patient Expectations About Treatment

A provider's competence and warmth make a provider more credible, believable, and/or persuasive (101), which may boost the impact of the expectations they set about treatment. A doctor who is competent (e.g., conducts a thorough exam, seems knowledgeable) will appear as a more reputable source of medical information. Thus, the patient may be more likely to internalize this competent doctor's message about a treatment's efficacy. Likewise, when a doctor is warm (e.g., is friendly, calls the patient by name), the patient may feel more relaxed, at ease, and like they are in good hands. The patient may then be more receptive to what the doctor has to say, view the doctor as trustworthy, and believe expectations set about the efficacy of treatment to a greater extent. A warm provider may also appear to better understand the patient, and thus enhance this patient's confidence that the provider has chosen a course of treatment that will work for them as an individual. Patients may thus listen to and trust explanations of warm and competent providers to a greater degree, and accordingly be more influenced by them physiologically (102–104).

Competent and warm providers may thus be better able to set specific, individualized expectations that are more meaningful, helpful, and relevant for patients. When expectations resonate with patients more, they increase healing to a greater degree (105). Similarly, competent and warm providers may also more effectively set expectations about patients' own role in their health management. For example, one study examining enhanced provider interactions included provider comments such as "You can really make a difference in your cold by taking care of yourself" (82, 83). Such a statement may have no potency if a provider seems to lack understanding of medicine and/or of a particular patient's needs and abilities, but may be particularly believable coming from a provider who is seen as competent and warm. As another example, warm and competent providers may also be more skilled at reassuring patients in the course of treatment by providing information clearly and confidently, and providing concern that seems authentic. This could positively impact patient expectations by, for example, resolving uncertainty (106, 107). Furthermore, a recent study shows that even without medication, physician reassurance can help patients feel better by reducing symptoms and speeding healing (108). Through such processes, competent and warm providers may more effectively leverage the healing that is evoked by setting patients' expectations about treatment.

Competence and Warmth Activate Conditioned Patient Responses

Competent and warm providers may more effectively leverage strategies that boost conditioned responses (109), including diagnostic rituals such as the physical exam. Further, competent and warm providers may simply *feel* more like a healer to the patient, thus leading the patient to experience greater conditioned responses. We thus theorize that warm and competent providers may activate conditioned patient responses because they are more effective at engaging in healing rituals that produce conditioned responses, and because patients may experience a greater conditioned response to these providers themselves.

It has been widely acknowledged that healing rituals can lead to conditioned placebo responses (10, 12, 100, 110). Even normal, everyday procedures that rely on only basic medical competence, such as taking a patient's height, weight, and blood pressure, can become conditioned stimuli for healing in a clinical context (105). However, there is likely great variation in how effectively different providers utilize healing rituals. Warmer, more competent providers may more effectively engage in rituals that produce conditioned healing responses in patients. For example, the physical exam may not only lead to more and better information with which to heal patients, it is likely that the "laying of hands" in the physical exam is healing in and of itself (111–113). Likewise, research on the meaning of touch for patients with cancer found that nurses' touch conveyed confidence to these patients, and this confidence in turn increased positive patient expectations and hope of recovery (114). But touch can also be aversive for some patients—if a provider is not warm and competent, then these rituals could backfire. Providers who are competent and warm—who are socially and emotionally skilled and able to quickly gauge what their patients prefer—may be better able to utilize medical rituals effectively, particularly rituals involving touch. Indeed, provider warmth and competence may be crucial in the success of these rituals, as these dimensions may be the difference between a ritualistic experience that boosts healing and one that is off-putting for the patient.

Research also supports the hypothesis that a competent and warm provider may activate or amplify conditioned patient responses. Some research suggests that providers who seemed more like an expert or fit certain stereotypes about a doctor were able to enhance response to a treatment regardless of whether they used a placebo or active acupuncture treatment (115). Providers who are competent and warm may thus seem more like a good doctor or a trustworthy expert, which could bolster a conditioned response to seeing such a provider. While participants in past research have been shown to display conditioned responses to doctors who better fit stereotypical images of doctors (i.e., White male doctors), as medicine grows ever-more diverse, aspects of the provider, such as warmth and competence, may rise up in place of physical attributes to produce conditioned responses in patients. We are not aware of any research that directly assesses the impact of provider competence and warmth on conditioning, and future research should investigate how qualities of the provider may amplify or otherwise influence the effects of conditioned healing.

Summary

We have proposed that competence and warmth play a key role in placebo effects by strengthening expectations and conditioning during medical treatment. Of course, being complex psychological phenomena, provider competence and warmth likely impact placebo response in many other ways, including by reducing stress and anxiety, increasing positive emotions, influencing physiology directly, and by beneficially impacting behavioral mechanisms such as adherence, motivation, and adoption of healthier behaviors (82, 83, 101, 116–123). Indeed, past research and theory have suggested that provider competence and warmth can set off a cascade of physiological changes in the body, including "endogenous neurotransmitters, hormones, and immune regulators that mimic the expected or conditioned pharmacological effects" (124). But given the known importance of expectations and conditioning for placebo effects and the attention paid to these mechanisms in the placebo literature (3), we have restricted our discussion to these mechanisms and encourage future research and theory on other mechanisms.

HOW CAN PROVIDERS DELIBERATELY LEVERAGE COMPETENCE AND WARMTH IN CLINICAL CARE?

In order to leverage competence and warmth in healthcare, we need to first understand what these qualities look like from a patient perspective and how they might reasonably be enacted from a provider perspective. To this end, we asked both patients and providers to describe their healthcare experiences. Their responses capture patients' and providers' impressions of how competence and warmth can be demonstrated in clinical encounters.

Provider Competence and Warmth From a Patient Perspective

To find out what provider competence and warmth look like to patients and how providers might embody this in real-world settings, we asked participants to describe healthcare experiences in open-ended responses.

Participants first answered two questions in which they imagined what positive qualities and behaviors a good doctor would demonstrate:

1. Imagine what a good doctor would be like. What good things would this doctor do?
2. What good qualities would this doctor have?

Then, participants reflected on their own experiences. Participants first responded yes or no to whether they had ever seen a good doctor, and yes or no to whether they had ever seen a bad doctor. If respondents answered yes to one or both questions, they were asked, respectively:

3. What was good about this doctor? and/or
4. What was bad about this doctor?

These questions allowed us to assess qualities and actions drawn from both patients' own positive or negative interactions with providers and patients' ideal interactions with providers.

In total, 334 American participants between age 25 and 87 (51.2% women, M_{age} = 43.10, SD_{age} = 14.09) responded to the survey, which was administered by Survey Sampling International (SSI). Participants came from a variety of racial/ethnic backgrounds [29.6% White/Caucasian, 24.9% Asian/Pacific Islander, 23.4% Black/African-American, 22.2% Hispanic/Latino (a)] and socioeconomic backgrounds (41.0% college education, 28.8% some college education, 21.0% high school or less). Detailed survey methods are described in previous publications (125).

Following similar procedures to previous research (125), the authors generated a coding scheme including five categories related to a provider's competence and four categories related to a provider's warmth (see **Table 9** for a description and examples of each category).

Two research assistants who were blind to hypotheses coded a randomly selected 20% of participant responses (N = 67 each) by

TABLE 9 | Competence and warmth demonstrations and examples from patients.

Category		
Competence/"gets it": *Related to a provider's effectiveness at diagnosing and treating disease/symptoms of disease and encouraging healthy habits*		
Subcategory	**Description**	**Examples**
"Medically knowledgeable" (general knowledge)	The doctor is medically knowledgeable, knows current research and practices, intelligent, well-educated.	What good qualities would this doctor have? "Good education" "Up to date with newer medical studies" What good things would this doctor do? "Be smart" "Keep me well informed about newest developments" What was good about this doctor? "He had a good knowledge of his field." "Gives proper treatment" What was bad about this doctor? "Incompetent" "Could not explain the importance of a balanced nutrition"
"Keeps at it" (thoroughness)	The doctor has an attention to detail, is thorough, covers all alternatives, has a good work ethic.	What good qualities would this doctor have? "Looks at any and all alternatives" "Would honestly do everything he can to help me" What good things would this doctor do? "Check me out thoroughly" "Would follow-up on small concerns" What was good about this doctor? "Attention to detail" "She was thorough." What was bad about this doctor? "Very rushed" "Not interested in your illness, just what prescriptions do you need"
"Understands my health" (patient-specific medical knowledge)	The doctor knows your health history, has experience with patients like you (e.g., demographically, or with particular conditions).	What good qualities would this doctor have? "Experience treating similar people" "Know my medical record for all appointments" What good things would this doctor do? "Know your body, habits, and family history" "Personalized patient care" What was good about this doctor? "Knows about my health" "Knew our family history" What was bad about this doctor? "Never had a patient who exhibited similar symptoms" "Ignoring available information about my history"
"Has seen it" (experience)	The doctor has a lot and/or a variety of medical experience, has been practicing medicine for many years, has seen a lot of patients and treated a lot of medical conditions generally, knows their skill set/limitations.	What good qualities would this doctor have? "Very experienced" "Not attempt any treatment beyond that which he is skilled" What good things would this doctor do? "Know the area of his practice" "Refers you to specialist as needed What was good about this doctor? "He knows what he's talking about." "If can't help, finds someone who can"
"Walks the walk" (role modeling)	The doctor maintains their own physical and mental health.	What good qualities would this doctor have? "Practices a healthy lifestyle themselves" "A great role model" What good things would this doctor do? "Eat healthy" What was good about this doctor? "Practiced what he preached"

TABLE 9 | Continued

Category		
Warmth/"gets me": *Related to a provider' viewing and/or treating the patient as a social being, including acknowledging their perspective about life and/or health*		
"Is nice to me" (general warmth)	The doctor is friendly, open, caring, empathetic, respectful, has people skills.	What good qualities would this doctor have? "Care about what is wrong with you" "A warm smile" What good things would this doctor do? "Have empathy" "Not get irritated or mean when I need help" What was good about this doctor? "Was very nice" "Had genuine concern for my well-being" What was bad about this doctor? "Disrespectful and rude" "Lack of compassion"
"Hears me" (active listening)	The doctor has good interpersonal skills, listens carefully, makes patient feel at ease, treats patient as an equal.	What good qualities would this doctor have? "Listens to your concerns" "Easy to talk to" What good things would this doctor do? "Talk to me like I am an intelligent person" "He listens and believes me" What was good about this doctor? "Good people skills and great communicator" "Listened to what I was saying" What was bad about this doctor? "Didn't talk to me" "Inability to listen"
"In it for the right reasons" (passion for people)	The doctor practices medicine to help people, loves what they do.	What good qualities would this doctor have? "A people person who really cares about people" "Passionate about what they do" What was good about this doctor? "Good heart for the people" "Loved their job" What was bad about this doctor? "Was not humanitarian"
"Takes the patient's perspective" (patient-specific warmth)	The doctor knows who the patient is and treats them as an individual, understands the patient's personal life, background, culture, worries, values, etc., thinks about a patient's individual goals, needs, and perspectives.	What good qualities would this doctor have? "Do not treat you just as a patient but as a person" "Interested in me as an individual" What good things would this doctor do? "Try to relate to me on a personal level so I feel comfortable with any diagnosis they give" "Cares about you as a person" What was good about this doctor? "Asked questions about what was going on in my life" "Treated me as a person, not an illness" What was bad about this doctor? "Didn't take the time to get to know me" "Didn't bother treating me like a human"

indicating whether participants mentioned this category (1) or did not mention this category (0) for each of the four questions. Coders first coded 20% of the responses and then discussed and reconciled any discrepancies before coding the 80% of responses (N = 100 each). Inter-rater agreement before coders began coding the full sample was acceptable (Cohen's kappas > 0.70 for all categories). Data and scripts for analysis are provided at https://osf.io/5jxqy/.

Table 9 depicts the different ways patients have experienced various forms of competence and warmth in their interactions with providers. These data illustrate that there is a rich variety of ways in which providers can demonstrate competence and warmth to their patients. Of course, providers do not need to embody all of these qualities or perform all of these actions. **Table 9** is not meant to be a checklist for effective medical care, but rather a rolodex of possible tools providers could employ to bolster competence and warmth. Ultimately, what appears to matter for healthcare is that patients perceive a provider as "getting it" and "getting me," and there are many routes to these same ends.

Competence and Warmth in Providers' Own Words

In addition to patient perspectives, we turned to medical providers to understand what competence and warmth actually look like in clinical practice. During focus groups in four Primary Care clinics, care team members were asked to generate ways they signal competence and warmth to patients. We collected responses from approximately 100 care team members, including physicians, medical assistants, nurses, and clinic staff.

Responses were collected during a larger training session, which also explained competence and warmth in the "gets it" and "gets me" framework. Providers were then asked: "How do you signal to patients that you get both 'it' and 'them'?" Providers listed at least one example of how they signal competence to patients (getting "it") and at least one example of how they signal warmth to patients (getting "them"). Providers' responses were coded and grouped into thematically similar strategies. **Table 10** lists the overarching strategies that emerged from providers' responses, and displays exemplary quotes for each category in providers' own words.

Importantly, as with **Table 9**, **Table 10** is not meant to suggest that providers adopt all of these strategies. Rather, **Table 10** suggests a multitude of ways in which providers could bolster patient perceptions of competence and warmth, allowing providers to flexibly choose strategies that resonate with them and/or their patients' needs. Providers' responses span a wide range of behaviors, suggesting that everyone on the care team can bring their own unique strengths to signaling competence and warmth in clinical encounters. Critically, since these responses were generated from all members of the care team, they encompass ways each person in a healthcare clinic could signal competence and warmth to patients, whether their role is as a physician interacting with patients intimately or a scheduler who only interacts with patients by phone. Providers can thus take away from these responses what is most useful and actionable for them given the particular demands and resources of their healthcare context.

While some of these behaviors are basic, intuitive practices (e.g., eye contact), others require the cooperation of multiple medical team members (e.g., consistent messaging to patients). Some require greater investments of time and effort, such as researching personalized treatments beforehand and asking patients about their concerns. However, there are also many strategies that require only intention, not additional time, such as calling patients by name, greeting them warmly, and projecting confidence. Further, even the more effort-intensive demonstrations of competence and warmth may save providers more time in the long-term by fully addressing patients' needs.

SUMMARY AND FUTURE DIRECTIONS

By framing patient–provider interactions in terms of provider competence and warmth, we have capitalized on decades of research in social perception to begin to unpack how and why patient–provider interactions can boost placebo response. We have also begun to identify ways providers can leverage competence and warmth to deliberately increase the strength of placebo response. The competence/warmth framework simplifies the complex patient–provider interaction, organizing dozens of behaviors and qualities into two key dimensions that can be bolstered through a variety of routes. It thus suggests to clinicians and researchers alike what to focus on to enhance patient–provider interaction quality and suggests many practical ways to leverage the power of the patient–provider relationship to boost placebo effects. It is our hope that the framework of competence and warmth will provide researchers and practitioners alike with a theoretical grounding from which to understand what aspects of the patient–provider interaction are most critical for improving various outcomes of medical care.

Further, we have illustrated how this framework is present in both placebo and medical literature, as evident in the way studies alter patient–provider interactions and how patient–provider interactions are assessed. This framework thus unites literature on social perception, placebo research, and medical research. In addition, considering the influence of competence and warmth could help generate novel ideas about the mechanisms through which patient–provider interactions may boost placebo effects. We have proposed that competence and warmth make a provider seem more credible and foster patients' belief in them and their statements, and thus enhance the impact of treatment expectations. We have also proposed that a provider's competence and warmth strengthen conditioned responses to providers and to medical rituals. There are a variety of other possible mechanisms through which a provider's competence and warmth may influence placebo effects and patient health more broadly (e.g., reducing anxiety).

It is likely that the qualities of competence and warmth foster other benefits in patient–provider interactions beyond enhancing patients' placebo response. For example, a provider's competence and warmth may establish trust between patients and providers. Indeed, competence and warmth emerge as core dimensions in literature on the social perception of trust (126, 127). Prerequisites of trust include *ability*, or "skills, competencies, and characteristics that enable a party to have influence within some specific domain," and *benevolence*, or "the extent to which a trustee is believed to want to do good to the trustor, aside from an egocentric profit motive" (127), dimensions that also map onto the competence/warmth framework. The possible relationship between competence, warmth, and trust in the healthcare context should be explored. Focusing on showcasing competence and warmth to patients could offer providers a more tangible route through which to establish trust than abstract recommendations to "get patients to trust you." Demonstrations of competence and warmth may be especially important for building trust in cross-race, cross-gender, and cross-socioecomonic status interactions, where trust may be absent or more challenging to build.

The guiding framework of competence and warmth inspires many open questions and serves as a guide for future research. One question is the degree to which competence and warmth are separable in medicine. A recent study found that behaviors often used to cultivate perceptions of warmth (e.g., eye contact) bolstered perceptions of *both* warmth and competence (128). In a medical context, perhaps especially when patients are anxious about very personal concerns, "getting me" may be critical to whether a provider seems to "get it." Likewise, the degree to which signals of warmth and competence *via* verbal, *vs.* non-verbal, *vs.* environmental cues evoke perceptions of these qualities is an open question. In addition, the universality of different experimental manipulations of warmth and competence is uncertain. For example, Kraft-Todd and colleagues (128) found

TABLE 10 | Competence and warmth strategies and examples from the healthcare team.

Category		
Competence/"gets it": *Related to a provider's* effectiveness at diagnosing and treating disease/symptoms of disease; a provider's understanding of diagnosis, prognosis, and treatment*		
Strategy	**Description**	**Examples**
"Review ahead of time"	The provider reviews relevant information on the patient, potential options, procedures, and treatments before the medical encounter in order to prepare.	Review medically-relevant information "Make sure you are familiar with the topics you discuss" "Have a couple of options in mind for therapy/plan before appointment" Review patient condition "Briefly reviewing chart before visit so patients feel that you are updated with their recent health changes/specialist views" "Not asking questions easily seen by chart review" "Reference things in the patient's chart to demonstrate that I've familiarized myself with their case"
"Encourages questions"	The provider encourages the patient to ask questions and have questions answered.	"State that you understand & address questions about their disease/treatment" "Ask if and answer any questions the patient has"
"Provide explanations"	The provider, upon hearing the questions and concerns of the patient, provides clear and informative answers.	"Very informational" "Explaining carefully"
"Share helpful information"	The provider shares information to inform the patient on their own role and experience, on the medical conditions and procedures, and on the medical institution. The patient thus feels well-informed and part of the decision-making process.	Share about the provider's role and experience "Relate their situation to another similar situation I've worked on and resolved" "Say, 'I've seen this many times'" "Explain my role and how I can help them" Share medically-relevant information "Explain rationale for treatment, including previous patient experiences" "Explain procedures in detail with examples" "When going over I advise patient on appropriate time frames for things they are due for and the importance of health maintenance." "Pull up supporting evidence; online resources to help guide our decisions" Share about medical institution "Knowledge of the hospital success measurements" "Use (name of institution) and our excellence, resources for context"
"Personalize medical care"	The provider understands the unique context and history of the patient, catering to their specific needs when providing medical care.	"Say, 'There are lots of ways to achieve improvement, and I/we want to find one(s) that fit you best'" "Say, '"As part of your (name of clinic) care team, we are looking for a personalized approach for you'"
"Be transparent"	The provider demonstrates honesty and transparency when faced with questions they do not have the answers to. They show a commitment to learning the answers and following up with the patient.	"If you don't know how to address something, instead of making something up, validate and give direction" "I admit when I'm not sure or don't know and offer continued research or collaboration with MD" "Being open about areas of ambiguity in outcomes/diagnoses/management/follow-up plan"
"Show confidence"	The provider conveys confidence in their role, work, experience, and surrounding environment.	"Provide statements with confidence, meaning not to be too wishy-washy about it" "Have my routine and comfortably complete it; confident in my environment" "Confidence in delivery of assessment & preparation for it"
"Have familiarity with procedures"	The provider is prepared and comfortable with the medical procedures performed.	"Keep arm elevated during blood pressure" "How relaxed you are while performing a procedure" "Take their weight, height, vitals" "Do procedures calmly/don't seem flustered"
"Appear presentable"	The provider presents themselves and their environment as being put-together.	"Wear professional clothes" "Keep the room clean" "Organized exam room for regular visits & for procedures"
"Collaborate well with team"	The provider holds an understanding of how they are one piece of a medical care team, leveraging their team members to contribute to the same goals.	"Everyone giving the same message & on the same page" "Say, 'I'm part of a team of ___ here to serve you and be sure you get the best care'" "Collaboration with peers" "Say, 'Dr. __ is the best!'"

TABLE 10 | Continued

Category		
Warmth/"gets me": *Related to a provider viewing and/or treating the patient as a social being, including acknowledging their perspective about life and/or health; a provider's understanding about the patient's goals, needs, and concerns*		
Strategy	**Description**	**Examples**
"Greet effectively"	The provider understands the importance of starting the encounter off on the right foot to make patients feel valued.	Introduction of provider "Introducing myself at beginning of visit" Communicate through body language "Greeting the patient with a smile and a handshake" "Nonverbal cues—eye contact, smile—when opening the encounter" "Open the door for them" "Ask, 'what brings you in to see your doctor?' with eye contact" Use patient's name "Always greet by preferred name and gender" "Call them by their first name with a huge smile on my face"
"Use intentional body language"	The provider's body language and nonverbal cues communicate that the patient is the focus of attention.	"Always smiling at patient" "During the first few minutes of connecting, make eye contact with patient and not computer" "Empathetic touch when upset" "Sit down when talking to patient"
"Form personal connection with patient"	The provider cares for the patient as a whole person, showing curiosity for and investment into their lives beyond the context of the medical encounter.	"Opening and closing each visit with brief small talk" "Ask about holiday plans and family details" "Say, 'I'm so glad to see you today'" "Establish rapport by asking personal questions" "Judicious sharing of personal information"
"Remember past details about patient"	The provider forms a relationship with the patient over the long-term, thoughtfully referencing previous encounters and details.	"Know something of major significance about their lives (e.g., going through a divorce" "Talk about a previous subject discussed during last appointment" "Say name of patient, family members, pets"
"Value patient's needs"	The provider prioritizes the patient's needs, concerns, and perspective. They are able to give space for the patient to express themselves and then respond to demonstrate that the patient has been heard.	Listen "Actively listening to their concerns" "Listen generously; use silence" "Repeat my understanding of what patient says" Be attuned to patient's needs "Know their health care goals" "Ask them what their thoughts are about the proposed treatment" "Anticipate patient's need by asking before leaving room"
"Convey empathy"	The provider empathizes with where the patient is coming from and conveys that they are alongside the patient as support.	"Regardless of their reason for visit, I always tell the patient, 'Don't worry, we will take care of you today!'" "Use 'we' to show that we are in this together" "Validate their feelings and expressions of concern" "Use cultural intelligence and respect"

**For this table, "providers" refers to the entire care team at several Primary Care clinics, and thus includes physicians, medical assistants, nurse practitioners, front desk staff, behavioral health specialists, and pharmacists.*

that a provider wearing a white coat did not enhance perceptions of their competence; indeed, evidence on whether professional attire affects perceptions of competence is largely mixed (129–132). Another interesting question for future research is whether the impact of more general qualities of warmth (e.g., general friendliness, eye contact) and competence (e.g., general medical knowledge, articulateness) differs from the impact from patient-specific qualities of warmth (e.g., asking a patient questions about their personal life) and competence (e.g., demonstrating knowledge of a patient's family history) (see examples in **Table 1**).

While we have proposed that warmth and competence work in conjunction to promote healing, certain contexts, patients, and circumstances may render either warmth or competence more impactful. Cultural expectations and individual personalities or desires likely play a role in both whether patients value warmth or competence more as well as how patients prefer their providers to express warmth and competence (133–135). For example, some of the behaviors patients and providers associated with warmth reviewed in this paper (e.g., calling a patient by their first name) may backfire in other cultural contexts. Different medical problems may also lend themselves more to warmth or competence; warmth might be especially important when dealing with a chronic illness that needs to be managed over time, while competence may be seen as more critical during surgery and for setting broken bones (136).

Regarding questions about the role of patient–provider relationships in placebo effects, the greatest need seems to be for rigorous research that separates the impact of provider interaction style (i.e., providers who are competent and/or warm) from the impact of explicitly set positive expectations. Future studies could help unpack whether and how provider competence and warmth boost the impact of expectations, as well as how setting expectations might boost patient perceptions of provider warmth and competence. This article hypothesizes mechanisms for how provider warmth and competence can boost placebo response, but future empirical research is needed to assess the validity of these hypotheses in research and clinical practice.

We hope that understanding and leveraging the competence and warmth framework will allow us to better address some of the most pressing problems in healthcare. For example, a wealth of literature suggests that minority populations in the U.S. have worse health outcomes (137). Recent authors suggest that differences in placebo response may be at least partially responsible for some of these disparities (138). Deliberately and effectively leveraging warmth and competence could potentially help healthcare providers diminish these gaps. Particularly as research suggests that cultural or racial matches between providers and patients lead to improved healthcare outcomes, warmth and competence may be one way to bridge the divide between providers and patients of different cultural, racial, and socioeconomic backgrounds, as it remains unfeasible to ensure that each patient is seen by a provider who matches his or her cultural background (135). Future research could explore these exciting possibilities.

It is our hope that the theory outlined in this article will spur novel research in these areas. Understanding how, when, and why provider qualities such as warmth and competence boost placebo response will not only further our comprehension of placebo effects, but will also help the medical field deliberately harness important mechanisms of placebo response that can be taken advantage of ethically alongside active medication and treatment. By distilling the complex qualities and behaviors of effective healthcare providers into warmth and competence, we hope this framework can help researchers and practitioners alike to more clearly understand how to practically and purposefully leverage the patient–provider relationship to boost placebo effects and improve healing.

AUTHOR CONTRIBUTIONS

LH and KL analyzed the data and drafted the manuscript and AC provided critical revisions. All authors listed have made a substantial, direct, and intellectual contribution to the work, and approved it for publication.

FUNDING

AC is supported by NIH/NCCIH Grant #DP2AT009511. AC and LH are supported by a grant from the Robert Wood Johnson Foundation. KL holds a Stanford Interdisciplinary Graduate Fellowship—Anonymous Donor.

ACKNOWLEDGMENTS

The authors would like to thank Michelle Chang, Isaac Handley-Miner, Matthew Bernstein, and Rina Horii for their contributions to the manuscript.

REFERENCES

1. Thomas KB. The placebo in general practice. *Lancet* (1994) 344(8929):1066–7. doi: 10.1016/S0140-6736(94)91716-7
2. Miller FG, Kaptchuk TJ. The power of context: reconceptualizing the placebo effect. *J R Soc Med* (2008) 101(5):222–5. doi: 10.1258/jrsm.2008.070466
3. Petrie KJ, Rief W. Psychobiological mechanisms of placebo and nocebo effects: pathways to improve treatments and reduce side effects. *Annu Rev Psychol* (2019) 70:599–625. doi: 10.1146/annurev-psych-010418-102907
4. Finniss DG, Kaptchuk TJ, Miller F, Benedetti F. Biological, clinical, and ethical advances of placebo effects. *Lancet* (2010) 375(9715):686–95. doi: 10.1016/S0140-6736(09)61706-2
5. Benedetti F, Maggi G, Lopiano L, Lanotte M, Rainero I, Vighetti S, et al. Open versus hidden medical treatments: the patient's knowledge about a therapy affects the therapy outcome. *Prev Treat* (2003) 6(1):ArtID 1a. doi: 10.1037/1522-3736.6.1.61a
6. Colloca L, Lopiano L, Lanotte M, Benedetti F. Overt versus covert treatment for pain, anxiety, and Parkinson's disease. *Lancet Neurol* (2004) 3(11):679–84. doi: 10.1016/S1474-4422(04)00908-1
7. Kam-Hansen S, Jakubowski M, Kelley JM, Kirsch I, Hoaglin DC, Kaptchuk TJ, et al. Altered placebo and drug labeling changes the outcome of episodic Migraine attacks. *Sci Transl Med* (2014) 6(218):218ra5. doi: 10.1126/scitranslmed.3006175
8. Vachon-Presseau E, Berger SE, Abdullah TB, Huang L, Cecchi GA, Griffith JW, et al. Brain and psychological determinants of placebo pill response In chronic pain patients. *Nat Commun* (2018) 9(1):3397. doi: 10.1038/s41467-018-05859-1
9. Price DD, Milling LS, Kirsch I, Duff A, Montgomery GH, Nicholls SS. An analysis of factors that contribute to the magnitude of placebo analgesia in an experimental paradigm. *Pain* (1999) 83(2):147–56. doi: 10.1016/S0304-3959(99)00081-0
10. Kaptchuk TJ, Kelley JM, Conboy LA, Davis RB, Kerr CE, Jacobson EE, et al. Components of placebo effect: randomised controlled trial in patients with irritable bowel syndrome. *BMJ* (2008) 2008:999–1003. doi: 10.1136/bmj.39524.439618.25
11. Howe LC, Goyer JP, Crum AJ. Harnessing the placebo effect: exploring the influence of physician characteristics on placebo response. *Health Psychol* (2017) 36(11):1074–82. doi: 10.1037/hea0000499
12. Czerniak E, Bigeon A, Ziv A, Karnieli-Miller O, Weiser M, Alon U, et al. Manipulating the placebo response in experimental pain by altering doctor's performance style. *Front Psychol* (2016) 7:874. doi: 10.3389/fpsyg.2016.00874

13. Fuentes J, Armijo-Olivo S, Funabashi M, Miciak M, Dick B, Warren S, et al. Enhanced therapeutic alliance modulates pain intensity and muscle pain sensitivity in patients with chronic low back pain: an experimental controlled study. *Phys Ther* (2014) 94(4):477–89. doi: 10.2522/ptj.20130118
14. Fiske ST, Cuddy AJC, Glick P. Universal dimensions of social cognition: warmth and competence. *Trends Cogn Sci* (2007) 11(2):77–83. doi: 10.1016/j.tics.2006.11.005
15. Cuddy AJC, Glick P, Beninger A. The dynamics of warmth and competence judgments, and their outcomes in organizations. *Res Organ Behav* (2011) 31:73–98. doi: 10.1016/j.riob.2011.10.004
16. Roussos G, Dunham Y. The development of stereotype content: the use of warmth and competence in assessing social groups. *J Exp Child Psychol* (2016) 141:133–44. doi: 10.1016/j.jecp.2015.08.009
17. Judd CM, James-Hawkins L, Yzerbyt V, Kashima Y. Fundamental dimensions of social judgment: understanding the relations between judgments of competence and warmth. *J Pers Soc Psychol* (2005) 89(6):899–913. doi: 10.1037/0022-3514.89.6.899
18. Cuddy AJC, Fiske ST, Glick P. Warmth and competence as universal dimensions of social perception: the stereotype content model and the BIAS Map. *Adv Exp Soc Psychol* (2008) 40:61–149. doi: 10.1016/S0065-2601(07)00002-0
19. Fiske ST, Cuddy AJC, Glick P, Xu J. A model of (often mixed) stereotype content: Competence and warmth respectively follow from perceived status and competition. *J Pers Soc Psychol* (2002) 82(6):878–902. doi: 10.1037//0022-3514.82.6.878
20. Abele AE, Cuddy AJC, Judd CM, Yzerbyt VY. Fundamental dimensions of social judgment. *Eur J Soc Psychol* (2008) 38:1063–5. doi: 10.1002/ejsp.574
21. Rosenberg S, Nelson C, Vivekananthan PS. A multidimensional approach to the structure of personality impressions. *J Pers Soc Psychol* (1968) 9(4):283–94. doi: 10.1037/h0026086
22. Wojciszke B. Multiple meanings of behavior: construing actions in terms of competence or morality. *J Pers Soc Psychol* (1994) 67(2):222–32. doi: 10.1037/0022-3514.67.2.222
23. Wojciszke B, Dowhyluk M, Jaworski M. Moral and competence-related traits: how do they differ? *Polish Psychol Bull* (1998) 29:283–94.
24. Cuddy AJC, Fiske ST, Glick P. The BIAS Map: behaviors from intergroup affect and stereotypes. *J Pers Soc Psychol* (2007) 92(4):631–48. doi: 10.1037/0022-3514.92.4.631
25. Wojciszke B, Abele AE, Baryla W. Two dimensions of interpersonal attitudes: liking depends on communion, respect depends on agency. *Eur J Soc Psychol* (2009) 39(6):973–90. doi: 10.1002/ejsp.595
26. Wojciszke B, Abele AE. The primacy of communion over agency and its reversals in evaluations. *Eur J Soc Psychol* (2008) 38(7):1139–47. doi: 10.1002/ejsp.549
27. Abele AE, Wojciszke B. Agency and communion from the perspective of self Versus others. *J Pers Soc Psychol* (2007) 93(5):751–63. doi: 10.1037/0022-3514.93.5.751
28. Ambady N, Rosenthal R. Half a minute: predicting teacher evaluations from thin slices of nonverbal behavior and physical attractiveness. *J Pers Soc Psychol* (1993) 64(3):431–41. doi: 10.1037//0022-3514.64.3.431
29. Ambady N, Rosenthal R. Thin slices of expressive behavior as predictors of interpersonal consequences: a meta-analysis. *Psychol Bull* (1992) 111(2):256–74. doi: 10.1037/0033-2909.111.2.256
30. Ambady N, Hallahan M, Rosenthal R. On judging and being judged accurately in zero-acquaintance situations. *J Pers Soc Psychol* (1995) 69(3):518–29. doi: 10.1037/0022-3514.69.3.518
31. Willis J, Todorov A. First impressions. *Psychol Sci* (2006) 17(7):592–8. doi: 10.1111/j.1467-9280.2006.01750.x
32. Cogsdill EJ, Todorov AT, Spelke ES, Banaji MR. Inferring character from faces: a developmental study. *Psychol Sci* (2014) 25(5):1132–9. doi: 10.1177/0956797614523297
33. Ambady N, LaPlante D, Nguyen T, Rosenthal R, Chaumeton N, Levinson W. Surgeons' tone of voice: a clue to malpractice history. *Surgery* (2002) 132(1):5–9. doi: 10.1067/msy.2002.124733
34. Carli LL, LaFleur SJ, Loeber CC. Nonverbal behavior, gender, and influence. *J Pers Soc Psychol* (1995) 68(6):1030–41. doi: 10.1037/0022-3514.68.6.1030
35. Knutson B. Facial expressions of emotion influence interpersonal trait inferences. *J Nonverbal Behav* (1996) 20(3):165–82. doi: 10.1007/BF02281954
36. Fiske ST, Xu J, Cuddy AC, Glick P. (Dis)respecting versus (dis)liking: status and interdependence predict ambivalent stereotypes of competence and warmth. *J Soc Issues* (1999) 55(3):473–89. doi: 10.1111/0022-4537.00128
37. Hojat M, Gonnella J, Nasca T, Mangione S, Vergare M, Magee M. Physician empathy: definition, components, measurement, and relationship to gender and specialty. *Am J Psychiatry* (2002) 159:1563–9. doi: 10.1176/appi.ajp.159.9.1563
38. Halpern J. What is clinical empathy? *J Gen Intern Med* (2003) 18:670–4. doi: 10.1046/j.1525-1497.2003.21017.x
39. Decety J, Fotopoulou A. Why empathy has a beneficial impact on others in medicine unifying theories. *Front Behav Neurosci* (2015) 8:1–11. doi: 10.3389/fnbeh.2014.00457
40. Engel GL. The need for a new model: a challenge for biomedicine. *Science* (1977) 196(4286):129–36. doi: 10.1126/science.847460
41. McCormick J. Death of the personal doctor. *Lancet* (1996) 348(9028):667–8. doi: 10.1016/S0140-6736(96)03512-X
42. Smith RC, Hoppe RB. The patient's story: integrating the patient- and physician-centered approaches to interviewing. *Ann Intern Med* (1991) 115(6):470–7. doi: 10.7326/0003-4819-115-6-470
43. Bensing J. Bridging the gap: the separate worlds of evidence-based medicine and patient-centered medicine. *Patient Educ Couns* (2000) 39(1):17–25. doi: 10.1016/S0738-3991(99)00087-7
44. Brown J, Stewart M, McCracken E, McWhinney IR, Levenstein J. The patient-centered clinical method. 2. Definition and application. *Fam Pract* (1986) 3(2):75–9. doi: 10.1093/fampra/3.2.75
45. Grol R, De Maeseneer J, Whitfield M, Mokkink H. Disease-centred versus patient-centred attitudes: comparison of general practitioners in Belgium, Britain and the Netherlands. *Fam Pract* (1990) 7(2):100–3. doi: 10.1093/fampra/7.2.100
46. King A, Hoppe RB. "Best practice" for patient-centered communication: A Narrative review. *J Grad Med Educ* (2013) 5(3):385–93. doi: 10.4300/JGME-D-13-00072.1
47. Levenstein JH, McCracken EC, McWhinney IR, Stewart MA, Brown JB. The patient-centered clinical method: 1. A model for the doctor-patient interaction in family medicine. *Fam Pract* (1986) 3:24–30. doi: 10.1093/fampra/3.1.24
48. Sweeney KG, MacAuley D, Gray DP. Personal significance: the third dimension. *Lancet* (1998) 351(9096):134–6. doi: 10.1016/S0140-6736(97)06316-2
49. Mishler EG. *The discourse of medicine: Dialetics of medical interviews*. New Jersey: Ablex Publishing Corporation (1984).
50. Eddy DM. Anatomy of a decision. *JAMA* (1990) 263(3):441–3. doi: 10.1001/jama.263.3.441
51. Engel GL. How much longer must medicine's science be bound by a seventeenth century world view? *Psychother Psychosom* (1992) 57(1–2):3–16. doi: 10.1159/000288568
52. De Valck C, Bensing J, Bruynooghe R, Batenburg V. Cure-oriented versus care-oriented attitudes in medicine. *Patient Educ Couns* (2001) 45(2):119–26. doi: 10.1016/S0738-3991(00)00201-9
53. Van Dulmen S, Van Den Brink-Muinen A. Patients' preferences and experiences in handling emotions: a study on communication sequences in primary care medical visits. *Patient Educ Couns* (2004) 55(1):149–52. doi: 10.1016/S0738-3991(04)00300-3
54. Bensing J, Schreurs K, De Rijk A. The role of the general practitioner's affective behaviour in medical encounters. *Psychol Health* (1996) 11(6):825–38. doi: 10.1080/08870449608400278
55. Roter D, Larson S. The Roter interaction analysis system (RIAS): utility and flexibility for analysis of medical interactions. *Patient Educ Couns* (2002) 46(4):243–51. doi: 10.1016/S0738-3991(02)00012-5
56. Charon R. Narrative medicine: a model for empathy, reflection, profession, and trust. *JAMA* (2001) 286(15):1897–902. doi: 10.1001/jama.286.15.1897
57. Helman CG. Disease versus illness in general practice. *J R Coll Gen Pract* (1981) 31:548–52.
58. Kelm Z, Wormer J, Walter J, Feudtner C. Interventions to cultivate physician empathy: a systematic review. *BMC Med Educ* (2014) 14(1):219. doi: 10.1186/1472-6920-14-219
59. Zimmerman C, Piccolo LD, Bensing J, Bergvik S, De Haes H, Eide H, et al. Coding patient emotional cues and concerns in medical consultations: The Verona coding definitions of emotional sequences (VR-CoDES). *Patient Educ Couns* (2011) 82:141–8. doi: 10.1016/j.pec.2010.03.017

60. Hawthorne G, Sansoni J, Hayes L, Marosszeky N, Sansoni E. Measuring patient satisfaction with health care treatment using the Short Assessment of Patient Satisfaction measure delivered superior and robust satisfaction estimates. *J Clin Epidemiol* (2014) 67(5):527–37. doi: 10.1016/j.jclinepi.2013.12.010
61. Associates PG. Patient satisfaction with the outpatient experience: how does your organization measure up? *Healthc Exec* (2003) 18(3):94–5.
62. Zusman EE. HCAHPS replaces press ganey survey as quality measure for patient hospital experience. *Neurosurgery* (2012) 71(2):N21–4. doi: 10.1227/01.neu.0000417536.07871.ed
63. Risser NL. Development of an instrument to measure patient satisfaciton with nurses and nursing care in primary care settings. *Nurs Res* (1975) 24(1):45–52. doi: 10.1097/00006199-197501000-00011
64. Jenkinson C, Coulter A, Bruster S. The Picker Patient Experience Questionnaire: development and validation using data from in-patient surveys in five countries. *Int J Qual Health Care* (2002) 14(5):353–8. doi: 10.1093/intqhc/14.5.353
65. Wolf MH, Putnam SM, James SA, Stiles WB. The medical interview satisfaction scale: development of a scale to measure patient perceptions of physician behavior. *J Behav Med* (1978) 1(4):391–401. doi: 10.1007/BF00846695
66. Baker R. Development of a questionnaire to assess patients' satisfaction with consultations in general practice. *Br J Gen Pract* (1990) 40(341):487–90.
67. La Monica EL, Oberst MT, Madea AR, Wolf RM. Development of a patient satisfaction scale. *Res Nurs Health* (1986) 9(1):43–50. doi: 10.1002/nur.4770090108
68. Howe LC, Hardebeck EJ, Leibowitz KA, Crum AJ. Providers' demeanor impacts patient perceptions of visit length. *J Gen Intern Med* (2019) 34(2):182–3. doi: 10.1007/s11606-018-4665-6
69. Presson AP, Zhang C, Abtahi AM, Kean J, Hung M, Tyser AR. Psychometric properties of the Press Ganey outpatient medical practice survey. *Health Qual Life Outcomes* (2017) 15:32. doi: 10.1186/s12955-017-0610-3
70. Westbrook KW, Babakus E, Grant CC. Measuring patient-perceived hospital service quality: validity and managerial usefulness of HCAHPS scales. *Health Mark Q* (2014) 31(2):97–114. doi: 10.1080/07359683.2014.907114
71. Sitzia J. How valid and reliable are patient satisfaction data? An analysis of 195 studies. *Int J Qual Health Care* (1999) 11(4):319–28. doi: 10.1093/intqhc/11.4.319
72. Roter D, Hall J. Studies of doctor-patient interaction. *Annu Rev Public Health* (1989) 10:163–80. doi: 10.1146/annurev.pu.10.050189.001115
73. Krupat E, Frankel RM, Stein T, Irish J. The Four Habits Coding Scheme: validation of an instrument to assess clinicians' communiucation behavior. *Patient Educ Couns* (2006) 62:38–45. doi: 10.1016/j.pec.2005.04.015
74. Frankel RM, Stein T. Getting the most out of the clinical encounter: The Four Habits model. *Perm J* (1996) 3(3):79–88.
75. Ong LML, Visser MRM, Kruyver IPM, Bensing JM, Van Den Brink-Muinen A, Stouthard JML, et al. The Roter Interaction Analysis System (RIAS) in oncological consultations: psychometric properties. *Psychooncology* (1998) 7(5):387–401. doi: 10.1002/(SICI)1099-1611(1998090)7:5<387::AID-PON316>3.0.CO;2-G
76. Roter D 1991. The Roter Method of Interaction Process Analysis. RIAS Manual; 1991.
77. Cavaco A, Roter D. Pharmaceutical consultations in community pharmacies: utility of the Roter Interaction Analysis System to study pharmacist-patient communication. *Int J Pharm Pract* (2010) 18(3):141–8. doi: 10.1211/ijpp.18.03.0003
78. Hojat M, Louis DZ, Markham FW, Wender R. Physicians' empathy and clinical outcomes for diabetic patients. *Acad Med* (2011) 86(3):359–64. doi: 10.1097/ACM.0b013e3182086fe1
79. Di Blasi Z, Harkness E, Ernst E, Georgiou A, Kleijnen J. Influence of context effects on health outcomes: a systematic review. *Lancet* (2001) 357(9258):757–62. doi: 10.1016/S0140-6736(00)04169-6
80. Hojat M, Mangione S, Nasca TJ, Cohen MJM, Gonnella JS, Erdmann JB, et al. The Jefferson Scale of Physician Empathy: development and preliminary psychometric data. *Educ Psychol Meas* (2001) 61(2):349–65. doi: 10.1177/00131640121971158
81. Kane GC, Gotto JL, Mangione S, West S, Hojat M. Jefferson Scale of Patient's Perceptions of Physician Empathy: preliminary psychometric data. *Croat Med J* (2007) 48(1):81–6.
82. Rakel D, Barrett B, Zhang Z, Hoeft T, Chewning B, Marchand L, et al. Perception of empathy in the therapeutic encounter: effects on the common cold. *Patient Educ Couns* (2011) 85(3):390–7. doi: 10.1016/j.pec.2011.01.009
83. Barrett B, Rakel D, Chewning B, Marchand L, Rabago D, Brown R, et al. Rationale and methods for a trial assessing placebo, echinacea, and doctor-patient interaction in the common cold. *Explore (NY)* (2007) 3(6):561–72. doi: 10.1016/j.explore.2007.08.001
84. Moore PJ, Adler NE, Robertson PA. Medical malpractice: the effect of doctor-patient relations on medical patient perceptions and malpractice intentions. *West J Med* (2000) 173(4):244–50. doi: 10.1136/ewjm.173.4.244
85. Kelley JM, Kraft-Todd G, Schapira L, Kossowsky J, Riess H. The influence of the patient-clinician relationship on healthcare outcomes: a systematic review and meta-analysis of randomized controlled trials. *PLoS One* (2014) 9(4):e94207. doi: 10.1371/journal.pone.0094207
86. Butow P, Cockburn J, Girgis A, Bowman D, Schofield P, D'Este C, et al. Increasing oncologists' skills in eliciting and responding to emotional cues: evaluation of a communication skills training program. *Psychooncology* (2008) 17(3):209–18. doi: 10.1002/pon.1217
87. Girgis A, Cockburn J, Butow P, Bowman D, Schofield P, Stojanovski E, et al. Improving patient emotional functioning and psychological morbidity: evaluation of a consultation skills training program for oncologists. *Patient Educ Couns* (2009) 77(3):456–62. doi: 10.1016/j.pec.2009.09.018
88. Bieber C, Müller KG, Blumenstiel K, Schuller-Roma B, Richter A, Hochlehnert A, et al. Partizipative Entscheidungsfindung (PEF) mit chronischen Schmerzpatienten: Der Patient als Partner im medizinischen Entscheidungsprozess. *Bundesgesundheitsblatt Gesundheitsforschung Gesundheitsschutz* (2004) 47(10):985–91. doi: 10.1007/s00103-004-0914-4
89. Bieber C, Müller KG, Blumenstiel K, Hochlehnert A, Wilke S, Hartmann M, et al. A shared decision-making communication training program for physicians treating fibromyalgia patients: effects of a randomized controlled trial. *J Psychosom Res* (2008) 64(1):13–20. doi: 10.1016/j.jpsychores.2007.05.009
90. Cals JWL, Hopstaken RM, Butler CC, Hood K, Severens JL, Dinant GJ. Improving management of patients with acute cough by C-reactive protein point of care testing and communication training (IMPAC3T): study protocol of a cluster randomised controlled trial. *BMC Fam Pract* (2007) 8:15. doi: 10.1186/1471-2296-8-15
91. Cals JWL, Butler CC, Hopstaken RM, Hood K, Dinant GJ. Effect of point of care testing for C reactive protein and training in communication skills on antibiotic use in lower respiratory tract infections: cluster randomised trial. *BMJ* (2009) 338:b1374. doi: 10.1136/bmj.b1374
92. Zanna MP, Hamilton DL. Attribute dimensions and patterns of trait inferences. *Psychon Sci* (1972) 27(6):353–4. doi: 10.3758/BF03328989
93. Wojciszke B, Bazinska R, Jaworski M. On the dominance of moral categories in impression formation. *Pers Soc Psychol Bull* (1998) 24(12):1251–63. doi: 10.1177/01461672982412001
94. Ybarra O, Chan E, Park D. Young and old adults' concerns about morality and competence. *Motiv Emot* (2001) 25(2):85–100. doi: 10.1023/A:1010633908298
95. Wojciszke B, Pienkowski R, Maroszek A, Brycz H, Ratajczak M. Lay inferences of personality traits: the role of behaviour prototypicality and between-trait differences. *Eur J Soc Psychol* (1993) 23(3):255–72. doi: 10.1002/ejsp.2420230304
96. Abele AE, Hauke N, Peters K, Louvet E, Szymkow A, Duan Y. Facets of the fundamental content dimensions: agency with competence and assertiveness-communion with warmth and morality. *Front Psychol* (2016) 7:1810. doi: 10.3389/fpsyg.2016.01810
97. Peeters G. In search for a social-behavioral approach-avoidance dimension associated with evaluative trait meanings. *Psychol Belg* (2001) 41(4):187–203.
98. Dupree C, Fiske ST. *Self-presentation in interracial settings: the competence downshift by white liberals. J Pers Soc Psychol* (2019). Advance online publication. doi: 10.31234/osf.io/pv2ab
99. Lovallo W. The cold pressor test and autonomic function: a review and integration. *Psychophysiology* (1975) 12(3):268–82. doi: 10.1111/j.1469-8986.1975.tb01289.x
100. Montgomery GH, Kirsch I. Classical conditioning and the placebo effect. *Pain* (1997) 72(1–2):107–13. doi: 10.1016/S0304-3959(97)00016-X
101. Wampold BE. The therapeutic value of the relationship for placebo effects and other healing practices. *Int Rev Neurobiol* (2018) 139:191–210. doi: 10.1016/bs.irn.2018.07.019
102. Carvalho C, Caetano JM, Cunha L, Rebouta P, Kaptchuk TJ, Kirsch I. Open-label placebo treatment in chronic low back pain: a randomized

controlled trial. *Pain* (2016) 157(12):2766–72. doi: 10.1097/j.pain.0000000000000700
103. Kaptchuk TJ, Friedlander E, Kelley JM, Sanchez MN, Kokkotou E, Singer JP, et al. Placebos without deception: a randomized controlled trial in irritable bowel syndrome. *PLoS One* (2010) 5(12):e15591. doi: 10.1371/journal.pone.0015591
104. Locher C, Nascimento AF, Kirsch I, Kossowsky J, Meyer A, Gaab J. Is the rationale more important than deception? a randomized controlled trial of openlabel placebo analgesia. *Pain* (2017) 158(12):2320–8. doi: 10.1097/j.pain.0000000000001012
105. Zion SR, Crum AJ. Mindsets matter : a new framework for harnessing the placebo effect in modern medicine. *Int Rev Neurobiol* (2018) 138:137–60. doi: 10.1016/bs.irn.2018.02.002
106. Williams S, Weinman J, Dale J, Newman S. Patient expectations: what do primary care patients want from the GP and how far does meeting expectations affect patient satisfaction? *Fam Pract* (1995) 12(2):193–201. doi: 10.1093/fampra/12.2.193
107. Thomas KB. General practice consultations: is there any point in being positive? *Br Med J (Clin Res Ed)* (1987) 294(6581):1200–2. doi: 10.1136/bmj.294.6581.1200
108. Leibowitz KA, Hardebeck EJ, Goyer JP, Crum AJ. Physician assurance reduces patient symptoms in US adults: an experimental study. *J Gen Intern Med* (2018) 33(12):2051–2. doi: 10.1007/s11606-018-4627-z
109. Price DD, Finniss DG, Benedetti F. A comprehensive review of the placebo effect: recent advances and current thought. *Annu Rev Psychol* (2008) 59:565–90. doi: 10.1146/annurev.psych.59.113006.095941
110. Bąbel P, Bajcar EA, Adamczyk W, Kicman P, Lisińska N, Świder K, et al. Classical conditioning without verbal suggestions elicits placebo analgesia and nocebo hyperalgesia. *PLoS One* (2017) 12(7):e0181856. doi: 10.1371/journal.pone.0181856
111. Kugler J, Verghese A. The physical exam and other forms of fiction. *J Gen Intern Med* (2010) 25(8):756–7. doi: 10.1007/s11606-010-1400-3
112. Verghese A, Brady E, Kapur CC, Horwitz RI. The bedside evaluation: ritual and reason. *Ann Intern Med* (2011) 155(8):550–3. doi: 10.7326/0003-4819-155-8-201110180-00013
113. Barnett K. A theoretical construct of the concepts of touch as they relate to nursing. *Nurs Res* (1972) 21(2):102–10. doi: 10.1097/00006199-197203000-00002
114. Morales E. Meaning of touch to hospitalized Puerto Ricans with cancer. *Cancer Nurs* (1994) 17(6):464–9. doi: 10.1097/00002820-199412000-00003
115. White P, Bishop FL, Prescott P, Scott C, Little P, Lewith G. Practice, practitioner, or placebo? a multifactorial, mixed-methods randomized controlled trial of acupuncture. *Pain* (2012) 153(2):455–62. doi: 10.1016/j.pain.2011.11.007
116. Del Canale S, Louis DZ, Maio V, Wang X, Rossi G, Hojat M, et al. The relationship between physician empathy and disease complications: an empirical study of primary care physicians and their diabetic patients in Parma, Italy. *Acad Med* (2012) 87(9):1243–9. doi: 10.1097/ACM.0b013e3182628fbf
117. Crum AJ, Salovey P, Achor S. Rethinking stress: the role of mindsets in determining the stress response. *J Pers Soc Psychol* (2013) 104(4):716–33. doi: 10.1037/a0031201
118. Kim SS, Kaplowitz S, Johnston MV. The effects of physician empathy on patient satisfaction and compliance. *Eval Health Prof* (2004) 27(3):237–51. doi: 10.1177/0163278704267037
119. Jackson JL, Chamberlin J, Kroenke K. Predictors of patient satisfaction. *Soc Sci Med* (2001) 52(4):609–20. doi: 10.1016/S0277-9536(00)00164-7
120. Crum AJ, Corbin WR, Brownell KD, Salovey P. Mind over milkshakes: mindsets, not just nutrients, determine ghrelin response. *Health Psychol* (2011) 30(4):424–9. doi: 10.1037/a0023467
121. Schwarzer R. Perceived self-efficacy: self-efficacy and health behavior theories. *Measurement* (1997) 1:1–33.
122. Hilliard ME, Eakin MN, Borrelli B, Green A, Riekert KA. Medication beliefs mediate between depressive symptoms and medication adherence in cystic fibrosis. *Health Psychol* (2015) 34(5):496–504. doi: 10.1037/hea0000136
123. Derksen F, Bensing J, Lagro-Janssen A. Effectiveness of empathy in general practice: a systematic review. *Br J Gen Pract* (2013) 63(606):e76–84. doi: 10.3399/bjgp13X660814
124. Neumann M, Edelhäuser F, Kreps GL, Scheffer C, Lutz G, Tauschel D, et al. Can patient-provider interaction increase the effectiveness of medical treatment or even substitute it? an exploration on why and how to study the specific effect of the provider. *Patient Educ Couns* (2010) 80(3):307–14. doi: 10.1016/j.pec.2010.07.020
125. Conner AL, Boles DZ, Markus HR, Eberhardt JL, Crum AJ. Americans' health mindsets: content, cultural patterning, and associations with physical and mental health. *Ann Behav Med* (2019) 53(4):321–32. doi: 10.1093/abm/kay041
126. Schoorman FD, Mayer RC, Davis JH. An integrative model of organizational trust: past, present, and future. *Acad Manage Rev* (2007) 32(2):344–54. doi: 10.5465/amr.2007.24348410
127. Mayer RC, Davis JH, Schoorman FD. An integrative model of organizational trust. *Acad Manage Rev* (1995) 20(3):709–34. doi: 10.5465/amr.1995.9508080335
128. Kraft-Todd GT, Reinero DA, Kelley JM, Heberlein AS, Baer L, Riess H. Empathic nonverbal behavior increases ratings of both warmth and competence in a medical context. *PLoS One* (2017) 12(5):e0177758. doi: 10.1371/journal.pone.0177758
129. Siu FL, Haber M. Patient attitudes toward emergency physician attire. *J Emerg Med* (2005) 29(1):1–3. doi: 10.1016/j.jemermed.2004.12.014
130. Bearman G, Bryant K, Leekha S, Mayer J, Munoz-Price LS, Murthy R, et al. Healthcare personnel attire in non-operating-room settings. *Infect Control Hosp Epidemiol* (2014) 35(02):107–21. doi: 10.1086/675066
131. Michael Petrilli C, Mack M, Janowitz Petrilli J, Hickner A, Saint S, Chopra V. Understanding the role of physician attire on patient perceptions: a systematic review of the literature - Targeting attire to improve likelihood of rapport (TAILOR) investigators. *BMJ Open* (2015) 5(1):e006578. doi: 10.1136/bmjopen-2014-006578
132. Traeger AC, Skinner IW, Hübscher M, Henschke N, Moseley GL, McAuley JH. What you wear does not affect the credibility of your treatment: a blinded randomized controlled study. *Patient Educ Couns* (2017) 100(1):104–11. doi: 10.1016/j.pec.2016.08.009
133. Sims T, Tsai JL, Koopmann-Holm B, Thomas EAC, Goldstein MK. Choosing a physician depends on how you want to feel: the role of ideal affect in health-related decision making. *Emotion* (2014) 14(1):187–92. doi: 10.1037/a0034372
134. Sims T, Tsai JL. Patients respond more positively to physicians who focus on their ideal affect. *Emotion* (2015) 15(3):303–18. doi: 10.1037/emo0000026
135. Sims T, Koopmann-Holm B, Young HR, Jiang D, Fung H, Tsai JL. Asian Americans respond less favorably to excitement (vs. calm)-focused physicians compared to European Americans. *Cult Divers Ethn Minor Psychol* (2018) Jan24(1):1–14. doi: 10.1037/cdp0000171
136. Ashton-James CE, Levordashka A. When the wolf wears sheep's clothing: individual differences in the desire to be liked influence nonconscious behavioral mimicry. *Soc Psychol Pers Sci* (2013) 4(6):643–8. doi: 10.1177/1948550613476097
137. Centers for Disease Control and Prevention. Health, United States, 2015 With Special Feature on Racial and Ethnic Health Disparities. Health, United States. 2015.
138. Friesen P, Blease C. Placebo effects and racial and ethnic health disparities: an unjust and underexplored connection. *J Med Ethics* (2018) 44(11):774–81. doi: 10.1136/medethics-2018-104811

9

A Qualitative Systematic Review of Effects of Provider Characteristics and Nonverbal Behavior on Pain and Placebo and Nocebo Effects

Hojjat Daniali[1] *and Magne Arve Flaten*[2*]

[1] Department of Humanity Sciences, Shahed University, Tehran, Iran, [2] Department of Psychology, Norwegian University of Science and Technology, Trondheim, Norway

Correspondence:
Magne Arve Flaten
magne.a.flaten@ntnu.no

Background: Previous research has indicated that the sex, status, and nonverbal behaviors of experimenters or clinicians can contribute to reported pain, and placebo and nocebo effects in patients or research participants. However, no systematic review has been published.

Objective: The aim of this study was to investigate the effects of experimenter/clinician characteristics and nonverbal behavior on pain, placebo, and nocebo effects.

Methods: Using EmBase, Web of Knowledge, and PubMed databases, several literature searches were conducted to find studies that investigated the effects of the experimenter's/clinician's sex, status, and nonverbal behaviors on pain, placebo, and nocebo effects.

Results: Thirty-four studies were included, 20 on the effects of characteristics of the experimenter/clinician, 11 on the role of nonverbal behaviors, and 3 on the effects of both nonverbal behaviors and characteristics of experimenters/clinicians on pain and placebo/nocebo effects. There was a tendency for experimenters/clinicians to induce lower pain report in participants of the opposite sex. Furthermore, higher confidence, competence, and professionalism of experimenters/clinicians resulted in lower pain report and higher placebo effects, whereas lower status of experimenters/clinicians such as lower confidence, competence, and professionalism generated higher reported pain and lower placebo effects. Positive nonverbal behaviors (e.g., smiling, strong tone of voice, more eye contact, more leaning toward the patient/participant, and more body gestures) contributed to lower reported pain and higher placebo effects, whereas negative nonverbal behaviors (i.e., no smile, monotonous tone of voice, no eye contact, leaning backward from the participant/patient, and no body gestures) contributed to higher reported pain and nocebo effects.

Conclusion: Characteristics and nonverbal behaviors of experimenters/clinicians contribute to the elicitation and modulation of pain, placebo, and nocebo effects.

Keywords: contextual factors, experimenter characteristics, experimenter sex, clinician sex, nonverbal behavior, placebo effect, nocebo effect, pain

INTRODUCTION

The present qualitative review investigated whether the characteristics or nonverbal behavior (NB) of the person administrating painful stimulation affected pain or placebo/nocebo effects in the research participant. The placebo effect is a psychobiological response that may occur following the application of active and inactive interventions (1). Applying an inactive medication paired with positive information about its analgesic effects can reduce pain (2). Likewise, negative information can reverse the analgesic effect of the medication (3, 4) and is called a "nocebo effect" (5, 6). Classical conditioning (previous experience with a treatment) and verbal information about the efficacy of the treatment are involved in the induction of placebo effects and expectations, that a treatment will reduce a symptom (e.g., pain), mediate the effects of both processes (7, 8).

Expecting that a procedure will increase pain may elicit anxiety and increase pain, whereas expecting that a procedure will decrease pain may reduce anxiety and thus reduce pain (9–12). As noted, placebo effects are induced by verbal information and/or classical conditioning [e.g., Refs. (2, 4, 12–14)]. However, other factors can modulate the experience of pain and placebo and nocebo effects. Treatments, whether active or sham, are administered in a compound of situational elements such as medication features (e.g., color of a tablet), the healthcare setting (hospital or clinic layout), and the characteristics and behavior of the experimenter/clinician. Such subtle cues in the environment (7, 15, 16) can affect the treatment outcome. For instance, Levine and Gordon (17) used three different methods of administering an inert substance (injection by a person sitting beside the patient and giving suggestive information; injection by a person in an adjacent room; or an injection by a programmable machine) and showed that even subtle cues that suggest a painkiller was administered could elicit a placebo response.

This systematic review is aimed to focus on the fields of pain and placebo/nocebo effects, due to their large literature background. This review is to our knowledge the first investigation of whether cues such as characteristics and NBs of the experimenter or clinician can affect pain, and placebo and nocebo effects.

Experimenter/Clinician Characteristics

Characteristics of experimenters/clinicians such as sex or gender contribute to the report of pain (18–21). "Gender" refers to the societal definition of characteristics for each sex and consists of beliefs of proper behaviors including pain behaviors. "Sex" refers to biological sex (20, 22). In Western societies, the stereotypical male gender role is characteristically stoic and tries to impress women by their capability to tolerate pain, whereas the female role displays higher sensitivity to pain to induce protective behaviors in men (19). Characteristics of observers or providers can impact the experience of pain (22–25). For instance, Aslaksen et al. (25) indicated that, compared to males tested by a male experimenter, male participants who were tested by a female experimenter reported lower pain. The status of the experimenter/clinician, like the expertise, appearance, and professionalism, is another characteristic that may influence the report of pain or placebo effects (22, 26–31). For instance, Mercer et al. (32) reported that patients perceived clinicians wearing laboratory coats as more professional, whereas clinicians with informal clothes were rated less professional, compared to clinicians with laboratory clothes (29, 32, 33).

Experimenter or Clinician Nonverbal Behaviors

NB is present in almost all human interactions and conveys information that may modulate the verbal message. NB is behavior without a linguistic component (34) and refers to expression of thoughts and feelings through nonverbal expressions (35). NBs can be automatic (36) and may gain priority when there is an incongruity between nonverbal and verbal information (37). NB is divided into positive (NBs that convey a positive emotion, attitude, or relationship) and negative (NBs that convey a negative emotion, attitude, or relationship); and into micro-level (e.g., smiling, leaning forward, hand movement, eye contact, tone of voice, and body gesture) and macro-level behaviors (i.e., a collection of micro-level behaviors that conveys a psychological meaning such as dominance, confidence, or warmth) (38). NB contributes to building of relationships, provides signs about unspoken thoughts and emotions, and strengthens or contradicts verbal information (39). Also, the perception of NBs can be nonconscious and automatic (35, 40–43). Research suggests that NBs of experimenters/clinicians can modulate pain, and placebo/nocebo effects [e.g., Refs. (22, 44)]. For instance, Ambady and Gray (40) demonstrated that clinician's negative NBs, such as lack of smiling, a larger distance from patients, and looking away from them, contributed to decreased cognitive (focused attention and level of consciousness) and physical functioning (walking across a room and getting up from a chair) of patients. Another study indicated that negative NBs of clinicians impacted patient's health outcome as keeping a larger distance, and not looking at patients decreased the satisfaction with the consultation (45).

Thus, the characteristics and NBs of the experimenter/clinician can have consequences for health (3) and a review is therefore warranted. This review investigated 1a) whether experimenters'/clinicians' sex can impact pain and placebo/nocebo effects, 1b) whether the status of experimenters/clinicians influences pain and placebo/nocebo effects, and 2) whether experimenter/clinician NBs affect pain and placebo/nocebo effects.

METHODS

Search Procedure

Searches in the PubMed, EmBase, and ISI databases (Web of Knowledge) were conducted until September 10, 2018. **Table 1** shows the list of Boolean term combinations that were used to search in each database.

Data Extraction

Data were extracted by the first author (HD). The second author (MF) checked the extracted data. The searches resulted in 3,958 hits. Only experimental (i.e., a causal manipulation following

TABLE 1 | Search terms used for the database search.

	AND	OR
"Nonverbal"	"placebo"	"nocebo"
"Nonverbal"	"pain"	
"Nonverbal"	"hyperalgesia"	"analgesia"
"Contextual factor"	"placebo"	"nocebo"
"Contextual factor"	"pain"	
"Contextual factor"	"hyperalgesia"	"analgesia"
"Situational factor"	"placebo"	"nocebo"
"Situational factor"	"pain"	
"Situational factor"	"hyperalgesia"	"analgesia"
"Context"	"placebo"	"Nocebo"
"Context"	"pain"	
"Context"	"hyperalgesia"	"analgesia"
"Subtle cues"	"placebo"	"nocebo"
"Subtle cues"	"pain"	
"Subtle cues"	"hyperalgesia"	"analgesia"
"Nonspecific factors"	"placebo"	"nocebo"
"Nonspecific factors"	"pain"	
"Nonspecific factors"	"hyperalgesia"	"analgesia"
"Experimenter sex"	"placebo"	"nocebo"
"Experimenter sex"	"pain"	
"Experimenter sex"	"hyperalgesia"	"analgesia"
"Experimenter gender"	"placebo"	"nocebo"
"Experimenter gender"	"pain"	
"Experimenter gender"	"hyperalgesia"	"analgesia"
"Physician sex"	"placebo"	"nocebo"
"Physician sex"	"pain"	
"Physician sex"	"hyperalgesia"	"analgesia"
"Physician gender"	"placebo"	"nocebo"
"Physician gender"	"pain"	
"Physician gender"	"hyperalgesia"	"analgesia"
"Clinician sex"	"placebo"	"nocebo"
"Clinician sex"	"pain"	
"Clinician sex"	"hyperalgesia"	"analgesia"
"Clinician gender"	"placebo"	"nocebo"
"Clinician gender"	"pain"	
"Clinician gender"	"hyperalgesia"	"analgesia"
"Provider gender"	"placebo"	"nocebo"
"Provider gender"	"pain"	
"Provider gender"	"hyperalgesia"	"analgesia"
"Clinician sex"	"placebo"	"nocebo"
"Clinician sex"	"pain"	
"Clinician sex"	"hyperalgesia"	"analgesia"
"Experimenter style"	"placebo"	"nocebo"
"Experimenter style"	"pain"	
"Experimenter style"	"hyperalgesia"	"analgesia"
"Experimenter status"	"placebo"	"nocebo"
"Experimenter status"	"pain"	
"Experimenter status"	"hyperalgesia"	"analgesia"
"Experimenter characteristic"	"placebo"	"nocebo"
"Experimenter characteristic"	"pain"	
"Experimenter characteristic"	"hyperalgesia"	"analgesia"
"Physician status"	"placebo"	"nocebo"
"Physician status"	"pain"	
"Physician status"	"hyperalgesia"	"analgesia"
"Physician style"	"placebo"	"nocebo"
"Physician style"	"pain"	
"Physician style"	"hyperalgesia"	"analgesia"
"Physician characteristic"	"placebo"	"nocebo"
"Physician characteristic"	"pain"	
"Physician characteristic"	"hyperalgesia"	"analgesia"

a random assignment in an experiment or a control group), quasi-experimental (i.e., a manipulation without *a priori* random assignment), and correlational (i.e., a non-experimental method to measure the relationship between variables) studies that investigated the contribution of characteristics and/or NBs of experimenters/clinicians to placebo, nocebo, and pain were included. Studies with both humans and animals were included and the primary target outcomes were pain report and pain behavior (e.g., pain intensity, sensitivity, threshold, duration, tolerance, unpleasantness, and pain medication use). The secondary target outcomes were symptom severity, improvement rate, mood, quality of life, and treatment expectation. A placebo response was defined as the difference between a group or condition where placebo treatment was administrated with information that the placebo was a painkiller, and a natural history control group or condition where no treatment was provided. Studies were also included if equal amounts of medication were administrated to all participants/patients, but where different types of information (verbal and/or nonverbal) about the drug were presented to different conditions and groups. Studies that reported a placebo response only as the difference between a pretest and a posttest in the same group were excluded. Studies that reported the effects of contextual factors such as group or family membership (e.g., the role of NBs of mothers on children reports of pain), race and ethnicity (e.g., the effects of black experimenter's sex), etc., without distinction from other characteristic of experimenters/clinicians, were excluded. There were no restrictions regarding the target population of included studies. As the terms "Sex" and "Gender" are inconsistently used in studies, both terms were entered in searches, even though the present review focuses on the effects of sex. There is not a review protocol, but a list of the excluded studies is available by contacting the first author (HD) (**Figure 1**).

In line with previous studies [e.g., Refs. (38, 40)], positive NBs were defined as leaning forward, keeping less distance to the participant or patient, more body gestures, a friendly and warm voice, frequent eye contact, nodding, and smiling. Negative NBs were defined as leaning backward, increased distance to the participant/patient, less body gestures, a cold and flat tone of voice, looking away, and frowning. Thirty-four studies (20 experimental, 11 quasi-experimental, and 3 correlational studies) that reported the effect of experimenters/clinicians characteristics and/or NBs on placebo/nocebo effects or pain were included. Included studies were classified in two tables on the basis of the relativeness to whether characteristics (sex and status) (20 studies, **Table 2**) or NBs (11 studies, **Table 3**) of the experimenter/clinician. Additionally, three studies were included in both tables as they had investigated both NBs and characteristics of experimenters/clinicians. Studies were classified according to design, number of participants, sample (healthy participants, patients, or animals), type of provider (clinician or experimenter), characteristics (**Table 2**) or NB (**Table 3**), target outcome, and the result.

Bias Risk Assessment

In order to represent trustable outcomes, systematic reviews should acknowledge a number of risk of biases (74). Although there is not a protocol review, the aims of this study did

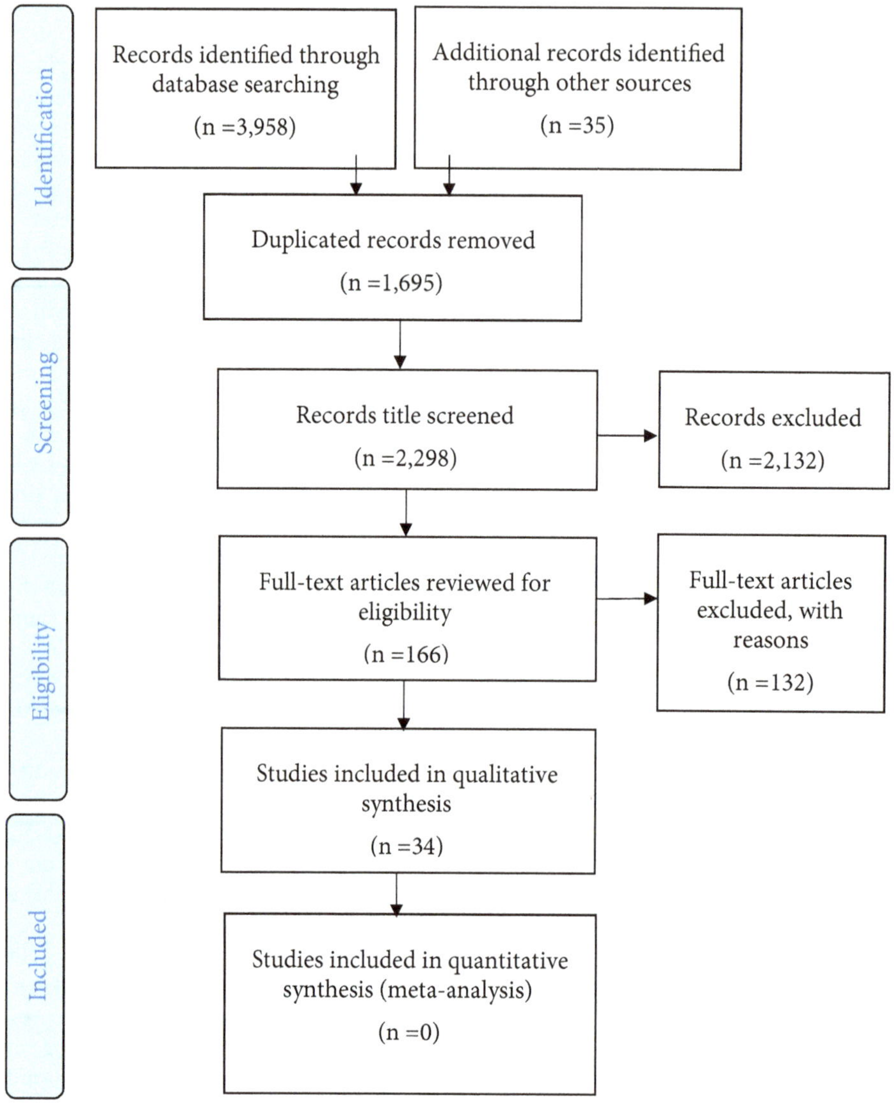

FIGURE 1 | PRISMA flow diagram of steps taken in this review.

not change throughout the study and the risk of reporting bias (i.e., changing the aims according to the nature of obtained findings) was avoided (74). To avoid the risk of evidence selection bias (lack of access to all of the accessible information), the references and citation lists (in google scholar) of all included studies were manually searched and studies that fulfilled the inclusion criteria were entered. Although there is no consensus on what tool to assess the risk of bias in different types of studies, the Cochrane risk of bias tool was used to evaluate the risk of bias in experimental studies that used random assignment and a control group (75). This tool provides a categorized qualitative judgment about the level of risk (high, low, or unknown) across a number of bias types, and includes random sequence generation (i.e., concerning randomization and random sampling), allocation concealment (i.e., hiding the nature of exposure and control groups from participants and personnel), blinding of participants and personnel, blinding of outcome assessment (e.g., the level of objectiveness in outcome assessments), incomplete outcome data (i.e., concerning the missing data and dropouts), selective reporting (i.e., reported and unreported findings), and other biases [for comprehensive information, see Ref. (75)]. To evaluate the risk of bias in quasi-experimental and correlational studies, the Risk of Bias Assessment tool for Non-randomized Studies (RoBANS) was used. RoBANS can be used to assess all study types except for randomized control trials and contains six domains for the risk of bias, which are the selection of participants, confounding variables (i.e., lack of clear distinction between dependent and independent variables), the measurement of exposure (e.g., reliability of measures and scales used), the blinding of outcome assessments, incomplete outcome

TABLE 2 | Studies investigating the role of the experimenter/clinician characteristics (sex and status).

Study	Design	N (Female)	Sample	Type of provider	Characteristics	Target outcome	Result
Egbert et al. (46)	Between subjects	97 (63)	Abdominal surgery patients	Clinicians	Status (confidence)	Narcotic usage, physical and emotional status, postoperative pain intensity	Confident clinicians induced less postoperative narcotics and a better physical and emotional condition.
Otto and Dougher (47)	Between subjects	80 (40)	Healthy participants	Experimenters (2 M and 2 F)	Experimenter sex	Pain intensity	No significant effect of experimenter sex
Levine and De Simone (19)	Mixed design	68 (33)	Healthy participants	Experimenters (1 M and 1 F)	Experimenter sex	Pain intensity	Female experimenters induced lower pain intensity in male subjects.
Feine et al. (48)	Between subjects	20 (20)	Healthy participants	Experimenters (1 F and 1 M)	Experimenter sex	Pain intensity	No significant effect
Bush et al. (49)	Between subjects	47 (24)	Orofacial pain patients	Experimenters (1 F and 1 M)	Experimenter sex	Pain intensity	No significant effect
Fillingim et al. (50)	Between subjects	209 (117)	Healthy participants	Experimenters (1 M and 1 F)	Experimenter and participant sex	Pain thresholds	Female experimenters induced higher pain thresholds in both male and female subjects.
Carter et al. (51)	Between subjects	80 (40)	Healthy participants	Experimenters (not reported)	Experimenter sex	Pain tolerance, electrocardiogram	Female experimenters induced lower electromyogram activity and higher pain tolerance in male and female subjects.
Kállai et al. (22)	Mixed design	160 (80)	Healthy participants	Experimenters (4 M and 4 F)	Status (professional or informal) Experimenter sex	Pain threshold, pain intensity, pain tolerance	Professional experimenters generated higher pain tolerance in participants. Experimenters induced higher pain tolerance in an opposite sex participant. Female experimenters induced higher pain intensity in male and female subjects.
Thorn et al. (52)	Correlation	219 (129)	Healthy participants	Experimenters (1 M and 1 F)	Experimenter sex	Pain intensity and tolerance	No significant effects.
Essick et al. (53)	Between subjects	34 (17)	Healthy participants	Experimenters (1 M and 1 F)	Experimenter sex	Pain sensitivity	No significant effect.
Gijsbers and Nicholson (54)	Between subjects	64 (32)	Healthy participants	Experimenters (1 M and 1 F)	Experimenter gender	Pain threshold	Female experimenters induced higher pain thresholds in male subjects.
Campbell et al. (26)	Between subjects	117 (117)	Healthy participants	Experimenters	Status (university professor or a graduate assistant)	Blood pressure response, pain tolerance, and unpleasantness	Professors generated higher blood pressure responsivity, higher pain tolerance, and lower pain unpleasantness in subjects.
Aslaksen et al. (25)	Mixed design	64 (32)	Healthy participants	Experimenters (3 M and 3 F)	Experimenter and participants gender	Pain intensity, heart rate, and skin conductance	Female experimenters induced lower pain reports in male subjects.
Williams et al. (55)	Correlation	70 (41)	Low back pain patients	Clinicians	Status (a clinician or an assistant)	Pain intensity recollection after an injection	Clinicians generated recalled-pain ratings in patients that correlated the ratings presented following the procedure. Assistants generated higher pain ratings than their original ratings.
Aslaksen and Flaten (56)	Within subjects	63 (32)	Healthy participants	Experimenters (4 M and 4 F)	Experimenter gender	Pain intensity, placebo, stress, arousal, mood	Male experimenters induced higher placebo responses in male subjects.

(Continued)

TABLE 2 | Continued

Study	Design	N (Female)	Sample	Type of provider	Characteristics	Target outcome	Result
Kaptchuk et al. (57)	Between subjects	262 (199)	Patients with IBS	Clinicians	Status (a placebo acupuncture augmented by confidence VS a placebo acupuncture alone—limited—and a waiting list)	Placebo, global improvement, adequate relief, symptom severity, quality of life	Confident clinicians generated higher global improvement, adequate relief of symptoms, better quality of life, and lower symptom severity scores in participants.
Weimer et al. (58)	Between subjects	64 (32)	Healthy participants	Experimenters (1 M and 1 F)	Experimenter sex	Placebo, nausea	No interaction between experimenter sex and placebo responses.
Vigil et al. (59)	Mixed design	352 (169)	Healthy participants	Experimenters (7 M and 7 F and 1 T)	Experimenter gender (and a transgendered experimenter with a feminine status), participant gender	Pain intensity	Male experimenters induced lower pain intensity in both male and female subjects. Transgendered experimenters induced higher pain intensity in female subjects.
Vigil and Alcock (60)	Correlation	199 (86)	Pain patients	Clinicians (not reported)	Experimenter gender	Pain intensity	Both sex patients presented higher pain levels to female clinicians.
Sorge et al. (61)	Mixed design	–	Mice	Experimenters (4 F and 4 M)	Experimenter sex	Facial grimacing as a pain behavior	Male experimenters induced less pain behaviors and more pain inhibition in rodents.
Vigil et al. (62)	Mixed design	132 (132)	Menstrual Pain patients	Clinicians (12 M and 7 F)	Clinician sex	Pain tolerance	Male clinicians induced higher pain tolerance in female patients.
Modić Stanke and Ivanec (27)	Mixed design	96 (69)	Healthy participants	Experimenters	Status (either a professor or a student)	Pain threshold	Professors generated higher pain thresholds in participants. Status influenced males more.
Howe et al. (44)	Between subjects	160 (80)	Healthy Participants	Experimenters	Status (high or low competence)	Placebo and nocebo effects (positive and negative expectations)	Competent experimenters enhanced the effects of positive expectations about a placebo cream on allergic responses.

Just for studies in which the effects of experimenter's/clinician's sex were investigated, the number of providers is presented; however, some studies have not reported this number. F, females; M, Males; T, transgendered; IBS, irritable bowel syndrome.

TABLE 3 | Studies investigating the role of the experimenter/clinician nonverbal behaviors.

Study	Design	N (Female)	Sample	Type of provider	Nonverbal behavior	Target outcome	Result
Egbert et al (46)*	Between subjects	97 (63)	Abdominal surgery patients	Clinicians	Enthusiasm and rapport	Narcotic usage, physical and emotional status, postoperative pain intensity	Enthusiastic clinicians induced less postoperative narcotics and a better physical and emotional condition.
Gryll and Katahn (63)*	Mixed design	160 (75)	Dental patients	Clinicians	Warm or neutral behavior of clinicians	Pain intensity, state anxiety	Enthusiastic messages generated lower pain intensity, less anxiety, and higher placebo effects in subjects.
Brown et al. (64)	Mixed design	101 (49)	Healthy participants	Experimenters	*Active support* (reassuring, encouraging, more understanding, more concern, more eye contact and body gestures), *passive supports* (small talk, few comments, trying to distract the participant, no eye contact or body gestures)	Pain intensity	Active and passive support of providers generated lower pain intensity compared to alone condition.
Kaptchuk et al. (57)	Between subjects	262 (199)	Patients with IBS	Clinicians	A placebo acupuncture *augmented* by a warm and friendly manner, active listening and empathy VS a placebo acupuncture alone (*limited*) and a waiting list	Placebo, global improvement, adequate relief, symptom severity, quality of life	Warm and friendly manner of clinicians generated higher global improvement, adequate relief of symptoms, better quality of life, and lower symptom severity scores in participants.
Verheul et al. (65)	Between subjects	30 (30)	Patients with menstrual pain	Clinicians	*Warm and empathic communication* (directing gaze and body posture toward participants) VS *cold and formal communication* (directing gaze and body posture away from participants).	State anxiety, affective state and outcome expectancies	Warm and empathic communication combined with positive expectations led to lower state anxiety. Affect-oriented communication style of providers influenced the positive and negative affects of participants.
Modić Stanke and Ivanec (66)	Mixed design	48 (48)	Healthy participants	Experimenters	Physical distance	Pain reports	No significant effects for the physical distance of unfamiliar observers on participants' pain reports.
Bohns and Wiltermuth (67)	Between subjects	89 (44)	Healthy participants	Experimenters	Personal space and tone of voice	Pain threshold	Preserving the personal space and speaking softly led to higher pain thresholds.
Valentini et al. (68)	Within subjects	27 (12)	Healthy participants	Experimenters	Observation of *facial expressions* with different emotional content (neutral, pain, and happy)	Pain intensity, placebo effect	Facial expressions (especially happy faces) boosted the placebo analgesia.
Ruben and Hall (69)	Within subjects	95 (55)	Healthy participants	Experimenters	*Nonverbally supportive provider* (friendly voice, leaning forward, open body posture, eye contact, nodding, and smiling) VS *nonverbally unsupportive provider* (rarely looking to camera, looking down frequently, folding arms, leaning back, distancing, cold tone of voice).	Judging the intensity of pain in the target (either with a supportive or a unsupportive clinician)	Nonverbally supportive experimenters generated more valid impressions of pain ratings and judges had higher accuracy in their pain assessment when viewing participants tested by supportive clinicians than subjects tested by nonverbally unsupportive clinicians.

(*Continued*)

TABLE 3 | Continued

Study	Design	N (Female)	Sample	Type of provider	Nonverbal behavior	Target outcome	Result
Ruben et al. (70)	Mixed design	205 (129)	Healthy participants	Experimenters	*High nonverbal support*: leaning forward, eye contact, nodding, smiling, gesturing, and using a warm voice tone; *low nonverbal support*: poor eye contact, looking down frequently, folded arms, leaning back, distancing from participants, and a cold voice tone.	Pain tolerance, pain intensity	Nonverbally supportive experimenters induced higher pain tolerance and a reduction in the expressed pain in participants, compared to less nonverbally supportive clinicians that induced lower pain tolerance in participants.
Czerniak et al. (71)	Between subjects	122 (46)	Healthy participants	Experimenters	*Performance status*: scenario A: sitting, minimal eye contact, lack of tactile interaction like shaking hands; scenario B: sitting and standing, frequent eye contact, tactile interaction.	Pain threshold and tolerance	Scenario B resulted in an increase in pain threshold compared to scenario A.
Howe et al. (44)	Between subjects	160 (80)	Healthy participants	Experimenters	*High warm communication* (more eye contact, more smile, less interpersonal distance), VS *low warm communication* (less eye contact, no smiles, more interpersonal distance).	Placebo and nocebo effects (positive and negative expectations)	Warmer experimenters enhanced the effects of positive expectations about a placebo cream on allergic responses. Less warm experimenters negated the effects of expectations about a placebo cream on allergic response.
Van Osch et al. (72)	Between subjects	293 (293)	Patients with menstrual pain	Clinicians	*Positive affect-oriented communication*: warm, emphatic; VS negative: cold, formal	Anxiety, mood, expectations, satisfaction	Positive affect-oriented communication reduced anxiety, negative mood, and increased satisfaction, whereas negative communication negated positive expectations and led to higher negative mood and anxiety.
He et al. (73)	Between subjects	89 (67)	Healthy participants	Experimenters	*Communication status*: *Warm*: strong tone, animated facial expressions, frequent eye contact, expressive hand gestures, open posture. *Neutral*: monotonous voice, neural facial expression, less frequent hand gesture, minimal eye contact.	Expectation of treatment outcome, motor coordination	Warm experimenters induced higher positive expectations of treatment outcome, more improvement in performance, and better balance and coordination, compared to neutral experimenters that induced lower positive expectations.

**The procedure of these studies are not well described, but it seems a "social interaction" factor that referred to a warm or neutral behavior of the provider was at play, and also a "pill administration message" factor that reffered to the content of the information about the pill. However, this last factor is confusing and we are not completely sure about what was actually manipulated.*

data, and selective outcome reporting. RoBANS is compatible with the Cochrane risk of bias tool and has a same qualitative judgment procedure [for more information, see Ref. (76)].

Using the Cochrane risk of bias assessment tool for experimental studies (75) and RoBANS for quasi-experimental and correlational studies (76), the risk of bias of the individual studies was judged by both authors and the second author (MF) synchronized the results in two tables (**Table 5** for Cochrane risk of bias assessment; and **Table 6** for the RoBANS; see the results).

RESULTS

A total of 34 studies were identified: 20 on the role characteristics, 11 on the role of NBs, and 3 studies on the role of both characteristics and NBs of the experimenters/clinicians.

Experimenter/Clinician Characteristics

Experimenter/Clinician Sex and the Participants' Pain

A total of 15 studies investigated whether the sex of the experimenter/clinician affected the pain report of research participants: Six studies showed a main effect of experimenter sex: three studies showed that male experimenters induced lower pain intensities than females did (22, 59, 60), and Sorge et al. (61) showed that male experimenters induced less pain behaviors and more pain inhibition in rodents. On the other hand, two studies reported that female experimenters induced lower pain intensities than males (50, 51). Nine studies reported no main effect for the sex of the experimenter/clinician (19, 25, 47–49, 52–54, 62) (**Table 2**).

Ten of these 15 studies investigated the interaction of experimenter and subject sex: Three studies showed that, compared to male experimenters, female experimenters induced higher pain thresholds (54), lower pain intensities (19, 25), and marginally significant lower pain unpleasantness (25) in male subjects. Two studies reported that, compared to female experimenters, male experimenters induced higher pain tolerance in female subjects (22, 62). On the other hand, five studies did not find a significant interaction of experimenter/clinician sex and participant sex on pain report (47, 50–53). The remaining four studies (48, 49, 59, 60) did not use subject sex as a dependent variable and thus could not investigate the interaction of experimenter/clinician sex and participant/patient sex. One study was on animals and was not relevant in this context (61) (**Table 2**).

In sum, there is no reliable tendency for a main effect of experimenter sex on pain. However, there is some evidence of an interactive effect, as 5 of 10 studies show that the experimenter induced less pain in a subject of the opposite sex (19, 22, 25, 54, 62) (**Table 2**).

Experimenter/Clinician Sex and Placebo/Nocebo Effects

Two studies investigated the role of experimenter/clinician sex on placebo/nocebo effects: Aslaksen and Flaten reported that, compared to female experimenters, male experimenters contributed to higher placebo responses in male subjects (56). However, Weimer et al. (58) who studied the effects of ginger and a placebo on nausea, reported no interaction between experimenter sex and placebo responses (**Table 2**; for a review, see **Table 4**).

In sum, there is no reliable tendency for the impact of experimenter sex on placebo effects (**Table 2**).

Experimenter/Clinician Status and Participants' Pain

Five studies investigated the effects of experimenter/clinician status on pain reports of research participants: Three studies showed that compared to lower professional status (a student or an assistant), higher-status (e.g., a faculty member or a professor) experimenters generated higher pain thresholds (27) and tolerance (22, 26) and lower pain unpleasantness (26). Williams and colleagues (55) reported that in comparison with research assistants, clinicians contributed to more accurate pain ratings (i.e., recollections of pain intensity following a surgery, correlated with pain ratings presented at the time of surgery) in low back pain patients. Also, Egbert et al. (46) reported that confident clinicians had patients with less usage of narcotics and in a better physical and emotional state than patients of less confident clinicians (**Table 2**).

In sum, all the five studies showed that higher professional status and higher confidence of experimenters/clinicians led to lower pain reports (22, 26, 27), more accurate pain ratings (55), and better physical and emotional state (46). No studies reported other effects of experimenter/clinician status on pain (**Table 2**).

Experimenter/Clinician Status and Placebo/Nocebo Effects

Two studies investigated the effects of the status of experimenters/clinicians on placebo/nocebo effects: Kaptchuk and colleagues (57) showed that, compared to less confident practitioners, more confident clinicians induced higher symptom relief, higher scores on a global improvement scale, and less symptom severity in patients with irritable bowel syndrome (IBS). Howe et al. (44) reported that competent experimenters (who made no mistakes throughout the experiment) induced higher placebo effects (**Table 2**).

To sum up, two studies revealed that confidence and competence status of experimenters/clinicians generated higher placebo effects (44, 57). No studies reported other effects of experimenter/clinician status on placebo effects (**Table 2**).

Nonverbal Behaviors

Experimenter/Clinician Nonverbal Behaviors and Participants' Pain

Seven studies investigated the effects of experimenters/clinicians NBs on the pain of research participants: Ruben et al. (70) showed that, compared to clinicians with negative NBs, clinicians with positive NBs induced higher pain tolerance and less pain expressions. In another study, Ruben and colleagues (69) showed that clinicians with positive NBs generated more accurate pain ratings (i.e., consistency between expressions of pain by subjects

TABLE 6 | Risk of Bias Assessment for quasi-experimental and correlational studies (RoBANS) of the effects of experimenters/clinicians characteristics and non-verbal behaviors on pain and placebo effects.

	1	2	3	4	5	6
Gryll and Katahn (63)	Low	Low	Low	Unclear	Low	Unclear
Otto et al. (47)	High	Low	High	High	Unclear	Unclear
Feine et al. (48)	Low	Low	Low	Unclear	Low	Unclear
Bush et al. (49)	Low	Low	High	Unclear	Unclear	Unclear
Fillingim et al. (50)	Low	Low	Low	Unclear	Low	Low
Thorn et al. (52)	Low	Unclear	High	Unclear	Unclear	Unclear
Essick et al. (53)	High	Low	High	Unclear	Low	Unclear
Campbell et al. (26)	Low	Low	Low	Unclear	Low	Low
Aslaksen et al. (25)	Low	Low	Unclear	Low	Low	Low
Williams et al. (55)	Low	Low	Low	Unclear	Low	Low
Aslaksen and Flaten (56)	Low	Low	Low	Low	Low	Low
Vigil and Alcock (60)	High	Low	Unclear	Unclear	Unclear	Unclear
Valentini et al. (68)	Low	Low	Unclear	Low	Low	Low
Vigil et al. (62)	Unclear	Low	Low	Low	Low	Unclear

Key
- Low risk of bias
- Unclear risk of bias
- High risk of bias

NUMBERS' DEFINITION:

1. Selection of participants
2. Confounding variables
3. Measurement of exposure
4. Blinding of outcome assessments
5. Incomplete outcome data
6. Selective outcome reporting

that this could be due to a response bias in males, so they were trying to impress female experimenters by reporting lower pain. Interestingly, Gijsbers and Nicholson (54) showed that by exaggerating the gender-related appearance and behaviors of female experimenters, the hypoalgesic effect of female experimenters on male subjects can be enlarged.

Two studies (22, 62) showed that male experimenter/clinicians induced lower pain reports in female subjects. This finding contradicts the conventional gender role assumptions that assumed a helpless state for females, in which they display higher pain to induce male protection. Kállai et al. (22) showed that females reported lower pain to male experimenters and concluded that females, as well as males, try to impress opposite sex experimenters by their ability to tolerate pain longer. This can be due to changes in the female gender role in contemporary societies in which more authority and power are granted for females.

A second explanation attributes the hypoalgesic effects of male experimenters on female subjects to the physiological aspects of females. Vigil et al. (62) tested two groups of high- and low-fertility females by male and female experimenters and showed that, compared to females who were tested by a female experimenter, high-fertility females who were tested by a male experimenter reported lower pain. This finding suggests that physiological factors can contribute to the lower pain reports of female subjects to male experimenters/clinicians. Also, this finding can partially explain why some studies [e.g., Ref. (25)] failed to observe a hypoalgesic effect of male experimenters on female subjects.

There was no reliable effect of experimenter/clinician sex on placebo analgesia (56, 58).

The Role of Experimenter/Clinician Status on Pain and Placebo Effects

Five studies showed that higher status of experimenters/ clinicians generated lower pain reports. Campbell et al. (26) demonstrated that subjects displayed higher blood pressure reactivity and pain tolerance to higher-status experimenters and concluded that increased blood pressure stimulated pressure receptors in the vasculature that also modulate the perception of pain (77–84). The stress induced by the higher-status experimenters may therefore lead to lower pain reports (26).

Two studies demonstrated that higher status of the experimenters/clinicians induced larger placebo effects. Howe et al. (44) showed that competent clinicians enhanced the effects of positive expectations and reduced subject's allergic responses. They suggested that outcome expectations, that are underlying factors for the placebo and nocebo effects, can be modulated by the warmth and competence of clinicians. Notably, Howe et al. (44) studied the effects of low-competence characteristics of clinicians on negative expectations, and did not observe a significant effect on negative expectations.

The Role of Experimenter/Clinician Nonverbal Behaviors on Pain and Placebo Effects

Six studies showed that positive NBs of experimenters/clinicians induced lower pain reports, and three studies showed that negative NBs resulted in higher pain reports. Pain is recognized as a stressor and most of painful situations induce stress and negative emotions (54, 85). Negative emotions and stress can increase the experience of pain [e.g., Refs. (56, 85)], whereas providing information about the forthcoming intervention and outcomes of a treatment may reduce the stress and negative emotions. As there can be uncertainty about the outcome of interventions (54, 85), participants/patients might use as much of accessible information as possible to gain knowledge about the efficacy of the intervention. NBs of experimenters/clinicians can be a substantial source of information for participants/patients (36, 69, 70). In this line, Ambady and Gray (40) showed that positive NBs of clinicians (e.g., facial expressiveness, nodding, and smiling) were associated with long-term improvements in cognitive and physical functioning of elderly patients. Previous studies have shown that clients can perceive the expectations of their providers [e.g., Refs. (36, 86)]. As interpersonal expectations are mostly communicated through NBs [e.g., Ref. (38)], positive NBs of experimenters/clinicians can be interpreted as a sign of satisfactory functioning or results and lead to decrease in negative emotions and subsequently lower pain reports, whereas negative NBs can be assumed as a sign of negative forthcoming results and lead to higher pain reports. In this line, Egbert et al. (46) showed that patients who were exposed to enthusiastic clinicians were in a better emotional state, and Gryll and Katahn (63) showed that enthusiasm by clinicians reduced negative emotions.

Seven studies showed that positive NBs of experimenters/ clinicians induced higher placebo effects, whereas negative NBs led to lower placebo effects and higher nocebo hyperalgesia. To explain the modulatory effects of NBs on placebo and nocebo effects, a similar perspective is taken. NBs may have a confirmatory (or contradictory) role for verbal information that is used to induce positive outcome expectations and placebo effects. So, positive NBs may have an additive value for the verbal information, e.g., that a tablet is a powerful pain killer, and negative NBs may contradict the verbal information and diminish the induction of placebo effects. In this line, Howe et al. (44) showed that positive NBs of clinicians enhanced the impact of positive expectations about the effects of an inert cream on allergic responses; and He et al. (73) showed that positive NBs of clinicians induced stronger positive expectations in a coordination and balance test. Expectations may also contribute to the modulation of emotions and stress. For instance, Verheul et al. (65) and Van Osch et al. (72) reported that positive NBs of clinicians enhanced positive outcome expectancies and reduced the state anxiety and negative mood, whereas negative NBs resulted in higher anxiety levels and expectations of longer pain duration.

Therefore, NBs may have an additive value for the role of verbal information in modulation of expectations, negative emotions, and stress, and hence lead to changes in amplitudes of placebo or nocebo effects. Several studies have reported failure to elicit a placebo effect [e.g., Refs. (58, 87)]. Uncontrolled NBs of experimenters/clinicians may partially account for such diversity in findings.

CONCLUSION

This qualitative review documented the contribution of experimenters/clinicians' sex, status, and NBs, as three factors capable of altering the perception of pain, and amplitude of placebo/nocebo effects and responses.

Sex, status, and NBs of experimenters/clinicians are interwoven in every laboratory and clinical setting and the present review shows that these factors can influence research results. The failure to control for the effects of characteristics and NBs of experimenters/clinicians can explain why placebo studies occasionally yield inconsistent or variable findings [e.g., Refs. (58, 87, 88)], or why the reliability of pain measurement is limited and doubted [e.g., Ref. (25)]. To gain a deeper understanding of the effects of such nonspecific factors, this review emphasizes the need to further investigate the contribution of characteristics and NBs of experimenters/clinicians in pain and placebo effects.

Recommendations for Future Research

Prospective investigations are encouraged to address the following gaps in current literature; first, to our knowledge, just two studies have investigated the separate effects of different NBs on pain and placebo effects (68, 73). Thus, future studies should specify what specific NBs (facial expressions, eye contact, nodding, physical distance, tone of voice, or body postures) that have the strongest impact on pain and placebo/nocebo effects; He et al. (73) showed that compared to physical distance and body posture, facial expressions and tone of voice had stronger effects on placebo effects. However, this finding should be replicated especially in prospective pain studies. Second, the interaction of NBs and sex of providers and subjects should be investigated to see whether NBs of experimenters can modulate the effects of sex or vice versa. Only one study has studied this and reported that positive NBs of experimenters induced lower pain reports in male subjects than in female subjects (70). Third, future studies should suggest how to control for the effects of NBs in research on pain and other symptoms. Indeed, this can only be achieved if we have more knowledge about the effects of each specific NB on pain or other symptoms. Fourth, studies could consider the effects of other genders (e.g., transgendered experimenters) on the experience of pain; to our knowledge, only one study has addressed this (59) and showed that compared to a male or female experimenter who acted in accordance with their sex, a biological male who acted in a feminine way induced higher pain reports in female subjects. Fifth, there might be an interaction between experimenters/clinician's sex and their status. Several studies have reported that for example, male providers were considered more credible (87); their status influenced male subjects more (27); male clinicians who were reputed for their expertise were more preferred over female clinicians; and female clinicians who were reputed for their interpersonal skills were preferred more by patients (30). The possible interaction of the status and the sex of the experimenters/clinicians should be taken into account to determine whether status can modulate the effects of sex or vice versa. According to our searches, only Kállai et al. (22) have tested both sex and status systematically, but unfortunately have not reported the interaction of sex and status of the experimenters. Lastly, the underlying mechanisms (e.g., expectations and emotions) of the effects of NBs and characteristics of experimenters/clinicians on pain and placebo effects are still unclear and should be investigated. More knowledge of these factors would be highly relevant in the training of health personnel.

LIMITATIONS

The present study contains a number of limitations that should be noted here. First is the qualitative nature of this study that hinders the generality of findings. Second is the heterogeneity of keywords used in different studies, which made it difficult to gain access to all related studies and may have caused to miss a few studies; however, to prevent this, several Boolean searches were conducted and also the reference and citation lists of included studies were checked. Third is the interpretation of the findings on the interaction of the experimenters'/clinicians' sex and subjects' sex. Of the included studies, five studies showed an interaction, and five studies did not find an interaction. Therefore, the findings on the interaction of the experimenter/clinician and participant's sex should be interpreted with caution. Fourth is the problem of confounding in some findings such as investigating the provider status and NBs simultaneously and without differentiation as in Kaptchuk et al. (57); or lack of clarity in methodological procedures such as absence of differentiation in providers' sex and status as in Campbell et al. [Ref. (26) or (87)]; or lack of differentiation between verbal and nonverbal components as in Gryll and Katahn (63). Such deficiencies limit the drawing of straightforward conclusions. Additionally, this systematic review did not comprise a review protocol, but authors tried to precisely characterize the scientific nature of this systematic review by determining *a priori* question and the procedure relevant to the questions.

AUTHOR CONTRIBUTIONS

MF planned the study. HD searched and extracted the articles and MF screened them. Both authors significantly contributed to the analyses of results, drafting of the manuscript, and preparation of the final draft.

FUNDING

The present research was funded by the Norwegian University of Science and Technology (NTNU).

REFERENCES

1. Savvas SM, Zelencich LM, Gibson SJ. Should placebo be used routinely for chronic pain in older people? *Maturitas* (2014) 79(4):389–400. doi: 10.1016/j.maturitas.2014.09.006
2. Flaten MA, Aslaksen PM, Finset A, Simonsen T, Johansen O. Cognitive and emotional factors in placebo analgesia. *J Psychosom Res* (2006) 61(1):81–9. doi: 10.1016/j.jpsychores.2005.12.004
3. Aslaksen PM, Lyby PS. Fear of pain potentiates nocebo hyperalgesia. *J Pain Res* (2015) 8:703. doi: 10.2147/JPR.S91923
4. Flaten MA, Simonsen T, Olsen H. Drug-related information generates placebo and nocebo responses that modify the drug response. *Psychosom Med* (1999) 61(2):250–5. doi: 10.1097/00006842-199903000-00018
5. Varelmann D, Pancaro C, Cappiello EC, Camann WR. Nocebo-induced hyperalgesia during local anesthetic injection. *Anesth Analg* (2010) 110(3):868–70. doi: 10.1213/ANE.0b013e3181cc5727
6. Carlino E, Benedetti F. Different contexts, different pains, different experiences. *Neuroscience* (2016) 338:19–26. doi: 10.1016/j.neuroscience.2016.01.053
7. Benedetti F. Placebo and the new physiology of the doctor-patient relationship. *Physiol Rev* (2013) 93(3):1207–46. doi: 10.1152/physrev.00043.2012
8. Benedetti F, Durando J, Vighetti S. Nocebo and placebo modulation of hypobaric hypoxia headache involves the cyclooxygenase-prostaglandins pathway. *Pain®* (2014) 155(5):921–8. doi: 10.1016/j.pain.2014.01.016
9. Flaten MA, Aslaksen PM, Lyby PS, Bjørkedal E. The relation of emotions to placebo responses. *Philos Trans R Soc Lond B Biol Sci* (2011) 366(1572):1818–27. doi: 10.1098/rstb.2010.0407
10. Al'Absi M, Flaten MA. Stress and pain: conclusions and future directions. In: Al'Absi M Flaten MA, editors. *The neuroscience of pain, stress, and emotion.* United States: Academic Press (2016). p. 283–9. doi: 10.1016/B978-0-12-800538-5.00013-3
11. Flaten M, Aslaksen P, Lyby P. Positive and negative emotion and placebo analgesia. In: Colloca L, Flaten MA, Meissner K, editors. *Placebo and pain: from bench to bedside.* United States: Academic Press (2013). p. 72–81. doi: 10.1016/B978-0-12-397928-5.00008-8
12. Colloca L. How placebo responses are formed. In: Colloca L, Flaten MA, Meissner K, editors. *Placebo and pain: from bench to bedside.* United States: Academic Press (2013). p. 137–48. doi: 10.1016/B978-0-12-397928-5.00014-3
13. Meissner K, Bingel U, Colloca L, Wager TD, Watson A, Flaten MA. The placebo effect: advances from different methodological approaches. *J Neurosci* (2011) 31(45):16117–24. doi: 10.1523/JNEUROSCI.4099-11.2011
14. Pollo A, Amanzio M, Arslanian A, Casadio C, Maggi G, Benedetti F. Response expectancies in placebo analgesia and their clinical relevance. *Pain* (2001) 93(1):77–84. doi: 10.1016/S0304-3959(01)00296-2
15. Di Blasi Z, Harkness E, Ernst E, Georgiou A, Kleijnen J. Influence of context effects on health outcomes: a systematic review. *Lancet* (2001) 357:757–62. doi: 10.1016/S0140-6736(00)04169-6
16. Kaptchuk TJ. The placebo effect in alternative medicine: can the performance of a healing ritual have clinical significance? *Ann Intern Med* (2002) 136(11):817–25. doi: 10.7326/0003-4819-136-11-200206040-00011
17. Levine JD, Gordon NC. Influence of the method of drug administration on analgesic response. *Nature* (1984) 312(5996):755. doi: 10.1038/312755a0
18. Robinson ME, Wise EA. Gender bias in the observation of experimental pain. *Pain* (2003) 104(1–2):259–64. doi: 10.1016/S0304-3959(03)00014-9
19. Levine FM, De Simone LL. The effects of experimenter gender on pain report in male and female subjects. *Pain* (1991) 44(1):69–72. doi: 10.1016/0304-3959(91)90149-R
20. Sanford SD, Kersh BC, Thorn BE, Rich MA, Ward LC. Psychosocial mediators of sex differences in pain responsivity. *J Pain* (2002) 3(1):58–64. doi: 10.1054/jpai.2002.xb30066
21. Weisse CS, Foster KK, Fisher EA. The influence of experimenter gender and race on pain reporting: does racial or gender concordance matter? *Pain Med* (2005) 6(1):80–7. doi: 10.1111/j.1526-4637.2005.05004.x
22. Kállai I, Barke A, Voss U. The effects of experimenter characteristics on pain reports in women and men. *Pain* (2004) 112(1-2):142–7. doi: 10.1016/j.pain.2004.08.008
23. Vervoort T, Goubert L, Eccleston C, Verhoeven K, De Clercq A, Buysse A, et al. The effects of parental presence upon the facial expression of pain: the moderating role of child pain catastrophizing. *Pain* (2008) 138(2):277–85. doi: 10.1016/j.pain.2007.12.013
24. Burns JW, Post KM, Smith DA, Porter LS, Buvanendran A, Fras AM, et al. Spouse criticism and hostility during marital interaction: effects on pain intensity and behaviors among individuals with chronic low back pain. *Pain* (2018) 159(1):25–32. doi: 10.1097/j.pain.0000000000001037
25. Aslaksen PM, Myrbakk IN, Høifødt RS, Flaten MA. The effect of experimenter gender on autonomic and subjective responses to pain stimuli. *Pain* (2007) 129(3):260–8. doi: 10.1016/j.pain.2006.10.011
26. Campbell TS, Holder MD, France CR. The effects of experimenter status and cardiovascular reactivity on pain reports. *Pain* (2006) 125(3):264–9. doi: 10.1016/j.pain.2006.06.002
27. Modić-Stanke K, Ivanec D. Pain threshold: measure of pain sensitivity or social behavior? *Psihologija* (2016) 49(1):37–50. doi: 10.2298/PSI1601037M
28. Testa M, Rossettini G. Enhance placebo, avoid nocebo: how contextual factors affect physiotherapy outcomes. *Man Ther* (2016) 24:65–74. doi: 10.1016/j.math.2016.04.006
29. Hush JM, Cameron K, Mackey M. Patient satisfaction with musculoskeletal physical therapy care: a systematic review. *Phys Ther* (2011) 91(1):25–36. doi: 10.2522/ptj.20100061
30. Bishop FL, Smith R, Lewith GT. Patient preferences for technical skills versus interpersonal skills in chiropractors and physiotherapists treating low back pain. *Fam Pract* (2012) 30(2):197–203. doi: 10.1093/fampra/cms066
31. O'keeffe M, Cullinane P, Hurley J, Leahy I, Bunzli S, O'sullivan PB, et al. What influences patient–therapist interactions in musculoskeletal physical therapy? Qualitative systematic review and meta-synthesis. *Phys Ther* (2016) 96(5):609–22. doi: 10.2522/ptj.20150240
32. Mercer E, MacKay-Lyons M, Conway N, Flynn J, Mercer C. Perceptions of outpatients regarding the attire of physiotherapists. *Physiother Can* (2008) 60(4):349–57. doi: 10.3138/physio.60.4.349
33. Petrilli CM, Mack M, Petrilli JJ, Hickner A, Saint S, Chopra V. Understanding the role of physician attire on patient perceptions: a systematic review of the literature—targeting attire to improve likelihood of rapport

(TAILOR) investigators. *BMJ Open* (2015) 5(1):e006578. doi: 10.1136/bmjopen-2014-006578
34. Bänziger T, Grandjean D, Scherer KR. Emotion recognition from expressions in face, voice, and body: the Multimodal Emotion Recognition Test (MERT). *Emotion* (2009) 9(5):691. doi: 10.1037/a0017088
35. DePaulo BM, Friedman HS. Nonverbal communication. In: Gilbert D, Fiske ST, Lindzey G, editors. *Handbook of social psychology*. 4th ed. New York: McGraw - Hill (1998). p. 3–40.
36. Belin P, Fillion-Bilodeau S, Gosselin F. The Montreal Affective Voices: a validated set of nonverbal affect bursts for research on auditory affective processing. *Behav Res Methods* (2008) 40(2):531–9. doi: 10.3758/BRM.40.2.531
37. Jacob H, Kreifelts B, Brück C, Nizielski S, Schütz A, Wildgruber D. Nonverbal signals speak up: association between perceptual nonverbal dominance and emotional intelligence. *Cogn Emot* (2013a) 27(5):783–99. doi: 10.1080/02699931.2012.739999
38. Ambady N, Bernieri FJ, Richeson JA. Toward a histology of social behavior: judgmental accuracy from thin slices of the behavioral stream. In: Zanna MP, editor. *Advances in experimental social psychology*. United States: Academic Press (2000). p. 201–71. doi: 10.1016/S0065-2601(00)80006-4
39. Silverman J, Kinnersley P. Doctors' non-verbal behaviour in consultations: look at the patient before you look at the computer. *Br J Gen Pract* (2010) 76–8. doi: 10.3399/bjgp10X482293
40. Ambady N, Gray HM. On being sad and mistaken: mood effects on the accuracy of thin-slice judgments. *J Pers Soc Psychol* (2002) 83(4):947. doi: 10.1037/0022-3514.83.4.947
41. Gilbert DT, Krull DS. Seeing less and knowing more: the benefits of perceptual ignorance. *J Pers Soc Psychol* (1988) 54(2):193. doi: 10.1037/0022-3514.54.2.193
42. Patterson ML, Stockbridge E. Effects of cognitive demand and judgment strategy on person perception accuracy. *J Nonverbal Behav* (1998) 22(4):253–63. doi: 10.1023/A:1022996522793
43. Calder AJ, Beaver JD, Winston JS, Dolan RJ, Jenkins R, Eger E, et al. Separate coding of different gaze directions in the superior temporal sulcus and inferior parietal lobule. *Curr Biol* (2007) 17(1):20–5. doi: 10.1016/j.cub.2006.10.052
44. Howe LC, Goyer JP, Crum AJ. Harnessing the placebo effect: exploring the influence of physician characteristics on placebo response. *Health Psychol* (2017) 36(11):1074. doi: 10.1037/hea0000499
45. Oliveira VC, Refshauge KM, Ferreira ML, Pinto RZ, Beckenkamp PR, Negrao Filho RF, et al. Communication that values patient autonomy is associated with satisfaction with care: a systematic review. *J Physiother* (2012) 58(4):215–29. doi: 10.1016/S1836-9553(12)70123-6
46. Egbert LD, Battit GE, Welch CE, Bartlett MK. Reduction of postoperative pain by encouragement and instruction of patients: a study of doctor-patient rapport. *N Eng J Med* (1964) 270(16):825–7. doi: 10.1056/NEJM196404162701606
47. Otto MW, Dougher MJ. Sex differences and personality factors in responsivity to pain. *Percept Mot Skills* (1985) 61(2):383–90. doi: 10.2466/pms.1985.61.2.383
48. Feine JS, Bushnell MC, Miron D, Duncan GH. Sex differences in the perception of noxious heat stimuli. *Pain* (1991) 44(3):255–62. doi: 10.1016/0304-3959(91)90094-E
49. Bush FM, Harkins SW, Harrington WG, Price DD. Analysis of gender effects on pain perception and symptom presentation in temporomandibular pain. *Pain* (1993) 53(1):73–80. doi: 10.1016/0304-3959(93)90058-W
50. Fillingim RB, Edwards RR, Powell T. The relationship of sex and clinical pain to experimental pain responses. *Pain®* (1999) 83(3):419–25. doi: 10.1016/S0304-3959(99)00128-1
51. Carter LE, McNeil DW, Vowles KE, Sorrell JT, Turk CL, Ries BJ, et al. Effects of emotion on pain reports, tolerance and physiology. *Pain Res Manage* (2002) 7(1):21–30. doi: 10.1155/2002/426193
52. Thorn BE, Clements KL, Ward LC, Dixon KE, Kersh BC, Boothby JL, et al. Personality factors in the explanation of sex differences in pain catastrophizing and response to experimental pain. *Clin J Pain* (2004) 20(5):275–82. doi: 10.1097/00002508-200409000-00001
53. Essick G, Guest S, Martinez E, Chen C, Mcglone F. Site-dependent and subject-related variations in perioral thermal sensitivity. *Somatosens Mot Res* (2004) 21(3-4):159–75. doi: 10.1080/08990220400012414
54. Gijsbers K, Nicholson F. Experimental pain thresholds influenced by sex of experimenter. *Percept Mot Skills* (2005) 101(3):803–7. doi: 10.2466/pms.101.3.803-807
55. Williams DA, Park KM, Ambrose KR, Clauw DJ. Assessor status influences pain recall. *J Pain* (2007) 8(4):343–8. doi: 10.1016/j.jpain.2006.10.005
56. Aslaksen PM, Flaten MA. The roles of physiological and subjective stress in the effectiveness of a placebo on experimentally induced pain. *Psychosom Med* (2008) 70(7):811–8. doi: 10.1097/PSY.0b013e31818105ed
57. Kaptchuk TJ, Kelley JM, Conboy LA, Davis RB, Kerr CE, Jacobson EE, et al. Components of placebo effect: randomised controlled trial in patients with irritable bowel syndrome. *Bmj* (2008) 336(7651):999–1003. doi: 10.1136/bmj.39524.439618.25
58. Weimer K, Schulte J, Maichle A, Muth ER, Scisco JL, Horing B, et al. Effects of ginger and expectations on symptoms of nausea in a balanced placebo design. *PLoS One* (2012) 7(11):e49031. doi: 10.1371/journal.pone.0049031
59. Vigil JM, Rowell LN, Alcock J, Maestes R. Laboratory personnel gender and cold pressor apparatus affect subjective pain reports. *Pain Res Manage* (2014) 19(1):e13–8. doi: 10.1155/2014/213950
60. Vigil JM, Alcock J. Tough guys or sensitive guys? Disentangling the role of examiner sex on patient pain reports. *Pain Res Manage* (2014) 19(1):e9–12. doi: 10.1155/2014/531396
61. Sorge RE, Martin LJ, Isbester KA, Sotocinal SG, Rosen S, Tuttle AH, et al. Olfactory exposure to males, including men, causes stress and related analgesia in rodents. *Nat Methods* (2014) 11(6):629. doi: 10.1038/nmeth.2935
62. Vigil JM, DiDomenico J, Strenth C, Coulombe P, Kruger E, Mueller AA, et al. Experimenter effects on pain reporting in women vary across the menstrual cycle. *Int J Endocrinol* (2015) 2015:1–8. doi: 10.1155/2015/520719
63. Gryll SL, Katahn M. Situational factors contributing to the placebo effect. *Psychopharmacology* (1978) 57(3):253–61. doi: 10.1007/BF00426747
64. Brown JL, Sheffield D, Leary MR, Robinson ME. Social support and experimental pain. *Psychosom Med* (2003) 65(2):276–83. doi: 10.1097/01.PSY.0000030388.62434.46
65. Verheul W, Sanders A, Bensing J. The effects of physicians' affect-oriented communication style and raising expectations on analogue patients' anxiety, affect and expectancies. *Patient Educ Couns* (2010) 80(3):300–6. doi: 10.1016/j.pec.2010.06.017
66. Modić Stanke K, Ivanec D. Social context of pain perception: the role of other people's presence and physical distance. *Rev Psychol* (2010) 17(1):69–74. https://hrcak.srce.hr/70663
67. Bohns VK, Wiltermuth SS. It hurts when I do this (or you do that): posture and pain tolerance. *J Exp Soc Psychol* (2012) 48(1):341–5. doi: 10.1016/j.jesp.2011.05.022
68. Valentini E, Martini M, Lee M, Aglioti SM, Iannetti G. Seeing facial expressions enhances placebo analgesia. *Pain®* (2014) 155(4):666–73. doi: 10.1016/j.pain.2013.11.021
69. Ruben MA, Hall JA. Healthcare providers' nonverbal behavior can lead patients to show their pain more accurately: an analogue study. *J Nonverbal Behav* (2016) 40(3):221–34. doi: 10.1007/s10919-016-0230-3
70. Ruben MA, Blanch-Hartigan D, Hall JA. Nonverbal communication as a pain reliever: the impact of physician supportive nonverbal behavior on experimentally induced pain. *Health Commun* (2016) 32(8):970–6. doi: 10.1080/10410236.2016.1196418
71. Czerniak E, Biegon A, Ziv A, Karnieli-Miller O, Weiser M, Alon U, et al. Manipulating the placebo response in experimental pain by altering doctor's performance style. *Front Psychol* (2016) 7:874. doi: 10.3389/fpsyg.2016.00874
72. Van Osch M, van Dulmen S, van Vliet L, Bensing J. Specifying the effects of physician's communication on patients' outcomes: a randomised controlled trial. *Patient Educ Couns* (2017) 100(8):1482–9. doi: 10.1016/j.pec.2017.03.009
73. He X, Sun Q, Stetler C. Warm communication style strengthens expectations and increases perceived improvement. *Health Commun* (2018) 33(8):939–45. doi: 10.1080/10410236.2017.1322482
74. Drucker AM, Fleming P, Chan AW. Research techniques made simple: assessing risk of bias in systematic reviews. *J Invest Dermatol* (2016) 136(11):e109–14. doi: 10.1016/j.jid.2016.08.021
75. Higgins JP, Altman DG, Gøtzsche PC, Jüni P, Moher D, Oxman AD, et al. The Cochrane Collaboration's tool for assessing risk of bias in randomised trials. *Bmj* (2011) 343:d5928. doi: 10.1136/bmj.d5928

76. Kim SY, Park JE, Lee YJ, Seo HJ, Sheen SS, Hahn S, et al. Testing a tool for assessing the risk of bias for nonrandomized studies showed moderate reliability and promising validity. *J Clin Epidemiol* (2013) 66(4):408–14. doi: 10.1016/j.jclinepi.2012.09.016
77. Geary DC, Vigil J, Byrd-Craven J. Evolution of human mate choice. *J Sex Res* (2004) 41(1):27–42. doi: 10.1080/00224490409552211
78. Ghione S. Hypertension-associated hypalgesia: evidence in experimental animals and humans, pathophysiological mechanisms, and potential clinical consequences. *Hypertension* (1996) 28(3):494–504. doi: 10.1161/01.HYP.28.3.494
79. France CR. Decreased pain perception and risk for hypertension: considering a common physiological mechanism. *Psychophysiology* (1999) 36(6):683–92. doi: 10.1111/1469-8986.3660683
80. Brody S, Rau H. Behavioral and psychophysiological predictors of self-monitored 19 month blood pressure change in normotensives. *J Psychosom Res* (1994) 38(8):885–91. doi: 10.1016/0022-3999(94)90075-2
81. Droste C, Kardos A, Brody S, Greenlee MW, Roskamm H, Rau H. Baroreceptor stimulation: pain perception and sensory thresholds. *Biol Psychol* (1994) 37(2):101–13. doi: 10.1016/0301-0511(94)90025-6
82. Dworkin BR, Elbert T, Rau H, Birbaumer N, Pauli P, Droste C, et al. Central effects of baroreceptor activation in humans: attenuation of skeletal reflexes and pain perception. *Proc Natl Acad Sci* (1994) 91(14):6329–33. doi: 10.1073/pnas.91.14.6329
83. Rau H, Brody S, Larbig W, Pauli P, Vöhringer M, Harsch B, et al. Effects of PRES baroreceptor stimulation on thermal and mechanical pain threshold in borderline hypertensives and normotensives. *Psychophysiology* (1994) 31(5):480–5. doi: 10.1111/j.1469-8986.1994.tb01051.x
84. Edwards L, Ring C, McIntyre D, Carroll D. Modulation of the human nociceptive flexion reflex across the cardiac cycle. *Psychophysiology* (2001) 38(4):712–8. doi: 10.1111/1469-8986.3840712
85. Edwards L, McIntyre DA, Carroll D, Ring C, Martin U. The human nociceptive flexion reflex threshold is higher during systole than diastole. *Psychophysiology* (2002) 39(5):678–81. doi: 10.1111/1469-8986.3950678
86. Rosenthal R, Rubin DB. Interpersonal expectancy effects: the first 345 studies. *Behav Brain Sci* (1978) 1(3):377–86. doi: 10.1017/S0140525X00075506
87. Flaten MA, Bjørkedal E, Lyby PS, Figenschau Y, Aslaksen PM. Failure to find a conditioned placebo analgesic response. *Front Psychol* (2018) 9. doi: 10.3389/fpsyg.2018.01198
88. Jacob H, Brück C, Domin M, Lotze M, Wildgruber D. I can't keep your face and voice out of my head: neural correlates of an attentional bias toward nonverbal emotional cues. *Cereb Cortex* (2013b) 24(6):1460–73. doi: 10.1093/cercor/bhs417

10

Re-evaluation of Significance and the Implications of Placebo Effect in Antidepressant Therapy

Marko Curkovic [1], Andro Kosec [2] and Aleksandar Savic [1,3]*

[1] Department for Diagnostics and Intensive Care, University Psychiatric Hospital Vrapce, Zagreb, Croatia, [2] Department of Otorhinolaryngology and Head and Neck Surgery, University Hospital Center Sestre Milosrdnice, Zagreb, Croatia, [3] Department of Psychiatry, University of Zagreb School of Medicine, Zagreb, Croatia

Keywords: depression, antidepressants, placebo, placebo effect, efficacy, randomized controlled trials

***Correspondence:**
Marko Curkovic
markocurak@gmail.com

INTRODUCTION

Placebo was conceived as an epistemological tool to control for incidental factors that could influence investigated outcomes (1, 2). As a phenomenon, placebo has been conceptualized in many different ways, both theoretically and practically, although a generally accepted definition is still to be devised (3). In clinical research setting it is, however, helpful to distinguish placebo response from placebo effect. Placebo response is considered to be the composite change observed in individuals after administration of placebo, consisting of different aspects, such as natural course of the disease and methodological artifacts, as well as the placebo effect itself (4, 5). Placebo effect would therefore be the change observed in individuals after controlling for natural course of the disorder, methodological aspects, and the effect linked to treatment-specific features (i.e., antidepressant verum) (1). In other words, placebo responses may or may not include placebo effect as genuine psychobiosocial effect that is usually attributed to various features of treatment situation and contexts (5). Recent findings consistently show a modest average effect (a mean effect size of $d = 0.30$) of antidepressants above placebo in short-term treatment of adult depression (6, 7). This could be interpreted as strong evidence of a modest effect. Whether this effect on outcome measures, that are rather limited and subjective, is clinically meaningful remains an open question (8). Issues of true long-term efficacy, safety and cost-effectiveness of antidepressant drugs still loom over the horizon (8–11). Still, these recent findings pose interesting questions, since similarly consistent findings have been published showing a large and highly variable placebo effect in studies aiming to prove true efficacy of antidepressants (12, 13). In other words, participants in antidepressant studies that are receiving, at least from a theoretical point, a supposedly inherently neutral intervention (one that should be lacking known, relevant, and specific features), show substantial and consistent improvement across different study designs and contexts.

CONTEXT

Double blind randomized placebo-controlled trials (DBRPCT) have long been considered to be the golden standard for determining true efficacy of an intervention. As such, DBRPCTs are based on the logic that reflects the basic premises of scientific epistemology: it allows a certain degree of control over factors that could influence outcomes of interest, but at the current point is not a subject of scientific inquiry (3). Randomization, blinding, and placebo control groups allow for probabilistic balancing of these unspecific factors, and prevent intentional or accidental influence from study participants and investigators (14). Consequently, it is assumed that true effect of intervention could be extracted based on the "additivity assumption"—true effect is one that is present only within the last remaining uncontrolled therapeutic features, and therefore attributed to the intervention being investigated.

Such a design, created for a very specific purpose, has its shortcomings that have been widely discussed [for more comprehensive discussion consider (14) and related commentaries]. In order for a DBRPCT to be internally valid (able to fulfill its explanatory purpose), a certain degree of deviation from external validity is required, causing loss of similarity to the targeted model—clinical practice (14, 15). Placebo in DBRPCTs was initially conceived as a procedure that allows blinding, removing the influences of study participants and investigators. It seems, however, that placebo consistently influences outcomes above and beyond its anticipated boundaries (1, 16, 17). Although we aim to constrain "human factor," certain aspects of human nature evade such attempts. Human subjects, inherently vulnerable because of the nature of their medical condition, are systematically and consistently reacting to a more or less specific set of internal and external cues, creating a "genuine" placebo effect. While placebo effect may be a valuable and legitimate object of research, one should be careful not to overgeneralize this term, since a tendency to erroneously characterize everything and anything as a placebo effect can be seen [for more detailed discussion consider (18)]. In other words, as previously mentioned, genuine placebo effect should be distinguished from methodological artifacts that exert certain influence on outcomes, such as natural course of the investigated condition, spontaneous variation in symptoms, and various sources of research bias (2, 18, 19). It seems that genuine placebo effect exercises a greater influence in its own right than any of above mentioned factors, and as such is neither inert nor unspecific. It is responsible for physical changes and effects in individuals that are specific and somewhat related to the investigated condition and/or effects of "true" treatment (1, 2, 16, 19, 20). The placebo effect is considered to be an adaptive process that emerges from contextual and individual features within a treatment situation, and as such is driven by underlying biological, psychological and social components that are not mutually exclusive [for further details consider: (1, 21)]. As such, the placebo effect may contradict the additivity assumption, influencing outcomes conjointly or even independently from the investigated intervention (1). Therefore, an "interactive" assumption has been proposed, acknowledging that underlying mechanisms that yield a therapeutic response interact in a complex manner (1, 22).

RECENT FINDINGS

Findings suggest that placebo effect in antidepressant trials is a genuine entity, and as such may be distinguished from methodological artifacts that are also exhibiting a substantial influence on outcomes (23–25). While recent findings suggest that antidepressants show therapeutic efficacy and effectiveness, it seems that placebo effect may be one of the key driving forces of their effect. Moreover, it has been suggested that as much as 88% of antidepressants efficacy could be attributed to the placebo effect (8). In other words, antidepressants would in that case have little additional specific effect beyond the placebo effect. Furthermore, recent analyses found that a subset of 17% of individuals with depression could exhibit "clinically significant advances" with placebo relative to antidepressants (26). Similarly, earlier findings suggested that 20% of individuals with depression could have a worse disease trajectory with antidepressant than with placebo therapy (27).

Moderators and mediators of placebo and antidepressant effects have been thoroughly investigated and reviewed [more thoroughly discussed in: (28, 29)]. Unbalanced studies group randomization and effect modulation by baseline severity have been previously singled out as most consistent and robust findings. It may seem intuitive that baseline severity of depression influences responses to any given intervention, and it has long been argued that as depression is more severe, placebo effects are less prominent, while response rates to antidepressants remain stable (28, 30). This concept was recently dismissed, as antidepressants or placebo intervention seems to be equally (in)effective across the whole depression severity spectrum (31, 32). Interestingly, recent findings even suggest that placebo response rates seem to be similar in persistent depressive disorder (defined as all forms of depressive conditions that persist for at least 2 years) compared to episodic depression (33). The probability of receiving placebo (unbalanced group randomization) has been repeatedly and firmly correlated with the antidepressants' response (12, 29, 34). This relationship has a linear gradual effect, with efficacy of antidepressants increasing as we move from greater toward lower probability of receiving placebo. So, antidepressant response rates are significantly higher in comparator trials than in DBRPCT. This finding is usually interpreted as implicit evidence that both placebo and treatment effects could be based on patient expectations (that could obviously be positive and/or negative) (12). Nonetheless, it has been shown that expectations (conceptualized as perceived treatment assignment) significantly change during studies while retaining their relative predictive power (35). What participants believe may be more important than what they actually receive as an intervention, making a false but sincerely held belief more important that actual intervention. Some advancement has been made in predicting antidepressant and placebo responses and/or responsiveness in research and clinical practice. Although certain neurobiological features, clinical and socio-demographic characteristics of patients have been highlighted as possible outcome predictors, low sensitivity and high intra- and inter-individual variability remain an issue (26, 36–38). Placebo responsiveness, and to lesser account antidepressant responsiveness remain highly and complexly variable on all levels.

DOES PLACEBO EFFECT HAVE AN EFFECT ABOVE AND BEYOND THAT OF ANTIDEPRESSANTS?

Many questions are still unanswered regarding characteristics, mechanisms and definition of the placebo response and effect. Line of research dealing with those issues could be referred to as "placebo explanatory research," and depression and psychiatry disorders in general could be seen as particularly fertile ground for these inquiries (1, 2, 16, 24, 25, 29). For example, open-label placebo administration with full disclosure, seems to yield similar antidepressant therapeutic effects as the traditionally administered ones (39). On the other hand, antidepressants compared with active placebos that imitate some side-effects showed no significant advantage (40). Thus, expectation related placebo effects may be driven by unblinding properties of side-effects, and further diminishing antidepressants' signaling potential (extricating true efficacy).

We consider "antidepressant explanatory research" as one being primarily oriented toward proving true antidepressants efficacy. Within this approach, it has been recently argued that the placebo control group should be completely omitted, as diverse variability of placebo effects seems to undermine internal validity making studies fundamentally invalid and uninterpretable (7, 12). Proponents of keeping the placebo control group, propose methodological and analytical approaches that aim to control and manage placebo effects [further details may be found in: (1, 41, 42)]. One of the underlying assumptions is that "placebo responders" influence outcomes blurring the antidepressants' signaling potential. Hence, different methods, such as placebo run-in phase could be applied in order to eliminate these obstacles. This approach should be considered ethically and methodologically erroneous as there is no evidence that such a stable trait exists. Just the opposite, it seems that placebo responsiveness emerges from complex interrelationship between stable and situational traits [recently elaborated in: (19)]. Furthermore, it could be argued that reduction of placebo responsiveness will further reduce antidepressants responsiveness (25). Similar logic is applied within the approach of risk modeling where "risk participants" (disproportionately contributing to the outcome) and/or "non-responders" (not prone to react regardless of assigned intervention) are further dealt in identify and mitigate manner (1, 42). All of these strategies may be considered pragmatic, as there is great pressure to reduce ineffectual research. There are other strategies that tackle different possible sources of error by manipulating study context, design, conduct and analysis with primary aim to enhance studies' internal validity, antidepressants' signal detection potential and yield more historically reliable response rates (1, 2, 16, 20, 25, 28, 41–43). However, these strategies tend to increase internal validity at the expense of external validity, and as such seem more like a harm reduction strategies than as true advancement of our understanding of the complex underlying phenomena (14, 18, 25, 44, 45). Following this line of argumentation, solutions could include introduction of an independent study investigator and the concept of "cold standardization"—a virtual, computer driven standardized recruitment, admission of interventions and assessment of study participants. Such an approach would have potential to eliminate some features of intrapersonal healing that has been singled out as possibly one of the major contributors to the placebo effect, tackle widespread issue of inadequate blinding and other sources of investigator or study-staff related biases (14). Although such (still hypothetical) computerized study investigator could standardize study recruitment, administration and assessment procedures, it would not be resistant to other sources of bias. One could even imagine that participants' expectations in such a setting would change in previously unimaginable directions (either by certain therapeutic potential of this interaction or properties of interventions itself, such as side effect profile). Although here being used as extreme argument on how one could possibly further strengthen studies internal validity, such an approach could be also used in order to distinguish specific features underlying placebo and/or therapeutic effects (serving a more pragmatic purpose).

Alternatively, "antidepressant pragmatic research" would steer toward comprehending complex interactions of specific and/or unspecific features that are contributing to a therapeutic effect. We should not try to simply manage placebo effects, but direct our attention to its understanding through rigorous initial planning, assessment, reporting and sharing of all data possibly linked to the therapeutic response as well as non-response (1, 17, 19, 20, 43, 44). In other words disentangling of the placebo enigma seems to carry the potential of being the royal road to answering presumably the most important question at hand: which elements of the intervention, and in what proportion, are the ones relieving the suffering? In that sense, inclusion of an additional study arm in which the primary aim is to reach the maximum possible efficiency through any means necessary could be labeled as "warm standardization" (25). Again, different means could be used for that purpose, for example harnessing and maximizing expectations or even including additional specific interventions (such as some form of specific psychotherapy—being previously conceived as inherently expectation modulatory treatment) (46). Finally, as placebo is a relational phenomenon that significantly differs from context to context, all known moderators and mediators of placebo effect (from its physical characteristics to informed consent process) should be rigorously reported (1, 2, 16, 17, 43). Factors that affect treatment outcomes need to be evidenced, extrapolated, weighted, agglomerated, and discussed having in mind that acquiring scientifically grounded knowledge is an iterative, cumulative process. Currently, novel analytical tool, such as computational methods allow us to amplify robustness of other data rich sources, such as electronic health records, while searching for the structures of causality that could be more rooted in real world estimates of certain interventions safety, efficacy and effectiveness (14, 45, 47–49).

AUTHOR CONTRIBUTIONS

MC provided and constructed initial idea of the manuscript. MC, AS, and AK co-authored and edited the manuscript.

REFERENCES

1. Enck P, Bingel U, Schedlowski M, Rief W. The placebo response in medicine: minimize, maximize or personalize? *Nat Rev Drug Discov.* (2013) 12:191–204. doi: 10.1038/nrd3923
2. Enck P, Klosterhalfen S, Weimer K, Horing B, Zipfel S. The placebo response in clinical trials: more questions than answers. *Philos Trans R Soc Lond B Biol Sci.* (2011) 366:1889–95. doi: 10.1098/rstb.2010.0384
3. Howick J. The relativity of 'placebos': defending a modified version of Grünbaum's definition. *Synthese.* (2017) 194:1363–96. doi: 10.1007/s11229-015-1001-0
4. Kelley JM. Lumping and splitting: toward a taxonomy of placebo and related effects. *Int Rev Neurobiol.* (2018) 139:29–48. doi: 10.1016/bs.irn.2018.07.011
5. Blease C. Conceptual consensus in placebo studies: Lessons from the philosophy of science. *Perspect Biol Med.* (2018) 61:412–30. doi: 10.1353/pbm.2018.0053
6. Jakobsen JC, Katakam KK, Schou A, Hellmuth SG, Stallknecht SE, LethMoller K, et al. Selective serotonin reuptake inhibitors versus placebo in patients with major depressive disorder. A systematic review with meta-analysis and trial sequential analysis. *BMC Psychiatry.* (2017) 17:58. doi: 10.1186/s12888-016-1173-2
7. Cipriani A, Furukawa TA, Salanti G, Chaimani A, Atkinson LZ, Ogawa Y, et al. Comparative efficacy and acceptability of 21 antidepressant drugs for the acute treatment of adults with major depressive disorder: a systematic review and network meta-analysis. *Lancet.* (2018) 391:1357–1366. doi: 10.1016/S0140-6736(17)32802
8. Hengartner MP, Plöderl M. Statistically significant antidepressant-placebo differences on subjective symptom-rating scales do not prove that the drugs work: effect size and method bias matter! *Front Psychiatry.* (2018) 9:517. doi: 10.3389/fpsyt.2018.005
9. Rudorfer MV. Recent findings of the comparative efficacy and tolerability of antidepressants for major depressive disorder: do we now know what to prescribe? *CNS Drugs.* (2018) 32:807. doi: 10.1007/s40263-018-0563-z
10. Fava GA, Benasi G, Lucente M, Offidani E, Cosci F, Guidi J. Withdrawal symptoms after serotonin-noradrenaline reuptake inhibitor discontinuation: systematic review. *Psychother Psychosom.* (2018) 87:195–203. doi: 10.1159/000491524
11. Carvalho AF, Sharma MS, Brunoni AR, Vieta E, Fava GA. The safety, tolerability and risks associated with the use of newer generation antidepressant drugs: a critical review of the literature. *Psychother Psychosom.* (2016) 85:270–88. doi: 10.1159/000447034
12. Salanti G, Chaimani A, Furukawa TA, Higgins JPT, Ogawa Y, Cipriani A, et al. Impact of placebo arms on outcomes in antidepressant trials: systematic review and meta-regression analysis. *Int J Epidemiol.* (2018) 47:1454–64. doi: 10.1093/ije/dyy076
13. Furukawa TA, Cipriani A, Atkinson LZ, Leucht S, Ogawa Y, Takeshima N, et al. Placebo response rates in antidepressant trials: a systematic review of published and unpublished double-blind randomised controlled studies. *Lancet Psychiatry.* (2016) 3:1059–66. doi: 10.1016/S2215-0366(16) 30307-8
14. Deaton A, Cartwright N. Understanding and misunderstanding randomized controlled trials. *Soc Sci Med.* (2017) 210:2–21. doi: 10.1016/j.socscimed.2017.12.005
15. Rothwell PM. External validity of randomised controlled trials: "to whom do the results of this trial apply?" *Lancet.* (2005) 365:82–93. doi: 10.1016/S0140-6736(04)17670-8
16. Enck P, Klosterhalfen S, Weimer K. Unsolved, forgotten, and ignored features of the placebo response in medicine. *Clin Ther.* (2017) 39:458–68. doi: 10.1016/j.clinthera.2016.11.016
17. Evers AWM, Colloca L, Blease C, Annoni M, Atlas LY, Benedetti F, et al. Implications of placebo and nocebo effects for clinical practice: expert consensus. *Psychother Psychosom.* (2018) 87:204–10. doi: 10.1159/000490354
18. Fava GA, Guidi J, Rafanelli C, Rickels K. The clinical inadequacy of the placebo model and the development of an alternative conceptual model. *Psychother Psychosom.* (2017) 86:332–40. doi: 10.1159/000480038
19. Carlino E, Vase L. Can knowledge of placebo and nocebo mechanisms help improve randomized clinical trials? *Int Rev Neurobiol.* (2018) 138:329–57. doi: 10.1016/bs.irn.2018.01.012
20. Kube T, Rief W. Are placebo and drug-specific effects additive? Questioning basic assumptions of double-blinded randomized clinical trials and presenting novel study designs. *Drug Discov Today.* (2017) 22:729–35. doi: 10.1016/j.drudis.2016.11.02240
21. Zion SR, Crum AJ. Mindsets Matter: A new framework for harnessing the placebo effect in modern medicine. *Int Rev Neurobiol.* (2018) 138:137–60. doi: 10.1016/bs.irn.2018.02.002
22. Kirsch I. Are drug and placebo effects in depression additive? *Biol Psychiatry.* (2000) 47:733–5. doi: 10.1016/S0006-3223(00)00832-5
23. Leuchter AF, Hunter AM., Tartter M, Cook IA. Role of pill-taking, expectation and therapeutic alliance in the placebo response in clinical trials for major depression. *Br J Psychiatry.* (2014) 205:443–9. doi: 10.1192/bjp.bp.113.140343
24. Mora MS, Nestoriuc Y, Rief W. Lessons learned from placebo groups in antidepressant trials. *Philos Trans R Soc Lond B Biol Sci.* (2011) 366:1879–88. doi: 10.1098/rstb.2010.0394
25. Rief W, Barsky AJ, Bingel U, Doering BK, Schwarting R, Wöhr M, et al. Rethinking psychopharmacotherapy: the role of treatment context and brain plasticity in antidepressant and antipsychotic interventions. *Neurosci Biobehav Rev.* (2016) 60:51–64. doi: 10.1016/j.neubiorev.2015.11.008
26. Webb CA, Trivedi MH, Cohen ZD, Dillon DG, Fournier JC, Goer F, et al. Personalized prediction of antidepressant v. placebo response: evidence from the EMBARC study. *Psychol Med.* (2018) 1–10. doi: 10.1017/S0033291718001708
27. Gueorguieva R, Mallinckrodt C, Krystal JH. Trajectories of depression severity in clinical trials of duloxetine insights into antidepressant and placebo responses. *Arch Gen Psychiatry.* (2011) 68:1227–37. doi: 10.1001/archgenpsychiatry.2011.132
28. Fava M, Evins AE, Dorer DJ, Schoenfeld DA. The problem of the placebo response in clinical trials for psychiatric disorders: culprits, possible remedies, and a novel study design approach. *Psychother Psychosom.* (2003) 72:115–27. doi: 10.1159/000069738
29. Weimer K, Colloca L, Enck P. Placebo effects in psychiatry: mediators and moderators. *Lancet Psychiatry.* (2015) 2:246–57. doi: 10.1016/S2215-0366(14)00092-3
30. Kirsch I, Moore TJ, Scoboria A, Nicholls SS. The emperor's new drugs: an analysis of antidepressant medication data submitted to the U.S. food and drug administration. *Prev Treat.* (2002) 5:23. doi: 10.1037/1522-3736.5.1.523a
31. Rabinowitz J, Werbeloff N, Mandel FS, Menard F, Marangell L, Kapur S. Initial depression severity and response to antidepressants v. placebo: patient level data analysis from 34 randomised controlled trials. *Br J Psychiatry.* (2016) 209:427–8. doi: 10.1192/bjp.bp.115.173906
32. Furukawa TA, Maruo K, Noma H, Tanaka S, Imai H, Shinohara K, et al. Initial severity of major depression and efficacy of new generation antidepressants: individual participant data meta-analysis. *Acta Psychiatr Scand.* (2018) 137:450–8. doi: 10.1111/acps.12886
33. Meister R, Jansen A, Harter M, Nestoriuc Y, Kriston L. Placebo and nocebo reactions in randomized trials of pharmacological treatments for persistent depressive disorder. A meta-regression analysis. *J Affect Disord.* (2017) 215:288–98. doi: 10.1016/j.jad.2017.03.024
34. Papakostas GI, Fava M. Does the probability of receiving placebo influence clinical trial outcome? A meta-regression of double-blind, randomized clinical trials in MDD. *Eur Neuropsychopharmacol.* (2009) 19:34–40. doi: 10.1016/j.euroneuro.2008.08.009
35. Laferton J, Vijapura S, Baer L, Clain AJ, Cooper A, Papakostas G, et al. Mechanisms of perceived treatment assignment and subsequent expectancy effects in a double blind placebo controlled RCT of major depression. *Front Psychiatry.* (2018) 9:424. doi: 10.3389/fpsyt.2018.00424
36. Iniesta R, Malki K, Maier W, Rietschel M, Mors O, Hauser J, et al. Combining clinical variables to optimize prediction of antidepressant treatment outcomes. *J Psychiatr Res.* (2016) 78:94–102. doi: 10.1016/j.jpsychires.2016.03.016
37. Trivedi MH, South C, Jha MK, Rush AJ, Cao J, Kurian B, et al. A novel strategy to identify placebo responders: prediction index of clinical and biological markers in the EMBARC trial. *Psychother Psychosom.* (2018) 87:285–95. doi: 10.1159/000491093
38. De Vries Y, Roest A, Bos E, Burgerhof J, Van Loo H, De Jonge P. Predicting antidepressant response by monitoring early improvement of

individual symptoms of depression: Individual patient data meta-analysis. *Br J Psychiatry.* (2019) 214:4–10. doi: 10.1192/bjp.2018.122

39. Kelley JM, Kaptchuk TJ, Cusin C, Lipkin S, Fava M. Open-label placebo for major depressive disorder: a pilot randomized controlled trial. *Psychother Psychosom.* (2012) 81:312–4. doi: 10.1159/000337053
40. Moncrieff J, Wessely S, Hardy R. Active placebos versus antidepressants for depression. *Cochrane Database Syst Rev.* (2004) 1:CD003012. doi: 10.1002/14651858.CD003012.pub2
41. Enck P, Klosterhalfen S, Zipfel S. Novel study designs to investigate the placebo response. *BMC Med Res Methodol.* (2011) 11:90. doi: 10.1186/1471-2288-11-90 41
42. Kessels R, Mozer R, Bloemers J. Methods for assessing and controlling placebo effects. *Stat Methods Med Res.* (2017) 1:962280217748339. doi: 10.1177/0962280217748339
43. Ćurković M, Košec A, Savić A. The meaning and influence of time-related dropout dynamics in antidepressant studies: reassessing current approaches. *Psychother Psychosom.* (2019). 1–2. doi: 10.1159/000 496498
44. Ioannidis JPA. Randomized controlled trials: often flawed, mostly useless, clearly indispensable: a commentary on Deaton and Cartwright. *Soc Sci Med.* (2018) 210:53–6. doi: 10.1016/j.socscimed.2018.04.029
45. Horwitz RI, Hayes-Conroy A, Caricchio R, Singer BH. From evidence based medicine to medicine based evidence. *Am J Med.* (2017) 130:1246–50. doi: 10.1016/j.amjmed.2017.06.012.
46. Rief W, Shedden-Mora MC, Laferton JAC, Auer C, Petrie K, Salzmann S, et al. Preoperative optimization of patient expectations improves long-term outcome in heart surgery patients: results of the randomized controlled PSY-HEART trial. *BMC Med.* (2017) 15:4. doi: 10.1186/s12916-016-0767-3.
47. Frieden TR. Evidence for health decision making-beyond randomized, controlled trials. *N Engl J Med.* (2017) 377:465–75. doi: 10.1056/NEJMra1614394.
48. Gillan CM, Whelan R. What big data can do for treatment in psychiatry. *Curr Opin Behav Sci.* (2017) 18:34–42. doi: 10.1016/j.cobeha.2017.07.003
49. Dwyer DB, Falkai P, Koutsouleris N. Machine learning approaches for clinical psychology and psychiatry. *Annu Rev Clin Psychol.* (2018) 14:91–118. doi: 10.1146/annurev-clinpsy-032816-045037

Optimizing Expectations *via* Mobile Apps: A New Approach for Examining and Enhancing Placebo Effects

Piotr Gruszka[1], Christoph Burger[2,3] and Mark P. Jensen[4]*

[1] Mental Health Research and Treatment Center, Faculty of Psychology, Ruhr-Universität Bochum, Bochum, Germany, [2] Department of Basic Psychological Research and Research Methods, Faculty of Psychology, University of Vienna, Vienna, Austria, [3] Department of Applied Psychology: Work, Education and Economy, Faculty of Psychology, University of Vienna, Vienna, Austria, [4]Department of Rehabilitation Medicine, University of Washington, Seattle, WA, United States

***Correspondence:**
Piotr Gruszka
piotr.gruszka@rub.de

There is growing interest in interventions that enhance placebo responses in clinical practice, given the possibility that this would lead to better patient health and more effective therapy outcomes. Previous studies suggest that placebo effects can be maximized by optimizing patients' outcome expectations. However, expectancy interventions are difficult to validate because of methodological challenges, such as reliable blinding of the clinician providing the intervention. Here we propose a novel approach using mobile apps that can provide highly standardized expectancy interventions in a blinded manner, while at the same time assessing data in everyday life using experience sampling methodology (e.g., symptom severity, expectations) and data from smartphone sensors. Methodological advantages include: 1) full standardization; 2) reliable blinding and randomization; 3) disentangling expectation effects from other factors associated with face-to-face interventions; 4) assessing short-term (days), long-term (months), and cumulative effects of expectancy interventions; and 5) investigating possible mechanisms of change. Randomization and expectancy interventions can be realized by the app (e.g., after the clinic/lab visit). As a result, studies can be blinded without the possibility for the clinician to influence study outcomes. Possible app-based expectancy interventions include, for example, verbal suggestions and imagery exercises, although a large number of possible interventions (e.g., hypnosis) could be evaluated using this innovative approach.

Keywords: placebo, expectancy, intervention, app, mobile, smartphone, expectation

INTRODUCTION

There is an increased interest in understanding the effects of placebo interventions and the mechanisms underlying these effects. While basic research has led to a better understanding of psychobiological mechanisms underlying placebo effects by means of strictly controlled experiments (1), applied research has focused on elucidating the factors contributing to placebo effects in clinical practice (2). Some of these studies have been extensively covered in the media, reflecting the interest in placebo effects among the general public. A number of researchers have emphasized the potential of maximizing placebo effects in clinical practice to optimize treatment outcomes (3–5).

Despite recent progress, research in this area faces several unsolved methodological challenges and awaits broader validation. Similarly, as is the case in psychotherapy trials, blinding is extremely difficult to achieve when delivering placebo interventions (6). As a result, it has been challenging to estimate the true effects of placebos separately from the effects of experimenter bias. It is therefore crucial to develop new methods to assess placebo effects.

This paper aims to highlight several methodological advantages of using mobile apps in the area of placebo research. Methodological advantages include full standardization and more reliable blinding, randomization, and allocation concealment. By delivering expectancy interventions *via* apps, researchers can disentangle expectancy effects due to the intervention from effects induced by the patient–researcher (or patient–practitioner) interaction, allowing for the control of experimenter bias (7). Further, combining app-based placebo interventions with experience sampling offers several opportunities for addressing important research questions, such as investigating the impact of placebo interventions on symptom trajectories and on changes in expectations. Additionally, subjective ratings can be potentially complemented by objective data gathered through smartphone sensors and mobile-based experiments. Validated apps can be used for treatment delivery to a large number of people.

Traditional Definition of Placebo Effects

The term *placebo effect* was first described as a set of positive changes that occur after an inert or inactive treatment (i.e., placebo) was administered to patients (1). Placebo effects are usually associated with so-called blinded randomized controlled trials (RCTs), where placebos—in the form of inert pills, injection, or sham procedures that resemble the active treatments—are administered to study participants in a control group. In order to be considered specifically effective (i.e., beyond the effects of placebos), active treatments are required to outperform placebos in these trials. Optimally, study participants, researchers, study clinicians, data collectors, outcome adjudicators, and data analysts are blinded in RCTs, in order to ensure that differences between active treatments and placebos are not confounded by potential biasing factors such as experimenter effects or participants' expectations (7–9).

Problems and Inconsistencies Inherent in the Traditional Definition of Placebo Effects

There are, however, several problems with the abovementioned traditional definition of the placebo effect. First, by defining it as the global response to a placebo treatment, this definition combines the genuine placebo response with other confounding factors, such as natural course or fluctuations in the outcome variable, regression to the mean, the effects of additional treatment(s), observer bias, and subsiding adverse effects of any previous treatments (10, 11). Furthermore, associating placebo effects with RCTs has led to an understanding of placebo effects as (mostly) a vehicle for testing the effectiveness of treatments, such as pharmacological substances, and not otherwise of much interest. As a result, many view placebo effects as something that should be controlled, rather than investigated or used to improve health and function (12).

Second, putting the placebo itself and its inertness into the focus of the definition has led to significant confusion and controversy regarding the placebo effect (e.g., how is it possible for an inert treatment to have genuine effects?). This has resulted in a rather negative connotation being attributed to placebo effects; they are often thought to be fictitious, nonexistent, or only for the gullible [for focus group results, see Ref. (13)]. Furthermore, placebo effects are often considered unworthy and unscientific (14).

As a result of these problems, there have been various attempts to make a case for abandoning the concept of placebo effect (15) and to propose new concepts [e.g., "context effects" (12), "meaning responses" (16)]. Because the concept of placebo is deeply entrenched in the literature, proposed alternative labels and concepts have not been adopted. We have therefore decided to continue using the term *placebo effect* in this paper. However, in order to reconcile this concept with the current evidence, a reconceptualization of this concept is in order [also see Ref. (11)]. In short, the focus should not be on the placebo itself but on the mechanisms underlying the placebo effects. Consistent with this idea, Gliedman and colleagues stated over 60 years ago that the "so-called placebo effect should be looked upon as an epiphenomenon of complicated psychological processes, which are far more important than the disarmingly simple means utilized for its realization" (17).

Reconceptualization of Placebo Effects

Placebo effects have been found to originate from psychobiological mechanisms in those who respond to placebos (1). Both conscious expectancies and unconscious conditioning mechanisms are assumed to be major contributing factors to placebo responses (1, 18). Previous research has shown that patients' expectations of clinical benefits play a major role in placebo effects by triggering distinct neurobiological systems that then shape the therapeutic outcomes (3, 11, 19).

When focusing on the underlying mechanism of expectancy learning, it becomes clear that placebo responses are omnipresent in clinical practice—even when no placebo is administered. When active treatments are administered, patients' responses are determined not only by specific effects of the treatments themselves but also by the patients' outcome expectations, as well as their possible interaction. This can be easily demonstrated by the so-called "open–hidden" paradigm, which has shown that treatments are more effective when they are given when the patients are present and fully aware of them (i.e., they are able to form expectations) than when they are given in a hidden manner and without patients' knowledge (11).

A large and growing literature has demonstrated that expectancy-driven placebo effects are a genuine phenomenon that occurs not only after the administration of inert but also of active treatments, and that contributes substantially to the success of many active medical treatments (1). Such effects are potentially relevant in clinical practice because they might lead to better patient health and more effective therapy outcomes.

In fact, several studies have shown a positive association between optimistic outcome expectations of patients and favorable therapeutic improvements for a variety of conditions and symptoms, such as disability after surgical interventions (19), hypertension (20, 21), depression (22), anxiety (23, 24), other psychiatric disorders (25), and pain (26).

However, some researchers are less optimistic about the clinical value of placebo effects. Hróbjartsson and Gøtzsche, for example, questioned the clinical relevance of placebos in their meta-analyses (27, 28) and argued that placebos can affect only subjective outcomes such as pain but not objective health parameters. Other researchers, however, note that placebos can improve objective outcomes such as peripheral health parameters and immune responses (29, 30).

Expectancy Interventions: Modifying Patients' Expectations to Improve Clinical Outcome

Recently, there has been increased interest in interventions that optimize placebo effects to improve clinical outcomes in routine medical care (1, 2, 31, 32). Previous research has established that interventions targeting outcome expectations have been shown to relieve patients' symptoms such as pain [for a meta-analysis, see Ref. (26)]. These expectancy interventions usually consist of brief procedures, such as verbal suggestions or imagery interventions, and can be implemented by clinicians in their routine clinical practice. There has been a growing interest in examining the effects of both verbal suggestions and imagery to increase patients' outcome expectations, which are then thought to enhance treatment outcomes. Such interventions have been used as part of hypnotic treatments for more than a century (33, 34). In fact, evidence indicates that expectancies are mediators of the effects of suggestions both in placebo interventions and in hypnosis (35).

Given that expectancy interventions have been shown to improve symptoms, one could argue that there is an ethical obligation to encourage their widespread implementation and application. This would raise the question regarding how such interventions can be most effectively delivered in order to reach as many patients as possible. Even if the intervention's benefit is small, it still could be considered a valuable public health intervention if it reaches a high number of people with few adverse effects.

Methodological Challenges in Validating Clinician-Delivered Expectancy Interventions

Despite the potential of placebo interventions for improving health outcomes, a number of researchers have noted that the efficacy of placebo interventions, such as expectancy interventions, has not been adequately validated. This lack of validation is due to the as-yet-unresolved challenges in placebo research (36, 37), such as the inability to achieve the basic prerequisites for rigorous validity testing of placebo interventions.

One critical precondition is the blinding of the person delivering the interventions. In placebo research—as is also the case in face-to-face psychotherapy trials—reliable blinding of the intervention is extremely challenging. When clinicians are delivering expectancy interventions (e.g., suggesting that pain will decrease soon), they are aware of doing so because delivering the intervention per se is a conscious social act. Thus, they cannot be blinded to treatment allocation or the type of interventions they are delivering. One can envision a variety of ways that this awareness could lead to additional conscious or unconscious changes in the clinicians' behaviors (e.g., preferential treatment) or verbal/nonverbal communication (e.g., more friendly and reassuring manner) that go beyond the expectancy intervention alone. This lack of blinding may, and probably does, result in experimenter bias (7, 38, 39), which can then contribute to spurious effects or overestimation of effect sizes. Although one might try to blind experimenters or study clinicians by not telling them about study hypotheses, their beliefs and assumptions about the intervention they are delivering can still bias outcomes.

One potential approach to understand the impact of interaction patterns on placebo effects is to manipulate factors within the patient–provider interaction. For example, Kaptchuk and colleagues (40) showed in a single-blind three-arm RCT of 262 patients with irritable bowel syndrome (IBS) that factors such as warmth, empathy, active listening, and indirect suggestions ("I have had much positive experience treating IBS and look forward to demonstrating that acupuncture is a valuable treatment in this trial") affected outcomes. It makes sense that factors such as clinicians' warmth, empathy, active listening, or suggestions have positive effects on clinical outcomes, given that similar aspects are at the heart of person-centered psychotherapy (congruence, unconditional positive regard, empathy) and hypnosis (suggestions) (41–46). However, the conclusions that can be drawn from the Kaptchuk et al. (40) and other similar studies are limited because they are generally conducted unblinded. As a result, it is not possible to conclude whether the outcomes are due to these nonspecific clinician factors (e.g., warm, friendly interaction, expectancy manipulation through verbal suggestion) that are a part of how the intervention is delivered, due to experimenter bias (e.g., differential treatment of patients beyond the actual intervention depending on their experimental condition), or both [for a review on the effects of nonverbal behaviors of experimenters on placebo effects in research participants, see Ref. (47)].

Further challenges for the rigorous evaluation of expectancy interventions are response sets, such as acquiescence bias (i.e., the patient or participant wishing to please the experimenter). It is also difficult to disentangle the impact of patient–provider interactions from other response biases. It has been shown, for example, that patients have a higher tendency for response bias when they are experiencing a warm patient–provider interaction (36). Thus, a patient might report a decrease in symptom severity to please the clinician, although it might not reflect an actual change in subjective experience.

In conventional settings, expectancy interventions are delivered by clinicians. These settings almost always involve biases such as those mentioned above. This crucially limits the interpretation of the results. These biasing effects may be an even bigger hindrance for placebo research in children and adolescents, as children are more suggestible than adults (48) and thus might be more easily influenced by experimenter or response bias.

ADVANTAGES OF USING MOBILE APPS FOR PLACEBO RESEARCH

There has been an increased interest in apps in the field of medicine and psychology in recent years. Mobile apps are being used more and more frequently by researchers, clinicians, and patients and have the potential to revolutionize different aspects of medical and psychotherapeutic care (49–54). However, to the best of our knowledge, apps have not been systematically used to examine or deliver placebo-boosting interventions. Thus, the field could potentially profit from technological advances in the area of smartphones.

We propose in this paper that the use of mobile apps can lead to many advantageous developments in both placebo research and clinical practice: i) using smartphones can help to solve problems inherent in validating placebo-boosting interventions such as expectancy manipulations; ii) mobile apps can be used to gain a better understanding of placebo mechanisms in everyday life; and iii) once placebo-boosting interventions have been successfully validated, apps can be used as an effective way to deliver these interventions as an adjunct to therapy sessions or as a stand-alone tool to a large number of people (see **Figure 1**).

Validating Placebo-Boosting Interventions

In light of difficulties in reproducing major findings in psychological and medical science (55–58) in recent years,

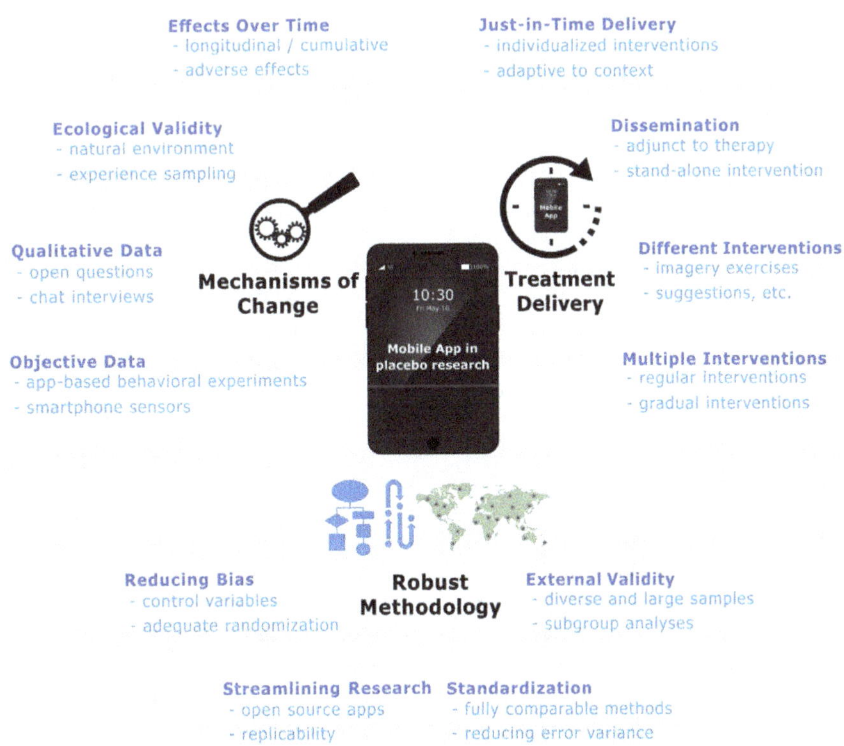

FIGURE 1 | Schematic overview of advantages of app-based expectancy interventions.

the area of placebo research might profit from innovative methodological advances. App-based studies offer several methodological advantages enabling more robust research, which can play an important role in improving the scientific status of expectancy interventions, potentially enabling them to be introduced into mainstream medicine (1).

One of the advantages of app-based expectancy interventions relates to the fact that they can be fully standardized. In the past, expectancy manipulations used different protocols and were conducted in different settings and with different samples. Thus, differences in outcomes may be related not only to different outcome measures and types of illnesses (29, 59) but also to different protocols, settings, clinicians, samples, sampling procedures, and methodological standards.

To address these issues, app-based interventions can take advantage of full standardization, thereby reducing heterogeneity. They can also ensure adherence to key characteristics of high-quality trials such as adequate randomization and allocation concealment, by performing these tasks objectively and reliably within the app. This can be achieved by placing importance on the right timing; that is, randomization and allocation concealment can be performed by the app after the clinic or lab visit (where the patient or study participant can be introduced to the app) so that it is impossible for inadequate group allocation or blinding to impact the experimenter or clinician and his or her interaction with the study participant. Alternatively, patients might use the app fully remotely without any contact at all with experimenters or clinicians. As it has been shown that trials with inadequate or unclear allocation concealment exaggerate subjective outcome effects (8, 60), the use of apps could potentially increase the reliability of effect size estimates.

By making the apps open-source, independent researchers could use them at minimal cost to conduct fully identical replications. Although innovative placebo interventions [e.g., open-label placebos (61, 62)] have been tested in recent years, identical replications of these studies are lacking. Given that effect sizes in psychology are, on average, only half the initial size when replicated (56), identical replications are crucial for validating expectancy interventions. Providing app-based expectancy interventions as open-source software may potentially reduce costs by streamlining research (63), thereby increasing the quality of conducted studies (64).

The standardization that results from the use of app-based expectancy interventions would lead to smaller heterogeneity and more precise replications. Thus, studies will be fully comparable and could be easily aggregated in prospective meta-analyses (65), leading to large and meaningful sample sizes, a key characteristic of robust research (66, 67). This would also allow investigators to quantify the influence of sample procedures and sample characteristics on trial outcomes and replication rates.

In addition, by standardizing expectancy interventions and increasing sample sizes, variance will be reduced. This could enable researchers to investigate the impact of expectancy interventions in different samples. Thus, conducting highly standardized app-based experimental interventions in different samples and cultures can lead to a better understanding of interpersonal and intercultural differences in expectations (68). This might lead to more precise predictions of placebo effects and to the development of more effective culturally sensitive expectancy interventions. As most research is conducted in Western, educated, industrialized, rich, and democratic (WEIRD) (69) samples, app-based expectancy interventions offer the potential of gathering data in more diverse and representative samples if uploaded to an app store or used as an add-on to established treatments.

Crucially, experimenter bias can be limited by disentangling patients' expectations from the patient–provider interaction. By delivering expectancy interventions within the app, expectations can be studied in isolation, disentangled from the effects of the patient–provider interaction. As such, expectancy interventions can be delivered at home, after seeing the clinician, thereby eliminating experimenter biases (7, 39), or even fully remotely if the app is uploaded to an app store.

Gaining Insights Into Placebo Mechanisms in Everyday Life

Ecological Validity

Further, app-based expectancy interventions offer the potential to deliver interventions with high ecological validity in patients' everyday life. Thus, effects from the lab can be extended to the natural surroundings of patients, thereby increasing the potential usefulness of interventions (64). Apps also offer the opportunity of combining experience sampling procedures with expectancy interventions. Although the advantages of experience sampling methodology have been discussed in the area of psychiatry before [e.g., Ref. (70)], to our knowledge, this methodology has not yet been applied to placebo research. Experience sampling is a method for assessing momentary thoughts, feelings, and symptoms and is usually employed several times per day over consecutive days (71, 72). This structured diary method can be easily implemented in mobile apps. It offers the possibility to assess symptom trajectories in everyday life as well as underlying mechanisms, thereby increasing ecological validity.

Investigating symptom trajectories over time could enable researchers to cluster study participants into different types of responders (73). Gueorguieva and colleagues (74), for example, have investigated trajectories of depression severity in clinical trials of duloxetine showing that placebo-treated patients were characterized by different trajectories than responders and nonresponders in the antidepressant-treated subsample. Moreover, it may be possible to differentiate study participants based on early or late responses. Simons and colleagues (75) have classified response trajectories of children with chronic pain after intensive pain rehabilitation treatment into early treatment responders, late treatment responders, and nonresponders.

In addition, more intensive daily experience sampling would enable researchers to investigate the variability in symptoms within and between persons following expectancy interventions. Apps might potentially enable researchers also to gather information on adverse events and long-term data after expectancy interventions. Thereby it would be possible to answer an important research question that has not yet been adequately addressed: Do expectancy interventions lead to long-lasting changes or only temporary improvement? Thus, this type of research has the potential to elucidate a much more in-depth understanding of placebo effects in everyday life.

Experience sampling might be used to assess not only symptom fluctuations but also changes in symptom expectations. Mun and colleagues (76) have, for example, investigated pain expectations in a sample of 231 individuals with rheumatoid arthritis showing that pain expectations are a reliable predictor of pain. As expectations are at the heart of placebo effects, the assessment and fluctuation of symptom expectations will add to a more precise understanding of placebo effects and a better understanding of expectations and their formation over time.

The assessment of symptoms and expectations *via* apps can be complemented by open questions and other qualitative assessments (e.g., interviews *via* smartphone chats about daily experiences) to investigate the impact of not only expectancy interventions but also daily experiences such as social interactions on symptom trajectories and expectations. A detailed understanding of these processes will enable a more precise prediction of placebo effects and will offer new avenues for individualized expectancy interventions.

Assessment of Objective Data

Subjective data on symptom and expectation trajectories can be complemented with data obtained through smartphone sensors. Smartphone sensors can provide researchers with data about social interactions, daily activities (e.g., physical activity and sleep quality), and mobility patterns (77, 78). Researchers targeting chronic pain could, for example, investigate how expectancy interventions affect physical activity, sleep quality, or social interactions.

Apps also offer the possibility of running behavioral experiments on smartphones. Thus, experiments from the lab could be conducted on smartphones. Free popular experimental software such as PsychoPy[1] is now also available for mobile devices (79, 80), potentially enabling researchers to conduct these experiments with minimal costs. A promising approach might be to develop experiments to phenotype beliefs underlying changes in expectations or to employ existing implicit measures such as the implicit association test (IAT) (81) for that purpose.

Although some researchers have argued that placebo effects lead only to an improvement in parameters that depend on subjective patient ratings (28), others came to more favorable conclusions (29). Thus, it seems crucial to find alternative ways of assessing objective data following expectancy interventions in order to resolve this issue. Smartphones and other mobile devices offer several efficient ways for doing so by assessing different types of behavioral measures in an unobtrusive way without putting additional burden on study participants.

Treatment Delivery

Multiple or Repeated Interventions

Apps also can be used to deliver multiple or repeated expectancy interventions, thereby potentially increasing their efficacy. One could, for example, deliver different weekly expectancy interventions and assess their impact on symptom trajectories through the use of experience sampling. This might potentially enable researchers to investigate cumulative effects of repeated expectancy interventions. As some patients show *cognitive immunization strategies* [strategies to weaken or eliminate expectation violation or, in other words, strategies to reduce cognitive dissonance between suggested information and individual beliefs, (82, 83)], it might be necessary to deliver expectancy interventions gradually or to individualize them according to patient beliefs, person characteristics, and symptom trajectories for them to take effect.

Just-in-Time Adaptive Expectancy Interventions

A precise understanding of symptom and expectation trajectories complemented with behavioral data through smartphone sensors might pave the way for the development of just-in-time adaptive expectancy interventions (JITAEIs). Just-in-time adaptive interventions (JITAIs) relate to interventions that are adapted to the status or context of an individual over time (84–87). As every person has individual beliefs, it is likely that individualized interventions will have higher efficacy. Psychotherapy research has shown, for example, that resistant patients profit more from nondirective therapy than from directive approaches (88). Thus, patients with more rigid health beliefs, which make them more resistant to change, could potentially profit more from indirect suggestions ("Many patients profited from the app before") or imagery exercises (e.g., imagining healthy future self) than from direct suggestions ("You will profit from this app"). Suggestions as part of expectancy interventions might therefore be delivered based on symptom changes, patients' beliefs and needs, other personal characteristics, and data from smartphone sensors. Thus, if patients have strong beliefs about their condition (as assessed by questionnaires) and have not shown symptom improvements for several weeks, they might be offered indirect suggestions, such as, "Some patients did not seem to profit from the app in the beginning, some were even frustrated. Often, however, their symptoms did in fact improve, bit by bit." Less resistant patients, who report early improvements in symptom reduction, might be given more direct suggestions such as, "You have used the app for one week now. Your pain has already decreased. You will experience your pain decreasing even further in the coming weeks." Thus, the app may be programmed in such a way as to accommodate the patients' symptom ratings, other personal characteristics, and objective data gathered through smartphone sensors to deliver individualized expectancy interventions.

Treatment Dissemination

Once an expectancy intervention is found to be effective for producing changes in reported symptoms, clinical implementation of that intervention may prove challenging, given the significant limitations on clinicians' time. Apps could potentially be used to deliver highly standardized expectancy interventions without posing an unnecessary burden on busy clinicians. Thus, app-based expectancy interventions might be used either as an add-on to existing medical and psychotherapeutic procedures or even as a stand-alone intervention.

[1] https://www.psychopy.org/

TABLE 1 | Summarized advantages of app-based expectancy interventions.

Validating placebo-boosting interventions	
Full standardization	Fully standardized placebo interventions are fully comparable, result in smaller heterogeneity, and can be easily aggregated, leading to large and meaningful sample sizes; this will enable investigating predictors of placebo responses in subgroups of patients.
Adequate randomization and blinding	Randomization can be conducted within the app, thereby ensuring adequate randomization and allocation concealment. Interventions can be delivered in the absence of the clinician, thereby ensuring reliable blinding.
Open-source apps	Releasing app-based expectancy interventions as open-source might enable other research groups and clinicians to conduct similar studies with little costs, thereby enabling easy-to-implement replications.
More diverse samples	Apps enable conducting expectancy interventions in more diverse samples and different cultures.
Limiting experimenter bias	Expectations can be studied in isolation from the effects of the patient–provider interaction, allowing disentangling patient expectations from effects of the patient–provider interaction.
Gaining insights into placebo mechanisms in everyday life	
Ecological validity	Symptom and expectation trajectories can be studied in everyday life, thereby increasing ecological validity and enabling individualized expectancy interventions.
Adverse events	Questions about adverse events can be easily integrated into apps, thus allowing gathering data on potential short- and longer-term adverse events due to expectancy interventions.
Long-term and cumulative effects	Long-term and cumulative effects of expectancy interventions can be assessed *via* experience sampling.
Qualitative data	Apps can be used to gather qualitative data (open questions, chat interviews) on the impact of expectancy interventions to understand the formation of expectations.
Objective data	Subjective patient ratings can be complemented with objective data by using behavioral experiments on smartphones and gathering data from smartphone sensors.
Treatment delivery	
Multiple interventions	The effectiveness of app-based expectancy interventions can be increased by delivering them multiple times.
Just-in-time adaptive expectancy interventions	App-based expectancy interventions can be individualized and delivered just in time to fit individual beliefs, personal characteristics, symptom trajectories, and objective data.
Treatment dissemination	App-based expectancy interventions can be uploaded to app stores and delivered as an add-on to existing medical and psychotherapeutic procedures or as a stand-alone intervention.

DISCUSSION

The present paper introduces a novel approach of delivering expectancy interventions (e.g., verbal suggestions, imagery exercises) aimed at boosting placebo effects through mobile apps. Because this approach does not involve an attendant person (e.g., an experimenter or clinician) to deliver the expectancy intervention, expectancy-driven components of the intervention can be disentangled from social interaction–driven components. Such an approach can answer questions such as what aspect of the placebo effect is driven by changes in expectancies. Moreover, this approach can help us to better understand the patient populations for whom such interventions may be most effective.

Previous studies have already shown that verbal suggestions delivered by technology (i.e., audio players) are effective in improving clinical symptoms in patients. For example, playing recorded hypnosis audio tracks, consisting of verbal suggestions (also used to elicit imagery), has been shown to be effective in reducing pain [e.g., Refs. (89, 90)]. These studies, however, did not use mobile apps to deliver the verbal suggestions and thus did not exploit the full potential of available technology. Nevertheless, the findings support the approach presented in this paper as promising.

As expectancy interventions have been used primarily in experimental research in relation to an active or placebo treatment [oral, injection, cutaneous, or other; see Ref. (26)], their implementation in clinical settings may be inspired by clinical hypnosis research. Clinical hypnosis has a long history of using verbal suggestions for symptom improvement (33, 34), with several journals focusing solely on hypnosis (e.g., *American Journal of Clinical Hypnosis*, *International Journal of Clinical and Experimental Hypnosis*). Bringing both fields together—research on clinical hypnosis and placebo research—may be particularly fruitful for developing more effective expectancy interventions. Thus, we think that new expectancy interventions for mobile apps would greatly profit from research in both the clinical hypnosis and placebo research fields. However, possible app-based expectancy interventions are not limited to verbal suggestions and imagery exercises, as a large number of expectancy interventions could be delivered and evaluated using this innovative approach.

We have described several advantages of app-based expectancy interventions (see **Table 1** for an overview). This approach makes it possible to investigate placebo effects independent of the patient–provider interaction, thereby overcoming some of the inherent methodological challenges associated with placebo interventions. Highly standardized app-based expectancy interventions can lead to more robust research by enabling researchers to replicate findings more easily. Apps also can be used to phenotype placebo responses longitudinally, while investigating mechanisms of change. Researchers can integrate behavioral experiments into their apps and gather data from smartphone sensors for this purpose. This could allow researchers to predict placebo responses more precisely, helping scientists gain insights into short-term, long-term, and cumulative effects of expectancy interventions as well as adverse events. Further, app-based expectancy interventions can be individualized and delivered just in time.

This approach has significant potential for both research and clinical practice. If simple app-based interventions aimed at improving outcome expectations (e.g., verbal suggestions or imagery exercises) lead to symptom relief, they could be widely applied to optimize patient treatment. Such approaches could be used to support medical treatment more efficiently (e.g., reducing dose of medication without diminishing effects, improving outcome effects without having to raise medication dose) or even be a viable alternative to medication when the anticipated adverse effects might outweigh the benefits of drug use (91). In the field of pediatrics, where medications may have long-term side effects on children's brain development, reducing the pharmacological load might be even more relevant. Improving outcome expectations could also translate into better patient adherence and compliance (32) and reduced feelings of helplessness and hopelessness.

However, since no effectiveness data on different forms of app-based expectancy interventions are currently available, it will take further empirical research efforts to understand the kinds of expectancy interventions that are most effective under what conditions and for what populations. Eventually, it will be necessary to conduct studies with large samples to investigate precise predictors of placebo responses taking into account various data sources, including data from smartphone sensors, app-based experiments, as well as biological data. These studies will provide important information for individualizing interventions, which could subsequently be delivered just in time.

Some limitations of this approach need to be acknowledged. The first limitation refers to the fact that mobile apps cannot replace the provider–patient relationship, which is considered an important factor of placebo effects and clinical outcomes. Rather, their strength lies in their ability to systematically study expectation effects separately from social interaction effects. App-based approaches might be of special interest for i) patients who do not want to disclose their problems to clinicians and ii) patients with a high affinity for smartphones and new technology, such as children and adolescents (92). They may also be used as an add-on or aftercare to medical/psychotherapeutic procedures.

The second limitation refers to legal, ethical, and privacy-related aspects of app-based treatments. Apps that aim to treat medical conditions are considered medical devices and need to adhere to relevant regulations, such as the European Medical Device Regulation or the Food and Drug Administration (FDA) regulation in the US before entering the market (93, 94). Furthermore, using medical apps in research potentially leads to challenges relating to consent and privacy (47). The fact that the legal situations regarding medical privacy vary between countries further complicates the matter (95). Several recommendations have been made to address ethical issues, data privacy, and data security concerns, which should be considered while developing mobile apps (96–99).

The introduction of app-based interventions also comes with technological challenges. First, although there are currently only two major operating systems available for smartphones (Android and iOS), new versions of these operating systems are released continuously. Most manufacturers also provide modified versions of Android, resulting in potential compatibility issues. In addition, manufacturers provide smartphones and other mobile devices with a plethora of different hardware specifications, including different screen sizes and screen resolutions. Thus, software developers not only need to ensure that the apps run on different operating systems but also need to program them with different screen sizes, screen resolutions, and hardware specifications in mind.

Second, it has been proposed that interventions that are delivered through a mobile device might lead to heightened expectations of a high-tech treatment among patients with high affinity for their digital devices. This phenomenon has been termed "digital placebo" (100). It has been argued that trials with such app-delivered interventions have to be complemented with an active placebo control group that also involves an app (101, 102) in order to distinguish the specific effects of the app-delivered interventions from digital placebo effects.

Further, the use of mobile technology and the Internet might be contraindicated for individuals prone to Internet addiction (103). These individuals might not profit from such apps and therefore should be assigned to other treatment modalities. Also, different operating systems or smartphone technologies in general might represent confounders that could bias the results. For example, the majority of the population in Europe uses Android smartphones, whereas there is a higher proportion of iPhone users in the US. There might also be sociodemographic differences between Android and iOS users (104).

Finally, we want to point out the importance of future research efforts to focus on translational aspects of their findings. It is well established that many findings from studies evaluating the efficacy of behavioral and health promotion interventions have not been put into (clinical) practice. It has been pointed out that an important reason for this gap between research results and evidence-based practice may lie in the tendency of the current research culture to neglect issues of external validity (105, 106). To address this important issue, Glasgow and colleagues argue that researchers should pay attention to issues of moderating variables (external validity) in both efficacy and effectiveness studies (107). These issues also have been shown to be present in smartphone-enhanced health research, as mobile health intervention studies tend to neglect the reporting of validity indicators, including indicators of external validity (108). Although there may be practical constraints, the usefulness of future research efforts (64) might benefit from quality criteria available from published best practice standards [e.g., Consolidated Standards of Reporting Trials of Electronic and Mobile HEalth Applications and onLine TeleHealth, CONSORT-EHEALTH (109)] and evaluation frameworks [e.g., RE-AIM framework: reach, efficacy/effectiveness, adoption, implementation, maintenance (105, 110)]. These criteria might be used at different stages throughout the research process (reviewing of literature, planning, conducting, reporting) as a guide to maximize internal and external validity. These criteria include, among others, reports on sample representativeness, research setting and delivery agents, theoretical framework, the development process, source code, accessibility and features/functionalities of the app, information on instructions/reminders/prompts, sustainability of effects, and potential conflicts of interest.

Once the above-described issues have been adequately tackled and the external validity of apps addressed, the use of apps and big data could potentially open up completely new avenues of research and contribute to truly personalized and more effective treatments. We have only touched upon some of the possibilities of smartphone technology in the area of placebo research. There will be many more approaches to come in the future, which we cannot even imagine right now.

AUTHOR CONTRIBUTIONS

PG, CB, and MJ conceived and designed the paper. PG and CB wrote the first draft of the manuscript. PG, CB, and MJ wrote the final version.

FUNDING

The authors acknowledge support by the DFG Open Access Publication Funds of the Ruhr-Universität Bochum.

REFERENCES

1. Petrie KJ, Rief W. Psychobiological mechanisms of placebo and nocebo effects: pathways to improve treatments and reduce side effects. *Annu Rev Psychol* (2019) 70:599–625. doi: 10.1146/annurev-psych-010418-102907
2. Evers AWM, Colloca L, Blease C, Annoni M, Atlas LY, Benedetti F, et al. Implications of placebo and nocebo effects for clinical practice: expert consensus. *Psychother Psychosom* (2018) 87:204–10. doi: 10.1159/000490354
3. Enck P, Bingel U, Schedlowski M, Rief W. The placebo response in medicine: minimize, maximize or personalize? *Nat Rev Drug Discov* (2013) 12:191–204. doi: 10.1038/nrd3923
4. Darnall BD, Colloca L. Optimizing placebo and minimizing nocebo to reduce pain, catastrophizing, and opioid use: a review of the science and an evidence-informed clinical toolkit. *Int Rev Neurobiol* (2018) 139:129–57. doi: 10.1016/bs.irn.2018.07.022
5. Kube T, Glombiewski JA, Rief W. Using different expectation mechanisms to optimize treatment of patients with medical conditions: a systematic review. *Psychosom Med* (2018) 80:535–43. doi: 10.1097/PSY.0000000000000596
6. Locher C, Gaab J, Blease C. When a placebo is not a placebo: problems and solutions to the gold standard in psychotherapy research. *Front Psychol* (2018) 9:2317. doi: 10.3389/fpsyg.2018.02317
7. Sackett DL. Bias in analytic research. *J Chronic Dis* (1979) 32:51–63. doi: 10.1016/B978-0-08-024907-0.50013-4
8. Wood L, Egger M, Gluud LL, Schulz KF, Altman DG, Ju P, et al. Empirical evidence of bias in treatment effect estimates in controlled trials with different interventions and outcomes: meta-epidemiological study. *BMJ* (2008) 336:601. doi: 10.1136/bmj.39465.451748.AD
9. Moher D, Hopewell S, Schulz KF, Montori V, Gøtzsche PC, Devereaux PJ, et al. CONSORT 2010 explanation and elaboration: updated guidelines for reporting parallel group randomised trials. *BMJ* (2010) 340:c869. doi: 10.1136/bmj.c869
10. Kienle GS, Kiene H. The powerful placebo effect: fact or fiction? *J Clin Epidemiol* (1997) 50:1311–8. doi: 10.1016/S0895-4356(97)00203-5
11. Finniss DG, Kaptchuk TJ, Miller F, Benedetti F. Placebo effects: biological, clinical and ethical advances. *Lancet* (2010) 375:686–95. doi: 10.1016/S0140-6736(09)61706-2
12. Di Blasi Z, Harkness E, Ernst E, Georgiou A, Kleijnen J. Influence of context effects on health outcomes: a systematic review. *Lancet* (2001) 357:757–62. doi: 10.1016/S0140-6736(00)04169-6
13. Bishop FL, Aizlewood L, Adams AEM. When and why placebo-prescribing is acceptable and unacceptable: a focus group study of patients' views. *PLoS One* (2014) 9:e101822. doi: 10.1371/journal.pone.0101822
14. Kaptchuk TJ, Miller FG. Placebo effects in medicine. *N Engl J Med* (2015) 373:8–9. doi: 10.1056/NEJMp1504023
15. Traeger AC, Kamper SJ. The effect of nothing? Time to abandon the concept of placebo. *Pain* (2017) 158:1179. doi: 10.1097/j.pain.0000000000000884
16. Hutchinson P, Moerman DE. The meaning response, "placebo," and methods. *Perspect Biol Med* (2018) 61:361–78. doi: 10.1353/pbm.2018.0049
17. Gliedman LH, Nash EH, Imber SD, Stone AR, Frank JD. Reduction of symptoms by pharmacologically inert substances and by short-term psychotherapy. *Arch Gen Psychiatry* (1958) 79:345–51. doi: 10.1001/archneurpsyc.1958.02340030109018
18. Benedetti F, Pollo A, Lopiano L, Lanotte M, Vighetti S, Rainero I. Conscious expectation and unconscious conditioning in analgesic, motor, and hormonal placebo/nocebo responses. *J Neurosci* (2003) 23:4315–23. doi: 10.1523/JNEUROSCI.23-10-04315.2003
19. Rief W, Shedden-Mora M, Laferton JA, Auer C, Petrie KJ, Salzmann S, et al. Preoperative optimization of patient expectations improves long-term outcome in heart surgery patients: results of the randomized controlled PSY-HEART trial. *BMC Med* (2017) 15:4. doi: 10.1186/s12916-016-0767-3
20. Wilhelm M, Winkler A, Rief W, Doering BK. Effect of placebo groups on blood pressure in hypertension: a meta-analysis of beta-blocker trials. *J Am Soc Hypertens* (2016) 10:917–29. doi: 10.1016/j.jash.2016.10.009
21. Agras WS, Horne M, Taylor CB. Expectation and the blood-pressure-lowering effects of relaxation. *Psychosom Med* (1982) 44:389–95. doi: 10.1097/00006842-198209000-00006
22. Rutherford BR, Wager TD, Roose SP. Expectancy and the treatment of depression: a review of experimental methodology and effects on patient outcome. *Curr Psychiatry Rev* (2010) 6:1–10. doi: 10.2174/157340010790596571
23. Keefe JR, Amsterdam J, Li QS, Soeller I, Derubeis R, Mao JJ. Specific expectancies are associated with symptomatic outcomes and side effect burden in a trial of chamomile extract for generalized anxiety disorder. *J Psychiatr Res* (2017) 84:90–7. doi: 10.1016/j.jpsychires.2016.09.029
24. Brown LA, Wiley JF, Wolitzky-taylor K, Roy-Byrne P, Sherbourne C, Stein MB, et al. Changes in self-efficacy and outcome expectancy as predictors of anxiety outcomes from the CALM study. *Depress Anxiety* (2014) 31:678–89. doi: 10.1002/da.22256
25. Noble LM, Douglas BC, Newman SP. What do patients expect of psychiatric services? A systematic and critical review of empirical studies. *Soc Sci Med* (2001) 52:985–98. doi: 10.1016/S0277-9536(00)00210-0
26. Peerdeman KJ, Van Laarhoven AIM, Keij SM, Vase L, Rovers MM, Peters ML, et al. Relieving patients' pain with expectation interventions: a meta-analysis. *Pain* (2016) 157:1179–91. doi: 10.1097/j.pain.0000000000000540
27. Hróbjartsson A, Gøtzsche PC. Placebo interventions for all clinical conditions. *Cochrane Database Syst Rev* (2010). doi: 10.1002/14651858.CD003974.pub3
28. Hróbjartsson A, Gøtzsche PC. Is the placebo powerless? An analysis of clinical trials comparing placebo with no treatment. *N Engl J Med* (2001) 344:1594–602. doi: 10.1056/NEJM200105243442106
29. Meissner K, Distel H, Mitzdorf U. Evidence for placebo effects on physical but not on biochemical outcome parameters: a review of clinical trials. *BMC Med* (2007) 5:3. doi: 10.1186/1741-7015-5-3
30. Schedlowski M, Enck P, Rief W, Bingel U. Neuro-bio-behavioral mechanisms of placebo and nocebo responses: implications for clinical trials and clinical practice. *Pharmacol Rev* (2015) 67:697–730. doi: 10.1124/pr.114.009423
31. Bishop FL, Coghlan B, Everitt H, Little P, Holmes MM, Seretis D, et al. What techniques might be used to harness placebo effects in non-malignant pain? A literature review and survey to develop a taxonomy. *BMJ Open* (2017) 7:e015516. doi: 10.1136/bmjopen-2016-015516
32. Faria V, Linnman C, Lebel A, Borsook D. Harnessing the placebo effect in pediatric migraine clinic. *J Pediatr* (2014) 165:659–65. doi: 10.1016/j.jpeds.2014.06.040

33. Spiegel D. Mesmer minus magic: hypnosis and modern medicine. *Int J Clin Exp Hypn* (2002) 50:397–406. doi: 10.1080/00207140208410113
34. Green JP, Laurence J-R, Lynn SJ. Hypnosis and psychotherapy: from Mesmer to mindfulness. *Psychol Conscious Theory Res Pract* (2014) 1:199–212. doi: 10.1037/cns0000015
35. Kirsch I. Hypnosis and placebos: response expectancy as a mediator of suggestion effects. *An Psicol* (1999) 15:99–110.
36. Hróbjartsson A. What are the main methodological problems in the estimation of placebo effects? *J Clin Epidemiol* (2002) 55:430–5. doi: 10.1016/S0895-4356(01)00496-6
37. Hróbjartsson A, Kaptchuk TJ, Miller FG. Placebo effect studies are susceptible to response bias and to other types of biases. *J Clin Epidemiol* (2011) 64:1223–9. doi: 10.1016/j.jclinepi.2011.01.008
38. Doyen S, Klein O, Pichon CL, Cleeremans A. Behavioral priming: it's all in the mind, but whose mind? *PLoS One* (2012) 7:e29081. doi: 10.1371/journal.pone.0029081
39. Rosenthal R, Rubin DB. Interpersonal expectancy effects: the first 345 studies. *Behav Brain Sci* (1978) 1:377–86. doi: 10.1017/S0140525X00075506
40. Kaptchuk TJ, Kelley JM, Conboy LA, Davis RB, Kerr CE, Jacobson EE, et al. Components of placebo effect: randomised controlled trial in patients with irritable bowel syndrome. *BMJ* (2008) 336:999. doi: 10.1136/bmj.39524.439618.25
41. Cornelius-White JHD, Kanamori Y, Murphy D, Tickle E. Mutuality in psychotherapy: a meta-analysis and meta-synthesis. *J Psychother Integr* (2018) 28:489–504. doi: 10.1037/int0000134
42. Farber BA, Suzuki JY, Lynch DA. Positive regard and psychotherapy outcome: a meta-analytic review. *Psychotherapy* (2018) 55:411–23. doi: 10.1037/pst0000171
43. Kolden GG, Wang C-C, Austin SB, Chang Y, Klein MH. Congruence/genuineness: a meta-analysis. *Psychotherapy* (2018) 55:424–33. doi: 10.1037/pst0000162
44. Elliott R, Bohart AC, Watson JC, Murphy D. Therapist empathy and client outcome: an updated meta-analysis. *Psychotherapy* (2018) 55:399–410. doi: 10.1037/pst0000175
45. Oakley DA, Halligan PW. Hypnotic suggestion: opportunities for cognitive neuroscience. *Nat Rev Neurosci* (2013) 14:565–76. doi: 10.1038/nrn3538
46. Jensen MP. Hypnosis for chronic pain management: a new hope. *Pain* (2009) 146:235–7. doi: 10.1016/j.pain.2009.06.027
47. Daniali H, Flaten MA. A qualitative systematic review of effects of provider characteristics and nonverbal behavior on pain, and placebo and nocebo effects. *Front Psychiatry* (2019) 10:242. doi: 10.3389/fpsyt.2019.00242
48. Ceci SJ, Bruck M. Children's suggestibility: characteristics and mechanisms. *Adv Child Dev Behav* (2006) 34:247–81. doi: 10.1016/S0065-2407(06)80009-1
49. Silva BMC, Rodrigues JJPC, de la Torre Díez I, López-Coronado M, Saleem K. Mobile-health: a review of current state in 2015. *J Biomed Inform* (2015) 56:265–72. doi: 10.1016/j.jbi.2015.06.003
50. Marcolino MS, Oliveira JAQ, D'Agostino M, Ribeiro AL, Alkmim MBM, Novillo-Ortiz D. The impact of mHealth interventions: systematic review of systematic reviews. *JMIR Mhealth Uhealth* (2018) 6:e23. doi: 10.2196/mhealth.8873
51. Neubeck L, Lowres N, Benjamin EJ, Freedman SB, Coorey G, Redfern J. The mobile revolution—using smartphone apps to prevent cardiovascular disease. *Nat Rev Cardiol* (2015) 12:350–60. doi: 10.1038/nrcardio.2015.34
52. Miller G. The smartphone psychology manifesto. *Perspect Psychol Sci* (2012) 7:221–37. doi: 10.1177/1745691612441215
53. Aboujaoude E. Telemental health: why the revolution has not arrived. *World Psychiatry* (2018) 17:277–8. doi: 10.1002/wps.20551
54. Hollis C, Morriss R, Martin J, Amani S, Cotton R, Denis M. Technological innovations in mental healthcare: harnessing the digital revolution. *Br J Psychiatry* (2015) 206:263–5. doi: 10.1192/bjp.bp.113.142612
55. Wen H, Wang H, He X, Wu C. On the low reproducibility of cancer studies. *Natl Sci Rev* (2018) 5:619–24. doi: 10.1093/nsr/nwy021
56. Open Science Collaboration. Estimating the reproducibility of psychological science. *Science* (2015) 349:aac4716. doi: 10.1126/science.aac4716
57. Ioannidis JPA. Why most published research findings are false. *PLoS Med* (2005) 2:e124. doi: 10.1371/journal.pmed.0020124
58. Shrout PE, Rodgers JL. Psychology, science, and knowledge construction: broadening perspectives from the replication crisis. *Annu Rev Psychol* (2018) 69:487–510. doi: 10.1146/annurev-psych-122216-011845
59. Benedetti F. Placebo effects: from the neurobiological paradigm to translational implications. *Neuron* (2014) 84:623–37. doi: 10.1016/j.neuron.2014.10.023
60. Pildal J, Hróbjartsson A, Jørgensen KJ, Hilden J, Altman DG, Gøtzsche PC. Impact of allocation concealment on conclusions drawn from meta-analyses of randomized trials. *Int J Epidemiol* (2007) 36:847–57. doi: 10.1093/ije/dym087
61. Park LC, Covi L. Nonblind placebo trial: an exploration of neurotic patients' responses to placebo when its inert content is disclosed. *Arch Gen Psychiatry* (1965) 12:336–45. doi: 10.1001/archpsyc.1965.01720340008002
62. Kaptchuk TJ, Friedlander E, Kelley JM, Sanchez MN, Kokkotou E, Singer JP, et al. Placebos without deception: a randomized controlled trial in irritable bowel syndrome. *PLoS One* (2010) 5:e15591. doi: 10.1371/journal.pone.0015591
63. Eisenstein EL, Collins R, Cracknell BS, Podesta O, Reid ED, Sandercock P, et al. Sensible approaches for reducing clinical trial costs. *Clin Trials* (2008) 5:75–84. doi: 10.1177/1740774507087551
64. Ioannidis JPA. Why most clinical research is not useful. *PLOS Med* (2016) 13:e1002049. doi: 10.1371/journal.pmed.1002049
65. Liberati A, Altman DG, Tetzlaff J, Mulrow C, Gøtzsche PC, Ioannidis JPA, et al. The PRISMA statement for reporting systematic reviews and meta-analyses of studies that evaluate health care interventions: explanation and elaboration. *J Clin Epedimiol* (2009) 62:e1ee34. doi: 10.1016/j.jclinepi.2009.06.006
66. Simons DJ. The value of direct replication. *Perspect Psychol Sci* (2014) 9:76–80. doi: 10.1177/1745691613514755
67. Zwaan RA, Etz A, Lucas RE, Donnellan MB. Making replication mainstream. *Behav Brain Sci* (2018), 41:e120. doi: 10.1017/S0140525X17001972
68. Ventriglio A, Magnifico G, Borraccino L, Rinaldi A, Ventriglio A, Magnifico G, et al. Placebo and cultural responses. *Nord J Psychiatry* (2018) 72:S33–S35. doi: 10.1080/08039488.2018.1525637
69. Henrich J, Heine SJ, Norenzayan A. The weirdest people in the world? *Behav Brain Sci* (2010) 33:61–135. doi: 10.1017/S0140525X0999152X
70. van Winkel M, Wichers M, Collip D, Jacobs N, Derom C, Thiery E, et al. Unraveling the role of loneliness in depression: the relationship between daily life experience and behavior. *Psychiatry* (2017) 80:104–17. doi: 10.1080/00332747.2016.1256143
71. Myin-Germeys I, Oorschot M, Collip D, Lataster J, Delespaul P, van Os J. Experience sampling research in psychopathology: opening the black box of daily life. *Psychol Med* (2009) 39:1533–47. doi: 10.1017/S0033291708004947
72. van Berkel N, Ferreira D, Kostakos V. The experience sampling method on mobile devices. *ACM Comput Surv* (2017) 50:93. doi: 10.1145/3123988
73. Shinohara K, Tanaka S, Imai H, Noma H, Maruo K, Cipriani A, et al. Development and validation of a prediction model for the probability of responding to placebo in antidepressant trials: a pooled analysis of individual patient data. *Evid Based Ment Health* (2019) 22:10–6. doi: 10.1136/ebmental-2018-300073
74. Gueorguieva R, Mallinckrodt C, Krystal JH. Trajectories of depression severity in clinical trials of duloxetine: insights into antidepressant and placebo responses. *Arch Gen Psychiatry* (2012) 68:1227–37. doi: 10.1001/archgenpsychiatry.2011.132
75. Simons LE, Sieberg CB, Conroy C, Randall ET, Shulman J, Borsook D, et al. Children with chronic pain: response trajectories after intensive pain rehabilitation treatment. *J Pain* (2018) 19:207–18. doi: 10.1016/j.jpain.2017.10.005
76. Mun CJ, Thummala K, Davis MC, Karoly P, Tennen H, Zautra AJ. Predictors and social consequences of daily pain expectancy among adults with chronic pain. *Pain* (2017) 158:1224–33. doi: 10.1097/j.pain.0000000000000903
77. Harari GM, Lane ND, Wang R, Crosier BS, Campbell AT, Gosling SD. Using smartphones to collect behavioral data in psychological science: opportunities, practical considerations, and challenges. *Perspect Psychol Sci* (2016) 11:838–54. doi: 10.1177/1745691616650285
78. Eagle N, Pentland AS. Reality mining: sensing complex social systems. *Pers Ubiquit Comput* (2006) 10:255–68. doi: 10.1007/s00779-005-0046-3
79. Ilixia Ltd. PsychoJs. (2018) Available at: https://github.com/psychopy/psychojs.
80. Peirce JW. PsychoPy—psychophysics software in Python. *J Neurosci Methods* (2007) 162:8–13. doi: 10.1016/j.jneumeth.2006.11.017

81. Greenwald AG, Mcghee DE, Schwartz JLK. Measuring individual differences in implicit cognition: the implicit association test. *J Pers Soc Psychol* (1998) 74:1464–80. doi: 10.1037//0022-3514.74.6.1464
82. Festinger L. *A theory of cognitive dissonance*. Stanford, USA: Stanford University (1957).
83. Rief W, Petrie KJ. Can psychological expectation models be adapted for placebo research? *Front Psychol* (2016) 7:1876. doi: 10.3389/fpsyg.2016.01876
84. Lei H, Nahum-Shani I, Lynch K, Oslin D, Murphy SA. A "smart" design for building individualized treatment sequences. *Annu Rev Clin Psychol* (2012) 8:21–48. doi: 10.1146/annurev-clinpsy-032511-143152
85. Nahum-Shani I, Smith SN, Spring BJ, Collins LM, Witkiewitz K, Tewari A, et al. Just-in-time adaptive interventions (JITAIs) in mobile health: key components and design principles for ongoing health behavior support. *Ann Behav Med* (2018) 52:446–62. doi: 10.1007/s12160-016-9830-8
86. Nahum-Shani I, Hekler EB, Spruijt-Metz D. Building health behavior models to guide the development of just-in-time adaptive interventions: a pragmatic framework. *Health Psychol* (2015) 34:1209–19. doi: 10.1037/hea0000306
87. Spruijt-Metz D, Wen CKF, O'Reilly G, Li M, Lee S, Emken BA, et al. Innovations in the use of interactive technology to support weight management. *Curr Obes Rep* (2015) 4:510–9. doi: 10.1007/s13679-015-0183-6
88. Beutler LE, Harwood TM, Michelson A, Song X, Holman J. Resistance/reactance level. *J Clin Psychol* (2011) 67:133–42. doi: 10.1002/jclp.20753
89. Rutten JMTM, Vlieger AM, Frankenhuis C, George EK, Groeneweg M, Norbruis OF, et al. Home-based hypnotherapy self-exercises vs individual hypnotherapy with a therapist for treatment of pediatric irritable bowel syndrome, functional abdominal pain, or functional abdominal pain syndrome: a randomized clinical trial. *JAMA Pediatr* (2017) 171:470–7. doi: 10.1001/jamapediatrics.2017.0091
90. Forbes A, MacAuley S, Chiotakakou-Faliakou E. Hypnotherapy and therapeutic audiotape: effective in previously unsuccessfully treated irritable bowel syndrome? *Int J Colorectal Dis* (2000) 15:328–34. doi: 10.1007/s003840000248
91. Powers SW, Coffey CS, Chamberlin LA, Ecklund DJ, Klingner EA, Yankey JW, et al. Trial of amitriptyline, topiramate, and placebo for pediatric migraine. *N Engl J Med* (2016) 376:115–24. doi: 10.1056/NEJMoa1610384
92. Naslund JA, Aschbrenner KA, Araya R, Marsch LA, Unützer J, Patel V, et al. Digital technology for treating and preventing mental disorders in low-income and middle-income countries: a narrative review of the literature. *Lancet Psychiatry* (2017) 4:486–500. doi: 10.1016/S2215-0366(17)30096-2
93. Shuren J, Patel B, Gottlieb S. FDA regulation of mobile medical apps. *JAMA* (2018) 320:337–8. doi: 10.1001/jama.2018.8832
94. Lang M. Heart rate monitoring apps: information for engineers and researchers about the new European Medical Devices Regulation 2017/745. *JMIR Biomed Eng* (2017) 2:e2. doi: 10.2196/biomedeng.8179
95. Dove ES, Phillips M. Privacy law, data sharing policies, and medical data: a comparative perspective. In: Gkoulalas-Divanis A, Loukides G, editors. *Medical data privacy handbook*. Cham: Springer (2015). p. 639–78. doi: 10.1007/978-3-319-23633-9_24
96. Torous J, Roberts LW. The ethical use of mobile health technology in clinical psychiatry. *J Nerv Ment Dis* (2017) 205:4–8. doi: 10.1097/NMD.0000000000000596
97. Torous J, Andersson G, Bertagnoli A, Christensen H, Cuijpers P, Firth J, et al. Towards a consensus around standards for smartphone apps and digital mental health. *World Psychiatry* (2019) 18:97–8. doi: 10.1002/wps.20592
98. Huckvale K, Prieto JT, Tilney M, Benghozi P, Car J. Unaddressed privacy risks in accredited health and wellness apps: a cross-sectional systematic assessment. *BMC Med* (2015) 13:214. doi: 10.1186/s12916-015-0444-y
99. Torous JB, Chan SR, Yellowlees PM, Boland R. To use or not? Evaluating ASPECTS of smartphone apps and mobile technology for clinical care in psychiatry. *J Clin Psychiatry* (2016) 77:e734–e738. doi: 10.4088/JCP.15com10619
100. Torous J, Firth J. The digital placebo effect: mobile mental health meets clinical psychiatry. *Lancet Psychiatry* (2016) 3:100–2. doi: 10.1016/S2215-0366(15)00565-9
101. Giosan C, Cobeanu O, Mogoaşe C, Szentagotai A, Mureşan V, Boian R. Reducing depressive symptomatology with a smartphone app: study protocol for a randomized, placebo-controlled trial. *Trials* (2017) 18:215. doi: 10.1186/s13063-017-1960-1
102. Arean PA, Hallgren KA, Jordan JT, Gazzaley A, Atkins DC, Heagerty PJ, et al. The use and effectiveness of mobile apps for depression: results from a fully remote clinical trial. *J Med Internet Res* (2016) 18:e330. doi: 10.2196/jmir.6482
103. Pawlikowski M, Nader IW, Burger C, Biermann I, Stieger S, Brand M. Pathological Internet use: it is a multidimensional and not a unidimensional construct. *Addict Res Theory* (2014) 22:166–75. doi: 10.3109/16066359.2013.793313
104. Pryss R, Reichert M, Schlee W, Spiliopoulou M, Langguth B, Probst T. Differences between Android and iOS users of the TrackYourTinnitus mobile crowdsensing mHealth platform. *Proc IEEE Symp Comput Med Syst* (2018), 411–6. doi: 10.1109/CBMS.2018.00078
105. Glasgow RE, Klesges LM, Dzewaltowski DA, Estabrooks P, Bull SS. The future of health behavior change research: what is needed to improve translation of research into health promotion practice? *Ann Behav Med* (2004) 27:3–12. doi: 10.1207/s15324796abm2701_2
106. Rothwell PM. Factors that can affect the external validity of randomised controlled trials. *PLoS Clin Trials* (2006) 1:e9. doi: 10.1371/journal.pctr.0010009
107. Glasgow RE, Lichtenstein E, Marcus A. Why don't we see more translation of health promotion research to practice? *Am J Public Health* (2003) 93:1261–67. doi: 10.2105/AJPH.93.8.1261
108. Blackman KCA, Zoellner J, Berrey LM, Alexander R, Fanning J, Hill JL, et al. Assessing the internal and external validity of mobile health physical activity promotion interventions: a systematic literature review using the RE-AIM framework. *J Med Internet Res* (2013) 15:e224. doi: 10.2196/jmir.2745
109. Eysenbach G, CONSORT-EHEALTH Group. CONSORT-EHEALTH: improving and standardizing evaluation reports of Web-based and mobile health interventions. *J Med Internet Res* (2011) 13:e126. doi: 10.2196/jmir.1923
110. Glasgow RE, Harden SM, Gaglio B, Rabin B, Smith ML, Porter GC, et al. RE-AIM planning and evaluation framework: adapting to new science and practice with a 20-year review. *Front Public Health* (2019) 7:64. doi: 10.3389/fpubh.2019.00064

12

Experimental Assessment of Nocebo Effects and Nocebo Side Effects: Definitions, Study Design and Implications for Psychiatry and Beyond

Kate Faasse[1], Suzanne G. Helfer[2], Kirsten Barnes[3], Ben Colagiuri[3] and Andrew L. Geers[4]*

[1] School of Psychology, University of New South Wales, Sydney, NSW, Australia, [2] Department of Psychology, Adrian College, Adrian, MI, United States, [3] School of Psychology, University of Sydney, Sydney, NSW, Australia, [4] Department of Psychology, University of Toledo, Toledo, OH, United States

***Correspondence:**
Kate Faasse
k.faasse@unsw.edu.au

Keywords: nocebo effect, side effects, experimental design, research methods—psychology, no treatment control

Interest in nocebo effects is increasing exponentially: a Google Scholar search for articles referencing *nocebo* in 1998 (20 years ago) yields 90 results, increasing to 449 in 2008 (10 years ago) and to 1600 in 2018. Increased attention has likely resulted from recognition of the prevalence and potential seriousness of nocebo effects in clinical contexts. It is estimated that up to 97% of reported pharmaceutical side effects are *not* caused by the drug itself but rather by nocebo effects and symptom misattribution (1). These nocebo effects can cause symptoms serious enough to require hospitalization and medical intervention (2). As a result of the increased recognition of the importance of nocebo effects, experimental research seeking to understand how nocebo effects are formed has also intensified.

As the literature on nocebo effects has expanded, additional methodological decision points arise for researchers in this area. In this article, we discuss a set of methodological issues that result from emerging approaches to studying nocebo effects, including distinctions between designs for standard nocebo effects versus nocebo side effects, the information provided by selecting different types of control groups in experimental designs, and the distinction between "true" nocebo effects and symptom misattribution. This discussion will focus on between-subjects designs, using examples of nocebo effects that are generated by verbal/written transmission of information. For each issue, we compare the different methodologies and seek to highlight the strengths and limitations of these approaches.

NOCEBO EFFECTS AND NOCEBO SIDE EFFECTS DESIGNS: DEFINITIONS

Definitions of the nocebo effect typically focus on the role of negative expectations in producing aversive outcomes [e.g., Refs. (3–7)]. In contrast, Faasse (8) extends this definition to incorporate past experience and other aspects of the treatment context. We would refine this further to define nocebo effects as unpleasant or adverse outcomes triggered by the treatment *context*, beyond any inherent pharmacological effects of the treatment itself. These nocebo effects are scientifically measurable effects caused by psychological processes including negative expectations, classical conditioning, and observational learning (9).

Although not always differentiated, there are two variants of nocebo effects that researchers examine: primary nocebo effects and nocebo side effects. Experimental designs that study *primary nocebo effects* focus on nocebo effects as the central "action" or primary negative outcome of a treatment/medical condition. Such outcomes have been described by Hahn (5, 6) as nocebo effects, where he distinguished these from what he called "placebo side effects," whereby a treatment intended primarily for benefit can cause harmful outcomes. As an example of a primary nocebo effect—when the potential adverse outcome is framed as the primary, or focal, effect of the treatment—Benedetti and colleagues (10) informed postoperative patients that a saline injection would increase pain, resulting in elevated pain. This design contrasts those of *nocebo side effect* experiments in which participants are informed of the main (typically beneficial) outcome of a treatment/condition, and also unpleasant outcomes that are ancillary to this main outcome. This conceptualization of nocebo side effects is similar to that of Barksy and colleagues (3) as a phenomenon occurring when placebo treatment results in unpleasant side effects. For example, Neukirch and Colagiuri (11) gave participants experiencing sleep difficulty an inert treatment to improve sleep—with or without the suggestion that it created a specific side effect (increased or decreased appetite). The results revealed that participants given the side-effect warning reported more changes in appetite—in the expected direction—than those not given the side-effect warning.

Notably, recent evidence suggests that primary nocebo and nocebo side effect manipulations do not produce equivalent results. Caplandies and colleagues (12) used an experimental design that compared the two nocebo effects and found that when headache pain was described as the *primary* effect of sham transcranial direct current stimulation (tDCS), headaches were significantly more likely to occur than when headache was described as a side effect of tDCS. These results indicate that nocebo effect instructions can produce different outcomes depending on whether the adverse effect is described as the primary effect or a side effect of treatment.

NOCEBO EFFECTS AND NOCEBO SIDE EFFECTS: EXPERIMENTAL DESIGN SELECTION

Making a clear distinction between a primary nocebo effect and a nocebo side effect design is valuable for several reasons. First, these two designs correspond to different clinical care circumstances. Primary nocebo effect designs relate to situations in which negative outcomes can occur without a concomitant benefit, such as when patients are given a warning about potential pain due to a medical condition (e.g., broken leg) or disease course (e.g., *rheumatoid arthritis*), which leads to increased negative expectations. In contrast, nocebo side effect designs are analogues of situations when there is a beneficial treatment that may also cause adverse effects. These designs have greater correspondence to medical treatments where treatment descriptions and instructions—including informed consent protocols, physician warnings, drug labels, and direct-to-consumer advertising—suggest that adverse outcomes can accompany a primary treatment benefit. Consequently, in the study of nocebo effects, researchers should decide between primary nocebo effect or nocebo side effect designs based on the applied circumstance they wish to understand.

A second reason for distinguishing between these two types of designs is that the pivotal mediating and moderating variables may diverge. Consider the case of moderating variables. When examining nocebo side effects, but not primary nocebo effects, variables such as number of side effects listed or their order could be critical moderators to assess. Additionally, it is possible that the contribution of different psychological mediators varies with these different designs. For example, primary nocebo effect designs emphasize adverse outcomes, whereas nocebo side effect designs emphasize the positive treatment effect as well as co-occurring adverse outcomes; because of this greater emphasis on negative outcomes, individuals in primary nocebo effect designs may devote more higher-order cognitive processes to thinking about the negative symptoms than individuals in the nocebo side effect designs (13). It should also be noted that nocebo side effects and placebo effects can, theoretically, co-exist within the same person, and the experience of benefits and unpleasant side effects may influence one another.

NOCEBO EFFECTS AND NOCEBO SIDE EFFECTS: CONTROL CONDITIONS

A second issue to consider is the appropriate control conditions for these designs. Here, we differentiate between several options.

No-treatment control group. It is widely accepted that when investigating the *placebo* effect, a placebo-treated group must be compared with an untreated control group in order to detect "true" rather than "perceived" placebo effects (14). The inclusion of an untreated comparison group allows researchers to distinguish between improvements *caused* by placebo administration and other factors that can result in apparent improvements, including natural history of the condition, Hawthorne effects, and regression to the mean. However, the importance of this distinction between "true" and "perceived" *nocebo* effects—and the inclusion of a no-treatment control group—is less well recognised (15).

We argue that no-treatment control groups are important for both primary nocebo and nocebo side effect designs. A simple laboratory procedure to test for true *nocebo* effects—both primary and side effects—would involve two conditions. In one condition, participants would take a sham treatment or undergo a sham procedure described as having either a primary or secondary (i.e., side effects) unpleasant outcome. In the other condition, participants would not get the nocebo treatment or procedure (i.e., they form the no-treatment control group), but undertake all other study components. An increase in the rate of unpleasant outcomes in the "treated" group would be indicative of a true nocebo effect—because comparing with the untreated control rules out natural history, Hawthorne effects, and regression to the mean, as alternative explanations.

Sham treatment/no-information control group. A second control condition that may be employed is one in which participants are given a treatment or procedure, but are not provided with information about possible unpleasant outcomes (primary or side effect; see **Table 1**). Thus, when a *sham treatment/no-information control group* is compared to a *sham treatment/*

TABLE 1 | Examples of control and experimental conditions in nocebo research, and information provided by these comparisons.

Control condition	Experimental condition	Information provided
No treatment	Sham treatment plus negative information about adverse outcomes	Evidence of "true" nocebo effect; no information about the role of information provision and subsequent expectations, or treatment context
Sham treatment with no information about adverse outcomes	Sham treatment plus negative information about adverse outcomes	Effect of information on nocebo outcomes, controls for effect of treatment administration; no evidence for "true" nocebo effect, participants may form own expectations in the absence of information about sham treatment
Sham treatment with standard information about adverse outcomes	Sham treatment with modified experimental information (typically employed to test strategies to *reduce* nocebo effects)	Effect of modified information presentation on nocebo outcomes; no evidence for "true" nocebo effect

negative information group, participants in both conditions engage in the treatment activity (12). This procedure keeps constant factors such as naturally occurring symptoms, treatment administration, and engagement in other experimental activities across the conditions. This control can be used for either primary nocebo or nocebo side effect studies and is useful for identifying the specific effect of the information provided. Some limitations of this control condition, however, are 1) because treatments or procedures are given without corresponding information about possible side effects or adverse outcomes, it has less ecological validity than the no-treatment control condition described above, and 2) the control group does not provide information on the generation of "true" nocebo effects, i.e., the magnitude of the overall nocebo effect compared to individuals with no treatment.

These two types of control conditions are not exhaustive. For example, as indicated in **Table 1**, other variations could include giving participants a treatment with "standard" or usual care information in order to test the effect of other information provision strategies, for example, standard information versus positive framing of information about adverse outcomes, which focuses on the proportion of patients who will *not* experience these unpleasant outcomes (16, 17). Of most importance, however, is that researchers consider carefully their hypotheses and relevance to clinical practice, consider which factor(s) differ between their chosen conditions, and utilize appropriate control conditions in experimental designs that will allow them to most appropriately test their research question. The control conditions described here are complementary rather than mutually exclusive, and we recommend that researchers consider including a no-treatment control as well as (for example) an information-related control condition. Finally, although this discussion has focused on designs using sham treatments, it is important to note that nocebo effects occur in response to active medical treatments too. In studies examining nocebo effects from active treatments, a no-treatment control condition is less likely to be helpful than an *active treatment/no-information control group*, which controls for the physiological effect of the treatment itself.

NOCEBO EFFECTS AND NOCEBO SIDE EFFECTS: MISATTRIBUTION

A third consideration in experimental designs to study nocebo effects and nocebo side effects is the role of symptom misattribution. In contrast to "true" nocebo effects, "perceived" nocebo effects are those symptoms that would have occurred regardless of treatment administration but are (mistakenly) attributed to the treatment. Misattribution is particularly relevant to the study of nocebo *side* effects, such as a where a patient is experiencing regular headaches, starts a new medication, and subsequently misattributes these headaches to the treatment. Although such misattributed symptoms are undoubtedly important in how patients view their treatments and influence their health care decisions, there are likely to be different processes underlying the development of misattributed and true nocebo side effects. When designing experimental studies to investigate true nocebo side effects, assessing baseline symptoms that may be subject to later misattribution and encouraging participants to report *all* symptoms experienced regardless of perceived cause may help to assess or reduce the influence of misattribution on results. If researchers wish to explicitly study misattribution, participants who receive an experimental treatment can be asked whether they believe their symptoms were *caused* by the treatment they received.

SUMMARY

Nocebo effects and nocebo side effects play an important role in the outcomes of medical care. Heightened recognition of their importance and increased experimental research seeking to understand how nocebo effects are formed have raised the need for consideration of the methodological decisions that researchers face in studying the nocebo effect. These decisions include whether to examine primary nocebo effects or nocebo side effects, appropriate control conditions, and differentiating true and perceived nocebo effects. Future research would benefit from careful selection of study design and assessment of nocebo outcomes. Such steps will contribute to generating a deeper understanding of how both primary nocebo effects and nocebo side effects develop.

AUTHOR CONTRIBUTIONS

AG and KF contributed to the conception of the work and wrote the first draft of the manuscript. All authors critically revised the manuscript for important intellectual content and provide approval for publication of the content.

FUNDING

KF is supported by an Australian Research Council Discovery Early Career Researcher Award (DE180100471); BC is supported by an Australian Research Council Discovery Early Career Researcher Award (DE160100864). The funder played no role in the conceptualization or preparation of this work. The researchers are independent from the funder.

REFERENCES

1. Mahr A, Golmard C, Pham E, Iordache L, Deville L, Faure P. Types, frequencies, and burden of nonspecific adverse events of drugs: analysis of randomized placebo-controlled clinical trials. *Pharmacoepidemiol Drug Saf* (2017) 26:731–41. doi: 10.1002/pds.4169
2. Reeves RR, Ladner ME, Hart RH, Burke RS. Nocebo effects with antidepressant clinical drug trial placebos. *Gen Hosp Psychiatry* (2007) 29(3):275–7. doi: 10.1016/j.genhosppsych.2007.01.010
3. Barsky AJ, Saintfort R, Rogers MP, Borus JF. Nonspecific medication side effects and the nocebo phenomenon. *Jama* (2002) 287(5):622–7. doi: 10.1001/jama.287.5.622
4. Colloca L. Nocebo effects can make you feel pain: negative expectancies derived from features of commercial drugs elicit nocebo effects. *Science (New York, N.Y.)* (2017) 358(6359):44. doi: 10.1126/science.aap8488
5. Hahn RA. The nocebo phenomenon: concept, evidence, and implications for public health. *Preventive Med* (1997) 26:607–11. doi: 10.1006/pmed.1996.0124
6. Hahn RA. Expectations of sickness: concept and evidence of the nocebo phenomenon. In: Kirsch I, editor. *How expectancies shape experience.* Washington, DC: American Psychological Association (1999). p. 333–56. doi: 10.1037/10332-014
7. Wager TD, Atlas LY. The neuroscience of placebo effects: connecting context, learning and health. *Nat Rev Neurosci* (2015) 16(7):403–18. doi: 10.1038/nrn3976
8. Faasse K. Nocebo effects in health psychology. *Austr Psychol* (2019) 1–13. doi: 10.1111/ap.12392
9. Colloca L. Placebo, nocebo, and learning mechanisms. In: Benedetti F, editor. *Placebo.*, vol. 225 Berlin Heidelberg: Springer-Verlag (2014). p. 17–35. doi: 10.1007/978-3-662-44519-8
10. Benedetti F, Amanzio M, Casadio C, Oliaro A, Maggi G. Blockade of nocebo hyperalgesia by the cholecystokinin antagonist proglumide. *Pain* (1997) 71(2):135–40. doi: 10.1016/S0304-3959(97)03346-0
11. Neukirch N, Colagiuri B. The placebo effect, sleep difficulty, and side effects: a balanced placebo model. *J Behav Med* (2015) 38(2):273–83. doi: 10.1007/s10865-014-9590-5
12. Caplandies FC, Colagiuri B, Helfer SG, Geers AL. Effect type but not attribute framing alters nocebo headaches in an experimental paradigm. *Psychol Consciousness Theor Res Pract* (2017) 4(3):259–73. doi: 10.1037/cns0000130
13. Geers AL, Briñol P, Petty RE. An analysis of the basic processes of formation and change of placebo expectations. *Rev Gen Psychol* (2018) 23:211–9. doi: 10.1037/gpr0000171
14. Ernst E, Resch KL. Concept of true and perceived placebo effects. *Bmj* (1995) 311(7004):551. doi: 10.1136/bmj.311.7004.551
15. Colloca L, Miller F. The nocebo effect and its relevance for clinical practice. *Psychosom Med* (2011) 73:598–603. doi: 10.1097/PSY.0b013e3182294a50
16. Barnes K, Faasse K, Geers A, Helfer S, Sharpe L, Colloca L, et al. Can positive framing reduce nocebo side effects? Current evidence and recommendation for future research. *Front Pharmacol* (2019) 10:167. doi: 10.3389/fphar.2019.00167
17. Faasse K, Huynh A, Pearson A, Geers A, Helfer S, Colagiuri B. The influence of side effect information framing on nocebo effects. *Ann Behav Med* (2018) 1–9. doi: 10.1093/abm/kay071

13

Placebo Effects in Psychotherapy: A Framework

Paul Enck* and Stephan Zipfel

Psychosomatic Medicine and Psychotherapy, Department of Internal Medicine VI, University Hospital Tübingen, Tübingen, Germany

***Correspondence:**
Paul Enck
paul.enck@uni-tuebingen.de

The issue of placebo response and the extent of its effect on psychotherapy is complex for two specific reasons: i) Current standards for drug trials, e.g., true placebo interventions, double-blinding, cannot be applied to most psychotherapy techniques, and ii) some of the "nonspecific effects" in drug therapy have very specific effects in psychotherapy, such as the frequency and intensity of patient–therapist interaction. In addition, different psychotherapy approaches share many such specific effects (the "dodo bird verdict") and lack specificity with respect to therapy outcome. Here, we discuss the placebo effect in psychotherapy under four aspects: a) nonspecific factors shared with drug therapy (context factors); b) nonspecific factors shared among all psychotherapy traditions (common factors); c) specific placebo-controlled options with different psychotherapy modalities; and d) nonspecific control options for the specific placebo effect in psychotherapy. The resulting framework proposes that the exploration and enumeration of context factors, common factors, and specific factors contributes to the placebo effects in psychotherapy.

Keywords: placebo effects, psychotherapy, control condition, placebo response, clinical trials

HISTORICAL ROOTS

Although the term "placebo" became commonplace medical language some time ago (1), it was not before the 1940s that placebo-controlled pharmacological trials became the standard in psychiatry and beyond (2). This rather restrictive use of the term for controlled trials was relinquished only recently in favor of a broader use in all therapeutic conditions, for differentiation between minimizing placebo effects in controlled trials, while maximizing it in daily routine (3, 4), and for harnessing the effect to improve the therapist–patient relationship (5).

Throughout this paper, we will use the terms "placebo effect" and "placebo response" (or "nocebo effect" and "nocebo response") in accordance with a recent expert opinion of the placebo research community (4): Placebo effect refers to a distinctive psychobiological phenomenon, while placebo response refers to the outcome of clinical trials, the amalgam of responses after receiving a placebo—bias in reporting, regression to mean, possibly also Hawthorne effects, and placebo effects (6).

However, psychotherapy and the placebo response share a specific and delicate relationship.

A response to placebo was soon recognized as an indication of a psychological rather than of a somatic/medical condition (7). Two "roots" of this early placebo research can be identified:

a) In the early 1950s, Stewart Wolff described the mechanisms (conditioning, expectation) by which placebo effects occurred and were strong, particularly with somatic symptoms such as pain and nausea (8, 9). At the same time, in psychiatry, particularly high placebo effects were observed in randomized controlled trials (RCT) with drugs in depression, anxiety, etc. (10), and among other things, the severity of the illness, duration of treatment, and previous therapies were causing this effect (11) [for a survey, see Weimer et al. (12)].

b) Around the same time, Jerome D. Frank noted that patients' and therapists' expectations influenced the outcome of psychotherapy (13) and speculated that suggestions (but not motivation) may play a role, as may the duration of therapy, specific-patient characteristics (which he called placebo reactors), and side effects may eliminate it. To distinguish between specific and nonspecific effects, Frank called for clearly defined control groups in psychotherapy also, regardless of its theoretical orientation.

Little has been achieved experimentally since then with regard to exploring placebo effects in psychotherapy, although the therapeutic options available have increased dramatically: psychodynamic psychotherapy, cognitive behavioral therapy (CBT), hypnotherapy, interpersonal psychotherapy, group therapy, couple and family therapy, mindfulness-based therapy (MBT), self-help programs (SHPs), phone- and internet-based therapies, health interventions, e.g., smartphone apps, and the like. The general and specific placebo effects of all of these should be examined. In the following sections, we will argue that of the many factors regarded as "nonspecific" in drug RCT, some should be considered as being specific in psychotherapy, while others remain nonspecific under all circumstances. As with drug therapy, however, not all nonspecific factors are attributable to a placebo effect; since response biases, statistical regression to the mean and spontaneous symptom variation account for some of the effects involved in both the drug and the placebo aspect of trials and therefore also influence psychotherapy. This concept is illustrated in **Figure 1**.

While most of the older and many recent publications on the placebo effect in psychotherapy avoid determining the size of the placebo effect in psychotherapy (14–18), unless they were claiming that the placebo concept cannot be applied to psychotherapy at all (15, 19), others argue that properly designed placebo (control) therapy may be as effective as psychotherapy (16). However, neither of these positions is helpful in planning a rational psychotherapy evaluation.

Instead, we will follow an argument raised by Blease (20, 21); according to which, there is general scientific consensus that the placebo concept exists, but unnecessary debate in placebo studies persists due to the failure to recognize this fact. In principle, the same underlying definitions for placebo response and placebo effect that apply in biomedical research interventions also apply to psychological interventions for which the concept "placebo" was not developed. The key difference lies in recognizing the serious challenges of placebo-controlled clinical trials for psychological treatments. It is therefore unnecessary to eliminate placebo concepts in psychological contexts, as proposed by Kirsch (15).

We will abstain from discussing the placebo concept of Grünbaum (22) for CBT for one simple reason: it was developed before the surge of empirical placebo research had begun in the 1990s (23) and thus cannot reflect current knowledge. Gaab (19) falls into the "Grünbaum trap" when arguing that psychotherapy is at risk of being misconstrued as "mere" placebo without such a discussion and that psychotherapists otherwise simply prescribe placebos. It is not without irony that Wampold (16) illustrates the concept with a contemporary drug example (antibiotics) but falls short (as do others) of explaining what contemporary "incidental constituents" of psychotherapy may be, adhering instead to Grünbaum´s 1986 definition.

A "Grünbaum trap" is what we call the outdated understanding of the placebo response in psychotherapy. It was developed as a seemingly timeless concept (applicable to all psychotherapies at all times, e.g., the "incidental constituents of psychotherapy" according to Grünbaum) when much of what determines the placebo response had already been identified, e.g., learning history and acute expectancies, which are no longer "incidental" in either drug therapy or psychotherapy.

Our subsequent arguments assume that—like drug RCT in similar conditions, when primary efficacy measures are

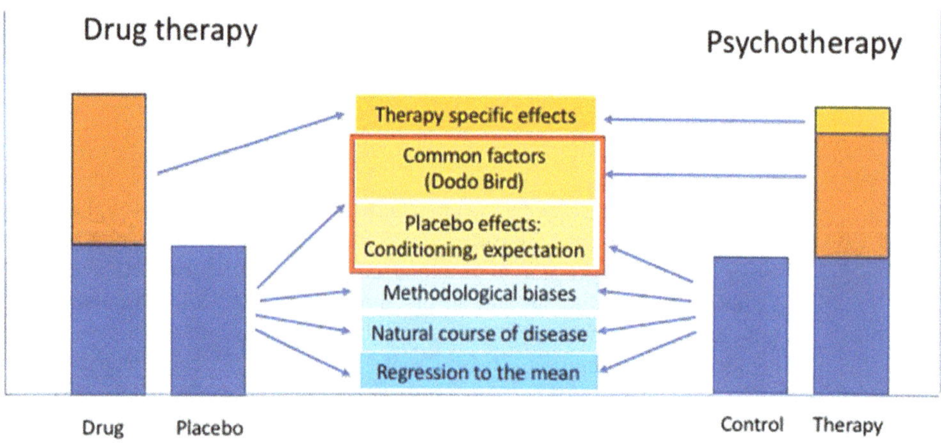

FIGURE 1 | Schematic relationship between shared and non-shared nonspecific factors contributing to the placebo response in drug and psychotherapy: factors that are part of the (nonspecific) placebo effect in drug therapy (e.g., therapist empathy, intensity of patient-therapist communication, etc.) become "common factors" across all psychotherapies [Rosenzweig's "Dodo Bird" (1936), or Lambert and Ogles' "common factors" (2004)], addition to a (small) specific effect of the different psychotherapy modalities that may be composed of a specific combination of the factors, as listed in **Table 1**.

patient-reported outcomes (PROs)—an average placebo response of around 40% may also be effective in psychotherapy, provided that optimal research conditions prevail; where this is not the case, the placebo response is liable to be higher. This position is supported by a more recent meta-analysis of psychotherapy trials in irritable bowel syndrome (IBS) with nearly 100 RCT of drug therapy and an average of 40% placebo response across all trials (24); six additional psychotherapy RCT also yielded an average placebo response of 40% (25).

This is similar to Lambert (26) who proposed that 40% of the effect of psychotherapy is attributable to factors beyond psychotherapy (or, in our terms, nonspecific effects: spontaneous variation, regression to the mean, biases) and a further 15% to the placebo effect (expectancy of improvement); in addition, 15% are thought to be due to the specifics of each psychotherapy modality, while the remaining 30% are common to all psychotherapies, the "dodo bird verdict" (27). These 30% "common factors" of all psychotherapies can be subdivided into "support factors," "learning factors," and "action factors," in accordance with Huibers and Cuijpers (28) (see **Table 1**).

While all these numbers may be variable with respect to their empirical base—from guesses to meta-analyses—they come surprisingly close to what has been reported from RCT across medicine (30) as well as from psychiatry (12) and in the range of what Henry K. Beecher had already estimated from the few clinical trials he had at his disposal in 1955 (7). Provided that PRO are in the focus, our current understanding is that at this level, placebo effects in drug therapy and in psychotherapy do not vary whatsoever in size and mechanism.

We will not elaborate further on the concept of these "common factors"—a detailed review and discussion is available in Lambert (26). An in-depth discussion of the control-group issue in psychological interventions can be found, among others, in Mohr et al. (31) and Guidi et al. (32).

TABLE 1 | Factors assumed to be common in all psychotherapies that may influence psychotherapy outcome. These can be classified in three groups and can—to different degrees—be effective in different psychotherapies, thus enabling different modes of psychotherapy to operate. Their sequential order (from left to right) is based on a concept by Lambert and Ogles (29) that is theory-driven and yet without empirical basis [concept according to Huibers and Cuijpers (28)].

Interaction factors	Process factors (Learning)	Process factors (Action)
Matching of patient/therapist:	*Emotional dimension:*	*Behavior:*
identification	accepting advice	practice
therapeutic alliance	affective experience	taking risks
therapist's expertise	assimilation of problems	facing fears
active participation of both	correction of emotionality	mastery efforts
structured communication	allowing emotionality	experiencing success
Positive relationship with:	*Cognitive dimension:*	*Behavioral regulation:*
Trust	Feedback	modeling
Empathy	Rationality	reality testing
acceptance	allowing insight	working through
reassurance	cognitive learning	cognitive mastery
genuineness	identifying expectations	predicting problems
release of tension	changing expectations	designing future solution
mitigation of isolation		

We will neither present nor discuss the vast body of evidence with regard to neurobiology and neurochemistry of the placebo response, but again refer to the literature, e.g., Fabrizio Benedetti´s book (33), and Luana Colloca´s reader (34, 35).

We will structure the following discussion using the analogy of drug therapy and aim to identify nonspecific effects in drug therapy that have either become specific or that have remained nonspecific in psychotherapy. We will discuss common problems of control for nonspecific effects across different psychotherapies as well as potentially specific problems in certain psychotherapies, as also illustrated in **Figure 1**. Finally, we will address placebo issues with a combination of drug and psychotherapy and discuss the relationship between placebo effects and the efficacy of psychotherapy.

NONSPECIFIC EFFECTS IN DRUG THERAPY WHICH BECOME SPECIFIC IN PSYCHOTHERAPY

Most RCT with drugs are keen to demonstrate that no center effects occurred, which otherwise could explain to some degree the efficacy of the drugs under investigation. In pivotal trials, such a center effect could potentially cause the requested indication to be declined by the approval authorities. It is of interest to note that in RCT before the 1990s, most studies were single-center trials in which such an effect was not even noticed. Furthermore, the qualification of trial doctors, the degree of their training, and their communication skills and empathy were rarely assessed or subsequently linked to treatment outcome. Age, sex, and other personal characteristics of the patients were not specifically taken into account, although it is well established that these factors may play a role in clinical routine (36) as well as in RCT, for both drug therapy (37) and psychotherapy (38). Rules of good clinical practice required independent raters and therapists, staff training, study monitoring, and strict adherence control (39).

Large multicenter trials produce higher placebo responses (40–42), presumably due to a lower standardization of recruitment [including recruitment biases (43)] and higher variability of therapist–patient interaction during the study. In agreement with this, more study visits are now clearly associated with higher placebo response rates in depression in both children (44) and adults (45), as well as in other areas of medicine, e.g., inflammatory (46) and functional bowel disorders (24).

Frequency and intensity of therapist–patient interaction are well-known factors determining the efficacy of psychotherapy (47). They may serve as an example of how nonspecific effects in drug therapy could become specific effects in psychotherapy, however common they may be for most psychotherapy modalities. This is why psychotherapy trials have always sought to standardize the amount of time spent with the patient as well as the communication between patient and therapist. Furthermore, while manuals harmonizing the content and interaction during therapy are standard in psychotherapy, such factors are now also deemed to be relevant in drug trials (48).

One prime example of a common but specific effect involved in psychotherapy is described in an open-label placebo study (49): To achieve an "augmented placebo response" in a sham-acupuncture trial in patients with IBS, acupuncturists were instructed to control their treatment behavior on the basis of a manualized script requesting intensified 20-min doctor–patient communication instead of the usual, standard acupuncture treatment. Many of the verbal instructions required "normal" therapist–patient communication behavior in a psychotherapy setting but may be rather atypical in drug therapy environments.

This procedure doubled the placebo response to sham acupuncture on most outcome measures.

NONSPECIFIC ELEMENTS IN DRUG THERAPY THAT REMAIN NONSPECIFIC IN PSYCHOTHERAPY

Of the small number of patient-centered predictors of the placebo response identified in RCT in psychiatry (12)—low severity of the disease, short disease duration, no treatment history, more recent trials—none were shown to be specifically relevant in psychotherapy, although it is open to speculation as to whether patients accepting psychotherapy as their primary treatment option are less severely affected, e.g., by depression, than patients accepting psychotropic drug therapy. In depression therapy in particular, younger age was associated with higher placebo response, but this may be due to shorter disease history and lower disease severity in children and adolescents than in adults (30, 50). These factors may lose their importance in all those cases in which a first-line drug therapy is not available.

Of the traditional therapist-centered variables tested (age, sex, theoretical orientation, and percentage of work time conducting therapy), only age was a significant demographic predictor of psychotherapy outcome in a univariate analysis, while in a multivariate analysis, interpersonal and social skills accounted for most of the outcome variance (51). While this casts doubts on the replicability of many psychotherapy RCT, it calls for more research into the role of researcher variables for therapy outcome (52): allegiance to theoretical concepts per se has been made responsible for most of the therapy outcomes (53).

It is, however, of relevance that, particularly in psychiatry—but not outside psychiatry, see Ref. (54)—an unbalanced randomization has been shown to drive the placebo effect: increased placebo effects were observed in depression (45, 55, 56), schizophrenia (57, 58), and psychosis (42) when more patients were randomized to active treatment than to (placebo) control. While this is usually carried out for ethical reasons (to leave the least number of patients untreated), it also serves in certain cases to test different drug dosages against one placebo arm.

Such designs are presumably also common in psychotherapy and may account for a substantial overall effect of the therapy: According to Papakostas and and Fava (55), a 10% increase in the probability of receiving active treatment (i.e., a 10% decrease in the probability of being assigned to the control condition) increases the probability of responding to active (drug) antidepressant therapy by 1.8% and to control (placebo) by 2.6%, in comparison with a 50:50 randomization scheme. When one active treatment is compared with another active treatment [comparative effectiveness research (CER)], the response was higher by a factor of 1.79 than in a placebo-controlled trial, solely brought about by the 100% certainty for patients that they would receive active antidepressant treatment (59).

COMMON CONTROL PROBLEMS IN ALL PSYCHOTHERAPY TRIALS AND THEIR ADVANTAGES AND PITFALLS

Different psychotherapy options share common features when it comes to standards as set down by RCT of drug therapy in psychiatry and psychosomatics, e.g., trial registration, power calculation, ethics approval, and informed consent are easily applicable to all. Others, such as monitoring of treatment progress and adherence control need to be adapted to the specific therapy in some cases, e.g., with internet-based therapies. In most cases, the design also required adaptation to specifics for certain therapy options (60).

The common denominator in all psychotherapy procedures is the inability to effectively blind treatment and control group assignment and to provide a "true" (by nature, ineffective) placebo treatment; among the many procedures that have been developed to secure blinding therapy assignment and to warrant equipoise (61), very few are applicable to psychotherapy (62). Both limitations have important consequences for the placebo response, as will be discussed later. Nevertheless, current guidelines for good clinical practice require independence of raters and diagnostic staff and their impartiality toward the intervention (39).

Ineffective Blinding

Blinding (of the patient) as well as double blinding (of both patient and therapist) is literally impossible, not only in psychotherapy but also with many other interventions such as manual or physical therapy. Even where apparently possible, e.g., in biofeedback and neurofeedback therapy where "false feedback" (signals from another patient, e.g., as "yoked control") is provided, patients will realize immediately whether they have been randomized to treatment or control. The situation mimics some of the circumstances encountered in therapies using technical tools, e.g., acupuncture, transcutaneous electric nerve stimulation, and transcranial magnetic stimulation where only those patients can be enrolled who had never experienced the "real" therapy before and who may possibly be hoodwinked (63).

In classical drug RCT, unblinding will have imminent consequences for efficacy. Deliberate unblinding of RTC is usually only carried out when severe safety concerns arise but may also occur incidentally when patients and/or doctors notice significant differences in reporting of adverse events (64); even meta-analyses can identify such involuntary unblinding (65). Such unblinding will enhance the response to active therapy and reduce the response to control, thus enlarging the treatment–control difference (66). However, when therapies with either double-blinded placebo-controlled drug interventions or unblinded but controlled psychotherapies for the same condition (depression) were compared, the meta-analysis showed a small but significant effect (drug–placebo difference) in favor of pharmacotherapy (67), indicating that (un-) blinding affects psychotherapy to a lesser degree than conventional drug RCT. Furthermore, patients who were obviously assigned to the control condition (irrespective of its form) will respond with disappointment (68), increased risk of dropping out (69, and potentially with nocebo effects (70), further contributing (via the "last value carried forward" requirement for intent-to-treat analysis of the trial data) to an overestimation of the efficacy of the active arm of the trial.

Blinding is particularly necessary with conventional crossover designs where each patient serves as his/her own control, thereby reducing the data variance and making RCT possible with considerably less patients than with a parallel-group design. However, crossover designs carry another risk: that of carry-over effects from one phase to the next. If the carry-over effect is based on the Pavlovian conditioning of responses (71), even the use of longer washout phases cannot prevent it from occurring.

Ineffective blinding and carry-over effects that cannot be washed out therefore constitute the two reasons why psychotherapeutic trials cannot employ a crossover design. The limitations of a parallel-group design, in particular higher between-subject data variance, had to be overcome by developing other design features to account for the missing "true placebo" in psychotherapy, predominantly "waiting list control" (WLC), and "treatment as usual" (TAU).

Waiting List Control

The fact that no "true placebo" is applicable in psychotherapy RCT does not imply that no placebo effect occurs, as discussed above in the case of CER: when psychotherapy is compared with another therapy, the placebo effect is not controlled for and can therefore no longer be quantified. It can, however, be assumed that some of the alternative control strategies in psychotherapy research also have enhancing placebo effects. This may specifically be true of WLC.

Like crossover studies, WLC reduces data variance on account of a lower within-subject than between-subject variability of data; in this case, however, all patients should have to wait (which is usually not the case). It is also argued that WLC may additionally serve as a control for spontaneous variation of symptoms, a condition that cannot be readily tested with any RCT: it is ethically questionable as to whether a "no treatment control" is acceptable unless the disease is of minor severity and no effective therapy is available. This is the most rigorous interpretation of the current position of the Declaration of Helsinki (72).

Three-arm trials (active, placebo, and no treatment), between 25% and 45% of the treatment effect—of either drug or psychotherapy—can be attributed to spontaneous variation (73), with highest effects in nausea (45%), smoking cessation (40%), depression (35%), phobia (34%), and acute pain (25%). The authors concluded that most of the placebo effects in these conditions are attributable to spontaneous variation of symptoms. However, Kirsch and Sapirstein concluded in their initial paper (74) that 25% of the improvement observed in the drug-treated group (for depression) was due to the active medication, 25% to natural history, and 50% to the placebo effect.

The use of WLC as an indicator of spontaneous variation is therefore misleading (patients are not naive but are promised effective treatment), and it would be more appropriate to install one of the novel designs that separate recruitment for a disease-monitoring study from recruitment for an intervention study, called Zelen design (75) or multiple cohort RCT (MCRCT) design (76) (for more details, see 77 and 78).

Since WLC are promising patient-effective treatment in the future, they may produce strong expectancy effects, probably enhancing the placebo response, even in the phase before the treatment actually commences: symptom improvement during waiting has been reported (79, 80)—similar to effects of run-in periods in drug trials (81)—and cannot be taken solely as indicative of spontaneous remission. Placebo-controlled trials are superior to WLC trials and induce greater symptom reduction (82), as do RCTS with a "no treatment" condition in comparison with WLC trials (70). Furthermore, this effect may rely on the duration of waiting, and standard rules for this have yet to be investigated. One way of doing so would be to install a "step-wedge approach" (83), where randomization between different waiting groups (periods of different length) is used to test a dose-response function of waiting and the point at which positive expectations (placebo effects) may turn into disappointment (nocebo effects) (70) and increased dropout rates (69).

Treatment as Usual

If being randomized to a WLC can induce hope (placebo) or disappointment (nocebo) depending on its length, being randomized to TAU, by dint of its name, is already suggestive of its nocebo effect, the implicit message being that "you get what everybody else gets with this disease, and this treatment is unsatisfactory; that is why we are testing the new one, to which you, unfortunately, have not been randomized." Unless this is a treatment-naive patient with a very short disease history [which is indicative of high placebo response rates in many conditions and with many therapies (12)], this also reminds him or her of previous unsatisfactory or unsuccessful therapies, which—as we know—contributes significantly to the efficacy of any novel therapies (84).

Being randomized to the active treatment arm rather than to TAU will therefore enhance the placebo effect by enabling patients to compare the ongoing therapy with (all) previously inefficient therapies. For this reason, they prefer to participate in the novel approach; being randomized to TAU is almost a verdict. A TAU approach therefore enhances the placebo effect in the active arm and induces nocebo effects in the control arm.

The only thing that we have learned for sure from placebo/nocebo research over the past 10 years is that words can be painful (85) and can induce nocebo effects (86, 87). TAU definitively hurts, and it would be better rephrased as "the best available and approved treatment" (BAAT) when compared with a novel approach, but this would not work without having a number of logistic repercussions for trial designs.

Firstly, the utmost standardization of the TAU/BAAT treatment used for control purposes would be required. However, this is usually not carried out in psychotherapy RCT involving TAU.

It is particularly complicated when patients are recruited from different clinical settings for treatment in a specialized center, but TAU is provided by the transferring therapist. It also generates a further methodological issue with regard to the selection of BAAT, when more than one is available on the market, in the region, or under prevailing restrictions, e.g., health insurance plans. It should be noted that control conditions, e.g., optimized treatment as usual (TAU-O) in psychotherapy trials [see for instance Refs. (88, 89)], face additional challenges, depending on the health care environment in which they were conducted. In Germany, by way of example, patients with a psychiatric or psychosomatic illness, e.g., anorexia nervosa, have access to inpatient, day-patient, and outpatient psychotherapy treatment. If these patients are randomized to the TAU-O arm, they have a choice with regard to a) the treatment setting, b) the treatment method (e.g., CBT or psychodynamic psychotherapy), c) the therapist, and d) the intensity or dosage of therapy. It is therefore also particularly important to discuss findings of studies on the background of the health care system in which they were conducted. These challenges are somewhat similar in CER, where divergent interests (drug companies, ethics boards, and patient representatives) may nominate different options as BAAT (90). Given the large number of different psychotherapeutic approaches to one disease, this may be impossible to achieve in RCT but perhaps in meta-analyses of RCT (91). Finally, if one novel treatment A is compared with the best (or one of the bests) treatment B, statistics cannot rely on A's superiority over B but should test A's non-inferiority in comparison with B, with the consequence that as many as a fourfold number of patients could be required to confirm this (92). Not to mention the fact that this generates an ethical paradox since, according to the Declaration of Helsinki, the smallest possible number of patients should be recruited for a trial, while all others should receive regular and adequate treatment (93).

Among the many design alternatives that have been developed to either explore and maximize the placebo response or to avoid or minimize it in drug RCT (3), the so-called preference design may indicate an alternative approach specifically relevant for psychotherapy (78). In short, patients can choose between two (or more) alternative therapies, e.g., drug or psychotherapy, and are assigned accordingly (94). Only those who have no clear preference will undergo randomization. The role of patients' preference (and its placebo effect) can be assessed *post hoc*, comparing those with a preference for the one therapy with those randomized to this therapy in each therapy arm.

Specific Control Problems with Specific Psychotherapy Modalities

Beyond these general problems of control conditions with global placebo and nocebo effects in psychotherapy RCT, specific psychotherapies generate specific problems related to control and adequate estimation of the placebo/nocebo effects. Much of what has recently been described as decisional framework for neurocognitive and behavioral intervention (60) applies to most other therapeutic options also.

The subsequent review of different psychotherapies that we discuss bears some arbitrary selection bias and may reflect a more traditional vision of the spectrum of psychotherapies available. However, the intention is to illustrate rather than to cover the variability of problems associated with specific psychotherapy modalities. Readers who feel neglected or overlooked are welcome to consider and outline the specifics of their own modus operandi in light of what has been discussed.

Psychodynamic Psychotherapy

As already observed by Frank (13), it is essential for any control strategy attempting to catch the placebo effect in psychotherapy RCT that it devotes the same interaction (time, number of contacts, and intensity of communication) between the patient and the therapist as is the case in the "active arm" of the therapy. He proposed the use of relaxation therapy as a control for psychodynamic therapy (PDT), but it may equally well be any other passive but interactive therapy. It should be borne in mind that, in most such cases, the control condition does not provide a clear measure of the placebo effect but simply another effective therapy. This will increase the pressure to demonstrate superiority of PDT over control while increasing the placebo effect in both arms. Recent approaches (52, 88) applied standardized diagnostic systems (e.g., operationalized psychodynamic diagnosis) to identify clear treatment foci on the basis of a psychodynamic approach (52, 88).

Cognitive Behavioral Therapy

Unlike psychodynamic psychotherapy (PDT), CBT approaches intrapersonal problems at an individualized rational (cognitive) or behavioral level on the basis of an extensive prior behavioral analysis. To adequately control for nonspecific effects, it is feasible that written information on putative cognitive and behavioral strategies that are independent of the patient's own history may provide a control strategy. Albeit this lacks the actual behavioral analysis that precedes the active part of the therapy, it is, nevertheless, part of it. Behavioral exercises and tasks, which may mimic some of the effects occurring, bear the risk of errors if not adequately structured to the patient´s pathology and therefore require careful monitoring.

Interpersonal Psychotherapy

Interpersonal psychotherapy, like CBT, is based on a very intimate knowledge and guidance of the patient's acute problems, and problem solving may therefore not tolerate "sham" interventions without becoming evident. Keeping an (electronic) diary may be a method of monitoring one's own problems in the absence of a therapist (95). MBT, self-aid programs, and educational programs may also provide a lower-level control for the attention received.

Mindfulness-Based Therapy

An increasing number of therapy studies have demonstrated the efficacy of MBT in somatoform disorders such as IBS. Meditation-based therapy is difficult to control for nonspecific effects. In some trials, validated self-aid programs are used for attention control (96) or "sham mindfulness meditation" (97).

Couple and Family Therapy

The nonspecific contribution of "proxies" toward therapy efficacy has been well established for children in medical therapy (98) but has rarely been assessed in adults (99). Experimentally, the placebo and the nocebo effects in both groups are affected by social models, be it peers, parents, or strangers (100, 101). The control strategies therefore become even more difficult when the "proxies" are part of the intervention, as is the case in pair and family therapy. Merrilees et al. (95) used event-contingent diaries about marital conflict situations to change marital interactions as a control strategy rather than conventional face-to-face family psychotherapy sessions.

Group Psychotherapy

The problem of "proxies" and "others" for the therapy progress and success of individual patients becomes even more virulent with group psychotherapy. One control strategy would be to run two (or more) groups in parallel, with all participants truly randomized to one of the groups, and to compare the group as well as the individual progress between the two. In addition, group processes could be monitored by applying group-specific outcome measures. A further control strategy could consist of using eHealth applications such as chatrooms, focus groups, self-aid guides, and blogs as controls (102).

Hypnotherapy

Nonspecific effects of hypnotherapy, whether general or in a disease-specific form such as gut-directed hypnotherapy (103), are probably best and most readily controlled by relaxation exercises and therapy, since these are similar with respect to the time spent (in a group setting as well as in individual therapy) and active/passive components. A comparison with mindfulness mediation (see previously), while perhaps advisable, has not yet been conducted.

Self-Help Programs

SHPs were initially developed as a control condition for more manualized therapies, especially in patients with somatoform disorders, such as the IBS (104). As they developed their own theoretical framework, and for economic reasons—providing professional help to more patients outside academic centers—many applications are now available, particularly in combination with web-based approaches (105).

E-Mental Health Approaches

The very recent development of phone- and internet-based therapies has spread across all psychotherapy modalities, from CBT to MBT and SHP, e.g., Refs. (106) and (107). Among the most widely used applications is Deprexis®, an internet-based CBT program for the treatment of depression (108, 109). Due to its high standardization, it can easily allow for the control of the effect of a variety of nonspecific factors such as age, sex/gender, race, and other therapist-based demographics, for style of communication (personalized versus neutral), for intensity of communication, e.g., with or without question and answer, feedback, chatroom activity, etc. By contrast, of the many smartphone health applications presently available (now numbering over 300,000), those with a psychotherapeutic approach still lack clear control strategies that would enable us to estimate the overall efficacy of their placebo effect (110). Using "virtual" doctors or therapists (111) in the future may enable us to exert a much better control of the nonspecific factors not only in psychotherapy but also in medical therapy in general (21, 112).

NONSPECIFIC SOLUTIONS FOR THE CONTROL OF THE SPECIFIC PLACEBO EFFECT IN PSYCHOTHERAPY

In a recent paper (60), we proposed a dynamic decision framework for choosing a control condition depending on the patient population and associated risks, i.e., the risk of the disease itself, placebo vs. nocebo responses in this population, and the armamentarium of available therapies with known efficacy for this patient group, as well as the trial stage. We argued that the choice of control group and its justification need to be taken into consideration, e.g., when comparing behavioral and pharmacological therapies. High participation risk studies should therefore choose among controls with high effect sizes favoring treatment (e.g., waiting list and TAU) that may require smaller sample sizes, while low-risk studies may opt for active comparators and minimal treatment control conditions [see Figures 1 and 2 in Ref. (60)].

Wampold characterizes three global strategies resulting from the need to control for nonspecific effects of psychotherapy: a) identifying single components of the psychotherapy under investigation and replacing them by components of another psychotherapy (tradition); b) dismantling, without replacing, one or more components of a specific psychotherapy; and c) using treatments that control for common factors such as education and counseling (16).

Neither strategy has produced convincing results when it comes to adequately controlling the placebo effect in psychotherapy and has (worst case) shown that the control therapies may be as effective as the therapy under investigation, e.g., Ref. (113). Another novel control strategy, known as "befriending" (114, 115), refers to professional (nurse-conducted) social contacts developed for patients with schizophrenia in the community (116). It may, however, fall into the same trap as others before it, in demonstrating that even the mildest form of patient–therapist communication can result in significant therapeutic effects (117) and may therefore be a specific control only for the specific group of patients for which it was developed.

The "Goldilocks placebo effect" (118) exploits something that has rarely been tested and compared in psychotherapy research, i.e., the provision of alternatives from which the patient may choose. Preference designs (94) allow patients to choose between alternative treatments when available (e.g., drug vs. psychotherapy, different psychotherapy options) prior to randomization. It also allows comparison of the efficacy in patient that preferred one treatment arm with patients that were randomized to this arm of the study. The role of preferences can also be included in the overall statistics when comparing both treatment effects (78). Although the use of preferences does not seem to affect the overall internal and external validity of trials (94) and the preferences themselves do not appear to play a role in the placebo response (119), the systematic evaluation of placebo data beyond acupuncture has not yet been carried out.

By way of comparison (antidepressant versus CBT) of treatment outcome (treatment–control difference, not of the placebo response) in patients with depression, patients in either arm who selected this treatment were found to respond better than those who were randomized to the same arm (120). The difference was even greater in CBT trials and was independent of depression severity and dropout rates. In a trial in patients with chronic widespread pain, participants could choose between four options (CBT, exercise, a combination of both, or TAU), and the treatment preference had no effect on treatment outcome, while improvement expectations did (121). Neither of the studies elaborated on the placebo effect size under preference–choice conditions.

The "Goldilocks principle," which refers to Goldilocks´ quote about her preferred porridge temperature as being "just right" in the popular fairytale "Goldilocks and the Three Bears" (Robert Southey 1837), has found many applications in science. The Goldilocks placebo effect study (118) takes things a step further and asks whether it is the number of options available rather than the option to select per se that determines the placebo effect, and that the effect is larger when this number is "just right" than when there are too many or too few options to choose from. While their example is taken from a choice between different alternative medicine remedy treatments (2, 12, or 38 Bach flower essences, where the middle option received the highest rating as well as the highest symptom improvement report), the principle may also apply to lower number of choice options. Whether it can explain the divergent results of the two preference studies cited previously (120, 121) remains open at this point, and more data are required before this principle can be applied to placebo effects in psychotherapy.

SOME SPECIFICS OF PSYCHOTHERAPY AND ITS EVALUATION

Unlike drug therapy, where drug–drug interactions appear to be a pharmaceutical problem only, and the placebo effects above (or below) both are identical, psychotherapy is often combined with drug therapy, albeit their interactions have rarely been investigated. An RCT with a combination of both cannot, therefore, easily answer the question as to the size of the placebo effect and the relative contribution of either component to it. In depression, for example, psychotherapy in combination with drug therapy (122) and vice versa (123) is more effective than psychotherapy or drug therapy alone. The question, however, remains unanswered. Direct comparison of drug and psychotherapy has shown no superiority of drug over psychotherapy (124), and assuming similar effect sizes of the placebo component under both conditions would not change this relationship. However, they cannot be taken as merely additive, and the superiority of the combination may be also a function of the individual patient's preference (120). Unless an RCT is conducted and evaluated that provides either drug therapy (or placebo) alone, or psychotherapy (or an appropriate control) alone, or both in any combination, we will presumably not be able to answer this question with sufficient accuracy. Such a study resembles similarity with a double-dummy design (125), and it can be combined with a "no treatment" control group, e.g., in a register trial (76). The same holds true of other combinations of psychotherapy, such as those with neuro-modulatory therapies and biofeedback approaches (126).

Finally, one issue that requires specific consideration is the fact that, in psychotherapy, the outcome measure is usually, if not invariably a measure of subjective PRO or expert-rated outcome, whereas in drug therapy, efficacy can often be measured with both PRO/expert-rated outcome and with biomarkers, or at least with the circulating or tissue-specific level of the applied drug. Since PRO are more susceptible to placebo response than biomarkers (127), approval authorities and expert boards usually require both as endpoints in RCTs. It would therefore be advantageous if psychotherapy research were able to develop the equivalent of a biomarker as an indicator of therapy success and as an adjunct measure of the size of the placebo response in psychotherapy in the future.

SUMMARY

Overestimation of the efficacy of interventions, not only in psychotherapy, is common to all medical subspecialties, as is the effort to minimize nonspecific treatment effects, among which the placebo effect has the poorest reputation. Unfortunately, as we have already shown previously, psychotherapy lacks a true placebo intervention, and some of the nonspecific effects in drug therapy, such as the empathy of the therapist and the quality of the patient–therapist communication, become quite specific effects in psychotherapy. On the other hand, many of the common control strategies in psychotherapy research, especially waiting list and TAU, tend to inflate these nonspecific effects at the expense of already reduced overall efficacy, be it specific for individual psychotherapy modalities or for a "common effect" of all of them.

Under these circumstances, the scientific community of placebo researcher should not seek exemption from the scientific rules of treatment evaluation that have been developed for drug therapy but rather seek specific strategies to control at least some of the elements of psychotherapy that are responsible for the placebo response. These strategies can either be specific to certain psychotherapy modalities (as we have discussed) or further develop common strategies for all, bearing the possibility of covering at least some of Grünbaum´s "incidental constituents" without attempting to identify and enumerate them all. For instance, changing the waiting-list control into a "step-wedge" design, evaluating the cohort multiple RCT design, or developing the preference design to a Goldilocks approach for psychotherapy are empirical ways of proceeding (78, 114, 115) and much more appropriate than reasoning why it is impossible to control placebo effect in psychotherapy or remonstrating that all of psychotherapy is only placebo.

Last but not least: Biomedicine has learned to accept that placebo/nocebo effects exist outside placebo-controlled trials in daily medicine, and they contribute to a large extent to the success or failure of patient treatment, sometimes even more so than the drugs available. It is now time for psychotherapists to accept them in their daily practice.

AUTHOR CONTRIBUTIONS

PE had the idea for the paper and conceptualized it. PE and SZ wrote the paper.

REFERENCES

1. Jutte R. The early history of the placebo. *Complement Ther Med* (2013) 21:94–7. doi: 10.1016/j.ctim.2012.06.002
2. Kaptchuk TJ. Intentional ignorance: a history of blind assessment and placebo controls in medicine. *Bull Hist Med* (1998) 72:389–433. doi: 10.1353/bhm.1998.0159
3. Enck P, Bingel U, Schedlowski M, Rief W. The placebo response in medicine: minimize, maximize or personalize? *Nat Rev Drug Discov* (2013) 12:191–204. doi: 10.1038/nrd3923
4. Evers AWM, Colloca L, Blease C, Annoni M, Atlas LY, Benedetti F, et al. Implications of placebo and nocebo effects for clinical practice: expert consensus. *Psychother Psychosom* (2018) 87:204–10. doi: 10.1159/000490354.
5. Colloca L, Miller FG. Harnessing the placebo effect: the need for translational research. *Philos Trans R Soc Lond B Biol Sci* (2011) 366:1922–30. doi: 10.1098/rstb.2010.0399
6. Schedlowski M, Enck P, Rief W, Bingel U. Neuro-bio-behavioral mechanisms of placebo and nocebo responses: implications for clinical trials and clinical practice. *Pharmacol Rev* (2015) 67:697–730. doi: 10.1124/pr.114.009423
7. Beecher HK. The powerful placebo. *J Am Med Assoc* (1955) 159:1602–6. doi: 10.1001/jama.1955.02960340022006
8. Wolf S. Effects of suggestion and conditioning on the action of chemical agents in human subjects; the pharmacology of placebos. *J Clin Invest* (1950) 29:100–9. doi: 10.1172/JCI102225
9. Wolf S. The pharmacology of placebos. *Pharmacol Rev* (1959) 11:689–704.
10. Loranger AW, Prout CT, White MA. The placebo effect in psychiatric drug research. *JAMA* (1961) 176:920–5. doi: 10.1001/jama.1961.03040240026010
11. Rickels K, Lipman R, Raab E. Previous medication, duration of illness and placebo response. *J Nerv Ment Dis* (1966) 142:548–54. doi: 10.1097/00005053-196606000-00006
12. Weimer K, Colloca L, Enck P. Placebo effects in psychiatry: mediators and moderators. *Lancet Psychiatry* (2015b) 2:246–57. doi: 10.1016/S2215-0366(14)00092-3
13. Frank JD. The influence of patients' and therapists' expectations on the outcome of psychotherapy. *Br J Med Psychol* (1968) 41:349–56. doi: 10.1111/j.2044-8341.1968.tb02043.x
14. Rosenthal D, Frank JD. Psychotherapy and the placebo effect. *Psychol Bull* (1956) 53:294–302. doi: 10.1037/h0044068
15. Kirsch I. Placebo psychotherapy: synonym or oxymoron? *J Clin Psychol* (2005) 61:791–803. doi: 10.1002/jclp.20126
16. Wampold BE, Minami T, Tierney SC, Baskin TW, Bhati KS. The placebo is powerful: estimating placebo effects in medicine and psychotherapy from randomized clinical trials. *J Clin Psychol* (2005) 61:835–54. doi: 10.1002/jclp.20129
17. Blease C, Kirsch I. The placebo effect and psychotherapy: implications for theory, research, and practice. *Psychol Conscious Theory Res Pract* (2016) 3:105–7. doi: 10.1037/cns0000094
18. Kirsch I, Wampold B, Kelley JM. Controlling for the placebo effect in psychotherapy: noble quest or tilting at windmills? *Psychol Conscious Theory Res Pract* (2016) 3:121–31. doi: 10.1037/cns0000065
19. Gaab J, Blease C, Locher C, Gerger H. Go open: a plea for transparency in psychotherapy. *Psychol Conscious Theory Res Pract* (2016) 3:175–98. doi: 10.1037/cns0000063
20. Blease C. Consensus in placebo studies: lessons from the philosophy of science. (2018a) 61:412–29. doi: 10.1353/pbm.2018.0053
21. Blease C. Psychotherapy and placebos: manifesto for conceptual clarity. *Front Psychiatry* (2018b) 9:379. doi: 10.3389/fpsyt.2018.00379
22. Grünbaum A. The placebo concept in medicine and psychiatry. *Psychol Med* (1986) 16:19–38. doi: 10.1017/S0033291700002506
23. Enck P, Horing B, Broelz E, Weimer K. Knowledge gaps in placebo research: with special reference to neurobiology. *Int Rev Neurobiol* (2018) 139:85–106. doi: 10.1016/bs.irn.2018.07.018
24. Ford AC, Moayyedi P. Meta-analysis: factors affecting placebo response rate in the irribowel syndrome. *Aliment Pharmacol Ther* (2010) 32:144–58. doi: 10.1111/j.1365-2036.2010.04328.x
25. Flik CE, Bakker L, Laan W, Van Rood YR, Smout AJ, De Wit NJ. Systematic review: the placebo effect of psychological interventions in the treatment of irritable bowel syndrome. *World J Gastroenterol* (2017) 23:2223–33. doi: 10.3748/wjg.v23.i12.2223
26. Lambert MJ. Maximizing psychotherapy outcome beyond evidence-based medicine. *Psychother Psychosom* (2017) 86:80–9. doi: 10.1159/000455170
27. Rosenzweig S. Some implicit common factors in diverse methods of psychotherapy. *Am J Orthopsychiatry* (1936) 6:412–5. doi: 10.1111/j.1939-0025.1936.tb05248.x
28. Huibers MJH, Cuijpers P. "Common (Nonspecific) Factors in Psychotherapy,". In: Cautin RL, Lilienfeld. SO, editors. *The Encyclopedia of Clinical Psychology*. New York: John WIley & Sons (2015). p. 681–6. doi: 10.1002/9781118625392.wbecp272
29. Lambert MJ, Ogles BM. The efficacy and effectiveness of psychotherapy. In: Lambert MJ, editor. Bergin and Garfield's handbook of psychotherapy and behavior change. 5th ed. New York: John Wiley & Sons (2004). p. 139–93.
30. Weimer K, Colloca L, Enck P. Age and sex as moderators of the placebo response - an evaluation of systematic reviews and meta-analyses across medicine. *Gerontology* (2015a) 61:97–108. doi: 10.1159/000365248
31. Mohr DC, Spring B, Freedland KE, Beckner V, Arean P, Hollon SD, et al. The selection and design of control conditions for randomized controlled trials of psychological interventions. *Psychother Psychosom* (2009) 78:275–84. doi: 10.1159/000228248
32. Guidi J, Brakemeier EL, Bockting CLH, Cosci F, Cuijpers P, Jarrett RB, et al. Methodological recommendations for trials of psychological interventions. *Psychother Psychosom* (2018) 87:276–84. doi: 10.1159/000490574
33. Benedetti F. *Placebo effects*. Oxord: Oxford University Press (2014). doi: 10.1093/acprof:oso/9780198705086.001.0001
34. Colloca L. Preface: The Fascinating Mechanisms and Implications of the Placebo Effect. *Int Rev Neurobiol* (2018a) 138:xv–xx. doi: 10.1016/S0074-7742(18)30027-8.
35. Colloca L. Preface: Part II: The Fascinating Mechanisms and Implications of the Placebo Effect. *Int Rev Neurobiol* (2018b)139:xvii–xxiii. doi: 10.1016/S0074-7742(18)30087-4.
36. Rakel DP, Hoeft TJ, Barrett BP, Chewning BA, Craig BM, Niu M. Practitioner empathy and the duration of the common cold. *Fam Med* (2009) 41:494–501.
37. Enck P, Klosterhalfen S, Kruis W. Determination of placebo effect in irritable bowel syndrome. *Dtsch Med Wochenschr* (2005) 130:1934–7. doi: 10.1055/s-2005-872605
38. Martens U, Caspari G, Rilk A, Hefner J, Teufel M, Klosterhalfen S, et al. Six-year follow-up of patients with functional bowel disorders, with and without

previous psychotherapy. *Psychosoc Med* (2010) 7:Doc06. doi: 10.3205/psm000068
39. Mentz RJ, Hernandez AF, Berdan LG, Rorick T, O'brien EC, Ibarra JC, et al. Good clinical practice guidance and pragmatic clinical trials: balancing the best of both worlds. *Circulation* (2016) 133:872–80. doi: 10.1161/CIRCULATIONAHA.115.019902
40. Bridge JA, Birmaher B, Iyengar S, Barbe RP, Brent DA. Placebo response in randomized controlled trials of antidepressants for pediatric major depressive disorder. *Am J Psychiatry* (2009) 166:42–9. doi: 10.1176/appi.ajp.2008.08020247
41. Yildiz A, Vieta E, Tohen M, Baldessarini RJ. Factors modifying drug and placebo responses in randomized trials for bipolar mania. *Int J Neuropsychopharmacol* (2011) 14:863–75. doi: 10.1017/S1461145710001641
42. Agid O, Siu CO, Potkin SG, Kapur S, Watsky E, Vanderburg D, et al. Meta-regression analysis of placebo response in antipsychotic trials, 1970-2010. *Am J Psychiatry* (2013) 170:1335–44. doi: 10.1176/appi.ajp.2013.12030315
43. Kobak KA, Kane JM, Thase ME, Nierenberg AA. Why do clinical trials fail? The problem of measurement error in clinical trials: time to test new paradigms? *J Clin Psychopharmacol* (2007) 27:1–5. doi: 10.1097/JCP.0b013e31802eb4b7
44. Rutherford BR, Sneed JR, Tandler JM, Rindskopf D, Peterson BS, Roose SP. Deconstructing pediatric depression trials: an analysis of the effects of expectancy and therapeutic contact. *J Am Acad Child Adolesc Psychiatry* (2011) 50:782–95. doi: 10.1016/j.jaac.2011.04.004
45. Mancini M, Wade AG, Perugi G, Lenox-Smith A, Schacht A. Impact of patient selection and study characteristics on signal detection in placebo-controlled trials with antidepressants. *J Psychiatr Res* (2014) 51:21–9. doi: 10.1016/j.jpsychires.2014.01.001
46. Jairath V, Zou G, Parker CE, Macdonald JK, Mosli MH, Alameel T, et al. Systematic review with meta-analysis: placebo rates in induction and maintenance trials of crohn's disease. *Aliment Pharmacol Ther* (2017) 45:1021–42. doi: 10.1111/apt.13973
47. Erekson DM, Lambert MJ, Eggett DL. The relationship between session frequency and psychotherapy outcome in a naturalistic setting. *J Consult Clin Psychol* (2015) 83:1097–107. doi: 10.1037/a0039774
48. Kobak KA. Inaccuracy in clinical trials: effects and methods to control inaccuracy. *Curr Alzheimer Res* (2010) 7:637–41. doi: 10.2174/156720510793499057
49. Kaptchuk TJ, Kelley JM, Conboy LA, Davis RB, Kerr CE, Jacobson EE, et al. Components of placebo effect: randomised controlled trial in patients with irritable bowel syndrome. *Bmj* (2008) 336:999–1003. doi: 10.1136/bmj.39524.439618.25
50. Weimer K, Gulewitsch MD, Schlarb AA, Schwille-Kiuntke J, Klosterhalfen S, Enck P. Placebo effects in children: a review. *Pediatr Res* (2013) 74:96–102. doi: 10.1038/pr.2013.66
51. Anderson T, Ogles BM, Patterson CL, Lambert MJ, Vermeersch DA. Therapist effects: facilitative interpersonal skills as a predictor of therapist success. *J Clin Psychol* (2009) 65:755–68. doi: 10.1002/jclp.20583
52. Leichsenring F, Steinert C. Replicability in psychotherapy research: uncontrolled risk factors and proposed measures. *Psychother Psychosom* (2016) 85:371–2. doi: 10.1159/000444858
53. Munder T, Brutsch O, Leonhart R, Gerger H, Barth J. Researcher allegiance in psychotherapy outcome research: an overview of reviews. *Clin Psychol Rev* (2013) 33:501–11. doi: 10.1016/j.cpr.2013.02.002
54. Elsenbruch S, Enck P. Placebo effects and their determinants in gastrointestinal disorders. *Nat Rev Gastroenterol Hepatol* (2015) 12:472–85. doi: 10.1038/nrgastro.2015.117
55. Papakostas GI, Fava M. Does the probability of receiving placebo influence clinical trial outcome? A meta-regression of double-blind, randomized clinical trials in mdd. *Eur Neuropsychopharmacol* (2009) 19:34–40. doi: 10.1016/j.euroneuro.2008.08.009
56. Sinyor M, Levitt AJ, Cheung AH, Schaffer A, Kiss A, Dowlati Y, et al. Does inclusion of a placebo arm influence response to active antidepressant treatment in randomized controlled trials? Results from pooled and meta-analyses. *J Clin Psychiatry* (2010) 71:270–9. doi: 10.4088/JCP.08r04516blu
57. Woods SW, Gueorguieva RV, Baker CB, Makuch RW. Control group bias in randomized atypical antipsychotic medication trials for schizophrenia. *Arch Gen Psychiatry* (2005) 62:961–70. doi: 10.1001/archpsyc.62.9.961
58. Mallinckrodt CH, Zhang L, Prucka WR, Millen BA. Signal detection and placebo response in schizophrenia: parallels with depression. *Psychopharmacol Bull* (2010) 43:53–72.
59. Rutherford BR, Sneed JR, Roose SP. Does study design influence outcome? The effects of placebo control and treatment duration in antidepressant trials. *Psychother Psychosom* (2009) 78:172–81. doi: 10.1159/000209348
60. Gold SM, Enck P, Hasselmann H, Friede T, Hegerl U, Mohr DC, et al. Control conditions for randomised trials of behavioural interventions in psychiatry: a decision framework. *Lancet Psychiatry* (2017) 4:725–32. doi: 10.1016/S2215-0366(17)30153-0
61. Boutron I, Guittet L, Estellat C, Moher D, Hrobjartsson A, Ravaud P. Reporting methods of blinding in randomized trials assessing nonpharmacological treatments. *PLoS Med* (2007) 4:e61. doi: 10.1371/journal.pmed.0040061
62. Button KS, Munafo MR. Addressing risk of bias in trials of cognitive behavioral therapy. *Shanghai Arch Psychiatry* (2015) 27:144–8. doi: 10.11919/j.issn.1002-0829.215042
63. Enck P, Klosterhalfen S, Zipfel S. Acupuncture, psyche and the placebo response. *Auton Neurosci* (2010) 157:68–73. doi: 10.1016/j.autneu.2010.03.005
64. Kim SE, Kubomoto S, Chua K, Amichai MM, Pimentel M. "Pre-cebo": an unrecognized issue in the interpretation of adequate relief during irritable bowel syndrome drug trials. *J Clin Gastroenterol* (2012) 46:686–90. doi: 10.1097/MCG.0b013e31825828a7
65. Shah E, Triantafyllou K, Hana AA, Pimentel M. Adverse events appear to unblind clinical trials in irritable bowel syndrome. *Neurogastroenterol Motil* (2014) 26:482–8. doi: 10.1111/nmo.12289
66. Berna C, Kirsch I, Zion SR, Lee YC, Jensen KB, Sadler P, et al. Side effects can enhance treatment response through expectancy effects: an experimental analgesic randomized controlled trial. *Pain* (2017) 158:1014–20. doi: 10.1097/j.pain.0000000000000870
67. Cuijpers P, Karyotaki E, Andersson G, Li J, Mergl R, Hegerl U. The effects of blinding on the outcomes of psychotherapy and pharmacotherapy for adult depression: a meta-analysis. *Eur Psychiatry* (2015) 30:685–93. doi: 10.1016/j.eurpsy.2015.06.005
68. Doering BK, Rief W, Petrie KJ. Lessons to be learned from placebo arms in psychopharmacology trials. *Handb Exp Pharmacol* (2014) 225:273–90. doi: 10.1007/978-3-662-44519-8_15
69. Cooper AA, Conklin LR. Dropout from individual psychotherapy for major depression: a meta-analysis of randomized clinical trials. *Clin Psychol Rev* (2015) 40:57–65. doi: 10.1016/j.cpr.2015.05.001
70. Furukawa TA, Noma H, Caldwell DM, Honyashiki M, Shinohara K, Imai H, et al. Waiting list may be a nocebo condition in psychotherapy trials: a contribution from network meta-analysis. *Acta Psychiatr Scand* (2014) 130:181–92. doi: 10.1111/acps.12275
71. Suchman AL, Ader R. Classic conditioning and placebo effects in crossover studies. *Clin Pharmacol Ther* (1992) 52:372–7. doi: 10.1038/clpt.1992.157
72. Association WM. World medical association declaration of helsinki: ethical principles for medical research involving human subjects. *JAMA* (2013) 310:2191–4. doi: 10.1001/jama.2013.281053
73. Krogsboll LT, Hrobjartsson A, Gotzsche PC. Spontaneous improvement in randomised clinical trials: meta-analysis of three-armed trials comparing no treatment, placebo and active intervention. *BMC Med Res Methodol* (2009) 9:1. doi: 10.1186/1471-2288-9-1
74. Kirsch I, Sapirstein G. Listening to prozac but hearing placebo: a meta-analysis of antidepressant medication. *Prev Treat* (1998) 1:0002a. doi: 10.1037//1522-3736.1.0002a
75. Zelen M. A new design for randomized clinical trials. *N Engl J Med* (1979) 300:1242–45. doi: 10.1056/NEJM197905313002203
76. Relton C, Torgerson D, O'cathain A, Nicholl J. Rethinking pragmatic randomised controlled trials: introducing the "cohort multiple randomised controlled trial" design. *BMJ* (2010) 340:c1066. doi: 10.1136/bmj.c1066
77. Fava GA, Tomba E, Tossani E. Innovative trends in the design of therapeutic trials in psychopharmacology and psychotherapy. *Prog Neuropsychopharmacol Biol Psychiatry* (2013) 40:306–11. doi: 10.1016/j.pnpbp.2012.10.014
78. Weimer K, Enck P. Traditional and innovative experimental and clinical trial designs and their advantages and pitfalls. *Handb Exp Pharmacol* (2014) 225:237–72. doi: 10.1007/978-3-662-44519-8_14

79. Hesser H, Weise C, Rief W, Andersson G. The effect of waiting: a meta-analysis of wait-list control groups in trials for tinnitus distress. *J Psychosom Res* (2011) 70:378–84. doi: 10.1016/j.jpsychores.2010.12.006
80. Huckert TF, Hank P, Krampen G. [Changes in psychopathological symptoms during the waiting period for outpatient psychotherapy]. *Psychother Psychosom Med Psychol* (2012) 62:301–9. doi: 10.1055/s-0032-1314837
81. Enck P, Vinson B, Malfertheiner P, Zipfel S, Klosterhalfen S. The placebo response in functional dyspepsia–reanalysis of trial data. *Neurogastroenterol Motil* (2009) 21:370–77. doi: 10.1111/j.1365-2982.2008.01241.x
82. Zhu Z, Zhang L, Jiang J, Li W, Cao X, Zhou Z, et al. Comparison of psychological placebo and waiting list control conditions in the assessment of cognitive behavioral therapy for the treatment of generalized anxiety disorder: a meta-analysis. *Shanghai Arch Psychiatry* (2014) 26:319–31. doi: 10.11919/j.issn.1002-0829.214173
83. De Allegri M, Pokhrel S, Becher H, Dong H, Mansmann U, Kouyate B, et al. Step-wedge cluster-randomised community-based trials: an application to the study of the impact of community health insurance. *Health Res Policy Syst* (2008) 6:10. doi: 10.1186/1478-4505-6-10
84. Hunter AM, Cook IA, Leuchter AF. Impact of antidepressant treatment history on clinical outcomes in placebo and medication treatment of major depression. *J Clin Psychopharmacol* (2010) 30:748–51. doi: 10.1097/JCP.0b013e3181faa474
85. Benedetti F, Lanotte M, Lopiano L, Colloca L. When words are painful: unraveling the mechanisms of the nocebo effect. *Neuroscience* (2007) 147:260–71. doi: 10.1016/j.neuroscience.2007.02.020
86. Hauser W, Hansen E, Enck P. Nocebo phenomena in medicine: their relevance in everyday clinical practice. *Dtsch Arztebl Int* (2012) 109:459–65. doi: 10.3238/arztebl.2012.0459
87. Bingel U, Placebo Competence Team. Avoiding nocebo effects to optimize treatment outcome. *JAMA* (2014) 312:693–4. doi: 10.1001/jama.2014.8342
88. Zipfel S, Wild B, Gross G, Friederich HC, Teufel M, Schellberg D, et al. Focal psychodynamic therapy, cognitive behaviour therapy, and optimised treatment as usual in outpatients with anorexia nervosa (ANTOP study): randomised controlled trial. *Lancet* (2014) 383:127–37. doi: 10.1016/S0140-6736(13)61746-8
89. Zipfel S, Herzog W, Kruse J, Henningsen P. Psychosomatic medicine in germany: more timely than ever. *Psychother Psychosom* (2016) 85:262–9. doi: 10.1159/000447701
90. Platt R, Kass NE, Mcgraw D. Ethics, regulation, and comparative effectiveness research: time for a change. *JAMA* (2014) 311:1497–8. doi: 10.1001/jama.2014.2144
91. Connolly Gibbons MB, Gallop R, Thompson D, Luther D, Crits-Christoph K, Jacobs J, et al. Comparative effectiveness of cognitive therapy and dynamic psychotherapy for major depressive disorder in a community mental health setting: a randomized clinical noninferiority trial. *JAMA Psychiatry* (2016) 73:904–11. doi: 10.1001/jamapsychiatry.2016.1720
92. Leon AC. Evolution of psychopharmacology trial design and analysis: six decades in the making. *J Clin Psychiatry* (2011) 72:331–40. doi: 10.4088/JCP.10r06669
93. Enck P, Klosterhalfen S, Weimer K, Horing B, Zipfel S. The placebo response in clinical trials: more questions than answers. *Philos Trans R Soc Lond B Biol Sci* (2011) 366:1889–95. doi: 10.1098/rstb.2010.0384
94. King M, Nazareth I, Lampe F, Bower P, Chandler M, Morou M, et al. Conceptual framework and systematic review of the effects of participants' and professionals' preferences in randomised controlled trials. *Health Technol Assess* (2005) 91–186:iii–iv. doi: 10.3310/hta9350
95. Merrilees CE, Goeke-Morey M, Cummings EM. Do event-contingent diaries about marital conflict change marital interactions? *Behav Res Ther* (2008) 46:253–62. doi: 10.1016/j.brat.2007.11.007
96. Gaylord SA, Whitehead WE, Coble RS, Faurot KR, Palsson OS, Garland EL, et al. Mindfulness for irritable bowel syndrome: protocol development for a controlled clinical trial. *BMC Complement Altern Med* (2009) 9:24. doi: 10.1186/1472-6882-9-24
97. Zeidan F, Johnson SK, Gordon NS, Goolkasian P. Effects of brief and sham mindfulness meditation on mood and cardiovascular variables. *J Altern Complement Med* (2010) 16:867–73. doi: 10.1089/acm.2009.0321
98. Liodden I, Sandvik L, Norheim AJ. Placebo by proxy - the influence of parental anxiety and expectancy on postoperative morbidities in children. *Forsch Komplementmed* (2015) 22:381–7. doi: 10.1159/000442565
99. Grelotti DJ, Kaptchuk TJ. Placebo by proxy. *BMJ* (2011) 343:d4345. doi: 10.1136/bmj.d4345
100. Vogtle E, Barke A, Kroner-Herwig B. Nocebo hyperalgesia induced by social observational learning. *Pain* (2013) 154:1427–33. doi: 10.1016/j.pain.2013.04.041
101. Colloca L, Benedetti F. Placebo analgesia induced by social observational learning. *Pain* (2009) 144:28–34. doi: 10.1016/j.pain.2009.01.033
102. Kramer JJ, Willemsen MC, Conijn B, Van Emst AJ, Brunsting S, Riper H. Effectiveness of a web-based self-help smoking cessation intervention: protocol of a randomised controlled trial. *BMC Public Health* (2009) 9:32. doi: 10.1186/1471-2458-9-32
103. Miller V, Carruthers HR, Morris J, Hasan SS, Archbold S, Whorwell PJ. Hypnotherapy for irritable bowel syndrome: an audit of one thousand adult patients. *Aliment Pharmacol Ther* (2015) 41:844–55. doi: 10.1111/apt.13145
104. Liegl G, Plessen CY, Leitner A, Boeckle M, Pieh C. Guided self-help interventions for irritable bowel syndrome: a systematic review and meta-analysis. *Eur J Gastroenterol Hepatol* (2015) 27:1209–21. doi: 10.1097/MEG.0000000000000428
105. Bernecker SL, Banschback K, Santorelli GD, Constantino MJ. A web-disseminated self-help and peer support program could fill gaps in mental health care: lessons from a consumer survey. *JMIR Ment Health* (2017) 4:e5. doi: 10.2196/mental.4751
106. Mohr DC, Cheung K, Schueller SM, Hendricks Brown C, Duan N. Continuous evaluation of evolving behavioral intervention technologies. *Am J Prev Med* (2013) 45:517–23. doi: 10.1016/j.amepre.2013.06.006
107. Heber E, Ebert DD, Lehr D, Cuijpers P, Berking M, Nobis S, et al. The benefit of web- and computer-based interventions for stress: a systematic review and meta-analysis. *J Med Internet Res* (2017) 19:e32. doi: 10.2196/jmir.5774
108. Schroder J, Bruckner K, Fischer A, Lindenau M, Kother U, Vettorazzi E, et al. Efficacy of a psychological online intervention for depression in people with epilepsy: a randomized controlled trial. *Epilepsia* (2014) 55:2069–76. doi: 10.1111/epi.12833
109. Fischer A, Schröder J, Vettorazzi E, Wolf OT, Pöttgen J, Lau S, et al. An online programme to reduce depression in patients with multiple sclerosis: a randomised controlled trial. *Lancet Psychiatry* (2015) 2:217–23. doi: 10.1016/S2215-0366(14)00049-2
110. Torous J, Firth J. The digital placebo effect: mobile mental health meets clinical psychiatry. *Lancet Psychiatry* (2016) 3:100–2. doi: 10.1016/S2215-0366(15)00565-9
111. Horing B, Newsome ND, Enck P, Babu SV, Muth ER. A virtual experimenter to increase standardization for the investigation of placebo effects. *BMC Med Res Methodol* (2016) 16:84. doi: 10.1186/s12874-016-0185-4
112. Giel KE, Leehr EJ, Becker S, Herzog W, Junne F, Schmidt U, et al. Relapse prevention via videoconference for anorexia nervosa - findings from the restart pilot study. *Psychother Psychosom* (2015) 84:381–3. doi: 10.1159/000431044
113. Baskin TW, Tierney SC, Minami T, Wampold BE. Establishing specificity in psychotherapy: a meta-analysis of structural equivalence of placebo controls. *J Consult Clin Psychol* (2003) 71:973–9. doi: 10.1037/0022-006X.71.6.973
114. Harris T, Brown GW, Robinson R. Befriending as an intervention for chronic depression among women in an inner city. 2: role of fresh-start experiences and baseline psychosocial factors in remission from depression. *Br J Psychiatry* (1999b) 174:225–32. doi: 10.1192/bjp.174.3.225
115. Harris T, Brown GW, Robinson R. Befriending as an intervention for chronic depression among women in an inner city. 1: randomised controlled trial. *Br J Psychiatry* (1999a) 174:219–24. doi: 10.1192/bjp.174.3.219
116. Turkington D, Sensky T, Scott J, Barnes TR, Nur U, Siddle R, et al. A randomized controlled trial of cognitive-behavior therapy for persistent symptoms in schizophrenia: a five-year follow-up. *Schizophr Res* (2008) 98:1–7. doi: 10.1016/j.schres.2007.09.026
117. Turkington D, Spencer H, Lebert L, Dudley R. Befriending: active placebo or effective psychotherapy? *Br J Psychiatry* (2017) 211:5–6. doi: 10.1192/bjp.bp.116.197467
118. Hafner RJ, White MP, Handley SJ. The goldilocks placebo effect: placebo effects are stronger when people select a treatment from an optimal number of choices. *Am J Psychol* (2018) 131:175–84. doi: 10.5406/amerjpsyc.131.2.0175
119. Prady SL, Burch J, Crouch S, Macpherson H. Insufficient evidence to determine the impact of patient preferences on clinical outcomes in

acupuncture trials: a systematic review. *J Clin Epidemiol* (2013) 66:308–18. doi: 10.1016/j.jclinepi.2012.09.011

120. Mergl R, Henkel V, Allgaier AK, Kramer D, Hautzinger M, Kohnen R, et al. Are treatment preferences relevant in response to serotonergic antidepressants and cognitive-behavioral therapy in depressed primary care patients? Results from a randomized controlled trial including a patients' choice arm. *Psychother Psychosom* (2011) 80:39–47. doi: 10.1159/000318772
121. Beasley MJ, Ferguson-Jones EA, Macfarlane GJ. Treatment expectations but not preference affect outcome in a trial of CBT and exercise for pain. *Can J Pain* (2017) 1:161–70. doi: 10.1080/24740527.2017.1384297
122. Karyotaki E, Smit Y, Holdt Henningsen K, Huibers MJ, Robays J, De Beurs D, et al. Combining pharmacotherapy and psychotherapy or monotherapy for major depression? A meta-analysis on the long-term effects. *J Affect Disord* (2016) 194:144–52. doi: 10.1016/j.jad.2016.01.036
123. Cuijpers P, Van Straten A, Warmerdam L, Andersson G. Psychotherapy versus the combination of psychotherapy and pharmacotherapy in the treatment of depression: a meta-analysis. *Depress Anxiety* (2009) 26:279–88. doi: 10.1002/da.20519
124. Cuijpers P, Andersson G, Donker T, Van Straten A. Psychological treatment of depression: results of a series of meta-analyses. *Nord J Psychiatry* (2011) 65:354–64. doi: 10.3109/08039488.2011.596570
125. Marusic A, Ferencic SF. Adoption of the double dummy trial design to reduce observer bias in testing treatments. *J R Soc Med* (2013) 106:196–8. doi: 10.1177/0141076813485350
126. Razza LB, Moffa AH, Moreno ML, Carvalho AF, Padberg F, Fregni F, et al. A systematic review and meta-analysis on placebo response to repetitive transcranial magnetic stimulation for depression trials. *Prog Neuropsychopharmacol Biol Psychiatry* (2018) 81:105–13. doi: 10.1016/j.pnpbp.2017.10.016
127. Hrobjartsson A, Gotzsche PC. Placebo interventions for all clinical conditions. *Cochrane Database Syst Rev* (2010) CD003974. doi: 10.1002/14651858.CD003974.pub3

14

Can a Brief Relaxation Exercise Modulate Placebo or Nocebo Effects in a Visceral Pain Model?

Sigrid Elsenbruch[1], *Till Roderigo*[1], *Paul Enck*[2] *and Sven Benson*[1*]

[1] *Institute of Medical Psychology and Behavioral Immunobiology, University Hospital Essen, Essen, Germany,* [2] *Department of Internal Medicine VI, University Hospital Tuebingen, Tuebingen, Germany*

***Correspondence:**
Sven Benson
sven.benson@uk-essen.de

Translational research aiming to elucidate mediators and moderators of placebo and nocebo effects is highly relevant. This experimental study tested effects of a brief progressive muscle relaxation (PMR) exercise, designed to alter psychobiological stress parameters, on the magnitude of placebo and nocebo effects in a standardized psychosocial treatment context. In 120 healthy volunteers (60 men, 60 women), pain expectation, pain intensity, and pain unpleasantness in response to individually-calibrated rectal distensions were measured with visual analog scales during a baseline. Participants were then randomized to exercise PMR (relaxation group: $N = 60$) or a simple task (control group: $N = 60$), prior to receiving positive (placebo), negative (nocebo) or neutral suggestions regarding an intravenous administration that was in reality saline in all groups. Identical distensions were repeated (test). State anxiety, salivary cortisol, heart rate, and blood pressure were assessed repeatedly. Data were analyzed using analysis of covariance, planned Bonferroni-corrected group comparisons, as well as exploratory correlational and mediation analyses. Treatment suggestions induced group-specific changes in pain expectation, with significantly *reduced* expectation in placebo and *increased* expectation in nocebo groups. PMR had no discernable effect on pain expectation, state anxiety or cortisol, but led to significantly lower heart rate and systolic blood pressure. Relaxation significantly interacted with positive treatment suggestions, which only induced placebo analgesia in relaxed participants. No effects of negative suggestions were found in planned group comparisons, irrespective of relaxation. Exploratory correlation and mediation analyses revealed that pain expectation was a mediator to explain the association between treatment suggestions and pain-related outcomes. Clearly, visceral pain modulation is complex and involves many cognitive, emotional, and possibly neurobiological factors that remain to be fully understood. Our findings suggest that a brief relaxation exercise may facilitate the induction of placebo analgesia by positive when compared to neutral treatment suggestions. They underscore the contribution of relaxation and stress as psychobiological states within the psychosocial treatment context—factors which clearly deserve more attention in translational studies aiming to maximize positive expectancy effects in clinical settings.

Keywords: placebo effect, nocebo effect, expectation, visceral pain, pain unpleasantness, stress, relaxation

INTRODUCTION

Although placebo research spans many medical disciplines, the pain field continues to drive conceptual, mechanistic, and clinical advances in placebo knowledge, providing fruitful opportunities of forward- and backward translation. Placebo analgesia constitutes one of the most fascinating and impressive examples of such translational research. Laboratory and preclinical studies in healthy populations and in patients with chronic pain conditions have elucidated the psychological and neurobiological mechanisms underlying placebo and nocebo effects (1, 2). The clinical potential offered by a transfer of this knowledge into treatment settings has been recognized within the pain field (3, 4) and beyond (5). This is underscored by trials supporting the efficacy of placebo interventions in patients with chronic low back pain (6, 7) and chronic visceral pain (8, 9). Facilitating placebo while minimizing nocebo effects may contribute to refining treatment approaches to provide patients with improved and more personalized patient care (10, 11). Toward this end, translational research aiming to optimize the efficacy of placebo interventions is highly relevant. In the context of chronic visceral pain and related gastrointestinal symptoms, the potential of placebo knowledge has been recognized but is far from fulfilled (12–14).

Various aspects of the psychosocial treatment context, including the setting (15), nature of the intervention, as well as the quality and quantity of patient-provider interactions (9, 16, 17), shape treatment expectations and thereby the presence and magnitude of placebo effects. Optimizing the psychosocial treatment context has the potential to improve the efficacy of placebo treatment, and to maximize the benefits of placebo-elements that are an inherent part of therapeutic interventions, including pharmacological treatments (4, 18). Interestingly, two laboratory studies in healthy volunteers support the idea that placebo analgesia can be enhanced with specific pharmacological interventions, i.e., the administration of vasopressin and oxytocin, respectively (19, 20). Whether behavioral approaches that target stress-related psychobiological factors are capable of facilitating placebo analgesia has not been tested. Herein, we explore for the first time the modulatory effects of a brief behavioral intervention, i.e., progressive muscle relaxation (PMR), on placebo and nocebo effects in a clinically-relevant model of visceral pain. The rationale was inspired by evidence supporting that *enhanced* stress [e.g., increased state anxiety (21–24), subjective stress levels (25–28), experimentally-induced fear (29), acute psychosocial stress (30)] moderates placebo and/or nocebo effects. As part of a larger experimental study (30), we herein implemented PMR aiming to test effects of *reduced* stress-related psychobiological factors on the magnitude of placebo and nocebo effects induced by treatment suggestions. Building on our earlier experimental studies on placebo/nocebo effects in the context of visceral pain (22, 30–33), we specifically aimed to test whether a brief relaxation exercise, carried out immediately prior to the delivery of deceptive positive (placebo), deceptive negative (nocebo), or truthful neutral (control) treatment suggestions, can facilitate placebo analgesia or reduce nocebo hyperalgesia in an established and clinically-relevant model of visceral pain in healthy volunteers. To explore if the effects of relaxation or treatment suggestions on outcomes were mediated by stress markers or expectations, we conducted correlational and mediation analyses.

MATERIALS AND METHODS

Participants

Healthy adults were recruited by local advertisements seeking volunteers for an experimental study on the modulation of visceral pain perception. We herein report on a total of $N = 120$ healthy volunteers (60 men, 60 women) who were randomized to a brief relaxation exercise or a control task on the experimental study day just prior to undergoing an established placebo/nocebo paradigm (see below, study design). Note that this study was conducted as part of a larger trial which also included an additional $N = 60$ volunteers who were randomized to a psychosocial stress protocol (data on the psychosocial stress and control groups have been reported in Roderigo et al. (30). Recruitment and screening procedures were accomplished with a total of $N = 219$ participants originally interested in the study. Reasons for non-participation were lack of interest, exclusion based on criteria specified below, and a high pain threshold that was above the herein applied safety cut-off for distensions at 55 mmHg. The study was conducted at Essen University Hospital with data collection between January 2015 and June 2016. The study protocol was approved by the local ethics committee (protocol number 13-5565-BO, approval date: August 28, 2013). All volunteers gave informed written consent in accordance with the Declaration of Helsinki and were paid for their participation.

Exclusion criteria included age <18 or >65 years, a body mass index (BMI) <18 or >30, any known medical or psychological conditions, current medication use (except thyroid medication, occasional over-the-counter drugs for minor allergies, benign headaches, etc.), current anxiety or depression symptoms above the published cut-off values on the Hospital Anxiety and Depression Scale (HADS) (34), current gastrointestinal (GI) symptoms suggestive of an undiagnosed GI condition (35), peri-anal tissue damage (e.g., painful hemorrhoids or fissures which may interfere with rectal balloon placement), and prior participation in any of our previous placebo studies. In an effort to reduce possible variability related to fluctuations of hormones across the female menstrual cycle, only women on hormonal contraceptives were recruited. All participants completed a comprehensive questionnaire battery, as detailed in Roderigo et al. (30). We herein characterized groups using the HADS (34) for symptoms of anxiety and depression, the trait version of the STAI (36) for trait anxiety, the TICS (screening scale) (37) for chronic perceived stress, and sum scores from a gastrointestinal (GI) symptom questionnaire (35) to assess frequency and severity of common upper and lower GI symptoms. Note that previous experience with any type of relaxation technique, including progressive muscle relaxation (PMR) was not an inclusion or exclusion criterion, however, it was required that volunteers were willing to complete a home-based PMR training program as part of the study, as detailed below.

Study Design and Procedures

During a 4-week period preceding the experimental study day, volunteers were instructed to complete a home-based, standardized training program in progressive muscle relaxation (PMR). This was done to achieve a large enough sample of individuals capable of completing a short relaxation exercise on the day of the study. In order to achieve proper blinding and randomization, all 180 participants underwent the training program. To do so, we selected a commercially available training manual that consisted of an illustrated book with an audio CD that contained guided training sessions. Note that the same audio-guided training CD was used by participants randomized to the brief relaxation group on the study day. Every volunteer—irrespective of possible prior experience with the PMR or other relaxation techniques—was instructed to start the training in the first week with two sessions of a long program that lasted ~40 min. Thereafter, participants could choose between the long version and a shorter 15-min. version in the remaining training weeks, but were required to practice at least twice per week. Participants recorded their practice in a training log, and at the end of the week (i.e., on Sundays) completed a standardized questionnaire assessing the number of training sessions (N), training duration (in minutes), perceived training efficacy (7-point Likert-scale ranging from "training worked not at all" to "training worked perfectly"), psychological distress (7-point Likert-scale ranging from "felt completely relaxed" to "felt extremely distressed") and various bodily symptoms (not reported here) for the past week. Together with each weekly questionnaire, participants collected morning saliva samples for analysis of the cortisol awakening response (CAR). In case of non-compliance (i.e., on average <2 training sessions per week) participants were encouraged to continue practicing for up to two additional weeks before the study day was scheduled. Note that questionnaire data and CAR were not acquired to verify the efficacy of PMR training (which is impossible given the absence of a control group that did not undergo training) but rather to provide sample characteristics for comparisons of groups that on the study day were randomized to brief relaxation exercise vs. a control task.

On the experimental study day, rectal sensory and pain thresholds were initially determined with a pressure-controlled barostat system (modified ISOBAR 3 device, G & J Electronics, Ontario, Canada), using well-established methodology [e.g., (22, 30–33, 38). During a BASELINE, each participant received a series of painful rectal distensions titrated individually to rectal threshold (6 distensions, duration each 30 s; pauses in-between 30 s). Participants were then randomized to relaxation (practice relaxation using the 15-min. audio-CD program, $N = 60$) or control intervention (engage in an easy cognitive activity, e.g., crosswords, reading a magazine, $N = 60$) while stratifying for sex. Immediately afterwards, participants were randomized to positive (placebo), negative (nocebo), or neutral treatment suggestions (details on suggestions below). This resulted in a total of 2 (relaxation, control) x 3 (positive, negative, neutral suggestions) experimental groups consisting of $N = 20$ participants per group. The series of rectal distensions using the same individualized pressures as during BASELINE was then repeated (TEST).

Treatment Suggestions and Blinding

We herein implemented previously used methodology to induce placebo and nocebo effects in this visceral pain model [e.g., (30, 33); for recent discussions of methodology aspects, see (13, 14)]. In this paradigm, deceptive or truthful treatment suggestions are delivered in combination with an i.v. administration that in reality contains saline. In placebo groups, volunteers receive positive treatment suggestions regarding pain relief induced by a spasmolytic drug (i.e., Butylscopolaminiumbromid). In nocebo groups, negative suggestions regarding increased pain sensitivity due to administration of an opioid antagonist (i.e., Naloxone) are delivered. In control groups, truthful information about saline are provided. These control groups (herein referred to as "neutral" groups to distinguish from the relaxation vs. control intervention group terminology) are an essential part of the study design as they allow a differentiation and separate analyses of placebo and nocebo effects, respectively, as well as controlling for effects of time (e.g., habituation), etc.

In order to achieve proper blinding and a randomization to treatment suggestions on the study day, all volunteers received deceptive information about all possible drug treatments during recruitment and informed consent, including detailed information about typical clinical uses, pharmacodynamics, and possible side effects. Blinding of the study team interacting with volunteers on the study day was accomplished as follows: The clinical psychologist responsible for recruitment and conducting the study protocol (relaxation, control) was blinded to subsequent treatment information, the physician who delivered treatment information was blinded to prior relaxation vs. control intervention, the female study nurse was fully blinded throughout the study day.

Pain-Related Measures

Primary outcome measures were overall perceived visceral pain intensity and pain unpleasantness, quantified with visual analogs scales (VAS, 0–100 mm, ends defined as none—very much). In addition, expected pain intensity was quantified with a VAS (0–100 mm, ends defined as none—very much) prior to BASELINE and TEST, respectively.

Additional Measures

State anxiety (STAI-S), salivary cortisol concentrations (see below), heart rate (Task Force Monitor, CNSystems Medizintechnik AG, Graz, Austria), and blood pressure were assessed repeatedly and are herein presented for a baseline (prior to first randomization to relaxation vs. control intervention), after treatment suggestions, and after the TEST series of distensions. Note that we chose not to additionally assess these stress-related measures in-between the intervention and delivery of treatment suggestions given concerns that this may disrupt or interfere with effects of relaxation on the subsequent experimental procedures.

Saliva samples were collected using Salivettes (Sarstedt, Nümbrecht, Germany). To assess the cortisol awakening

TABLE 3 | Stress parameters.

	Relaxation group (*N* = 60)	Control group (*N* = 60)	ANCOVA time effect[a]	ANCOVA group effect[a]	ANCOVA interaction[a]
SYSTOLIC BP (mmHg)					
BASELINE	122.2 ± 1.6	119.9 ± 1.6	$F = 2.41, p = 0.09$	$F = 0.21, p = 0.65$	$F = 9.22$, p<0.001
After treatment suggestion	120.0 ± 1.6	117.1 ± 1.4			
After TEST	117.9 ± 1.6***	120.5 ± 1.4			
DIASTOLIC BP (mmHg)					
BASELINE	80.7 ± 1.1	78.9 ± 1.2	$F = 0.13, p = 0.88$	$F = 0.16, p = 0.69$	$F = 0.40, p = 0.67$
After treatment suggestion	78.7 ± 1.0	77.9 ± 1.0			
After TEST	78.6 ± 1.1	77.9 ± 1.6			
HEART RATE (beats/min)					
BASELINE	67.2 ± 1.4#	63.1 ± 1.1#	$F = 0.72, p = 0.49$	$F = 1.88, p = 0.17$	$F = 8.10, p < 0.001$
After treatment suggestion	64.4 ± 1.4**	63.1 ± 1.1			
After TEST	63.6 ± 1.4***	64.2 ± 1.2			
SALIVARY CORTISOL (nmol/l)					
BASELINE	12.2 ± 1.2	11.2 ± 0.8	$F = 11.68, p < 0.001$	$F = 0.64, p = 0.43$	$F = 0.07, p = 0.94$
After treatment suggestion	10.2 ± 0.9***	9.1 ± 0.5***			
After TEST	9.8 ± 0.8***	8.7 ± 0.6***			
STAI STATE ANXIETY					
BASELINE	37.4 ± 1.0	38.1 ± 1.2	$F = 9.56, p < 0.001$	$F = 0.07, p = 0.79$	$F = 0.53, p = 0.58$
After treatment suggestion	35.5 ± 1.2	36.1 ± 1.0			
After TEST	31.5 ± 0.9***	33.1 ± 0.9*			

All data are shown as mean ± standard error of the mean, unless indicated otherwise. Stress parameters were repeatedly assessed, i.e., at BASELINE (prior to first randomization to relaxation vs. control intervention), after treatment suggestions, and after the series of distensions (TEST). BP, blood pressure; STAI, Spielberger State-Trait Anxiety Inventory (state version).

*[a]Results of analyses of covariances (ANCOVA) accounting for HADS anxiety scores. Incomplete/missing data: Incomplete STAI-S questionnaires: N = 3 relaxation group, N = 2 control group; technical errors with ECG signal for heart rate: N = 3 relaxation group, N = 6 control group. *p < 0.05, **p < 0.01, ***p < 0.001, results of Bonferroni-corrected paired t-tests comparing means vs. baseline within each experimental group. #p < 0.05, result of post-hoc computed Bonferroni-corrected ANCOVA, comparing relaxation and control group at distinct time points.*

decreases over time (salivary cortisol: $F = 11.68$, $p < 0.001, \eta_p^2 = 0.09$; state anxiety scores: $F = 9.56$, $p < 0.001$, $\eta_p^2 = 0.08$), however, without evidence of significant group × time interactions (salivary cortisol: $F = 0.07$, $p = 0.86$, $\eta_p^2 = 0.01$; state anxiety scores: $F = 0.53$, $p = 0.59$, $\eta_p^2 = 0.01$). No significant effects were observed for diastolic blood pressure.

Pain-Related Measures

Expected pain intensity (**Figure 1A**) was reduced by positive and increased by negative treatment suggestions ($F = 8.84, p < 0.001$, $\eta_p^2 = 0.14$, ANCOVA main effect of treatment information; $F = 32.25, p < 0.001$, $\eta_p^2 = 0.37$, ANCOVA interaction effect of time × treatment information). Pain expectation was not affected by relaxation, as indicated by the absence of significant main or interaction effects.

For perceived pain intensity (**Figure 1B**), there was a significant effect of treatment suggestions ($F = 4.38$, $p = 0.015$ $\eta_p^2 = 0.07$, time x suggestion interaction; $F = 3.70$, $p = 0.028$ $\eta_p^2 = 0.06$, main effect of suggestion), but no main effect of the intervention ($F = 0.01$, $p = 0.98$ $\eta_p^2 = 0.01$, time x intervention interaction; $F = 0.31$, $p = 0.58$ $\eta_p^2 = 0.01$, main effect of intervention) and no interaction effect ($F = 1.29$, $p = 0.29$ $\eta_p^2 = 0.02$, time × suggestion × intervention interaction). Planned comparisons of group means revealed significantly reduced perceived pain intensity at TEST due to positive compared to neutral suggestions in the relaxation groups ($F = 8.04$, $p = 0.008$, $\eta_p^2 = 0.19$), while a similar placebo effect was not observed in the control groups ($F = 0.44$, $p = 0.51$, $\eta_p^2 = 0.01$). Nocebo effects, tested by comparing groups with negative vs. neutral treatment suggestions, were not observed in either intervention group (relaxation: $F = 0.3$, $p = 0.57$, $\eta_p^2 = 0.01$; control: $F = 1.9$, $p = 0.17$, $\eta_p^2 = 0.05$).

For pain unpleasantness (**Figure 1C**), a significant interaction between intervention, treatment suggestions, and time ($F = 3.53$, $p = 0.032$, $\eta_p^2 = 0.06$), as well as a significant effect of treatment suggestions ($F = 4.41$, $p = 0.014$ $\eta_p^2 = 0.07$, time × suggestion interaction; $F = 3.21$, $p = 0.044$ $\eta_p^2 = 0.05$, main effect of treatment suggestion) emerged, while effects of the intervention were not significant ($F = 0.82$, $p = 0.37$, $\eta_p^2 = 0.01$, time × intervention interaction; $F = 0.37$, $p = 0.54$ $\eta_p^2 = 0.01$, main effect of intervention). Planned comparisons of group means revealed significantly reduced unpleasantness at TEST in response to positive when compared to neutral suggestions ($F = 7.8$, $p = 0.008$, $\eta_p^2 = 0.18$) in relaxation groups, but not in control groups ($F = 0.9$, $p = 0.34$, $\eta_p^2 = 0.02$). No significant effects of negative suggestions were observed (relaxation groups: $F = 0.02$, $p = 0.88$, $\eta_p^2 = 0.01$; control groups: $F = 0.63$, $p = 0.43$, $\eta_p^2 = 0.02$).

TABLE 4 | Stress parameters in all experimental groups.

		Relaxation group			Control group		
		Treatment suggestions			Treatment suggestions		
		Positive ($n = 20$)	Neutral ($n = 20$)	Negative ($n = 20$)	Positive ($n = 20$)	Neutral ($n = 20$)	Negative ($n = 20$)
Systolic BP (mmHg)	BASELINE	123.8 ± 2.9	122.6 ± 3.2	120.2 ± 2.5	120.4 ± 2.9	119.9 ± 2.0	119.3 ± 3.4
	After treatment suggestion	121.2 ± 2.6	119.5 ± 3.1	119.4 ± 2.6	117.4 ± 2.9	119.1 ± 2.0	114.9 ± 2.3
	After TEST	119.1 ± 2.9	118.3 ± 2.8	116.5 ± 2.5	119.6 ± 2.9	120.7 ± 2.3	121.4 ± 2.4
Diastolic BP (mmHg)	BASELINE	82.7 ± 1.7	80.1 ± 2.4	79.4 ± 1.6	76.9 ± 2.2	81.6 ± 1.9	78.4 ± 1.8
	After treatment suggestion	79.7 ± 1.6	78.5 ± 2.0	78.0 ± 1.7	77.8 ± 2.1	80.2 ± 1.6	75.9 ± 1.6
	After TEST	78.9 ± 2.0	79.1 ± 2.0	77.9 ± 1.6	74.3 ± 4.1	81.1 ± 1.8	78.2 ± 1.4
Heart rate (beats/min)	BASELINE	66.0 ± 1.8	68.7 ± 3.1	66.8 ± 2.2	62.2 ± 1.9	63.8 ± 2.2	63.3 ± 1.8
	After treatment suggestion	63.6 ± 1.9	66.4 ± 2.9	63.3 ± 2.3	62.3 ± 1.9	63.4 ± 2.1	63.5 ± 1.8
	After TEST	62.7 ± 1.8	65.4 ± 3.4	62.8 ± 1.9	64.2 ± 2.0	62.9 ± 2.6	65.4 ± 1.4
Salivary cortisol (nmol/l)	BASELINE	12.2 ± 1.5	12.2 ± 2.7	12.3 ± 1.8	10.6 ± 1.4	12.8 ± 1.6	10.3 ± 1.2
	After treatment suggestion	10.0 ± 1.3	10.1 ± 1.9	10.5 ± 1.8	8.6 ± 0.9	10.4 ± 1.1	8.4 ± 0.6
	After TEST	9.4 ± 1.1	9.8 ± 1.5	10.1 ± 1.7	7.7 ± 0.8	10.1 ± 1.3	8.2 ± 0.7
STAI State anxiety	BASELINE	36.0 ± 1.9	37.0 ± 1.7	39.3 ± 1.6	38.4 ± 2.4	38.3 ± 2.1	37.6 ± 1.9
	After treatment suggestion	33.4 ± 2.2	32.8 ± 1.5	40.5 ± 1.8	34.6 ± 1.8	34.9 ± 1.5	38.7 ± 2.0
	After TEST	30.8 ± 1.5	31.1 ± 1.2	32.7 ± 2.1	33.4 ± 1.2	31.9 ± 1.2	34.4 ± 1.9

Data shown here extend data shown in ***Table 3****. All data are shown as mean ± standard error of the mean. BP, Blood pressure; STAI, State Trait Anxiety Inventory.*

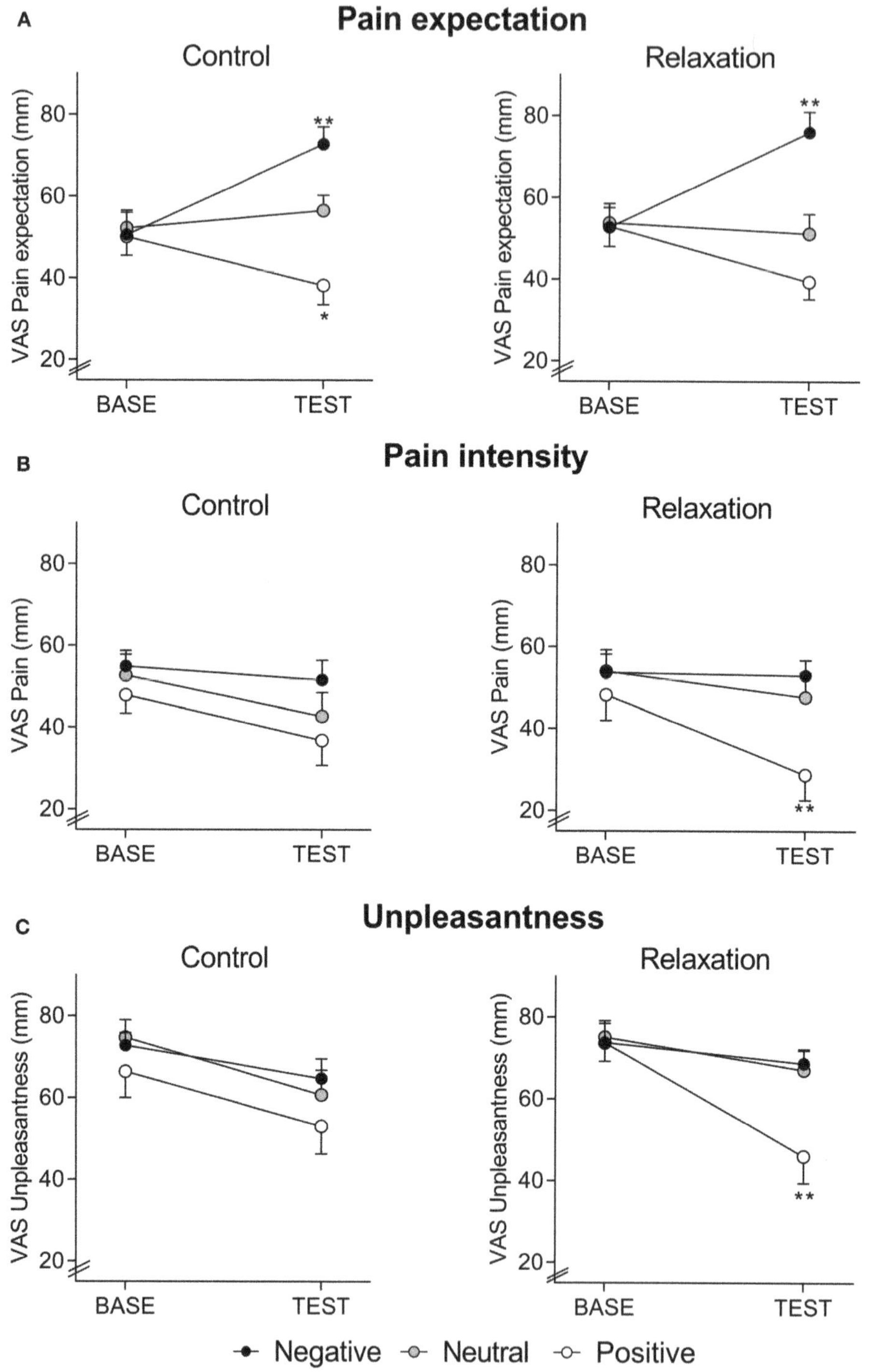

FIGURE 1 | Expected pain intensity **(A)**, perceived pain intensity **(B),** and perceived pain unpleasantness **(C)**, assessed with visual analog scale (VAS, 0–100 mm) at BASELINE and TEST, in groups receiving positive, neutral, or negative treatment information after relaxation (right panels) or control (left panels). Note that pain expectation was assessed before, whereas perceived pain intensity and unpleasantness were assessed after the series of distensions during BASELINE and TEST, respectively. For ANCOVA results, please see text. $^{*}p < 0.05$; $^{**}p < 0.01$ results of planned comparisons with Bonferroni-correction at TEST (for exact *p*-values, see text) comparing groups with positive information to groups with neutral information (to test for placebo effects) and groups with negative information to groups with neutral information (to test for nocebo effects) after either relaxation or control.

Exploratory Correlational and Mediation Analyses

To explore the role of pain expectation, we conducted correlational and mediation analyses both in the whole sample and in groups with positive suggestions (placebo groups) and negative suggestions (nocebo groups). In the whole sample of $N = 120$, pain expectation was significantly associated with both perceived pain intensity ($r = 0.58$, $p < 0.001$) and pain unpleasantness ($r = 0.38$, $p < 0.001$). In addition, pain expectation correlated with state anxiety ($r = 0.25$, $p = 0.007$), but not with other stress markers. No significant correlations between any other stress marker and pain outcomes were found (all $p > 0.05$, data not shown).

Within placebo groups ($N = 40$), pain expectation was positively correlated with perceived pain intensity ($r = 0.54$, $p < 0.001$, **Figure 2A**) and unpleasantness ($r = 0.32$, $p = 0.047$, **Figure 2B**). To explore if pain expectation mediated effects of positive treatment suggestions, we conducted mediation analyses on data from placebo and neutral suggestion groups ($N = 80$) after ensuring that positive associations remained significant in multiple regression analyses including treatment suggestions in addition to pain expectation as independent variables (data not shown). We found an indirect effect of pain expectation which mediated the association between treatment suggestions and pain intensity (**Figure 3A**) as well as unpleasantness (**Figure 3B**).

Within nocebo groups ($N = 40$), pain expectation was significantly associated pain intensity ($r = 0.53$, $p = 0.03$), but not with unpleasantness ($r = 0.25$, $p = 0.11$). The former association remained significant in multiple regression analyses including treatment suggestions in addition to pain expectation as independent variables (data not shown). To explore if pain expectation mediated effects of negative treatment suggestions, we conducted mediation analysis for pain intensity on data from nocebo and neutral suggestion groups ($N = 80$). We found an indirect effect of pain expectation which mediated the association between treatment suggestions and pain intensity (**Figure 3C**).

We conducted additional mediation analyses to explore if putative effects of relaxation vs. control on pain intensity or unpleasantness could be explained by pain expectation. In separate analyses within the placebo, nocebo, and control groups, we did not find evidence of direct or indirect effects of relaxation on pain outcomes (data not shown). This is in line with (1) the absence of significant effects of relaxation on expectations and (2) the non-significant correlations between stress markers and outcome variables.

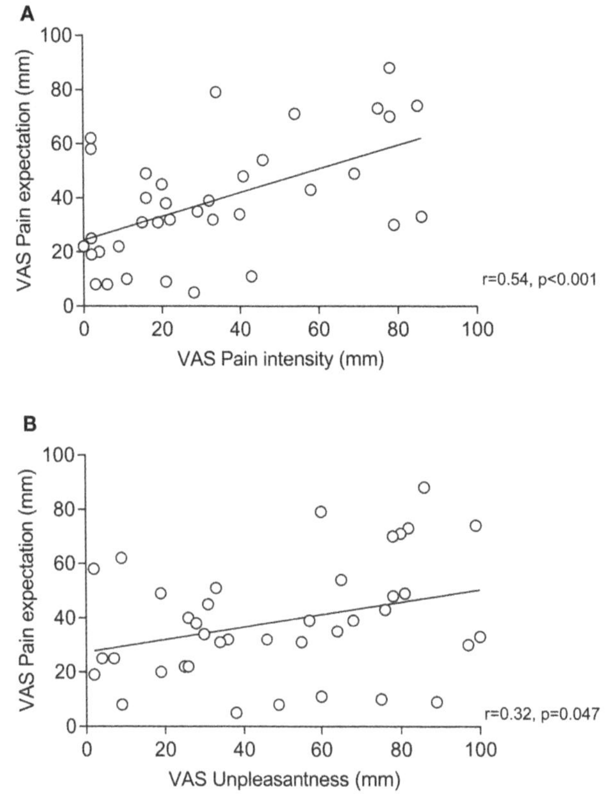

FIGURE 2 | Correlations (Pearson's r) between pain expectation and perceived pain intensity **(A)** and pain expectation and perceived pain unpleasantness **(B)** within groups receiving positive treatment suggestions (i.e., placebo groups).

DISCUSSION

This is the first study testing whether a behavioral intervention aimed at reducing acute stress parameters affects the response to positive and/or negative treatment suggestions in a clinically-relevant model of visceral pain. Our findings suggest that a brief relaxation exercise may facilitate the induction of placebo analgesia by positive when compared to neutral treatment suggestions. These findings extend evidence that placebo analgesia can be boosted with pharmacological interventions (19, 20). There are clearly many facets surrounding the psychosocial treatment context that ultimately determine the presence and magnitude of expectancy effects. Our results support the contribution of relaxation and stress as psychobiological states within the psychosocial treatment context—factors which clearly deserve more attention in translational studies aiming to maximize positive expectancy effects in clinical settings.

Healthy volunteers were randomized to a brief muscle relaxation exercise or a control task just prior to randomly receiving deceptive positive, deceptive negative, or truthful neutral treatment suggestions regarding an intravenous infusion that was in reality saline in all groups. These treatment suggestions induced group-specific changes in pain expectation, with *reduced* pain expectation in groups receiving positive suggestions of pain relief (i.e., placebo groups) and *increased* pain expectation in groups receiving negative suggestions of enhanced pain sensitivity (i.e., nocebo groups). While the relaxation exercise had no discernable effect on pain expectation, relaxation significantly interacted with positive treatment suggestions. Planned comparisons of group means showed significantly reduced pain intensity and lower pain unpleasantness after positive compared to neutral treatment suggestions only in the relaxation groups. In other words, positive treatment suggestions only induced placebo analgesia in relaxed participants, which

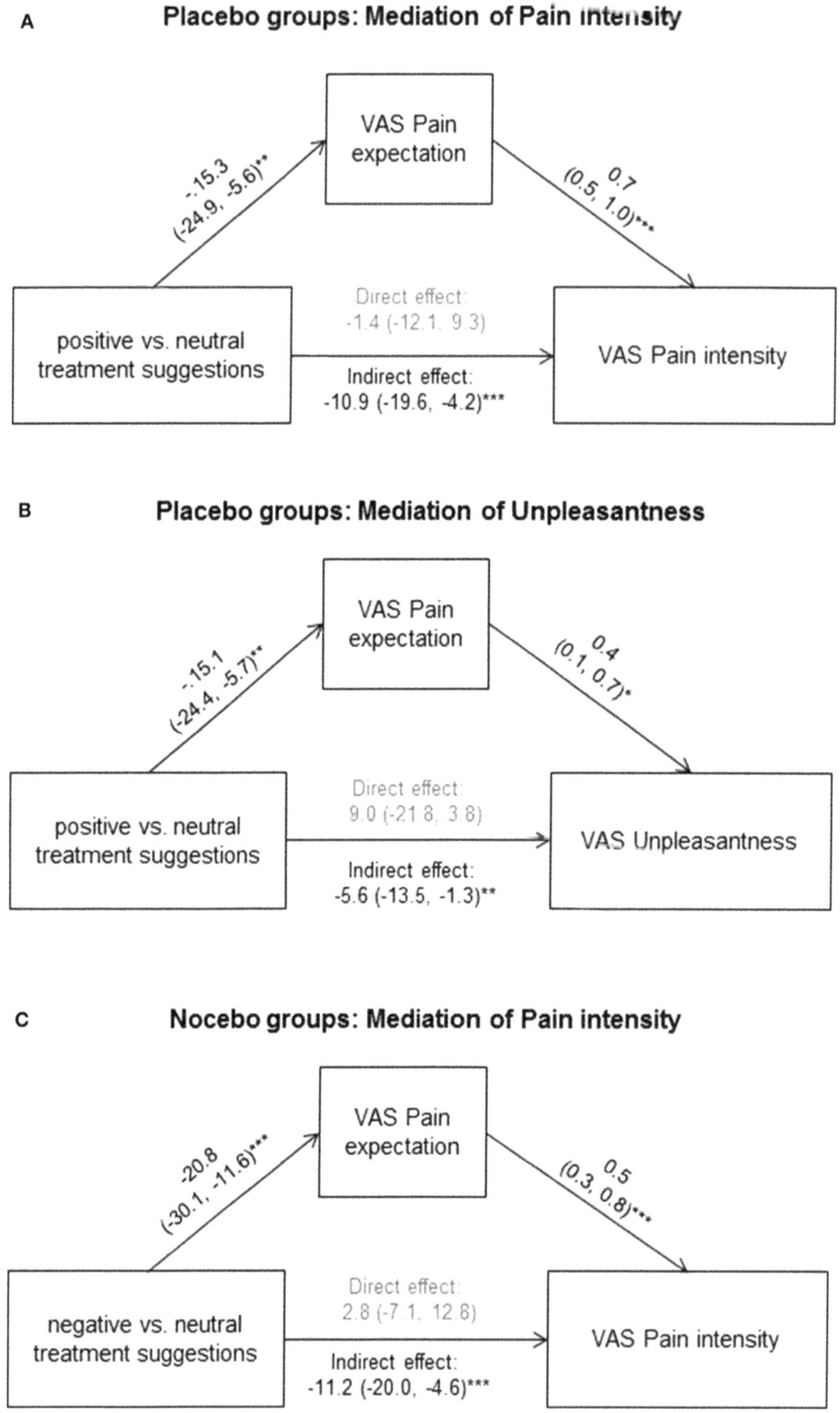

FIGURE 3 | To explore if pain expectation mediated effects of positive treatment suggestions, we conducted mediation analyses on data from placebo and neutral suggestion groups for pain intensity **(A)** and unpleasantness **(B)**, as well as on data from nocebo and neutral suggestion groups for pain intensity **(C)**. Standardized coefficients with 95% CIs are shown. $^{*}p < 0.05$; $^{**}p < 0.01$; $^{***}p < 0.001$.

is partly in line with our hypothesis assuming a facilitated placebo effect. On the other hand, relaxation had no discernable effect on groups receiving negative suggestions. Since no nocebo effects were observed in either relaxation or control group, we could not confirm our hypothesis that relaxation may reduce nocebo hyperalgesia.

We chose a brief relaxation exercise as behavioral intervention with the intention to acutely reduce stress parameters within a highly standardized psychosocial treatment context. This approach was conceptually and methodologically based on our earlier brain imaging work on the role of emotional context in visceral pain processing (38). It complements placebo/nocebo studies in the broader pain field aiming to discern effects of acute stress, state anxiety or fear (23, 25, 26, 28–30, 40) on placebo analgesia or nocebo hyperalgesia. In order to verify the efficacy of the intervention and to gain insight into possible mechanisms, we assessed several relevant stress markers reflecting different biopsychological aspects of stress. Brief relaxation significantly reduced systolic blood pressure and heart rate, supporting effects on the autonomic nervous system (ANS). On the other hand, no effects on state anxiety or cortisol concentrations were found. This could indicate that measures of ANS function (herein: heart rate and blood pressure) are more sensitive or responsive to short-term effects of PMR, at least in healthy individuals. However, it should be noted that cortisol and state anxiety significantly decreased in both groups, and that these measures could not be assessed immediately after the relaxation exercise for methodological considerations. Hence, effects on state anxiety or cortisol could be difficult to detect given reductions in both groups and may have been missed herein. Nevertheless, the ANS is increasingly appreciated in the context of pain modulation [e.g., (41)], especially in acute and chronic visceral pain as a key component of the brain axis (42–50). Within the placebo field, the ANS has been proposed as a primary mediator of peripheral placebo effects in conditioning models (51, 52). Placebo analgesia evokes complex effects within the cardiovascular system, including changes in heart rate and blood pressure (25, 53). Blood pressure and stress were found to mediate hyperalgesia after nocebo suggestions (27), and a recent study supports a role of autonomic arousal in the persistence of nocebo hyperalgesia (54). Interestingly, the same study (54) found no correlation between either self-reported anxiety or autonomic arousal and placebo analgesia/nocebo hyperalgesia. We also explored these relationships in our dataset, and found no correlations between placebo effects and stress markers. In fact, pain expectation was the only mediator we could identify to explain the association between treatment suggestions and pain-related outcomes. These results call for caution with respect to any speculation about stress-related mechanisms and underscore the need to further study possible moderators of placebo analgesia, especially emotional factors that have been proposed to play a role in placebo analgesia (55, 56). Clearly, visceral pain modulation is complex and involves many cognitive, emotional, and possibly neurobiological factors that remain to be fully understood.

This study has strengths and limitations. Strengths include the clinically-relevant visceral pain model, blinding procedures, the combination of different psychobiological measures for traits and states, and the inclusion of groups receiving positive, negative or neutral treatment suggestions within one study. The full factorial within-between study design goes beyond correlational approaches aiming to identify psychological mediators and moderators of placebo and nocebo effects. At the same time, final group *N*s are relatively small, posing limitations of statistical power, and risk of Type II error. This may for example explain why *post hoc* testing revealed a statistically significant reduction in pain expectation induced by positive vs. neutral suggestions only in the control but not in the relaxation group. Further, for reasons of feasibility and cost effectiveness, data from the control group were also used in Roderigo et al. (30), and there was also no additional control group that did not undergo prior relaxation training for feasibility reasons and to ensure blinding and randomization on the study day. We therefore cannot assess possible effects of prior relaxation training on measures obtained on the study day. While the absence of the brief PMR vs. control exercise effects on pain-related outcomes on the study day may be interpreted as evidence supporting a lack of relaxation effects on visceral pain, this would in our view be premature. First, we could not ascertain whether regular PMR exercise of 4 weeks did in fact induce changes in variables relevant to chronic stress. To do so was not our intention since this was not a treatment study but rather herein implemented in order to teach a sufficiently large number of study volunteers to perform PMR on the study day, aiming to realize a study design with proper randomization and blinding. We recruited a tightly-screened, healthy population of young individuals with comparatively low levels of chronic stress or stress-related symptom burden. Hence, our findings likely do not transfer to other populations at risk for stress-related health conditions or even patients with chronic pain, and should not be viewed as evidence for or against the potential clinical use of relaxation techniques in patients. In irritable bowel syndrome, for example, a recent meta-analysis (57) showed a clinical benefit of relaxation methods, and an older, more comprehensive Cochrane review (58) on relaxation therapy and stress management revealed medium effect sizes for symptom severity after 2–3 months, but inconsistent longer-term findings (after 6–12) months with regard to abdominal pain and quality of life. The lack of control group without prior relaxation training further limits our ability to test the possibility that the absence of nocebo effects could be explained by effect(s) of previous relaxation training. There are other methodological considerations regarding the absence of nocebo effects herein: Given clear effects of negative suggestions on expected pain intensity, we would argue that the nocebo manipulation did not "fail" *per se.* This is supported by positive correlations between pain expectation and intensity and to a smaller extent pain with unpleasantness, supporting the connection between negative pain-related expectations and ratings. Whether, negative expectations are more tightly "linked" with intensity than unpleasantness requires further study. Nocebo effects in visceral pain models have thus far not been studied outside of our group, and they may be more difficult to reliably elicit in the laboratory setting than placebo effects. It is conceivable that they can more effectively be induced in healthy individuals under conditions of heightened stress or arousal, e.g., in the scanner setting (33) that is *per se* stressful (59) or after acute psychosocial stress as shown in a separate arm of this study (30). Our nocebo paradigm relied exclusively on treatment suggestions, and the study was only powered to detect large effects. Combining suggestions with a learning experience (i.e., a preconditioning procedure consisting of the surreptitious increase/decrease of pain intensity prior to suggestions) may be more efficacious and enhance effect size (13, 22). Finally, our approach to utilize truthful information regarding i.v. administration of saline as a control (i.e., groups with "neutral suggestions") is essential to properly quantify placebo/nocebo effects and distinguish them from other effects, like habituation, sensitization, order effects, etc. At the same time, these "neutral" groups are not untreated and hence by definition not free of treatment-related expectations. This may also reduce the magnitude of expectancy effects when their detection essentially relies on group comparisons [for more detailed methodological considerations, see (13)].

Together, our data provide further evidence that psychological states may alter how individuals respond to treatment suggestions. They complement recent conceptual developments on how bodily symptoms are experienced (60), especially interoceptive symptoms (61) which are demonstrably particularly salient and unpleasant when compared to exteroceptive, somatic stimuli even at matched intensities (62). Inter-individual variability in the presence and magnitude of placebo and nocebo effects is likely not only moderated by individual traits, characteristics of the treatment, and patient-provider interactions, but also by the psychological state in which treatment expectations are formed. Our findings call for more research to unravel how psychological states and their neurobiological correlates contribute to inter-individual variability in expectancy effects on symptom perception. Further, these experimental data acquired in a clinically-relevant pain model pave the way toward translation into clinical populations implementing behavioral interventions that target patients' expectancies and (also) consider psychobiological states. Indeed, placebo and nocebo effects for interoceptive, visceral symptoms are relevant to the treatment of the large group of patients with functional gastrointestinal disorders like IBS (12), but studies are needed to test whether findings from healthy volunteers can be transferred to patients. The role of the psychobiological stress systems in the pathophysiology of these clinical conditions is undisputable, as is the importance of pain or symptom-related cognitive and emotional factors (12, 42, 63, 64). If indeed these very same systems (or one of these) impacts how treatment expectations are processed, the implications are broad both for clinical practice and treatment trials. Indeed, placebo research has impressively demonstrated the clinical potential offered by psychological interventions (1, 2, 11), especially in the context of pain (1, 4). Effort to transfer knowledge from mechanistic work to clinical routine (65) are built on evidence that placebo analgesia engages similar neurobiological mechanisms as those responsible for the efficacy of pharmacological analgesic treatment (11, 66), and effectively enhances the "pure" pharmacological effect of analgesics in experimental but also in clinical settings (1, 2, 4, 18). Together, these findings pave the way for future studies. Our findings provide a small, additional "piece of the puzzle," at minimum supporting that the recent statement "Implementation of successful treatment requires effective communication skills to improve patient acceptance, adherence and to optimize the patient provider relationship." (67) may need amendment to incorporate additional aspects of the psychosocial treatment context, including individual treatment expectations and psychobiological states.

AUTHOR CONTRIBUTIONS

SB and SE: planning of the study and acquisition of funding. TR and SB: conducting the study. TR, SB, SE, and PE: data analysis and interpretation. SE, SB, and PE: drafting of the manuscript. All authors: revision of the manuscript for critical intellectual content and approval of the final draft submitted. All authors agree to be accountable for all aspects of the work in ensuring that questions related to the accuracy or integrity of any part of the work are appropriately investigated and resolved.

FUNDING

Funded by a research grant (EL 236/8-2) from the German Research Foundation (Deutsche Forschungsgemeinschaft, DFG (FOR 1328). The DFG had no role in the study design, collection, analysis, interpretation of the data, or in the writing of the report.

ACKNOWLEDGMENTS

The authors express their gratitude to Dr. M. Schöls and M. Hetkamp for their support during data acquisition.

REFERENCES

1. Colloca L, Klinger R, Flor H, Bingel U. Placebo analgesia: psychological and neurobiological mechanisms. *Pain.* (2013) 154:511–4. doi: 10.1016/j.pain.2013.02.002
2. Schedlowski M, Enck P, Rief W, Bingel U. Neuro-bio-behavioral mechanisms of placebo and nocebo responses: implications for clinical trials and clinical practice. *Pharmacol Rev.* (2015) 67:697–730. doi: 10.1124/pr.114.009423
3. Colloca L, Enck P, DeGrazia D. Relieving pain using dose-extending placebos: a scoping review. *Pain.* (2016) 157:1590–8. doi: 10.1097/j.pain.0000000000000566
4. Klinger R, Colloca L, Bingel U, Flor H. Placebo analgesia: clinical applications. *Pain.* (2014) 155:1055–8. doi: 10.1016/j.pain.2013.12.007
5. Benedetti F. Placebo effects: from the neurobiological paradigm to translational implications. *Neuron.* (2014) 84:623–37. doi: 10.1016/j.neuron.2014.10.023

6. Carvalho C, Caetano JM, Cunha L, Rebouta P, Kaptchuk TJ, Kirsch I. Open-label placebo treatment in chronic low back pain: a randomized controlled trial. *Pain*. (2016) 157:2766–72. doi: 10.1097/j.pain.0000000000000700
7. Xiang Y, He JY, Li R. Appropriateness of sham or placebo acupuncture for randomized controlled trials of acupuncture for nonspecific low back pain: a systematic review and meta-analysis. *J Pain Res*. (2017) 11:83–94. doi: 10.2147/JPR.S152743
8. Kaptchuk TJ, Friedlander E, Kelley JM, Sanchez MN, Kokkotou E, Singer JP, et al. Placebos without deception: a randomized controlled trial in irritable bowel syndrome. *PLoS ONE*. (2010) 5:e15591. doi: 10.1371/journal.pone.0015591
9. Kaptchuk TJ, Kelley JM, Conboy LA, Davis RB, Kerr CE, Jacobson EE, et al. Components of placebo effect: randomised controlled trial in patients with irritable bowel syndrome. *BMJ*. (2008) 336:999–1003. doi: 10.1136/bmj.39524.439618.25
10. Bingel U, Placebo Competence Team. Avoiding nocebo effects to optimize treatment outcome. *JAMA*. (2014) 312:693–4. doi: 10.1001/jama.2014.8342
11. Enck P, Bingel U, Schedlowski M, Rief W. The placebo response in medicine: minimize, maximize or personalize? *Nat Rev Drug Discov*. (2013) 12:191–204. doi: 10.1038/nrd3923
12. Elsenbruch S, Enck P. Placebo effects and their determinants in gastrointestinal disorders. *Nat Rev Gastroenterol Hepatol*. (2015) 12:472–85. doi: 10.1038/nrgastro.2015.117
13. Elsenbruch S, Labrenz F. Nocebo effects and experimental models in visceral pain. In "Neurobiology of the Placebo Effect Part I". *Int Rev Neurobiol*. (2018) 138:285–306. doi: 10.1016/bs.irn.2018.01.010
14. Enck P, Chae Y, Elsenbruch S. Novel designs and paradigms to study the placebo response in gastroenterology. *Curr Opin Pharmacol*. (2017) 37:72–9. doi: 10.1016/j.coph.2017.10.003
15. Ulrich RS. View through a window may influence recovery from surgery. *Science*. (1984) 224:420–1. doi: 10.1126/science.6143402
16. He X, Sun Q, Stetler C. Warm communication style strengthens expectations and increases perceived improvement. *Health Commun*. (2018) 33:939–45. doi: 10.1080/10410236.2017.1322482
17. Suarez-Almazor ME, Looney C, Liu Y, Cox V, Pietz K, Marcus DM, et al. A randomized controlled trial of acupuncture for osteoarthritis of the knee: effects of patient-provider communication. *Arthritis Care Res*. (2010) 62:1229–36. doi: 10.1002/acr.20225
18. Bingel U, Wanigasekera V, Wiech K, Ni Mhuircheartaigh R, Lee MC, Ploner M, et al. The effect of treatment expectation on drug efficacy: imaging the analgesic benefit of the opioid remifentanil. *Sci Transl Med*. (2011) 3:70ra14. doi: 10.1126/scitranslmed.3001244
19. Colloca L, Pine DS, Ernst M, Miller FG, Grillon C. Vasopressin boosts placebo analgesic effects in women: a randomized trial. *Biol Psychiatry*. (2016) 79:794–802. doi: 10.1016/j.biopsych.2015.07.019
20. Kessner S, Sprenger C, Wrobel N, Wiech K, Bingel U. Effect of oxytocin on placebo analgesia: a randomized study. *JAMA*. (2013) 310:1733–5. doi: 10.1001/jama.2013.277446
21. Colloca L, Benedetti F. Nocebo hyperalgesia: how anxiety is turned into pain. *Curr Opin Anaesthesiol*. (2007) 20:435–9. doi: 10.1097/ACO.0b013e3282b972fb
22. Elsenbruch S, Schmid J, Bäsler M, Cesko E, Schedlowski M, Benson S. How positive and negative expectations shape the experience of visceral pain: an experimental pilot study in healthy women. *Neurogastroenterol Motil*. (2012) 24:914-e460. doi: 10.1111/j.1365-2982.2012.01950.x
23. Van Den Houte M, Van Oudenhove L, Bogaerts K, Van Diest I, Van den Bergh O. Endogenous pain modulation: association with resting heart rate variability and negative affectivity. *Pain Med*. (2018) 19:1587–96. doi: 10.1093/pm/pnx165
24. Woo KY. Unravelling nocebo effect: the mediating effect of anxiety between anticipation and pain at wound dressing change. *J Clin Nurs*. (2015) 24:1975–84. doi: 10.1111/jocn.12858
25. Aslaksen PM, Flaten MA. The roles of physiological and subjective stress in the effectiveness of a placebo on experimentally induced pain. *Psychosom Med*. (2008) 70:811–8. doi: 10.1097/PSY.0b013e31818105ed
26. Aslaksen PM, Lyby PS. Fear of pain potentiates nocebo hyperalgesia. *J Pain Res*. (2015) 8:703–710. doi: 10.2147/JPR.S91923
27. Aslaksen PM, Zwarg ML, Eilertsen HI, Gorecka MM, Bjørkedal E. Opposite effects of the same drug: reversal of topical analgesia by nocebo information. *Pain*. (2015) 156:39–46. doi: 10.1097/j.pain.0000000000000004
28. Bjørkedal E, Flaten MA. Expectations of increased and decreased pain explain the effect of conditioned pain modulation in females. *J Pain Res*. (2012) 5:289–300. doi: 10.2147/JPR.S33559
29. Lyby PS, Forsberg JT, Asli O, Flaten MA. Induced fear reduces the effectiveness of a placebo intervention on pain. *Pain*. (2012) 153:1114–21. doi: 10.1016/j.pain.2012.02.042
30. Roderigo T, Benson S, Schöls M, Hetkamp M, Schedlowski M, Enck P, et al. Effects of acute psychological stress on placebo and nocebo responses in a clinically relevant model of visceroception. *Pain*. (2017) 158:1489–98. doi: 10.1097/j.pain.0000000000000940
31. Elsenbruch S, Kotsis V, Benson S, Rosenberger C, Reidick D, Schedlowski M, et al. Neural mechanisms mediating the effects of expectation in visceral placebo analgesia: an fMRI study in healthy placebo responders and nonresponders. *Pain*. (2012) 153:382–90. doi: 10.1016/j.pain.2011.10.036
32. Schmid J, Langhorst J, Gaß F, Theysohn N, Benson S, Engler, H, et al. Placebo analgesia in patients with functional and organic abdominal pain: a fMRI study in IBS, UC and healthy volunteers. *Gut*. (2015) 64:418–27. doi: 10.1136/gutjnl-2013-306648
33. Schmid J, Theysohn N, Gaß F, Benson S, Gramsch C, Forsting M, et al. Neural mechanisms mediating positive and negative treatment expectations in visceral pain: a functional magnetic resonance imaging study on placebo and nocebo effects in healthy volunteers. *Pain*. (2013) 154:2372–80. doi: 10.1016/j.pain.2013.07.013
34. Herrmann-Lingen C, Buss U, Snaith RP. *Hospital Anxiety and Depression Scale (HADS) - Deutsche Version (2. Auflage)*. Bern: Hans Huber (2005).
35. Lacourt TE, Houtveen JH, Doornen LJ, Benson S, Grigoleit JS, Cesko E, et al. Biological and psychological predictors of visceral pain sensitivity in healthy premenopausal women. *Eur J Pain*. (2014) 18:567–74. doi: 10.1002/j.1532-2149.2013.00397.x
36. Laux L, Glanzmann P, Schaffner P, Spielberger CD. *Das State-Trait-Angstinventar. Theoretische Grundlagen und Handanweisung*. Goettingen: Beltz (1981).
37. Schulz P, Schlotz W. The Trier Inventory for the Assessment of Chronic Stress (TICS): scale construction, statistical testing, and validation of the scale work overload. *Diagnostica*. (1999) 45:8–19. doi: 10.1026/0012-1924.45.1.8
38. Elsenbruch S, Rosenberger C, Bingel U, Forsting M, Schedlowski M, Gizewski ER. Patients with irritable bowel syndrome have altered emotional modulation of neural responses to visceral stimuli. *Gastroenterology*. (2010) 139:1310–9. doi: 10.1053/j.gastro.2010.06.054
39. Pruessner JC, Kirschbaum C, Meinlschmid G, Hellhammer DH. Two formulas for computation of the area under the curve represent measures of total hormone concentration versus time-dependent change. *Psychoneuroendocrinology*. (2003) 28:916–31. doi: 10.1016/S0306-4530(02)00108-7
40. Vase L, Robinson ME, Verne GN, Price DD. Increased placebo analgesia over time in irritable bowel syndrome (IBS) patients is associated with desire and expectation but not endogenous opioid mechanisms. *Pain*. (2005) 115:338–47. doi: 10.1016/j.pain.2005.03.014
41. Fechir M, Breimhorst M, Kritzmann S, Geber C, Schlereth T, Baier B, et al. Naloxone inhibits not only stress-induced analgesia but also sympathetic activation and baroreceptor-reflex sensitivity. *Eur J Pain*. (2012) 16:82–92. doi: 10.1016/j.ejpain.2011.06.009
42. Boeckxstaens G, Camilleri M, Sifrim D, Houghton LA, Elsenbruch S, Lindberg G, et al. Fundamentals of neurogastroenterology: physiology/motility – sensation. *Gastroenterology*. (2016) 2016:S0016-5085(16)00221-3. doi: 10.1053/j.gastro.2016.02.030
43. Botha C, Farmer AD, Nilsson M, Brock C, Gavrila AD, Drewes AM, et al. Preliminary report: modulation of parasympathetic nervous system tone influences oesophageal pain hypersensitivity. *Gut*. (2015) 64:611–7. doi: 10.1136/gutjnl-2013-306698
44. Eckberg DL. Sympathovagal balance: a critical appraisal. *Circulation*. (1997) 96:3224–32. doi: 10.1161/01.CIR.96.9.3224
45. Farmer AD, Coen SJ, Kano M, Naqvi H, Paine PA, Scott SM, et al. Psychophysiological responses to visceral and somatic pain in functional chest

pain identify clinically relevant pain clusters. *Neurogastroenterol Motil.* (2014) 26:139–48. doi: 10.1111/nmo.12245
46. Farmer AD, Coen SJ, Kano M, Paine PA, Shwahdi M, Jafari J, et al. Psychophysiological responses to pain identify reproducible human clusters. *Pain.* (2013) 154:2266–76. doi: 10.1016/j.pain.2013.05.016
47. Frokjaer JB, Bergmann S, Brock C, Madzak A, Farmer AD, Ellrich J, et al. Modulation of vagal tone enhances gastroduodenal motility and reduces somatic pain sensitivity. *Neurogastroenterol Motil.* (2016) 28:592–8. doi: 10.1111/nmo.12760
48. Gabella G. *Autonomic Nervous System, eLS.* New York, NY: John Wiley & Sons, Ltd. (2001).
49. Mazurak N, Seredyuk N, Sauer H, Teufel M, Enck P. Heart rate variability in the irritable bowel syndrome: a review of the literature. *Neurogastroenterol Motil.* (2012) 24:206–16. doi: 10.1111/j.1365-2982.2011.01866.x
50. Pellissier S, Dantzer C, Canini F, Mathieu N, Bonaz B. Psychological adjustment and autonomic disturbances in inflammatory bowel diseases and irritable bowel syndrome. *Psychoneuroendocrinology.* (2010) 35:653–62. doi: 10.1016/j.psyneuen.2009.10.004
51. Meissner K. Placebo responses on cardiovascular, gastrointestinal, and respiratory organ functions. *Handb Exp Pharmacol.* (2014) 225:183–203. doi: 10.1007/978-3-662-44519-8_11
52. Ober K, Benson S, Vogelsang M, Bylica A, Günther D, Witzke O, et al. Plasma noradrenaline and state anxiety levels predict placebo response in learned immunosuppression. *Clin Pharmacol Ther.* (2012) 91:220–6. doi: 10.1038/clpt.2011.214
53. Pollo A, Vighetti S, Rainero I, Benedetti F. Placebo analgesia and the heart. *Pain.* (2003) 102:125–33. doi: 10.1016/s0304-3959(02)00345-7
54. Colagiuri B, Quinn VF. Autonomic arousal as a mechanism of the persistence of nocebo hyperalgesia. *J Pain.* (2018) 19:476–86. doi: 10.1016/j.jpain.2017.12.006
55. Flaten MA, Aslaksen PM, Lyby PS, Bjørkedal E. The relation of emotions to placebo responses. *Philos Trans R Soc Lond B Biol Sci.* (2011) 366:1818–27. doi: 10.1098/rstb.2010.0407
56. Flaten MA. Pain-related negative emotions and placebo analgesia. *Handb Exp Pharmacol.* (2014) 225:81–96. doi: 10.1007/978-3-662-44519-8_5
57. Ford AC, Lacy BE, Harris LA, Quigley EMM, Moayyedi P. Effect of antidepressants and psychological therapies in irritable bowel syndrome: an updated systematic review and meta-analysis. *Am J Gastroenterol.* (2019) 114:21–39. doi: 10.1038/s41395-018-0222-5
58. Zijdenbos IL, de Wit NJ, van der Heijden GJ, Rubin G, Quartero AO. Psychological treatments for the management of irritable bowel syndrome. *Cochrane Database Syst Rev.* (2009) 2009:Cd006442. doi: 10.1002/14651858.CD006442.pub2
59. Vachon-Presseau E, Martel MO, Roy M, Caron E, Albouy G, Marin MF, et al. Acute stress contributes to individual differences in pain and pain-related brain activity in healthy and chronic pain patients. *J Neurosci.* (2013) 33:6826–33. doi: 10.1523/JNEUROSCI.4584-12.2013
60. Van den Bergh O, Witthöft M, Petersen S, Brown RJ. Symptoms and the body: taking the inferential leap. *Neurosci Biobehav Rev.* (2017) 74:185–203. doi: 10.1016/j.neubiorev.2017.01.015
61. Petersen S, von Leupoldt A, den Bergh OV. Interoception and the uneasiness of the mind: affect as perceptual style. *Front Psychol.* (2015) 6:1408. doi: 10.3389/fpsyg.2015.01408
62. Koenen LR, Icenhour A, Forkmann K, Pasler K, Theysohn N, Forsting M, et al. Greater fear of visceral pain contributes to differences between visceral and somatic pain in healthy women. *Pain.* (2017) 158:1599–608. doi: 10.1097/j.pain.0000000000000924
63. Elsenbruch S, Enck P. The stress concept in gastroenterology: from Selye to today. *F1000Res.* (2017) 6:2149. doi: 10.12688/f1000research.1 2435.1
64. Enck P, Azpiroz F, Boeckxstaens G, Elsenbruch S, Feinle-Bisset C, Holtmann G, et al. Functional dyspepsia. *Nat Rev Dis Primers.* (2017) 3:17081. doi: 10.1038/nrdp.2017.81
65. Brody H, Miller FG. Lessons from recent research about the placebo effect–from art to science. *JAMA.* (2011) 306:2612–3. doi: 10.1001/jama.2011.1850
66. Wager TD, Atlas LY. The neuroscience of placebo effects: connecting context, learning and health. *Nat Rev Neurosci.* (2015) 16:403–18. doi: 10.1038/nrn3976
67. Drossman DA, Tack J, Ford AC, Szigethy E, Törnblom H, Van Oudenhove L. Neuromodulators for functional GI disorders (disorders of gut-brain interaction): a Rome Foundation Working Team Report. *Gastroenterology.* (2017) 2017:S0016-5085(17) 36718-5.

15

Placebo and Nocebo Effects in Cognitive Neuroenhancement: When Expectation Shapes Perception

Alexander Winkler and Christiane Hermann*

Department of Clinical Psychology and Psychotherapy, Justus-Liebig-University, Giessen, Germany

Correspondence:
Alexander Winkler
Alexander.Winkler@psychol.uni-giessen.de

Objective: The number of students using prescription drugs to improve cognitive performance has increased within the last years. There is first evidence that the expectation to receive a performance-enhancing drug alone can result in improved perceived and actual cognitive performance, suggesting a substantial placebo effect. In addition, expecting a placebo can result in lower perceived and actual cognitive performance, suggesting a nocebo effect. Yet, the underlying mechanisms of these effects remain to be elucidated. The aim of our study was to investigate whether the expectation of receiving a performance-increasing drug or a performance-impairing drug leads to changes in actual and perceived cognitive performance, compared to a control group without expectation manipulation.

Methods: A total of $N = 75$ healthy adults were recruited for an experiment to "try cognitive performance-modulating drugs." A participant's actual cognitive performance (alertness, working memory, sustained attention, and divided attention) using the standardized test of attentional performance (TAP) as well as their performance expectation were assessed. Participants were randomly assigned in equal numbers to either receiving a placebo performance increasing nasal spray ("Modafinil") or a nocebo performance impairing nasal spray ("Vividrin®") or no nasal spray (natural history). After placebo/nocebo nasal spray administration, cognitive performance was reassessed. Subsequent to the second assessment, participants rated their perceived change in cognitive performance, as well as adverse symptoms.

Results: Unlike hypothesized, a positive or negative performance expectation did not result in changes in actual performance, corresponding to the induced expectation. Participants in the placebo-Modafinil group rated their perceived change in cognitive performance subsequent to the application of the nasal spray significantly better (d = 1.16) compared to the nocebo-Vividrin® group. Additionally, participants who expected to receive Modafinil felt less tired than participants in the Vividrin® group (d = 0.96).

Conclusion: Manipulation of performance expectation affects the perceived change in performance and tiredness, but not the actual cognitive performance in healthy adults. This may explain why college students use such drugs despite their little impact on actual cognitive functioning.

Keywords: placebo, nocebo, neuroenhancement, expectation, cognitive, performance, drugs

INTRODUCTION

The number of students using prescription drugs to improve cognitive performance without medical indication has increased over the last years, in spite of the potential risks associated with this use (1). Prevalence rates of non-medical stimulant use of 8.3% (lifetime) and 5.9% (past-year) in a sample of 4,580 US college students (2), 4.3% (lifetime) in a representative sample of 1,128 adults in the German population (3), and a lifetime prevalence rate of 6.5% among Australian university students (4) have been reported

Intriguingly, findings about the actual cognitive enhancement effects of stimulants in non-clinical populations are heterogeneous, suggesting a limited benefit at best (5–7). For example, Ilieva et al. (8) demonstrated that, in healthy participants, a dose of mixed-amphetamine salts enhanced the perceived, but not the actual cognitive ability, suggesting that pharmacological neuroenhancement may exclusively boost the subjective perception of cognitive performance. Interestingly, even if actual performance is improved after drug intake, this might at least partially be accounted for by performance expectation (9). Using a balanced placebo design, Cropsey et al. (9) compared the pharmacological versus expectancy effects of mixed amphetamine salts on cognitive performance in college students. Administered amphetamine salts enhanced cognitive performance in only 2 of 31 subtests of a neuropsychological test battery. Expected administration of the stimulant medication yielded improved perceived and actual cognitive performance, regardless of the group allocation (placebo vs. mixed amphetamine salts) (9). Likewise, Dawkins et al. (10) were able to show that expected caffeine intake improved attention regardless of whether students had consumed caffeinated or decaffeinated coffee in a balanced placebo design.

Aside from studies assessing placebo effects using mixed amphetamine salts (8, 9), caffeine (10, 11), or nicotine (12), studies investigating placebo and nocebo effects on cognitive neuroenhancement have either relied on administering placebo pills or used various psychological interventions (e.g., verbal suggestions) in order to manipulate performance expectation.

Among the studies utilizing placebo pills to manipulate performance expectation, only few studies have directly addressed whether placebo administration is effective in inducing cognitive neuroenhancement measured subjectively and/or objectively. Looby and Earleywine (13) showed that the expectation to receive methylphenidate enhances subjective arousal, but neither perceived nor actual cognitive performance. In fact, such an expectation even tended to impair cognitive performance (13). Szemerszky et al. (14) reported a detrimental effect of a placebo pill on perceived performance in a 14-min vigilance task when the pill was given together with information about its (putative) negative cognitive effects (14). However, in this study, actual cognitive performance was not assessed. Furthermore, there was no increase in symptom reports in the nocebo group (14). Notably, only non-specific bodily symptoms (e.g., abdominal pain, headache, itching) were assessed. Moreover, participants were not specifically informed about potentials side effects of the pill, which was described as a mild sedative.

There are two studies suggesting a placebo effect on objective measures of cognitive performance (15, 16). For example, in healthy seniors, a 2-week intake of a placebo pill enhanced memory and attention performance in comparison to a no pill control condition (15). Interestingly, expectancy of improvement and actual improvement of cognitive performance were correlated, though small in magnitude. In two double-blind randomized-controlled experiments among university students, Colagiuri and Boakes (16) were able to demonstrate that participants who believed they had been allocated to the cognitive-enhancing drug group, due to false (positive) feedback given about their cognitive performance, performed better than those who believed they had been given a placebo.

In one of the very few studies manipulating performance expectation without pill administration, Fuhr and Werle (17) found neither an effect of a mental training based on verbal suggestion nor of the information about the effectiveness of the training on actual cognitive performance. In one of the few studies including both a placebo and a nocebo instruction, the expectation that a tone of a specific frequency will improve or impair cognitive performance strongly affected perceived, but not actual cognitive performance (18). Szemerszky et al. (14) demonstrated a negative effect of a sham magnetic field on perceived performance in a 14-min vigilance task. Unfortunately, actual cognitive performance was not assessed. Moreover, no change in symptom reports was noted (14). There are some studies supporting placebo effects on objective measures of cognitive performance (19–23). For example, sham subliminal presentation of the answers in a knowledge test improved the test scores in college students (20). Fluid intelligence was higher subsequent to a working memory training (1 h) in participants expecting an intelligence boost as compared to participants with no expectation regarding the outcome of the training (Foroughi et al., (21). Turi et al. (22) found a cognitive placebo effect on objective performance measures, but no effect on expectation and perceived performance, using a sham non-invasive brain stimulation technique. Colagiuri et al. (19) demonstrated both a placebo and a nocebo effect in a large sample of university students completing an implicit learning task while being exposed to an odor supposedly enhancing or impairing cognitive performance or having no effect at all. Participants given positive information responded faster; participants given negative information responded slower in cued reaction time trials as compared to the control group (19). Turi et al. (23) demonstrated that a sham non-invasive brain stimulation was able to increase (placebo condition) or decrease (nocebo condition) expected and perceived cognitive performance. Placebo and nocebo effects were also manifest in response accuracy in a reward-based learning performance test (23).

In sum, despite the heterogeneity of findings in the current literature, there is first evidence for placebo and nocebo effects on cognitive performance. However, the influence of such placebo and nocebo instructions has been directly compared only in very few studies [e.g., Ref. (18)]. Additionally, the influence of such placebo/nocebo expectations on cognitive performance has not consistently been evaluated both subjectively and objectively. In the present study, we used a randomized controlled parallel group design to evaluate the effects of expecting a performance-increasing drug (placebo) or a performance-impairing drug (nocebo) on change in performance expectation, actual and perceived cognitive performance, and adverse somatic symptoms ("side effects"), compared to a control group without expectation manipulation, in a sample of 75 college students. We hypothesized that participants in the placebo group would show a higher and participants in the nocebo group a lower performance expectation compared to the control group. We also hypothesized that, depending on the positive or negative performance expectation, perceived and actual performance in a standardized test battery of attention measures would be altered in comparison to the control condition. Additionally, we hypothesized that participants will specifically endorse those adverse symptoms that were described as the side effects of the drug in the drug information leaflet the participants received as part of the placebo/nocebo induction.

METHOD

Participants

Seventy-five participants, 49 females (65.3%) and 26 males (34.7%), between 18 and 37 years old (M = 22.7, SD = 3.8) participated. Participants were recruited between March and June 2018 *via* e-mail advertisement ["Brain doping—Healthy participants wanted for an experiment on nootropics (smart drugs)"] addressed to staff and students of a German university. As cover story, participants were told that the goal of the study was to assess short-term effects of cognitive-performance-modulating drugs using a new delivery route (nasal spray). Participants were told that they would be randomly assigned to either a group receiving a fast acting stimulant ("Modafinil") or a fast acting antiallergic agent ("Vividrin") or no medication at all. In addition, they were informed that their cognitive performance would be tested using a computer-based cognitive performance task before and after drug administration. Actually, participants in the Modafinil and the Vividrin group both received the same placebo nasal spray without active ingredient. Inclusion criteria were age between 18 and 65 years, and fluency in German. Exclusion criteria were allergies to any substances actually (chili and sesame) or purportedly (Modafinil, Vividrin®) used in the study, pregnancy or nursing, suffering from a known mental disorder or severe medical condition, and intake of psychopharmacological drugs or prescription drugs used for enhancing cognitive performance within the last month before participation. All inclusion and exclusion criteria were assessed *via* self-report in a phone screening. Participants gave written informed consent and were paid 10€ for their participation. The experiment was conducted according to the Declaration of Helsinki and the local ethics committee approved the study protocol (#2018-0001).

The sample size was based on an *a priori* power analysis using G*Power 3 software (24) for our main outcome, the actual objective performance. For the 3 × 2 ANOVA interaction effect between three groups and two test of attentional performance (TAP) assessments, a total sample of at least 72 participants would be needed to detect a small effect (f = .15) with 95% power, alpha at .05, and correlation between repeated measurements (estimated on the basis of retest reliability described in the TAP manual) of.80.

The participants were randomly assigned in equal numbers to the placebo-Modafinil, nocebo-Vividrin®, and a natural history group. We observed no significant differences between the three groups regarding age, sex, and previous experience with performance-enhancing drugs (see **Table 1**). After completion of the experiment, seven participants (9%; placebo-Modafinil: n = 2, nocebo-Vividrin®: n = 3, natural history: n = 2) reported that they had not believed the cover story. Since the number of non-believers was similar across groups, these participants were not excluded from statistical analyses.

Questionnaires and Self-Ratings

Subjective Performance Expectation

To assess participant's subjective performance expectation, we used the item "I will perform well in the task" to be rated on a seven-point Likert scale ranging from 1 (not agree at all) to 7 (totally agree). We assessed performance expectation online prior to each TAP assessment (see **Figure 1**).

Perceived Change in Cognitive Performance

Participants were asked to rate the perceived change in cognitive performance between the first and the second cognitive assessment ("How do you rate your cognitive performance now in comparison to the first assessment?") on a visual analog scale (VAS) ranging from 1 (worse) to 100 (better). The rating was assessed online after the second TAP assessment.

Adverse Symptoms/"Side Effects"

Subjectively perceived adverse symptoms and side effects of the purportedly administered drugs were assessed using the Generic Assessment of Side Effects Scale (GASE) (25). The original GASE entails 36 symptoms and covers the most frequently reported

TABLE 1 | Sample characteristics at baseline.

	Placebo-Modafinil (n = 25)	Nocebo-Vividrin® (n = 25)	Natural history (n = 25)	Group effect
Age in years, M (SD)	22.5 (4.0)	22.7 (4.0)	22.8 (3.7)	$F(2,72) = 0.043, p = .958$
Number females, n (%)	13 (52.0%)	19 (76.0%)	17 (68.0%)	$\chi^2(2) = 3.30, p = .192$
Previous experience with performance modulation drugs, n (%)	0.0 (0.0%)	1.0 (4.0%)	1.0 (4.0%)	$\chi^2(2) = 1.03, p = .598$

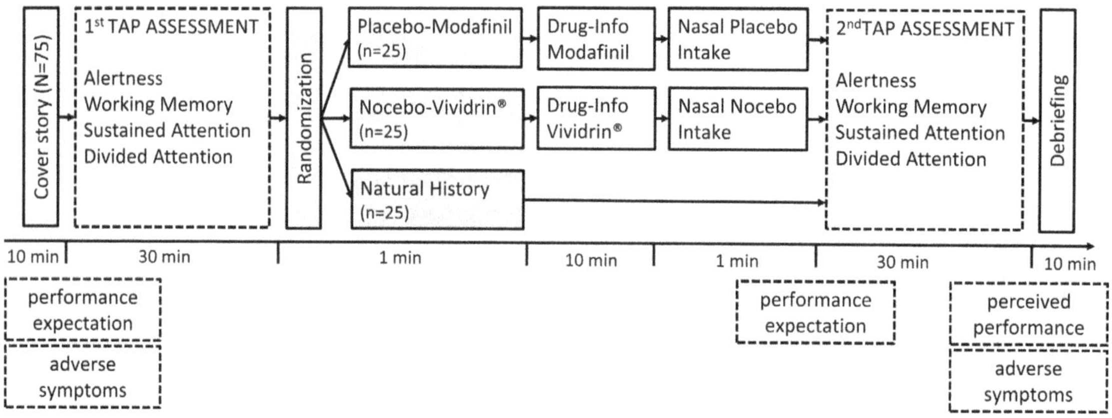

FIGURE 1 | Study design (see Methods for details) and outcome measurements (dashed frames) for the placebo–Modafinil (*n* = 25), nocebo-Vividrin® (*n* = 25), and natural history (*n* = 25) condition; TAP, Test of Attentional Performance.

side effects of medications in clinical trials. The severity of each symptom is rated on a four-point Likert scale ranging from "not present" (0) to "severe" (3). The GASE has good internal consistency (Cronbach's α = 0.89) and has been validated (25). For the purpose of our study, 12 adverse symptoms were taken from the original GASE such that they matched the potential side effects as described in the drug information leaflet given to the participants (Modafinil: headache, palpitations/irregular heartbeat, abdominal pain, fatigue/tiredness and irritability/nervousness; Vividrin®: bitter taste, nausea, skin rash/itching, feeling of weakness and drowsiness/exhaustion; both drugs: dizziness, irritation of nose or throat). We selected those adverse symptoms that could be expected to occur relatively quickly following acute administration of the drug and to fluctuate over the course of the experiment. We followed the recommendation of Rheker et al. (26) and assessed adverse symptoms twice, before the first TAP assessment (as baseline) and after the second TAP assessment, since complaints about minor bodily symptoms are extremely common in the general population (base rates up to 80%) (27, 28) and might easily be misattributed to the nasal spray intake.

Cognitive Performance

Cognitive performance was tested using the subtests Alertness, Working Memory, Sustained Attention, and Divided Attention of the computer-based TAP (29). The TAP is a well-established test battery for assessing various aspects of cognitive performance and is suitable for testing healthy subjects. For each TAP subtest, the test performance scores were determined according to the TAP manual (see **Table 2**). Alertness is tested by requiring participants to press a key as quickly as possible when they notice a cross on the monitor, which is displayed at randomly varying intervals (preceded or not preceded by a warning tone). Working Memory is tested by a modified N-1 back task, i.e., a sequence of numbers is presented on a computer screen, and participants are required to indicate whether or not the currently presented number matches the previously shown number or the one before. In the Sustained Attention test, a sequence of stimuli is presented on the monitor. Participants are required to press a key whenever the stimulus presented matches the preceding stimulus regarding one of two predetermined stimulus characteristics (color, shape, size, or filling). In the Divided Attention test, participants undergo a dual task, i.e., a visual ("press a key when a varying number of crosses on the monitor form a square") and an auditory task ("press a key when a tone occurs twice in a row within a high and low tone sequence"). For all subtests that were used, the maximum level of difficulty was selected, whenever different levels of difficulty were available. As displayed in **Figure 1**, the TAP was assessed before and after manipulation of participants' expectation.

Experimental Setup

In the current randomized controlled parallel group design study, the primary outcome was actual cognitive performance analyzed *via* a 2 × 3 mixed model ANOVA with the repeated factor time (first TAP assessment vs. second TAP assessment) and the between group factor group (placebo vs. nocebo vs. natural history). Secondary outcomes were performance expectation, perceived performance, and adverse symptoms. All participants underwent the first cognitive test battery (TAP) as baseline measurement (see **Figure 1**). Then, participants were randomly assigned to one of three groups (placebo-Modafinil, nocebo-Vividrin®, natural history). Participants allocated to the placebo-Modafinil group were informed that they will receive a stimulating drug that enhances cognitive performance and increases general alertness. Participants allocated to the nocebo-Vividrin® group were informed that they will receive a drug that dampens the activity of the central nervous systems and reduces alertness. Both groups actually received an active placebo nasal spray consisting of a mixture of sesame oil and capsaicin (0.0007%). Participants in the natural history group did not receive the nasal spray and were not further instructed regarding (potential) drug administration. Investigators were partially blinded to group allocation, since the participant leaflet for Modafinil or Vividrin® was handed to the participants in a closed envelope. Hence, the experimenter was unaware of whether the participant received the Modafinil or the Vividrin® instruction

TABLE 2 | Cognitive performance (TAP scores at 1st assessment and 2nd assessment) per group and group*time interaction.

TAP Subtest	Placebo-Modafinil (n = 25)				Nocebo-Vividrin® (n = 25)				Natural history (n = 25)				Group		Time		Group*time interaction	
	1st assessment		2nd assessment		1st assessment		2nd assessment		1st assessment		2nd assessment		$F(2,72)$	p	$F(1,72)$	p	$F(2,72)$	p
	M	SD	M	SD	M	SD	M	SD	M	SD	M	SD						
Alertness (without warning signal)																		
Median reaction time (ms)	235.3	33.7	237.7	34.5	231.2	27.0	235.3	31.4	241.0	49.5	240.0	45.8	0.27	.766	0.31	.578	0.21	.811
SD reaction time	32.9	17.5	44.2	27.7	34.6	22.0	39.4	22.9	33.8	16.2	41.6	23.9	0.04	.963	10.40	.002	0.57	.566
Alertness (with warning signal)																		
Median reaction time (ms)	232.6	33.7	231.1	37.5	226.7	20.8	227.2	24.7	236.7	39.3	232.0	44.5	0.33	.718	0.56	.458	0.35	.707
SD reaction time	29.7	13.6	35.6	20.9	32.9	14.1	36.5	20.0	33.6	15.6	36.8	23.6	0.16	.854	5.97	.017	0.24	.786
Number of lapses	1.24	0.72	1.16	0.62	1.16	0.69	1.08	0.81	1.24	0.93	1.20	0.50	0.27	.764	0.31	.577	0.01	.988
Number of Anticipations	0.44	0.71	1.28	1.59	0.76	1.05	1.32	1.75	0.56	1.08	1.52	2.02	0.18	.835	19.84	<.001	0.45	.639
Phasic Alertness (ms)	0.01	0.08	0.03	0.08	0.02	0.08	0.03	0.06	0.01	0.08	0.03	0.07	0.02	.981	3.18	.079	0.02	.978
Working Memory																		
Number of omissions	1.28	1.14	1.24	1.42	1.92	2.31	2.04	2.46	1.20	1.35	0.84	1.11	2.71	.073	0.25	.620	0.57	.569
Number of errors	1.36	1.38	0.80	1.08	0.88	1.01	0.76	0.93	1.20	1.19	0.48	0.65	0.74	.482	9.65	.003	1.43	.247
Sustained Attention																		
Number of omissions	7.60	7.11	8.36	7.45	7.60	5.69	9.16	7.42	7.88	5.88	8.04	6.77	0.03	.966	2.75	.101	0.66	.519
Number of errors	5.28	5.73	2.80	4.35	7.60	8.52	3.68	5.23	7.36	12.63	4.76	10.40	0.45	.642	27.12	<.001	0.64	.530
Divided Attention																		
Number of omissions	1.08	1.47	1.64	1.91	1.40	2.61	1.88	2.82	1.12	1.17	1.44	1.83	0.28	.755	3.65	.060	0.09	.915
Number of errors	0.96	1.40	0.84	1.86	1.04	1.37	0.92	1.12	0.80	0.91	0.52	0.71	0.56	.574	1.37	.245	0.13	.878

TAP, Test of Attentional Performance.

together with the nasal spray. For participants allocated to the natural history group, the experimenter was unblinded, since the participants were instructed to inform the experimenter that they were not supposed to take any nasal spray after reading the leaflet. After the information about the purported drug was given, participants in the placebo-Modafinil and nocebo-Vividrin® group received the active placebo nasal spray. Participants were instructed to wait for 60 s after the drug application in order to ensure good absorption before undergoing the second performance test. Subjective performance expectation was measured prior to each TAP assessment. The perceived change in performance was rated after the second TAP test. Adverse symptoms were assessed before the first TAP test and after the second TAP test. Participants assigned to the natural history group underwent the same procedure; however, they received no nasal spray (see **Figure 1**).

Study Procedure

Individuals interested in the study underwent a telephone screening to examine inclusion and exclusion criteria and to arrange a lab appointment. The participants were seated in a lab with the experimenter running the experiment from an adjacent room. The participants were monitored using a camera; they could communicate with the experimenter using a microphone at any time. After giving informed consent, participants completed the questionnaires online. Then they underwent the experiment (for details, see the section Experimental Setup). After completing the experiment, participants were asked to indicate whether or not they had believed the cover story, and they were then debriefed following a standardized protocol and were paid. The experiment lasted about 90 min in total.

Statistical Analysis

Statistical analyses were performed using IBM SPSS Statistics 23.0 for Windows (Chicago, SPSS, Inc.). Group differences in age, sex and previous experience with performance-enhancing drugs at baseline were analyzed using univariate analysis of variance (ANOVA) and chi-square tests.

Group differences regarding change in performance expectation over time were tested using a mixed design ANOVA with *time* (before and after expectation manipulation) as within subject and *group* (placebo-Modafinil, nocebo-Vividrin®, natural history) as between group factors. Significant group × time interaction effect was followed up by Bonferroni-corrected *post hoc* tests, mean differences (M_{diff}) are reported.

Group differences in perceived change of cognitive performance were tested using a univariate ANOVA, followed by Bonferroni-corrected *post hoc* tests; mean differences (M_{diff}) are reported.

To test for group differences in change of actual cognitive performance, we carried out mixed design ANOVAs with *time* (first and second TAP assessment) as repeated measures and *group* (placebo-Modafinil, nocebo-Vividrin®, natural history) as between-group factor for each TAP subtest performance score as dependent variable.

Group differences in drug-specific and unspecific adverse symptoms ("side effects") as described in the drug information leaflet assessed following the second TAP assessment were evaluated in an exploratory analysis using ANCOVAs for each item with symptom intensity prior to the first TAP assessment used as covariate, respectively. For this exploratory analysis, the family-wise error rate was set at .10. Bonferroni correction led to a *p*-value of .02 for single comparisons with respect to drug specific symptoms, and .05 as criterion for significance for single comparisons with respect to unspecific symptoms. Significant ANCOVAs were followed up by Bonferroni-corrected pairwise *post hoc* comparisons. Mean differences (M_{diff}) are reported.

Product-moment correlation analyses were conducted to test the relationship between change in performance expectation and perceived change in performance.

RESULTS

Performance Expectations and Actual Cognitive Performance

Performance Expectation

The mixed-measure ANOVA revealed a significant interaction effect between group and time [$F(2,72) = 8.74$, $p < .001$], a main effect of group [$F(2, 72) = 4.01$, $p = .022$], but no significant main effect of time. Follow-up tests revealed that the groups differed significantly in their performance expectation after expectation manipulation, but not at baseline (see **Figure 2**). Participants in the placebo-Modafinil group ($M = 5.4$, $SD = 0.23$) endorsed a significantly higher performance expectation than participants in the nocebo-Vividrin® ($M = 4.0$, $SD = 0.23$, $M_{diff} = 1.4$, $p < .001$, $d = 1.04$) and in the natural history group ($M = 4.2$, $SD = 0.23$, $M_{diff} = 1.2$, $p = .001$, $d = 1.45$), after expectation manipulation. There was no significant difference in performance expectation between the nocebo-Vividrin® and the natural history group ($M_{diff} = 0.2$, $p = 1.000$). Moreover, performance expectation increased significantly in the placebo-Modafinil group following the expectation manipulation ($M_{diff} = 0.72$, $p = .009$, $d = 0.64$), and it decreased significantly in the nocebo-Vividrin® group ($M_{diff} = -0.56$, $p = .039$, $d = -0.38$) and the natural history group ($M_{diff} = -0.72$, $p = .009$, $d = -0.86$).

Perceived Change in Performance Between First and Second Assessment TAP

The univariate ANOVA yielded a significant group main effect [$F(2,38) = 6.37$, $p = .004$]. As illustrated in **Figure 3**, Bonferroni-corrected *post hoc* tests revealed that the placebo-Modafinil group reported significantly greater improvement in performance than the nocebo-Vividrin® group ($M_{diff} = 22.91$, $p = .003$, $d = 1.16$). Neither the placebo-Modafinil group ($M_{diff} = 11.71$, $p = .190$, $d = 0.85$) nor the nocebo-Vividrin® group ($M_{diff} = -11.20$, $p = .207$, $d = 0.71$) differed from the natural history group with respect to perceived change in performance.

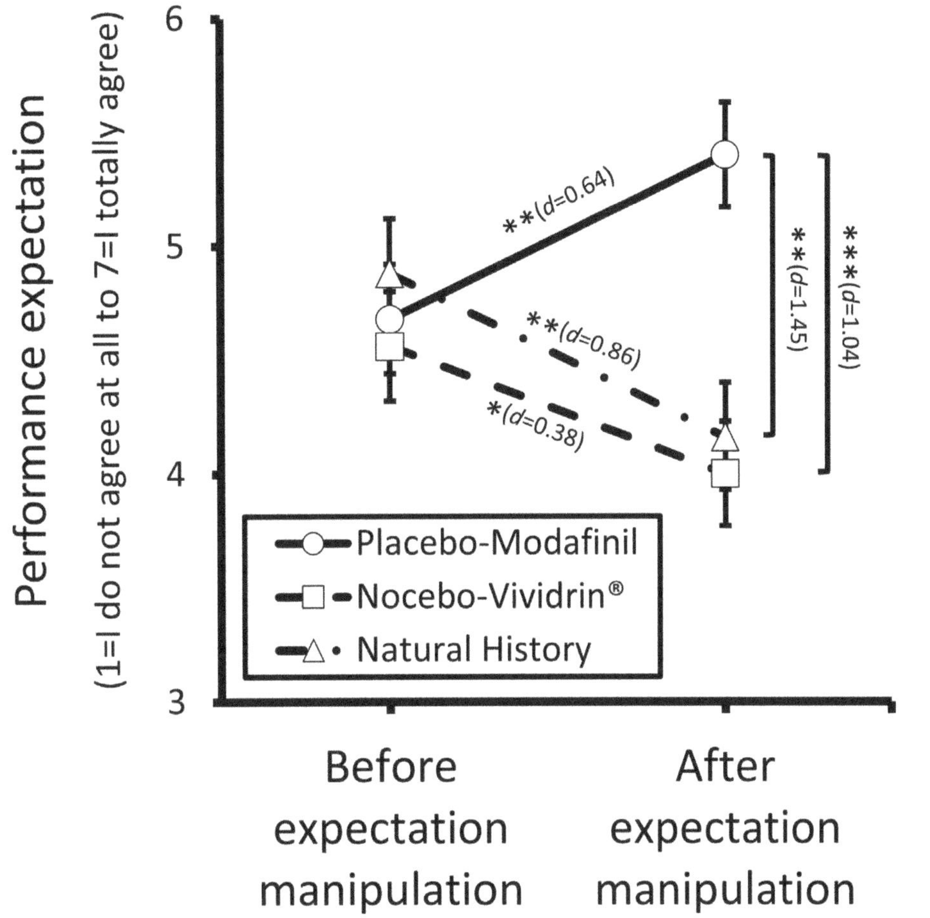

FIGURE 2 | Performance expectation ("I will perform well in the task") before the first TAP assessment and after expectation manipulation *via* drug information and nasal placebo intake. Error bars represent standard errors. *d* = Cohen's *d*. *p < .05. **p < .01. ***p < .001.

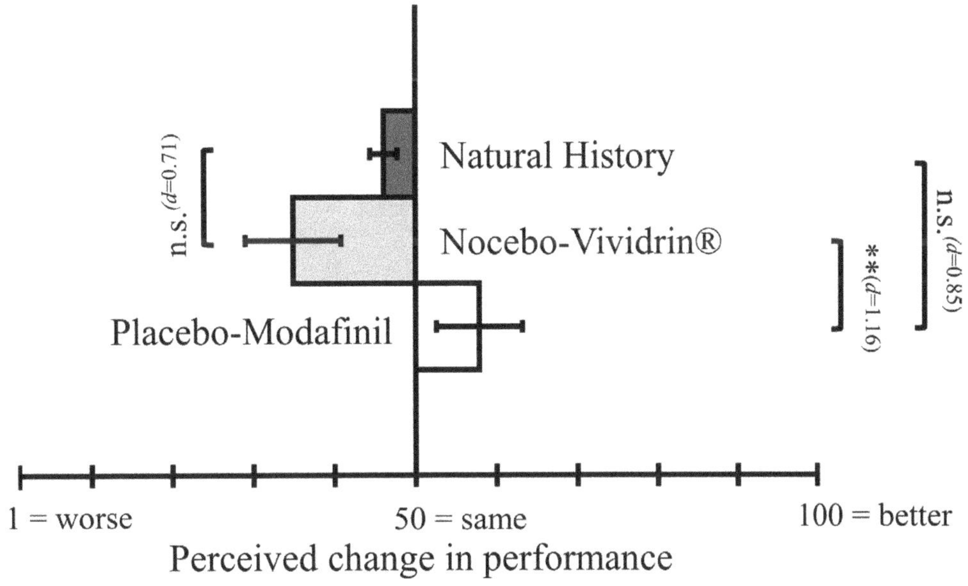

FIGURE 3 | Perceived change in performance ("How do you rate your cognitive performance now in comparison to the first assessment?") using a 1–100 VAS (1 = "worse"; 100 = "better"). Error bars represent standard errors. **p < .01.

Relationship Between Performance Expectation and Perceived Change in Performance

In the placebo-Modafinil and the nocebo-Vividrin® group combined, there was a significant positive correlation between performance expectation after placebo intake and perceived change in performance from the first assessment TAP to the second assessment TAP ($r = .47$, $p = .002$) as measured after the second assessment TAP.

Actual Cognitive Performance

There was no statistically significant interaction effect between group and time (first assessment vs. second assessment) for any of the TAP performance indices, as displayed in **Table 2**. Thus, there was no evidence for a differential effect of group allocation on actual cognitive performance. Moreover, no significant group main effects emerged. However, there were significant main effects for time, with respect to some subtests. Alertness without warning signal standard deviation reaction time [$F(1, 72) = 10.40$, $p = .002$, partial $\eta^2 = .126$], Alertness with warning signal standard deviation reaction time [$F(1, 72) = 5.97$, $p = .017$, partial $\eta^2 = .077$], and Alertness with warning signal number of anticipations [$F(1, 72) = 19.84$, $p < .001$, partial $\eta^2 = .216$] show higher values at the second assessment, respectively. Working Memory number of errors [$F(1, 72) = 9.65$, $p = .003$, partial $\eta^2 = .118$] and Sustained Attention number of errors [$F(1, 72) = 27.12$, $p < .001$, partial $\eta^2 = .274$] show lower values at the second assessment, respectively.

Adverse Symptoms ("Side Effects")

There was a significant difference in fatigue [$F(2,71) = 4.41$, $p = .016$] and irritation of nose or throat [$F(2,71) = 29.82$, $p < .001$] between groups after the second TAP assessment as revealed by ANCOVAs with symptom intensity prior to the first TAP assessment as covariate (see **Table 3**).

Fatigue. In comparison to participants in the nocebo-Vividrin® group, participants in the placebo-Modafinil group reported significantly less fatigue after placebo treatment ($M_{diff} = 0.84$, $p = .005$, $d = 0.96$). However, there was no significant difference between the natural history group and the placebo-Modafinil group ($M_{diff} = 0.52$, $p = .136$, $d = 0.56$) or nocebo-Vividrin® group ($M_{diff} = 0.32$, $p = .641$, $d = 0.36$), with respect to fatigue post second TAP assessment.

Irritation of nose and throat. In comparison to participants in the natural history group, participants in the placebo-Modafinil group ($M_{diff} = 0.92$, $p < .001$, $d = 2.02$) and the nocebo-Vividrin® group ($M_{diff} = 0.96$, $p < .001$, $d = 2.23$) reported significantly more irritation of their nose and throat after the placebo intervention.

TABLE 3 | Intensity of the 12 selected GASE adverse symptom items before 1st TAP assessment (baseline) and post 2nd TAP assessment.

	Placebo-Modafinil (n = 25)		Nocebo-Vividrin® (n = 25)		Natural history (n = 25)		Difference between groups post 2nd assessment (with pre 1st assessment as covariate)	
	Pre 1st assessment, M (SD)	Post 2nd assessment, M (SD)	Pre 1st assessment, M (SD)	Post 2nd assessment, M (SD)	Pre 1st assessment, M (SD)	Post 2nd assessment, M (SD)	$F(2,71)$	p
Placebo-Modafinil specific								
Headache	0.20 (0.41)	0.36 (0.57)	0.28 (0.46)	0.56 (0.65)	0.28 (0.54)	0.52 (0.65)	0.49	.616
Palpitations, irregular heartbeat	0.00 (0.00)	0.16 (0.62)	0.12 (0.44)	0.08 (0.28)	0.12 (0.33)	0.00 (0.00)	1.44	.243
Abdominal pain	0.04 (0.20)	0.00 (0.00)	0.20 (0.65)	0.28 (0.68)	0.04 (0.20)	0.04 (0.20)	2.45	.094
Fatigue (tiredness)	**0.64 (0.64)**	**0.92 (0.91)**	**0.92 (0.70)**	**1.76 (0.83)**	**1.00 (0.76)**	**1.44 (0.96)**	**4.41***	**.016**
Irritability, nervousness	0.24 (0.44)	0.16 (0.62)	0.32 (0.48)	0.20 (0.50)	0.40 (0.58)	0.08 (0.28)	0.83	.441
Nocebo-Vividrin® specific								
Bitter taste	0.12 (0.33)	0.12 (0.33)	0.00 (0.00)	0.32 (0.56)	0.04 (0.20)	0.08 (0.28)	2.67	.076
Nausea	0.00 (0.00)	0.00 (0.00)	0.00 (0.00)	0.08 (0.28)	0.00 (0.00)	0.04 (0.20)	1.03	.363
Skin rash or itching	0.08 (0.28)	0.04 (0.20)	0.12 (0.33)	0.08 (0.28)	0.12 (0.44)	0.12 (0.44)	0.75	.477
Feeling of weakness	0.08 (0.28)	0.12 (0.33)	0.12 (0.33)	0.44 (0.77)	0.20 (0.50)	0.28 (0.46)	2.14	.126
Drowsiness (exhaustion)	0.52 (0.59)	0.84 (0.94)	0.76 (0.66)	1.48 (0.77)	0.64 (0.64)	1.32 (0.85)	2.87	.063
Unspecific								
Dizziness	0.04 (0.20)	0.40 (0.71)	0.04 (0.20)	0.32 (0.56)	0.12 (0.33)	0.28 (0.46)	0.65	.525
Irritation of nose or throat	**0.16 (0.47)**	**1.00 (0.58)**	**0.24 (0.44)**	**1.04 (0.54)**	**0.08 (0.28)**	**0.08 (0.28)**	**29.82*****	**<.001**

GASE, Generic Assessment of Side Effects Scale, Bonferroni correction of the family wise error rate led to a p-value of .02 as criterion for significance with respect to the drug specific symptoms and .05 as criterion for significance with respect to unspecific symptoms.

$^*p < .02$, $^{***}p < .001$.

DISCUSSION

Our key finding is that manipulation of performance expectation *via* a placebo cognitive performance enhancing nasal spray affects the perceived change in performance and tiredness, but not the actual cognitive performance in healthy adults. Reasons for nonmedical use of prescription stimulants among university students are to improve concentration, to perform better in university (2), to "catch up with high achieving students," to increase the amount of work done under time constraint, to improve energy, and to "pull an all-nighter" (30). Therefore, the demonstrated placebo effect affecting subjective outcomes like perceived performance and tiredness could partially explain why these drugs are used despite potential risks and unclear benefit.

As hypothesized, the placebo-Modafinil group showed a significantly higher performance expectation after the expectation manipulation than the nocebo-Vividrin® and the natural history group. Although nearly all prior studies assumed that *a priori* performance expectation was changed by the intervention (e.g., administration of a placebo pill or verbal suggestion), the majority of these studies did not assess performance expectation directly after the intended expectation manipulation. Rather, the change in performance expectation was extrapolated based on a *post hoc* performance rating (9, 10, 14, 16–21). Clearly, *a priori* performance expectations and *a posteriori* performance ratings tap different aspects. Indeed, we observed only a moderate positive correlation between performance expectation after placebo intake and perceived change in performance (r = .47). Moreover, the few studies that directly assessed *a priori* performance expectation (13, 15) failed to report changes in performance expectation due to their intervention. Hence, it is unclear whether the intervention actually resulted in change in expectation. In the present study, we carefully assessed performance expectation prior and subsequent to the placebo instruction and observed a medium-sized (d = 0.64) increase in performance expectation within the placebo-Modafinil group.

Contrary to our hypothesis that a positive performance expectation would improve actual performance, there were no group differences in actual cognitive performance. This finding is consistent with the study of Looby and Earleywine (13), but inconsistent with the finding of an improvement in sustained attention in participants believing that they had received a cognitive-enhancing drug (16). Interestingly, in the latter study, performance expectation was induced by providing false feedback that participants had improved their performance by 20% due to the pill they had taken before in a blinded manner. Hence, based on their apparent change in performance, participants formed their belief about whether or not they had taken active pill or the placebo. As is long known, (perceived) mastery of a task has a strong effect on self-efficacy (31). In a similar vein, beliefs based on (seeming) changes in performance are likely to be more credible and powerful than verbal suggestion for the participants. This is also consistent with findings that verbal suggestion as compared to conditioning is associated with a smaller placebo effect (32). Oken et al. (15) also found an improvement of actual cognitive performance (memory and attention) after placebo pill intake. This may be explainable by the fact that Oken et al. (15) investigated performance-enhancing placebo effects in a sample of healthy seniors, 65–85 years of age. In elderly individuals, a placebo effect might manifest itself more easily because any ceiling effect is unlikely due to lower baseline levels of cognitive functions such as attention or memory. In line with such an interpretation, Oken et al. (15) reported that even in their sample of elderly, older participants demonstrated a greater benefit from placebo intake. Indeed, Oken et al. (15) relied on a neuropsychological assessment battery typically used for dementia screening (CERAD), whereas the TAP used in the current study is also sensitive for measuring high levels of cognitive functioning. Moreover, given the role of medication-related beliefs (33), a potential confounding influence could be that the attitude towards neuroenhancement as treatment for a cognitive deficit in elderly is quite different than the expected effects of drugs used for "brain doping" by healthy young adults.

As predicted, participants in the placebo-Modafinil group rated their perceived change in cognitive performance subsequent to the application of the nasal spray significantly better (d = 1.16) compared to the nocebo-Vividrin® group. Hence, an enhanced performance expectation affects the perceived change in performance, irrespective of any changes in actual cognitive performance. Similar observations, i.e., that performance expectation affects the perceived change in performance, but not the actual cognitive performance, have been made previously [e.g., Ref. (18)]. As outlined by Schwarz and Büchel (18), it is possible that objective measures of cognitive performance are generally not susceptible to expectancy manipulation. Those studies demonstrating an expectancy-induced change in objective performance (15, 16) are at odds with such an assumption. Alternatively, it is possible that only specific cognitive functions are susceptible to expectancy manipulation (e.g., tasks entailing a motivational component and/or tasks requiring great effort). Previous studies vary considerably with regard to the specific type of cognitive task used to evaluate changes in performance. For example, implicit learning task (19) or tests of fluid intelligence (21) have been used. Taking into account previous reports on changes in cognitive functioning due to administration of cognitive enhancers in healthy participants, we decided to focus on attention as a core cognitive function rather than complex cognitive functions (e.g., problem solving). We choose the TAP due to the broad range of functioning it allows to test. However, the TAP was developed to allow a differential diagnosis of attention deficits, based on reference data in the general population. Clearly, in our sample, there is no evidence for a potential ceiling effect. The mean T-values range between 46 and 57 for the different performance indices, indicating average cognitive performance in our healthy sample. At this point, it is far from being clear which method for expectation manipulation, e.g. sham subliminal presentation of information (20) or smelling an odor (19) or verbal suggestion, is particularly effective in yielding actual changes in performance. Moreover, it is unclear which aspects of cognitive functioning are susceptible to a placebo manipulation. Finally yet importantly, design differences (e.g., balanced placebo design vs. between group designs) could account for the heterogeneous results.

Contrary to our hypotheses, there was no difference in performance expectation between the nocebo-Vividrin® and the natural history group, indicating that the intended manipulation of the performance expectation had failed for the nocebo-Vividrin® group. Our results show that both groups, the nocebo-Vividrin® group ($d = -0.38$) and the natural history group ($d = -0.86$), showed a significant decrease in performance expectation compared to baseline with the effect sizes suggesting a larger drop. Possibly, participants in the natural history group, who were interested in participating in a study on brain doping as advertised, were disappointed that they were assigned to the control (natural history) group and therefore did not have the chance to try a smart drug, thus resulting in a nocebo effect. Participants in the nocebo-Vividrin® group may have underestimated the effects of Vividrin® due to its being administered as part of study on brain doping. Alternatively, participants may have had prior experiences with Vividrin®, which is a common anti-allergic substance, and, based on their own experience, did therefore not expect a deteriorated cognitive performance. As described above, the majority of studies did not directly assess performance expectation; hence, there are no previous findings on whether performance expectation is susceptible to negative manipulation in the same way as it is to positive manipulation.

We also attempted to evoke adverse symptoms consistent with the side effect profiles of the placebo/nocebo medications as listed in the drug information leaflets given to the participants. There was no evidence for a drug-specific side effect profile in either experimental group. Yet, the description of adverse symptoms is known to influence participants' perception of bodily symptoms (34). Fatigue was described as a potential side effect of Modafinil. Interestingly, participants in the placebo-Modafinil group felt less tired after the second TAP test than the nocebo-Vividrin® group. This suggests that describing Modafinil as a stimulating drug, which facilitates general alertness, overshadowed the listed side effects, especially given that fatigue as a side effect might seem counterintuitive for a stimulating drug. Moreover, since increased alertness and prolonged endurance when working are known reasons for nonmedical use of prescription stimulants (30), disregarding tiredness as an unwanted side effect could partly explain why these drugs are used despite potential risks and unclear benefit, especially if the effect could be evoked even by a medication without active component (a placebo).

There were no group differences regarding the other complaints, except for irritation of nose and throat, which is attributable to the capsaicin in the nasal spray, and therefore was reported significantly more often in the experimental groups as compared to the natural history group. Possibly, participants assumed that a single dose of the study medication would not lead to the side effects as described, but, based on previous experiences when taking medications, implicitly assumed that such side effect would primarily occur when regularly taking the same medication.

Limitations

First of all, we cannot rule out a certain self-selection bias of the participants such that we may have tested primarily individuals willing to try a cognitive-performance-modulating drug using a new route of delivery (see the cover story of the study) in an experimental setting and/or individuals with prior experience with such drugs. Additionally, due to the cover story, participants might have expected to get the chance of trying a performance-enhancing drug and were disappointed when they were allocated in the nocebo or natural history group, potentially leading to a reduced motivation and commitment.

Furthermore, our findings are limited to healthy adults. As stated by Fuhr and Werle (17), psychological interventions for enhancing cognitive performance might even be more effective for patients with impaired cognitive functioning, e.g., when suffering from an affective disorder. Patients might be more susceptible to expectancy manipulation and might benefit both subjectively and objectively, for example, due to better concentration, greater motivation, and higher perceived self-efficacy.

The approach to evoke adverse symptoms *via* information provided in the drug information leaflets may have not been optimal as they were described next to the drug action effects. Participants may have focused on the potentially desired effects and may have disregarded the adverse effects, especially if assuming, based on personal experience that "side effects" occur primarily when a drug is taken repeatedly.

We also cannot rule out that the placebo and the nocebo instruction might have been not fully equivalent since we referred to the substance name in the placebo condition (Modafinil), but used the trade name in the nocebo condition (Vividrin®). Given that Vividrin® is relatively well known, this might have triggered more expectations, thus confounding our expectancy manipulation.

In placebo/nocebo studies, in general, the situational context strongly influences study outcomes. Participants may have not fully believed that an actual drug, especially with negative effects on cognitive performance, would be applied at a department of psychology, especially with no physician being ostensibly involved.

Finally, it should be noted that attentional performance is just one facet of cognitive performance. However, unlike most previous studies, we used several tests of attentional performance rather than relying on just one or two tests. If performance expectancy primarily alters those cognitive functions entailing for example a strong motivational component, future studies should seek to use more comprehensive cognitive test batteries to elucidate which cognitive functions may be susceptible to performance expectancy effects.

To our knowledge, the present study is the first study investigating expectancy effects in pharmacological neuroenhancement including both placebo and nocebo instructions, assessing performance expectation directly after the intended manipulation and perceived change in cognitive performance, as well as cognitive measures. Additionally, it is the first study investigating drug-specific side effects of placebo- and nocebo-medication in the context of pharmacological neuroenhancement.

Conclusions

Manipulation of performance expectation affects the perceived change in performance and tiredness in healthy adults. This may explain why college students use such drugs despite their small, if any impact on actual cognitive functioning. Therefore, future studies should systematically assess the role of performance expectation, perceived change in performance, and tiredness in predicting future use of prescription drugs to improve cognitive performance. Future studies should also address whether enhancing placebo effects could be helpful in improving perceived or actual deficits in cognitive performance. This could stimulate clinical studies on utilizing placebo effects in clinical practice, for example, in patients suffering from affective disorders. Future studies should entail different cognitive tasks such that it can be determined what makes a cognitive task susceptible to expectancy manipulation. This holds the opportunity to elucidate the underlying mechanisms of such placebo/nocebo responses. With respect to the effect of nocebo responses on cognitive performance, our results suggest that demonstrating differences between a nocebo group (expectation manipulation intended to decrease performance expectation) and a natural history group seems to be challenging, due to potential nocebo effects within the natural history group. Nevertheless, in direct comparison with a placebo group (expectation manipulation intended to increase performance expectation) our data give evidence that a nocebo-intervention affects the perceived change in performance, irrespective of any changes in the actual cognitive performance. Future studies should apply alternative approaches to a natural history control group. Additionally maybe it would be beneficial to separate studies addressing placebo and nocebo effects in cognitive performance to avoid expectation violation of participants interested to try a pharmacological neuroenhancer and receiving no medication at all or a substance supposed to provoke the opposite effect.

The present findings add to the growing body of evidence that highlights the influence of prescription-stimulant-related expectancies on subjective outcomes but not cognitive performance. This finding implies that more information about the role of subjective expectations and the discrepancy between subjectively perceived and actual changes in cognitive performance needs to be communicated to the public in an attempt to modify beliefs held by (potential) users, thus possibly correcting individual beliefs about the benefit of such drugs.

ETHICS STATEMENT

This study was carried out in accordance with the recommendations of the local ethics committee of the faculty of psychology at Justus-Liebig-University Giessen, Germany with written informed consent from all subjects. All subjects gave written informed consent in accordance with the Declaration of Helsinki. The protocol was approved by the local ethics committee of the faculty of psychology at Justus-Liebig-University Giessen, Germany.

AUTHOR CONTRIBUTIONS

Both authors contributed to the conception and design of the study. AW and CH conducted the statistical analysis. AW wrote the first draft of the manuscript. Both authors approved the submitted version.

ACKNOWLEDGMENTS

We thank Tim Bartenschlager for his assistance in data acquisition.

REFERENCES

1. Swanson JM, Volkow ND. Increasing use of stimulants warns of potential abuse. *Nature* (2008) 453:586. doi: 10.1038/453586a
2. Teter CJ, McCabe SE, LaGrange K, Cranford JA, Boyd CJ. Illicit use of specific prescription stimulants among college students: prevalence, motives, and routes of administration. *Pharmacotherapy* (2006) 26:1501–10. doi: 10.1592/phco.26.10.1501
3. Bagusat C, Kunzler A, Schlecht J, Franke AG, Chmitorz A, Lieb K. Pharmacological neuroenhancement and the ability to recover from stress—a representative cross-sectional survey among the German population. *Subst Abuse Treat Prev Policy* (2018) 13:1–16. doi: 10.1186/s13011-018-0174-1
4. Lucke J, Jensen C, Dunn M, Chan G, Forlini C, Kaye S, et al. Non-medical prescription stimulant use to improve academic performance among Australian university students: prevalence and correlates of use. *BMC Public Health* (2018) 18:1–7. doi: 10.1186/s12889-018-6212-0
5. Repantis D, Schlattmann P, Laisney O, Heuser I. Modafinil and methylphenidate for neuroenhancement in healthy individuals: a systematic review. *Pharmacol Res* (2010) 62:187–206. doi: 10.1016/j.phrs.2010.04.002
6. Bagot KS, Kaminer Y. Efficacy of stimulants for cognitive enhancement in non-attention deficit hyperactivity disorder youth: a systematic review. *Addiction* (2014) 109:547–57. doi: 10.1111/add.12460
7. Ilieva IP, Hook CJ, Farah MJ. Prescription stimulants' effects on healthy inhibitory control, working memory, and episodic memory: a meta-analysis. *J Cognit Neurosci* (2015) 27:1069–89. doi: 10.1162/jocn_a_00776
8. Ilieva I, Boland J, Farah MJ. Objective and subjective cognitive enhancing effects of mixed amphetamine salts in healthy people. *Neuropharmacology* (2013) 64:496–505. doi: 10.1016/j.neuropharm.2012.07.021
9. Cropsey KL, Schiavon S, Hendricks PS, Froelich M, Lentowicz I, Fargason R. Mixed-amphetamine salts expectancies among college students: is stimulant induced cognitive enhancement a placebo effect? *Drug Alcohol Depend* (2017) 178:302–9. doi: 10.1016/j.drugalcdep.2017.05.024
10. Dawkins L, Shahzad F-Z, Ahmed SS, Edmonds CJ. Expectation of having consumed caffeine can improve performance and mood. *Appetite* (2011) 57:597–600. doi: 10.1016/j.appet.2011.07.011
11. Walach H, Schmidt S, Dirhold T, Nosch S. The effects of a caffeine placebo and suggestion on blood pressure, heart rate, well-being and cognitive performance. *Int J Psychophysiol* (2002) 43:247–60. doi: 10.1016/S0167-8760(01)00188-X
12. Harrell PT, Juliano LM. A direct test of the influence of nicotine response expectancies on the subjective and cognitive effects of smoking. *Exp Clin Psychopharmacol* (2012) 20:278–86. doi: 10.1037/a0028652
13. Looby A, Earleywine M. Expectation to receive methylphenidate enhances subjective arousal but not cognitive performance. *Exp Clin Psychopharmacol* (2011) 19:433–44. doi: 10.1037/a0025252

14. Szemerszky R, Dömötör Z, Berkes T, Köteles F. Attribution-based nocebo effects. Perceived effects of a placebo pill and a sham magnetic field on cognitive performance and somatic symptoms. *Int J Behav Med* (2016) 23:204–13. doi: 10.1007/s12529-015-9511-1
15. Oken BS, Flegal K, Zajdel D, Kishiyama S, Haas M, Peters D. Expectancy effect: impact of pill administration on cognitive performance in healthy seniors. *J Clin Exp Neuropsychol* (2008) 30:7–17. doi: 10.1080/13803390701775428
16. Colagiuri B, Boakes RA. Perceived treatment, feedback, and placebo effects in double-blind RCTs: an experimental analysis. *Psychopharmacology* (2010) 208:433–41. doi: 10.1007/s00213-009-1743-9
17. Fuhr K, Werle D. Mental training for better achievement: effects of verbal suggestions and evaluation (of effectiveness) on cognitive performance. *Front Psychiatry* (2018) 9:510. doi: 10.3389/fpsyt.2018.00510
18. Schwarz KA, Büchel C. Cognition and the placebo effect–dissociating subjective perception and actual performance. *PLoS One* (2015) 10:e0130492. doi: 10.1371/journal.pone.0130492
19. Colagiuri B, Livesey EJ, Harris JA. Can expectancies produce placebo effects for implicit learning? *Psychon Bull Rev* (2011) 18:399–405. doi: 10.3758/s13423-010-0041-1
20. Weger UW, Loughnan S. Mobilizing unused resources: using the placebo concept to enhance cognitive performance. *Q J Exp Psychol* (2013) 66:23–8. doi: 10.1080/17470218.2012.751117
21. Foroughi CK, Monfort SS, Paczynski M, McKnight PE, Greenwood PM. Placebo effects in cognitive training. *Proc Natl Acad Sci U S A* (2016)113 (27), 7470–4. doi: 10.1073/pnas.1601243113
22. Turi Z, Mittner M, Paulus W, Antal A. Placebo intervention enhances reward learning in healthy individuals. *Sci Rep* (2017) 7:1–15. doi: 10.1038/srep41028
23. Turi Z, Bjørkedal E, Gunkel L, Antal A, Paulus W, Mittner M. Evidence for cognitive placebo and nocebo effects in healthy individuals. *Sci Rep* (2018) 8:17443. doi: 10.1038/s41598-018-35124-w
24. Faul F, Erdfelder E, Lang A-G, Buchner A. G*Power 3: a flexible statistical power analysis program for the social, behavioral, and biomedical sciences. *Behav Res Methods* (2007) 39:175–91. doi: 10.3758/BF03193146
25. Rief W, Barsky AJ, Glombiewski JA, Nestoriuc Y, Glaesmer H, Braehler E. Assessing general side effects in clinical trials: reference data from the general population. *Pharmacoepidemiol Drug Saf* (2011) 20:405–15. doi: 10.1002/pds.2067
26. Rheker J, Rief W, Doering BK, Winkler A. Assessment of adverse events in clinical drug trials: identifying amitriptyline's placebo- and baseline-controlled side effects. *Exp Clin Psychopharmacol* (2018) 26(3):320–6. doi: 10.1037/pha0000194
27. Rief W, Hessel A, Braehler E. Somatization symptoms and hypochondriacal features in the general population. *Psychosom Med* (2001) 63:595–602. doi: 10.1097/00006842-200107000-00012
28. Hiller W, Rief W, Braehler E. Somatization in the population: from mild bodily misperceptions to disabling symptoms. *Soc Psychiatry Psychiatr Epidemiol* (2006) 41:704–12. doi: 10.1007/s00127-006-0082-y
29. Zimmermann P, Fimm B. *Testbatterie zur Aufmerksamkeitsprüfung (TAP).* Herzogenrath: PSY-TEST (2009).
30. Vargo EJ, Petroczi A. "It was me on a good day": exploring the smart drug use phenomenon in England. *Front Psychol* (2016) 7:1–12. doi: 10.3389/fpsyg.2016.00779
31. Bandura A. Self-efficacy mechanism in human agency. *Am Psychol* (1982) 37:122–47. doi: 10.1037/0003-066X.37.2.122
32. Colloca L, Benedetti F. Placebo analgesia induced by social observational learning. *Pain* (2009) 144:28–34. doi: 10.1016/j.pain.2009.01.033
33. Watkinson A, Chapman SCE, Horne R. Beliefs about pharmaceutical medicines and natural remedies explain individual variation in placebo analgesia. *J Pain* (2017) 18:908–22. doi: 10.1016/j.jpain.2017.02.435
34. Barsky AJ, Saintfort R, Rogers MP, Borus JF. Nonspecific medication side effects and the nocebo phenomenon. *JAMA* (2002) 287:622–27. doi: 10.1001/jama.287.5.622

16

Placebo Effect in the Treatment of Depression and Anxiety

*Irving Kirsch**

Harvard Medical School, Boston, MA, United States

***Correspondence:**
Irving Kirsch
ikirsch@bidmc.harvard.edu

The aim of this review is to evaluate the placebo effect in the treatment of anxiety and depression. Antidepressants are supposed to work by fixing a chemical imbalance, specifically, a lack of serotonin or norepinephrine in the brain. However, analyses of the published and the unpublished clinical trial data are consistent in showing that most (if not all) of the benefits of antidepressants in the treatment of depression and anxiety are due to the placebo response, and the difference in improvement between drug and placebo is not clinically meaningful and may be due to breaking blind by both patients and clinicians. Although this conclusion has been the subject of intense controversy, the current article indicates that the data from all of the published meta-analyses report the same results. This is also true of recent meta-analysis of all of the antidepressant data submitted to the Food and Drug Administration (FDA) in the process of seeking drug approval. Also, contrary to previously published results, the new FDA analysis reveals that the placebo response has not increased over time. Other treatments (e.g., psychotherapy and physical exercise) produce the same benefits as antidepressants and do so without the side effects and health risks of the active drugs. Psychotherapy and placebo treatments also show a lower relapse rate than that reported for antidepressant medication.

Keywords: placebo, nocebo, depression, anxiety, antidepressants

INTRODUCTION

The aim of this review is to evaluate the placebo effect in the treatment of anxiety and depression. On February 19, 2012, Leslie Stahl opened a segment of the CBS news program *60 Minutes* saying "The medical community is at war, battling over the scientific research and writings of a psychologist named Irving Kirsch. The fight is about antidepressants and Kirsch's questioning of whether they work." By that time, I had co-authored three meta-analyses and a book concerning the placebo effect in the treatment of depression (1–4). Two of these meta-analyses (2, 3) were conducted on the data sent to the Food and Drug Administration (FDA) by the manufacturers of what at that time were the six most widely prescribed antidepressants—data that we obtained using the Freedom of Information Act. We found that although the people given antidepressants showed considerable improvement in the clinical trials submitted to the FDA by the manufacturers, so did the people given placebo, and the difference in outcome between drug and placebo was below the criterion for clinical meaningfulness used by the National Institute for Health and Care Excellence (NICE), the organization that sets treatment guidelines for the National Health Service in the United Kingdom.

There is now a crisis concerning the lack of replicability of many studies in psychology and medicine (5, 6). I am pleased to report that the antidepressant meta-analyses we published have not contributed to this crisis. There are now at least nine subsequent meta-analyses aimed at replicating or discrediting our studies (7–16). Some of these were restricted to changes on the

Hamilton Rating Scale for Depression (HAM-D), whereas others included data from a variety of scales. Some were conventional meta-analyses in which means and standard deviations were used to calculate effect sizes, whereas others were patient-level analyses. Although interpretations of the data varied from study to study, the results have been consistent across all of them. We had reported a mean drug-placebo difference of 1.80 points on the HAM-D and a standardized mean difference (SMD) of 0.32. The differences reported in the replications ranged from 1.62 to 2.56 HAM-D points, with SMD effect sizes ranging from 0.23 to 0.34. To put this into perspective, the NICE criteria for clinical significance of antidepressant-placebo differences are three points on the HAM-D or SMDs of at least 0.50, corresponding to what Cohen (17) proposed as a moderate effect size.

Special attention is due to the preliminary results of a patient-level meta-analysis reported by Stone et al. (15). Marc Stone is the Deputy Director for Safety at the Division of Psychiatric Products of the FDA. He and his colleagues reported a patient-level analysis of the data from all randomized placebo-controlled trials of antidepressants in the treatment of Major Depressive Disorder that had been submitted to the FDA between 1979 and 2016. The similarity in outcome between what the Stone et al. data and those that my colleagues and I had reported in 2002 and 2008 is astounding. We had reported a drug response of 10.1 points on the HAM-D and a placebo response of 8.3 point—a drug-placebo difference of 1.8 points. In Stone et al.'s comprehensive analysis of the data from the 73,178 patients in the 228 trials submitted to the FDA, the drug response was 10.1 points, the placebo response was 8.3 points—yielding a drug-placebo difference of 1.80 points on the 17-item HAM-D, exactly what my colleagues and I reported in our analysis of the FDA data for the six antidepressants that we evaluated (2).

Antidepressants are also used to treat anxiety disorders. Might they be more effective in treating anxiety than in treating depression? My colleagues and I have assessed that issue in a meta-analysis of the effects of paroxetine in treating anxiety disorders (18). We chose to limit our analysis to paroxetine so that we could assess a complete dataset of unpublished pre- and post-marketing trials, as well as those that had been published. As part of a 2004 lawsuit settlement, GlaxoSmithKline was required to post online the results of all clinical trials involving its drugs on its Clinical Trial Register (19). Examining these data, we found a drug-placebo effect size (SMD) of 0.27, similar to those reported for antidepressants in the treatment of depression. In a subsequent study, Roest et al. (20) analyzed data obtained from the FDA for premarketing trials of nine second-generation antidepressants in the treatment of anxiety disorders. They reported an SMD of 0.33, similar to that reported by Sugarman and colleagues for paroxetine (18) and to those reported in the meta-analyses of antidepressants in the treatment of depression cited above. Subsequently, Sugarman and colleagues (21) replicated the Roest et al. study and found an SMD of 0.34 across all antidepressants and all anxiety disorders, with individual effect sizes ranging from 0.26 to 0.39. Thus, antidepressants are no better in treating anxiety disorders than they are in treating depression.

The impact of placebo factors in the treatment of anxiety can also be seen in a study by Faria et al. (22). Participants diagnosed with social anxiety disorder (SAD) were treated with an selective seratonin reuptake inhibitor (SSRI) (escitalopram). Approximately half of the patients were accurately informed that they were taking an SSRI. The others were told that they were being given an active placebo (i.e., a drug that produces side effects but has no therapeutic effect on the condition being treated). Telling patients that they were being treated by an active medication doubled its effectiveness on a continuous measure of anxiety and tripled the response rate.

Critics have noted that the criteria proposed for clinical significance by NICE (3 points on the HAM-D or SMDs of at least 0.50) are arbitrary (23), and they are correct. The NICE criteria are as arbitrary as the criterion of $p < .05$ for statistical significance, the use of a 50% reduction in symptoms as a criterion of a clinical response, and the use of a HAM-D score below 8 as the criterion of remission. Given that the conventional cutoffs for statistical significance are arbitrary, as are those for assessing clinical "response" and "remission," why would we expect the criteria for the clinical significance of drug-placebo differences to be any less arbitrary?

Nevertheless, Joanna Moncrieff and I (24) have proposed empirically derived criteria for the clinical significance of antidepressant-placebo differences. We used published data from a large patient-level analysis (25) of the correspondence between changes on the HAM-D and the Clinical Global Impressions-Improvement (CGI-I) scale, a scale that rates improvement on a scale of 1 (very much improved) through 4 (no change) to 7 (very much worse). This analysis revealed that an improvement of three points on the HAM-D (SMD = 0.375) is equivalent to a clinician rating "no change" on the CGI-I. A CGI-I rating of "minimally improved" corresponds to a HAM-D difference of 7 points (SMD = 0.873), and a rating of "much improved" corresponds to a 14-point HAM-D difference (SMD = 1.75). None of the meta-analyses have reported drug-placebo differences that come close to reaching the criterion for CGI-I ratings of minimal improvement, even among the most severely depressed patients.

Many depressed patients report substantial improvement after taking antidepressant medication, as do psychiatrists when describing their outcomes. How are we to reconcile this with the consistent finding that the differences between the response to antidepressants and placebos are vanishingly small? The answer is the placebo response. Although drug–placebo differences in outcome are equivalent to no difference at all, both drug and placebo responses can be substantial. The improvement of 8.3 points following placebo treatment and 10.1 points on the active drugs reported by Kirsch et al. (3) and Stone et al. (15) corresponds to CGI-I ratings between minimally improved and much improved. It is only the 1.8-point difference that corresponds to a CGI-I rating of no change. Thus, the clinically meaningful improvement seen following prescriptions of antidepressants is largely to the placebo response (i.e., the placebo effect, regression toward the mean, and spontaneous remission).

The failure to find meaningful differences between antidepressants and placebos has been blamed on increasing placebo responses over the years (26), and some meta-analyses have shown increases in both the placebo response and the drug response over time [e.g., Ref. (27)]. However, the comprehensive analysis of all trials submitted to the FDA from 1979 to 2016 tells a different story (15). The placebo response was 8.3 HAM-D points in both 1979 and 2016, with little variation between those dates. There was a small decrease (0.8 points) in the drug–placebo difference over time, but this was due to a 0.8-point decrease in the drug response (from 10.7 points in 1979 to 9.9 points in 2016), rather than an increase in the placebo response.

PLACEBO EFFECTS VERSUS PLACEBO RESPONSES

In 1965, Fisher and colleagues (28, pp. 57–58) noted that "a clinical response following treatment (*drug response*) is not synonymous with an effect which can be attributed to the treatment (*drug effect*)." In 1998, Kirsch and Sapirstein (4) extended this distinction to placebo responses and effects, and in 2018, a group of 29 internationally recognized placebo researchers published a "consensus statement," in which they endorsed the view that "the placebo and nocebo response includes all health changes that result after administration of an inactive treatment (i.e., differences in symptoms before and after treatment), thus, including natural history and regression to the mean. The *placebo and nocebo effect* refers to the changes specifically attributable to placebo and nocebo mechanisms" (29, p. 206). The meta-analyses described above indicate a strong placebo response, but with one exception: they do not assess the placebo effect.

In the one exception (4), Guy Sapirstein and I assessed the placebo effect by comparing the placebo response in drug trials to changes observed in no-treatment natural-history control conditions in psychotherapy studies. We found that 25% of the drug response was duplicated in the no-treatment groups, and 75% of the drug response was found in the placebo groups. Thus, the placebo effect was 50% of the drug response—double the drug effect and also double the response found in the no-treatment controls. It was a genuine placebo effect.

A limitation of our study was that data in the no-treatment groups and data in the placebo groups came from different studies. That limitation has been overcome in a clinical trial reported by Leuchter and his colleagues (30). This was a three-arm study, in which depressed patients were randomized to either antidepressant plus supportive care, placebo plus supportive care, or supportive care alone. Mean HAM-D improvement was 10.05 points in the antidepressant group and 7.59 in the placebo group, but only 1.37 in the supportive care only group. As in the Kirsch and Sapirstein study, the response in the placebo group was mostly a genuine placebo effect and not simply due to spontaneous improvement or regression toward the mean.

IS THERE A DRUG EFFECT AT ALL?

Although the difference between antidepressant and placebo is not clinically meaningful, it is statistically significant. Can we interpret that small but statistically significant difference as a genuine drug? Although that cannot be ruled out, there is another possibility. Clinical trials in which patients and/or their doctors or other outcome raters are asked to judge whether the patient was given an active drug or a placebo are consistent in showing that those judgements are very accurate. This indicates that the trials are not really double-blind. Numerous studies have shown that when patients know they are getting a drug, they are more responsive to the drug than when they know they might be getting a placebo (31–35). This indicates a placebo effect component in the drug response. Similarly, the placebo response is reduced when people know they might be getting a placebo than when they are led to believe that they are getting the active drug (31, 36). Therefore, the small drug–placebo difference in outcome might be due to the increased response in the drug group and decreased responding in the placebo group produced by what participants are told about the trials.

In 1986, Rabkin and her colleagues (1986) published a study in which doctors and their depressed patients who had been randomized to imipramine, phenelzine, or placebo were asked to guess the group to which the patients had been assigned. Overall, 78% of patients and 87% of the doctors accurately identified whether the patients had been given an active drug or a placebo. As shown in **Figure 1**, patients randomized to active drug groups were especially successful in breaking blind, whereas those receiving placebo seem to be merely guessing. In contrast, doctors showed high levels of accuracy in identifying group assignment for patients in the placebo groups as well as those in the drug groups. Furthermore, this pattern of results has been replicated successfully in subsequent studies (38–41), indicating that they are reliable. Rabkin et al. concluded that "in view of these findings we recommend that investigators routinely record and report doctor and patient opinions about treatment assignment in randomized trials, preferably both early in the trial and at the end" (p. 86). Unfortunately, this recommendation has been largely ignored.

Given these exceptionally high rates of breaking blind, the next question is whether this phenomenon is associated with the outcome of clinical trials. In 2013, Baethge and colleagues (42) reported the results of a meta-analysis addressing this issue. In 47 clinical trials of psychiatric disorders in which blinding was assessed, the correlation between patient accuracy and the drug–placebo effect size was .51 ($p = .002$) and that between rater accuracy and effect size was .55 ($p = .067$). Thus, the greater the likelihood of breaking blind, the greater the drug–placebo difference.

However, there is an interpretive problem with respect to understanding the direction of causality in the data on accuracy of judgements of group assignment. In most of the studies in which blinding was assessed, the assessment was made near the end of the trial. Thus, it is possible that breaking blind is a consequence rather than a cause of drug–placebo differences. However, some of the data reported by Rabkin et al. (37) indicate that breaking blind is not solely a consequence of the patients' responses to treatment. **Figure 2** displays the accuracy of judgements separately for patients who responded to treatment and those who did not. Of particular interest is the ability of both patients and doctors to accurately guess group assignment of nonresponders in the drug group. Seventy-four percent of nonresponders who received an active drug judged themselves to

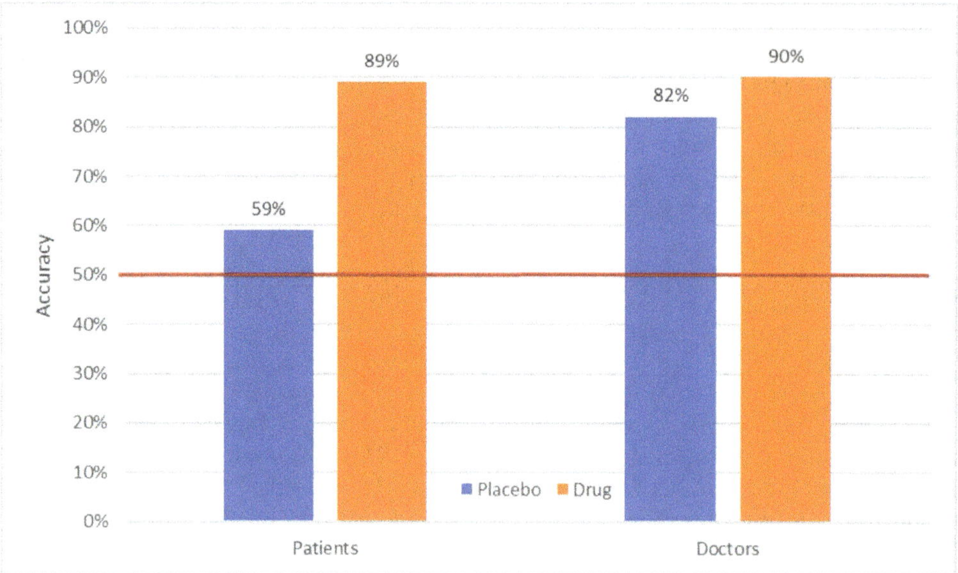

FIGURE 1 | Accuracy of patient and doctor "guesses" as a function of actual treatment (37).

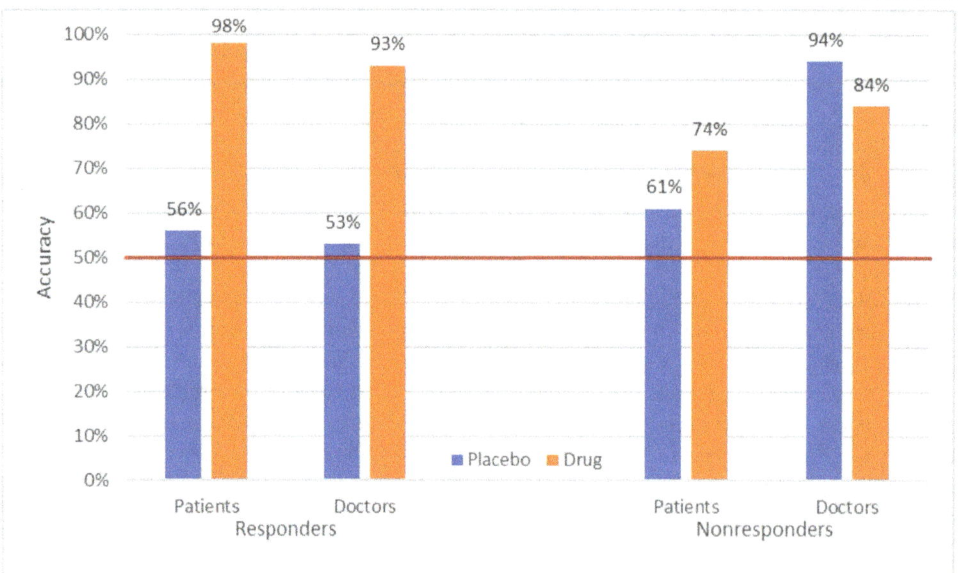

FIGURE 2 | Accuracy of patient and doctor "guesses" as a function of actual treatment and patient response (37).

be on the drug, as did 84% of their doctors. Furthermore, almost half of responders to placebo guessed they were on placebo. Although this would be expected by chance guessing, it indicates that the improvement experienced by these placebo responders did not lead them to think they were taking an active medication. Taken together, these data indicate that although response to treatment influences patients' and doctors' judgements of treatment assignment, it does not fully explain the accuracy of those judgements.

I and others (1, 43, 44) have hypothesized that the presence of side effects is responsible for breaking blind. As part of the informed consent processes, patients in clinical trials are told that they might receive a placebo. They are also told that the medication under investigation has side effects, and they are told exactly what the known side effects are. Now placebos can also generate side effects, a phenomenon known as the nocebo effect, but they do so to a much lesser degree than active medications (45). This difference in side effects might lead patients in clinical trials, as well as the clinicians who rate their improvement, to figure out to which group they have been randomized. To the extent that this occurs, the trial is not really double-blind. In this section, I describe data indicating that patients in clinical trials often do break blind and that breaking blind affects the outcomes of the trials.

Studies have shown mixed results for the hypothesis and drug–placebo differences are associated with reported side effects (46–51). However, side effects may be only one of the cues leading participants in clinical trials to break blind. Joanna Moncrief (52) has hypothesized that people learn how to recognize the sometimes subtle changes produced by medications without necessarily reporting symptoms that would be listed as a side effect on the checklists used to assess them.

Two studies conducted by Aimee Hunter and colleagues at UCLA provide indirect support for this hypothesis (53, 54). In each of these studies, depressed patients in clinical trials were grouped according to whether they had ever been on antidepressants before. As displayed in **Figure 3**, there were virtually no differences at all between drug and placebo among patients who had never been taken antidepressants before. In contrast, among those with prior experience, drug–placebo differences were both significant and substantially larger than those reported in other clinical trials, whereas the combined differences for antidepressant-experienced and antidepressant-naive participants are in the same range of other clinical trials. Taken together, the data from both studies strongly suggest that prescriptions for antidepressants should not be given to depressed people who have never taken them before.

WHAT IS TO BE DONE?

How then shall we treat depression? One suggestion that has been made to me informally is to prescribe antidepressants as active placebos. An active placebo is a pharmacologically active substance that does not have specific activity for the condition being treated. Antidepressant medications have little or no pharmacological effects on depression or anxiety, but they do elicit a substantial placebo effect. Could we not use them as a means of capitalizing on the power of placebo?

The problem with this suggestion is that treatment decisions need to be based on an assessment of risks, as well as benefits. The risks of antidepressant treatment include suicidal and violent aggressive behavior in adolescents and young adults; stroke, death from all causes, falls and fractures, and epileptic seizures in the elderly; and sexual dysfunction, withdrawal symptoms, diabetes, deep vein thrombosis, and gastrointestinal and intracranial bleeding in everyone else (55–62). One might argue that these risks might be worth taking for an effective treatment of severe depression, but are they worth risking for a treatment that has no benefit at all over placebo for first-time users?

A second possibility would be to prescribe placebos. They are safe and effective, with relatively few nocebo side effects and no health risks. The problem with prescribing placebos rests with the commonly held assumption that to be effective in clinical practice, placebos have to be presented deceptively as active medications. This assumption has been reported to be false in recent clinical trials [reviewed in Ref. (63)]. In these studies, placebos were presented non-deceptively as placebos with no active ingredients. How could this ever work? The answer is that it was accompanied by a rationale in which it was explained that placebos have been found effective to the condition being treated, that it has been found to involve Pavlovian conditioning, and that it might therefore be effective in treating the person's condition. This rationale has been found to be critical for the success of the open-label placebo (OLP) intervention (64). Additional OLP trials with larger samples, longer duration, and blinded assessors are warranted.

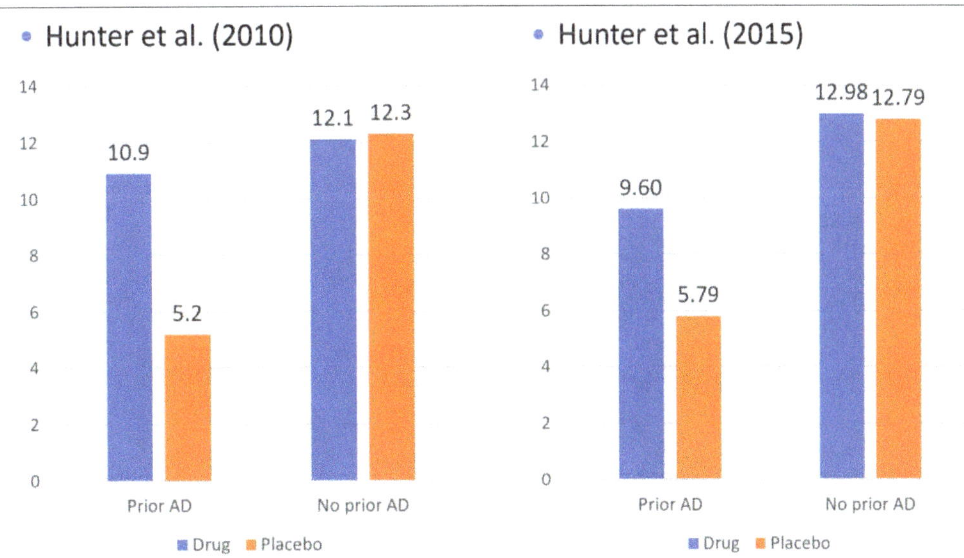

FIGURE 3 | Drug-placebo differences as a function of prior antidepressant use.

Unfortunately, only one of the studies assessing OLPs involved the treatment of depression, and that one, although showing promising results, was only a small pilot (65). However, there are many other treatments that equal antidepressants in terms of degree of symptom reduction (66–69). These include psychotherapy, physical exercise, acupuncture, omega-3, homeopathy, tai chi, qigong, and yoga. We do not know the mechanisms of these alternative treatments, and their efficacy may be at least partly due to expectancy, but they are certainly safer than antidepressant medication.

The long-term advantage of psychotherapy over medication has been shown in a number of studies [reviewed in Ref. (70)]. Whereas short-term outcomes were equivalent between the two treatments, long-term outcomes were significantly better for patients who had received psychotherapy than for those who had received medication. Additionally, the National Institute of Mental Health (NIMH) Treatment of Depression Collaborative Research Program reported relapse rates of 36% and 33% for cognitive behaviour therapy and interpersonal therapy, respectively, compared with a 50% relapse rate for antidepressant medication (71). However, the rate of relapse for patients who had recovered on placebo was 33%, the same as that for psychotherapy. There are two take-home messages from these data. First, it dispels the myth that placebo responses are short-lived. Second, it raises the questions of whether psychotherapy reduces relapse or medication increases it (72).

Support for the hypothesis that antidepressant medication increases the risk of relapse comes from other studies comparing antidepressant and placebo treatment for depression and anxiety disorders. Consistent with the NIMH data, a 2011 meta-analysis reported a relapse rate of 25% for depressed patients successfully treated with placebo compared to relapse rates ranging from 42% to 57% among those treated with various antidepressants (73). A direct test of the effect of antidepressants and psychotherapy on the risk of relapse comes from a study on the treatment of panic disorder (74). The study compared the 6-month relapse rates for patients who had been treated with a tricyclic antidepressant (imipramine), cognitive behavior therapy (CBT), or the two combined. The results, displayed in **Figure 4**, indicate that the risk of relapse following imipramine was more than double that following CBT. However, the addition of the antidepressant to imipramine completely erased that benefit. Similarly, physical exercise as a treatment for depression has been shown to have a much lower relapse rate than SSRIs, but that benefit disappears when the two treatments are combined (75).

These studies reveal another benefit of including placebos in clinical trials of medication. They can reveal situations in which the treatment does more harm than good for the condition being treated. For example, placebos have outperformed antipsychotic medication (haloperidol and risperidone) in the treatment of delirium in palliative care patients and aggression in intellectually disabled adults (76, 77). Similarly, placebo was significantly better than a combination of chondroitin and glucosamine in the treatment of knee osteoarthritis (78) and showed similar superiority in a trial of nutraceuticals in the treatment of depression (79).

Given these data, I suggest that the following principles be used in treatment selection. When treatments are equally effective, recommend the safest. When they are equally safe, let the patient choose which he or she prefers. Before making this choice, however, patients should be accurately informed of the potential harms of antidepressant medication (e.g., increased risk of relapse, suicidality, gastrointestinal and intracranial bleeding, deep vein thrombosis, pulmonary embolism, diabetes, stroke, epilepsy, and death from all causes), as well as the finding that all of these treatments appear to be equally effective in the short term but that psychotherapy and physical exercise might be more effective than antidepressants in the long run.

AUTHOR CONTRIBUTIONS

IK wrote the article.

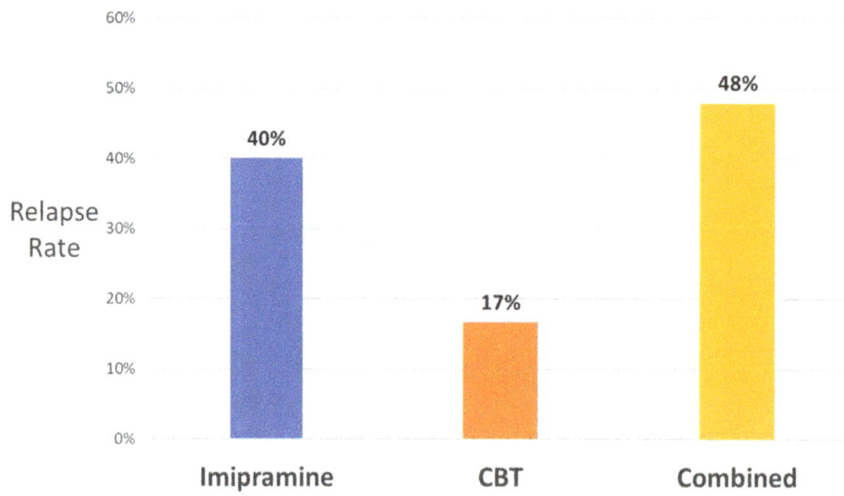

FIGURE 4 | Six-month relapse rates in panic disorder for patients who had been treated with imipramine or placebo, with or without CBT (74).

REFERENCES

1. Kirsch I. *The emperor's new drugs: exploding the antidepressant myth*. New York: basic books (2010).
2. Kirsch I, Deacon BJ, Huedo-Medina TB, Scoboria A, Moore TJ, Johnson BT. Initial severity and antidepressant benefits: a meta-analysis of data submitted to the Food and Drug Administration. *PLoS Med* (2008) 5. doi: 10.1371/journal.pmed.0050045
3. Kirsch I, Moore TJ, Scoboria A, Nicholls SS. The emperor's new drugs: an analysis of antidepressant medication data submitted to the U.S. Food and Drug Administration. *Prev Treat* (2002) 5(1):23. Retrieved from http://ezproxy.lib.uconn.edu/login?url=http://search.ebscohost.com/login.aspx?direct=true&db=pdh&AN=pre-5-1-23a&site=ehost-liveirving.kirsch{{{at}}}uconn.edu. doi: 10.1037/1522-3736.5.1.523a
4. Kirsch I, Sapirstein G. Listening to Prozac but hearing placebo: a meta-analysis of antidepressant medication. In: Kirsch I, editor. *How expectancies shape experience*. American Psychological Association (1999). p. 303–20. doi: 10.1037/10332-012
5. Ioannidis JPA. Contradicted and initially stronger effects in highly cited clinical research. *JAMA* (2005) 294(2):218–28. doi: 10.1001/jama.294.2.218
6. Open science collaboration. Estimating the reproducibility of psychological science. *Science* (2015) 349(6251):aac4716. Retrieved from http://science.sciencemag.org/content/349/6251/aac4716.abstract. doi: 10.1126/science.aac4716
7. Cipriani A, Furukawa TA, Salanti G, Chaimani A, Atkinson LZ, Ogawa Y, et al. Comparative efficacy and acceptability of 21 antidepressant drugs for the acute treatment of adults with major depressive disorder: a systematic review and network meta-analysis. *Lancet* (2018) 391(10128):1357–66. doi: 10.1016/S0140-6736(17)32802-7
8. Fountoulakis KN, Möller HJ. Efficacy of antidepressants: a re-analysis and re-interpretation of the Kirsch data. *Int J Neuro-Psychopharmacol* (2011) 14(3):405. doi: 10.1017/S1461145710000957
9. Fournier JC, DeRubeis RJ, Hollon SD, Dimidjian S, Amsterdam JD, Shelton RC, et al. Antidepressant drug effects and depression severity: a patient-level meta-analysis. *J Am Med Assoc* (2010) 303(1):47–53. doi: 10.1001/jama.2009.1943
10. Furukawa TA, Maruo K, Noma H, Tanaka S, Imai H, Shinohara K, et al. Initial severity of major depression and efficacy of new generation antidepressants: individual participant data meta-analysis. *Acta Psychiatr Scand* (2018) 137(6):450–8. doi: 10.1111/acps.12886
11. Gibbons RD, Hur K, Brown CH, Davis JM, Mann JJ. Benefits from antidepressants: synthesis of 6-week patient-level outcomes from double-blind placebo-controlled randomized trials of fluoxetine and venlafaxine. *Arch Gen Psychiatry* (2012) 69(6):572–9. doi: 10.1001/archgenpsychiatry.2011.2044
12. Jakobsen JC, Katakam KK, Schou A, Hellmuth SG, Stallknecht SE, Leth-Møller K, et al. Selective serotonin reuptake inhibitors versus placebo in patients with major depressive disorder. A systematic review with meta-analysis and trial sequential analysis. *BMC Psychiatry* (2017) 17(1):58. doi: 10.1186/s12888-016-1173-2
13. Khin NA, Chen YF, Yang Y, Yang P, Laughren TP. Exploratory analyses of efficacy data from major depressive disorder trials submitted to the US Food and Drug Administration in support of new drug applications. *J Clin Psychiatry* (2011) 72(4):464. doi: 10.4088/JCP.10m06191
14. NICE. Depression: management of depression in primary and secondary care. Clinical practice guideline No 23. (2004).
15. Stone M, Kalaria S, Richardville K, Miller B. Components and trends in treatment effects in randomized placebo-controlled trials in major depressive disorder from 1979 to 2016. Paper presented at the American Society of Clinical Psychopharmacology, Miami (2018).
16. Turner EH, Matthews AM, Linardatos E, Tell RA, Rosenthal R. Selective publication of antidepressant trials and its influence on apparent efficacy. *N Engl J Med* (2008) 358:252–60. doi: 10.1056/NEJMsa065779
17. Cohen J. A power primer. *Psychol Bull* (1992) 112(1):155–9. doi: 10.1037//0033-2909.112.1.155
18. Sugarman MA, Loree AM, Baltes BB, Grekin ER, Kirsch I. The efficacy of paroxetine and placebo in treating anxiety and depression: a meta-analysis of change on the hamilton rating scales. *PLoS One* (2014) 9(8):e106337. doi: 10.1371/journal.pone.0106337
19. Harris G. Maker of Paxil to release all trial results. *N Y Times* (2004).
20. Roest AM, de Jonge P, Williams CD, de Vries Y, Schoevers RA, Turner EH. Reporting bias in clinical trials investigating the efficacy of second-generation antidepressants in the treatment of anxiety disorders: a report of 2 meta-analyses. *JAMA Psychiatry* (2015) 72(5):500–10. doi: 10.1001/jamapsychiatry.2015.15
21. Sugarman MA, Kirsch I, Huppert JD. Obsessive-compulsive disorder has a reduced placebo (and antidepressant) response compared to other anxiety disorders: a meta-analysis. *J Affect Disord* (2017) 218(Supplement C):217–26. Retrieved from http://www.sciencedirect.com/science/article/pii/S0165032717303051. doi: 10.1016/j.jad.2017.04.068
22. Faria V, Gingnell M, Hoppe JM, Hjorth O, Alaie I, Frick A, et al. Do You Believe It? Verbal suggestions influence the clinical and neural effects of escitalopram in social anxiety disorder: a randomized trial. *EBioMedicine* (2017) 179–88. doi: 10.1016/j.ebiom.2017.09.031
23. Turner EH, Rosenthal R. Efficacy of antidepressants. *BMJ* (2008) 336(7643):516–7. Retrieved from http://www.bmj.com/content/336/7643/516.abstract. doi: 10.1136/bmj.39510.531597.80
24. Moncrieff J, Kirsch I. Empirically derived criteria cast doubt on the clinical significance of antidepressant-placebo differences. *Contemp Clin Trials* (2015) 43:60–2.
25. Leucht S, Fennema H, Engel R, Kaspers-Janssen M, Lepping P, Szegedi A. What does the HAMD mean? *J Affect Disord* (2013) 148(2–3):243–8. Retrieved from http://www.sciencedirect.com/science/article/pii/S0165032712008348. doi: 10.1016/j.jad.2012.12.001
26. Stahl SM, Greenberg GD. Placebo response rate is ruining drug development in psychiatry: why is this happening and what can we do about it? *Acta Psychiatr Scand* (2019) 139(2):105–7. doi: 10.1111/acps.13000
27. Walsh BT, Seidman SN, Sysko R, Gould M. Placebo response in studies of major depression: Variable, substantial, and growing. *JAMA* (2002) 287(14):1840–7. Retrieved from http://ezproxy.lib.uconn.edu/login?url=http://search.ebscohost.com/login.aspx?direct=true&db=psyh&AN=2002-12736-006&site=ehost-live. doi: 10.1001/jama.287.14.1840
28. Fisher S, Lipman RS, Uhlenhuth E, Rickels K, Park LC. Drug effects and initial severity of symptomatology. *Psychopharmacologia* (1965) 7(1):57–60. doi: 10.1007/BF00404165
29. Evers AWM, Colloca L, Blease C, Annoni M, Atlas LY, Benedetti F, et al. Implications of placebo and nocebo effects for clinical practice: expert consensus. *Psychother Psychosomatics* (2018) 87(4):204–10. doi: 10.1159/000490354
30. Leuchter AF, Hunter AM, Tartter M, Cook IA. Role of pill-taking, expectation and therapeutic alliance in the placebo response in clinical trials for major depression. *Br J Psychiatry* (2014) 443–9. Retrieved from http://bjp.rcpsych.org/content/early/2014/08/27/bjp.bp.113.140343.abstract. doi: 10.1192/bjp.bp.113.140343
31. Papakostas GI, Fava M. Does the probability of receiving placebo influence clinical trial outcome? A meta-regression of double-blind, randomized clinical trials in MDD. *Eur Neuropsychopharmacol* (2009) 19:34–40. doi: 10.1016/j.euroneuro.2008.08.009
32. Rutherford BR, Sneed JR, Roose SP. Does study design influence outcome? *Psychother Psychosomatics* (2009) 78(3):172–81. doi: 10.1159/000209348
33. Rutherford BR, Wall MM, Brown PJ, Choo T-H, Wager TD, Peterson BS, et al. Patient expectancy as a mediator of placebo effects in antidepressant clinical trials. *Am J Psychiatry* (2017) 174:135–42. doi: 10.1176/appi.ajp.2016.16020225
34. Sinyor M, Levitt AJ, Cheung AH, Schaffer A, Kiss A, Dowlati Y, et al. Does inclusion of a placebo arm influence response to active antidepressant treatment in randomized controlled trials? Results from pooled and meta-analyses. *J Clin.Psychiatry* (2010) 71:270–9. doi: 10.4088/JCP.08r04516blu
35. Sneed JR, Rutherford BR, Rindskopf D, Lane DT, Sackeim HA, Roose SP. Design makes a difference: a meta-analysis of antidepressant response rates in placebo-controlled versus comparator trials in late-life depression. *Am J Geriatr Psychiatry* (2008) 16(1):65–73. doi: 10.1097/JGP.0b013e3181256b1d
36. Rief W, Glombiewski JA. The hidden effects of blinded, placebo-controlled randomized trials: an experimental investigation. *Pain* (2012) 153(12):2473–7. doi: 10.1016/j.pain.2012.09.007
37. Rabkin JG, Markowitz JS, Stewart JW, McGrath PJ, Harrison W, Quitkin FM, et al. How blind is blind? Assessment of patient and doctor medication guesses

in a placebo-controlled trial of imipramine and phenelzine. *Psychiatry Res* (1986) 19:75–86. doi: 10.1016/0165-1781(86)90094-6

38. Chen JA, Papakostas GI, Youn S, Baer L, Clain AJ, Fava M, et al. Association between patient beliefs regarding assigned treatment and clinical response: reanalysis of data from the hypericum depression trial study group. *J Clin Psychiatry* (2011) 72(12):1669–76. doi: 10.4088/JCP.10m06453
39. Chen JA, Vijapura S, Papakostas GI, Parkin SR, Kim DJH, Cusin C, et al. Association between physician beliefs regarding assigned treatment and clinical response: re-analysis of data from the hypericum depression trial study group. *Asian J Psychiatry* (2015) 13:23–9. Retrieved from http://www.sciencedirect.com/science/article/pii/S1876201814002810. doi: 10.1016/j.ajp.2014.12.002
40. Hrobjartsson A, Emanuelsson F, Skou Thomsen AS, Hilden J, Brorson S. Bias due to lack of patient blinding in clinical trials. A systematic review of trials randomizing patients to blind and nonblind sub-studies. *Int J Epidemiol* (2014) 43:1272–83. doi: 10.1093/ije/dyu115
41. Margraf J, Ehlers A, Roth WT, Clark DB, Sheikh J, Agras WS, et al. How blind are double-blind studies? *J Consult Clin Psychol* (1991) 59(1):184–7. doi: 10.1037//0022-006X.59.1.184
42. Baethge C, Assall OP, Baldessarini RJ. Systematic review of blinding assessment in randomized controlled trials in schizophrenia and affective disorders 2000-2010. *Psychother Psychosomatics* (2013) 82(3):152–60. doi: 10.1159/000346144
43. Greenberg RP, Fisher S. Examining antidepressant effectiveness: findings, ambiguities, and some vexing puzzles. In: Fisher S, Greenberg RP, editors. *The limits of biological treatments for psychological distress: comparisons with psychotherapy and placebo*. Hillsdale, NJ: Lawrence Erlbaum (1989). p. 1–37.
44. Oronowicz-Jaśkowiak W, Bąbel P. Twenty years after 'listening to prozac but hearing placebo'. Do we hear placebo even louder? *Health Psychol Rep* (2019) 7(1):1–8. doi: 10.5114/hpr.2019.83383
45. Philipp M, Kohnen R, Hiller KO. Hypericum extract versus imipramine or placebo in patients with moderate depression: randomised multicentre study of treatment for eight weeks. *Br Med J* (1999) 319:1534–9. doi: 10.1136/bmj.319.7224.1534
46. Ashar YK, Cohen ZD, Chang LJ, Wager TD, Dimidjian S (2015). Side effects or main effects? Side effects predict treatment response in ADM and placebo treatment of MDD. paper presented at the association for behavioral and cognitive therapy, chicagno.
47. Barth M, Kriston L, Klostermann S, Barbui C, Cipriani A, Linde K. Efficacy of selective serotonin reuptake inhibitors and adverse events: meta-regression and mediation analysis of placebo-controlled trials. *Br J Psychiatry* (2016) 208(2):114–9. Retrieved from http://bjp.rcpsych.org/content/bjprcpsych/208/2/114.full.pdf. doi: 10.1192/bjp.bp.114.150136
48. Greenberg RP, Bornstein RF, Zborowski MJ, Fisher S, Greenberg MD. A meta-analysis of fluoxetine outcome in the treatment of depression. *J Nerv Ment Dis* (1994) 182:547–51. doi: 10.1097/00005053-199410000-00003
49. Laferton JAC, Vijapura S, Baer L, Clain AJ, Cooper A, Papakostas G, et al. Mechanisms of perceived treatment assignment and subsequent expectancy effects in a double blind placebo controlled RCT of major depression. *Front Psychiatry* (2018) 9:424. Retrieved from http://www.ncbi.nlm.nih.gov/pmc/articles/PMC6137256/. doi: 10.3389/fpsyt.2018.00424
50. Max MB, Schafer SC, Culnane M, Dubner R, Gracely RH. Association of pain relief with drug side effects in postherpetic neuralgia: a single-dose study of clonidine, codeine, ibuprofen, and placebo. *Clin Pharmacol Ther* (1988) 43(4):363–71. doi: 10.1038/clpt.1988.44
51. Shah E, Triantafyllou K, Hana A, Pimentel M. Adverse events appear to unblind clinical trials in irritable bowel syndrome. *Neurogastroenterol Motil* (2014) 26(4):482–8. doi: 10.1111/nmo.12289
52. Moncrieff J. *The myth of the chemical cure*. Basingstoke: Palgrave Macmillan (2008). doi: 10.1057/9780230589445
53. Hunter AM, Cook I, Tartter M, Sharma S, Disse G, Leuchter A. Antidepressant treatment history and drug-placebo separation in a placebo-controlled trial in major depressive disorder. *Psychopharmacology* (2015) 232(20):3833–40. doi: 10.1007/s00213-015-4047-2
54. Hunter AM, Cook IA, Leuchter AF. Impact of antidepressant treatment history on clinical outcomes in placebo and medication treatment of major depression. *J Clin Psychopharmacol* (2010) 30(6):748–51. doi: 10.1097/JCP.0b013e3181faa474
55. Andrews PW, Thomson JA, Amstadter A, Neale MC. Primum non nocere: an evolutionary analysis of whether antidepressants do more harm than good. *Front Psychol* (2012) 3. Retrieved from http://www.frontiersin.org/Journal/Abstract.aspx?s=413&name=evolutionary_psychology&ART_DOI=10.3389/fpsyg.2012.00117. doi: 10.3389/fpsyg.2012.00117
56. Braun C, Bschor T, Franklin J, Baethge C. Suicides and suicide attempts during long-term treatment with antidepressants: a meta-analysis of 29 placebo-controlled studies including 6,934 patients with major depressive disorder. *Psychother Psychosomatics* (2016) 85(3):171–9. doi: 10.1159/000442293
57. Coupland C, Dhiman P, Morriss R, Arthur A, Barton G, Hippisley-Cox J. Antidepressant use and risk of adverse outcomes in older people: population based cohort study. *BMJ* (2011) 343. doi: 10.1136/bmj.d4551
58. Fava GA, Benasi G, Lucente M, Offidani E, Cosci F, Guidi J. Withdrawal symptoms after serotonin-noradrenaline reuptake inhibitor discontinuation: systematic review. *Psychother Psychosomatics* (2018) 87(4):195–203. doi: 10.1159/000491524
59. Maslej MM, Bolker BM, Russell MJ, Eaton K, Durisko Z, Hollon SD, et al. The mortality and myocardial effects of antidepressants are moderated by preexisting cardiovascular disease: a meta-analysis. *Psychother Psychosomatics* (2017) 86(5):268–82. doi: 10.1159/000477940
60. Molero Y, Lichtenstein P, Zetterqvist J, Gumpert CH, Fazel S. Selective serotonin reuptake inhibitors and violent crime: a cohort study. *PLoS Med* (2015) 12(9):e1001875. doi: 10.1371/journal.pmed.1001875
61. Stone MB. In Search of a Pony. *Med Care* (2018) 56(5):375–81. doi: 10.1097/MLR.0000000000000895
62. Yuet WC, Derasari D, Sivoravong J, Mason D, Jann M. Selective serotonin reuptake inhibitor use and risk of gastrointestinal and intracranial bleeding. *J Am Osteopathic Assoc* (2019) 119(2):102–11. doi: 10.7556/jaoa.2019.016
63. Charlesworth JE, Petkovic G, Kelley JM, Hunter M, Onakpoya I, Roberts N, et al. Effects of placebos without deception compared with no treatment: a systematic review and meta-analysis. *J Evidence-Based Med* (2017) 10(2):97–107. doi: 10.1111/jebm.12251
64. Locher C, Frey Nascimento A, Kirsch I, Kossowsky J, Meyer A, Gaab J. Is the rationale more important than deception? A randomized controlled trial of open-label placebo analgesia. *Pain* (2017) 158(12):2320–8. Retrieved from http://journals.lww.com/pain/Fulltext/2017/12000/Is_the_rationale_more_important_than_deception__A.7.aspx. doi: 10.1097/j.pain.0000000000001012
65. Kelley JM, Kaptchuk TJ, Cusin C, Lipkin S, Fava M. Open-label placebo for major depressive disorder: a pilot randomized controlled trial. *Psychother Psychosom* (2012) 81:312–4.
66. Appleton KM, Sallis HM, Perry R, Ness AR, Churchill R. Omega-3 fatty acids for depression in adults. *Cochrane Database Syst Rev* (2015) 11. doi: 10.1002/14651858.CD004692.pub4
67. Khan A, Faucett J, Lichtenberg P, Kirsch I, Brown WA. A Systematic review of comparative efficacy of treatments and controls for depression. *PLoS One* (2012) 7(7):e41778. doi: 10.1371/journal.pone.0041778
68. Macías-Cortés E, Llanes-González L, Aguilar-Faisal L, Asbun-Bojalil J. Individualized homeopathic treatment and fluoxetine for moderate to severe depression in peri-and postmenopausal women (HOMDEP-MENOP study): a randomized, double-dummy, double-blind, placebo-controlled trial. *PLoS One* (2015) 10(3):e0118440. doi: 10.1371/journal.pone.0118440
69. Zou L, Yeung A, Li C, Wei G-X, Chen K, Kinser P, et al. Effects of meditative movements on major depressive disorder: a systematic review and meta-analysis of randomized controlled trials. *J Clin Med* (2018) 7(8):195. doi: 10.3390/jcm7080195
70. Cuijpers P, Hollon SD, van Straten A, Bockting C, Berking M, Andersson G. Does cognitive behaviour therapy have an enduring effect that is superior to keeping patients on continuation pharmacotherapy? A meta-analysis. *BMJ Open* (2013) 3(4):e002542. Retrieved from http://bmjopen.bmj.com/content/3/4/e002542.abstract. doi: 10.1136/bmjopen-2012-002542
71. Shea MT, Elkin I, Imber SD, Sotsky SM, Watkins JT, Collins JF, et al. Course of depressive symptoms over follow-up: findings from the National Institute of Mental Health Treatment of Depression Collaborative Research Program. *Arch Gen Psychiatry* (1992) 49(10):782–7. doi: 10.1001/archpsyc.1992.01820100026006
72. Hollon SD, Cohen ZD, Singla DR, Andrews PW. Recent developments in the treatment of depression. *Behavior Ther* (2019) 50(2):257–69. Retrieved from

http://www.sciencedirect.com/science/article/pii/S000578941930005X. doi: 10.1016/j.beth.2019.01.002

73. Andrews PW, Kornstein S, Halberstadt L, Gardner C, Neale MC. Blue again: Perturbational effects of antidepressants suggest monoaminergic homeostasis in major depression. *Front Psychol* (2011) 2. Retrieved from http://www.frontiersin.org/Journal/Abstract.aspx?s=413&name=evolutionarypsychology&ART_DOI=10.3389/fpsyg.2011.00159. doi: 10.3389/fpsyg.2011.00159
74. Barlow DH, Gorman JM, Shear MK, Woods SW. cognitive-behavioral therapy, imipramine, or their combination for panic disorder. *JAMA* (2000) 283:2529–36. doi: 10.1001/jama.283.19.2529
75. Babyak MA, Blumenthal JA, Herman S, Khatri P, Doraiswamy PM, Moore KA, et al. Exercise treatment for major depression: maintenance of therapeutic benefit at 10 months. *Psychosomatic Med* (2000) 62:633–8. doi: 10.1097/00006842-200009000-00006
76. Agar MR, Lawlor PG, Quinn S, Draper B, Caplan GA, Rowett D, et al. Efficacy of oral risperidone, haloperidol, or placebo for symptoms of delirium among patients in palliative care: a randomized clinical trial. *JAMA Internal Med* (2017) 177(1):34–42. doi: 10.1001/jamainternmed.2016.7491
77. Tyrer P, Oliver-Africano PC, Ahmed Z, Bouras N, Cooray S, Deb S, et al. Risperidone, haloperidol, and placebo in the treatment of aggressive challenging behaviour in patients with intellectual disability: a randomised controlled trial. *Lancet* (2008) 371:57–63. doi: 10.1016/S0140-6736(08)60072-0
78. Roman-Blas JA, Castañeda S, Sánchez-Pernaute O, Largo R, Herrero-Beaumont G, Group C. G. C. T. S., et al. Combined treatment with chondroitin sulfate and glucosamine sulfate shows no superiority over placebo for reduction of joint pain and functional impairment in patients with knee osteoarthritis: a six-month multicenter, randomized, double-blind, placebo-controlled clinical trial. *Arthritis Rheumatol* (2017) 69(1):77–85. doi: 10.1002/art.39819
79. Sarris J, Byrne GJ, Stough C, Bousman C, Mischoulon D, Murphy J, et al. Nutraceuticals for major depressive disorder- more is not merrier: an 8-week double-blind, randomised, controlled trial. *J Affect Disord* (2019) 245:1007–15. Retrieved from http://www.sciencedirect.com/science/article/pii/S0165032718314113. doi: 10.1016/j.jad.2018.11.092

17

Placebo and Nocebo Effects across Symptoms: From Pain to Fatigue, Dyspnea, Nausea and Itch

Fabian Wolters[1,2]*, *Kaya J. Peerdeman*[1,2] *and Andrea W.M. Evers*[1,2,3]

[1] *Health, Medical and Neuropsychology Unit, Institute of Psychology, Faculty of Social and Behavioral Sciences, Leiden University, Leiden, Netherlands,* [2] *Leiden Institute for Brain and Cognition, Leiden University, Leiden, Netherlands,* [3] *Department of Psychiatry, Leiden University Medical Center, Leiden, Netherlands*

Correspondence:
Fabian Wolters
f.wolters@fsw.leidenuniv.nl

Placebo and nocebo effects are, respectively, the helpful and harmful treatment effects that do not arise from active treatment components. These effects have thus far been researched most often in pain. It is not yet clear to what extent these findings from pain can be generalized to other somatic symptoms. This review investigates placebo and nocebo effects in four other highly prevalent symptoms: dyspnea, fatigue, nausea, and itch. The role of learning mechanisms (verbal suggestions, conditioning) in placebo and nocebo effects on various outcomes (self-reported, behavioral, and physiological) of these different somatic symptoms is explored. A search of experimental studies indicated that, as in pain, the combination of verbal suggestion and conditioning is generally more effective than suggestion alone for evoking placebo and nocebo effects. However, conditioning appears more and verbal suggestions less relevant in symptoms other than pain, with the exception of placebo effects on fatigue and nocebo effects on itch. Physiological measures, such as heart rate, lung function, or gastric activity, are rarely affected even when self-reported symptoms are. Neurobiological correlates are rarely investigated, and few commonalities appear across symptoms. Expectations generally predict placebo and nocebo effects for dyspnea and itch but seem less involved in fatigue and nausea. Individual characteristics do not consistently predict placebo or nocebo effects across symptoms or studies. In sum, many conclusions deriving from placebo and nocebo pain studies do appear to apply to other somatic symptoms, but a number of important differences exist. Understanding what type of learning mechanisms for which symptom are most likely to trigger placebo and nocebo effects is crucial for generalizing knowledge for research and therapies across symptoms and can help clinicians to optimize placebo effects in practice.

Keywords: placebo and nocebo effects, suggestion, conditioning, fatigue, dyspnea, nausea, itch, pain

INTRODUCTION

The placebo effect, the positive treatment outcomes that cannot be ascribed to active treatment components, has evolved from a nuisance in clinical trials to a phenomenon worth studying in its own right. Placebo effects can influence clinical outcomes in a meaningful way (1) and, under optimal conditions, achieve a large magnitude (2, 3). Moreover, placebo effects occur not just when a placebo is given, but can potentially enhance any active treatment that a patient receives (1, 4). Medical outcomes can be further influenced by the nocebo effect, where, instead of the positive effect in the case of placebo, harmful treatment side effects are evoked or increased, or positive treatment effects are reduced (5, 6).

Most of what we know about placebo and nocebo effects—their magnitude, their working mechanisms, their physiological and neurological correlates—comes from the study of these effects in pain. There are good reasons for this, as pain is well studied, is the most commonly reported somatic symptom (7), and can greatly influence quality of life (8). Pain also has the advantage that it is relatively easy to manipulate and control in laboratory settings: it can be tuned "up" and "down" by exposing the participant to different levels of a noxious stimulus such as heat, cold, or pressure. By contrast, other somatic sensations generally take more time to evoke (e.g., fatigue) or tend to last for a time even after the stimulus is removed (e.g., itch and nausea). This has led to a strong research tradition of studies on placebo analgesia and nocebo hyperalgesia to emerge in the last century, using the benefit of cumulative findings in comparable research settings to thoroughly investigate underlying mechanisms of these effects.

Placebo and nocebo effects play a role not just in pain, but in a wide range of conditions and symptoms. The available research indicates that the underlying mechanisms for these effects might differ per symptom (9). Accordingly, similar procedures might lead to very different results when symptoms are very different, such as pain and hormone levels (10), or to more comparable results when symptoms are more alike, such as pain and itch (11). Symptoms can differ on aspects such as conscious accessibility, the amount of cognitive control one can exert over it, what physiological systems they are connected to, and the related conditions and possible pathophysiological pathways [see, e.g., Ref. (12) for a comparison of itch and pain]. All of these factors can influence a symptom's susceptibility to placebo and nocebo effects or to learning mechanisms that cause them. The dominant position of pain in placebo and nocebo studies might give the impression that placebo and nocebo effects are only impactful for pain, or that they operate in other symptoms exactly as they do in pain. More importantly, knowing which findings generalize from pain to other symptoms could lead to more effective use of placebo and nocebo effects in both research and clinical practice.

While placebo and nocebo studies of symptoms other than pain are not as plentiful, some lines of research have a long history—for example, the placebo effect was studied in weightlifters and asthmatics in the early 1970s (13, 14). However, as in pain, these studies tend to focus only on a single symptom; there is very little comparative work that examines the similarities and differences between placebo and nocebo effects on pain and these other symptoms. The current review aims to help fill that gap. To facilitate the comparison with pain, we will focus on symptoms that share the features of being subjective, somatic, and commonly reported in the general population (7, 15–17) and that have been studied in the area of placebo and nocebo effects: fatigue, dyspnea, nausea, and itch. We will focus primarily on whether the learning mechanisms that have been established for pain function similarly for these other symptoms, with the status of research for each symptom separately being featured in the discussion. The focus will be on verbal suggestion and conditioning, as other learning mechanisms (such as observational learning) are rarely investigated in the included symptoms [although see Ref. (18) for an exception]. We will first see whether these learning mechanisms are similarly effective at inducing placebo and nocebo effects on fatigue, dyspnea, nausea, and itch as they are at affecting pain. After discussing these results, we will compare the selected symptoms with pain in terms of possible underlying mechanisms, specifically the role of expectations, and individual predictors of placebo and nocebo responses.

SEARCH STRATEGY AND SELECTION CRITERIA

We searched the scientific literature for experimental research on placebo and nocebo effects on subjective, somatic, and commonly reported symptoms other than pain. The included symptoms (and related search terms) were as follows: fatigue (mental fatigue, muscle fatigue), itch (pruritus, antipruritic), nausea (motion sickness, emetic, antiemetic), dizziness (vertigo, fainting), and dyspnea (asthma). These terms were entered in databases PubMed, PsycINFO, and Web of Science in combination with search terms for placebo and nocebo effects (placebo effect, placebo effects, nocebo, conditioning, operant conditioning, classical conditioning, verbal suggestion). Only those studies were included that either mentioned at least one of the included symptoms in the suggestion given to participants or included at least one of these symptoms as a self-reported outcome after a learning procedure featuring verbal suggestion or conditioning. Both studies that included healthy participants and those drawing participants from clinical samples were included. Only experimental laboratory studies were considered, since there are many possible reasons for symptom change in clinical trials and it is unclear whether the change in the placebo group (placebo *response*) is actually due to the placebo (placebo *effect*) or due to other factors such as natural history [see, e.g., Ref. 4)]. This process resulted in no relevant studies for dizziness, and thus this symptom was not further considered. Further studies were added by examining included studies for references and upon expert recommendation.

To answer the question whether expectations play a role in placebo and nocebo effects in fatigue, dyspnea, nausea, and itch, those studies that have explicitly examined participants' expectations were considered. To examine the question of which traits identify the placebo responder, the studies included based on the aforementioned criteria were scanned for individual characteristics used in moderation analyses. Only variables measured through questionnaires and gender were identified; no studies investigating, e.g., genetic factors were found. A brief summary of the results of included studies can be found in **Table 1**, while a detailed overview of every study is available as **Supplemental Material**.

TABLE 1 | Overview of results of included studies.

Learning mechanism	Symptom	Type of measure	Proportion positive results
Placebo—verbal suggestion	Fatigue	Self-reported	7/13
		Behavioral	10/11
		Physiological	1/5
	Dyspnea	Self-reported	3/5
		Behavioral	-
		Physiological	1/5
	Nausea	Self-reported	3/6
		Behavioral	0/2
		Physiological	0/4
	Itch	Self-reported	1/6
		Behavioral	-
		Physiological	0/6
Placebo—conditioning	Fatigue	Self-reported	1/2
		Behavioral	2/2
		Physiological	-
	Dyspnea	Self-reported	-
		Behavioral	-
		Physiological	-
	Nausea	Self-reported	6/7
		Behavioral	1/2
		Physiological	1/4
	Itch	Self-reported	2/2
		Behavioral	0/1
		Physiological	-
Nocebo—verbal suggestion	Fatigue	Self-reported	1/3
		Behavioral	1/2
		Physiological	0/1
	Dyspnea	Self-reported	3/5
		Behavioral	-
		Physiological	3/5
	Nausea	Self-reported	0/3
		Behavioral	1/1
		Physiological	0/1
	Itch	Self-reported	5/5
		Behavioral	1/1
		Physiological	2/2
Nocebo—conditioning	Fatigue	Self-reported	0/1
		Behavioral	1/1
		Physiological	-
	Dyspnea	Self-reported	8/8
		Behavioral	-
		Physiological	5/8
	Nausea	Self-reported	4/4
		Behavioral	2/2
		Physiological	0/1
	Itch	Self-reported	3/3
		Behavioral	0/1
		Physiological	-

Positive results: studies where a significant effect was found in the direction matching the verbal suggestion or learning procedure.

PLACEBO EFFECTS

In the prototypical experimental placebo analgesia study, participants are exposed to a painful stimulus, and then receive an inert treatment (the placebo) that is suggested to be an analgesic. This method is easily converted for use in other symptoms by changing the noxious stimulus; for example, instead of applying heat to induce pain, participants cycle on an ergometer to induce fatigue or sit in a rotation chair to induce nausea. The placebo itself is also adaptable: for instance, instead of an analgesic cream, a cream can be described as antiallergenic or an inert inhaler can be described as a bronchodilator. Some studies do not feature a separate inert medication, but directly suggest a change in the method or substance that induces the noxious sensation. For example, electrical stimulation can be described as very likely or very unlikely to cause itch.

Placebo effects can be evoked by only the verbal suggestion of symptom relief, but also by letting participants experience the reduction in stimulus intensity through a conditioning procedure. Meta-analyses have shown that in experimental studies investigating placebo mechanisms, verbal suggestions alone are on average rather effective at evoking placebo analgesia (3, 19). This analgesic placebo effect tends to be further enhanced when verbal suggestion and conditioning are combined (19–21). Conditioning can also be used to evoke placebo effects by itself, without verbal suggestions (21–24), but this is less often investigated in pain and even rarer in most other symptoms we discuss. Other learning mechanisms, such as letting the participant observe the effect in another person, are also rarely examined. Therefore, we will discuss first the effect of only verbal suggestions, and then all studies using conditioning, either paired with verbal suggestion or used by itself. Within each of these categories, fatigue, dyspnea, nausea, and itch are handled in order.

PLACEBO EFFECTS EVOKED THROUGH VERBAL SUGGESTIONS

Fatigue. A substantial number of studies have investigated the effect of a verbal suggestion of reduced fatigue or increased performance (25–38). In seven of the 13 studies, participants report a lower sense of fatigue while performing a motor task in the placebo condition than in a control condition (25, 28–30, 32, 33, 35). The lack of an effect in the remaining studies might be due to other factors, such as small sample size [Refs. (26, 38); 9 and 10, respectively] or the generic wording of the suggestion [not specifically directed toward fatigue (31, 34) or suggesting a 50/50 chance of placebo (27)]. Across all of the studies, participants also perform better; all but one study (37) find that participants either produced more power or continued a set performance for longer (26–33, 36, 38). Physiological indications of effort, such as blood lactate or heart rate, are often measured, but are not affected in most studies (28, 29, 33, 34, 38), even when the study found effects on fatigue or performance. A decreased readiness potential using EEG during repeated finger movements might indicate that placebo effects on fatigue and performance are caused by a central action in the preparatory phase of movement (35). Thus, overall, it seems that verbal suggestions are effective at reducing experienced fatigue and improving performance, but this is often not accompanied by the expected changes on physiological measures.

Dyspnea. Six studies, all using asthmatic participants, have investigated the placebo effect induced by a verbal suggestion on dyspnea (39–44). Three of the five studies that examined self-reported dyspnea report a decrease in symptoms (39, 42, 43). Participants in these studies first received a suggestion of bronchoconstriction (39, 42) or were denied their normal asthma medication (42, 43) before offering participants the placebo which was suggested to improve their breathing. The two studies that report non-significant findings on self-reported dyspnea (40, 44) tested the placebo without first inducing breathing problems. It is likely that a reduction of dyspnea is only expected or possible when it is clearly present in the first place. None of the studies found an effect on measures of lung function (39, 40, 42, 44), except Kemeny and colleagues (41), who did not examine self-reported dyspnea but found an improvement on airway reactivity after a placebo induction. No behavioral or neurological measures were collected. The tentative conclusion from these limited findings is that an existing feeling of dyspnea can be reduced by a verbal suggestion, but likely without accompanying physiological changes [which are themselves not strongly correlated to subjective asthma symptoms; see, e.g., Ref. (45)].

Nausea. Eight studies have examined the effect of suggestion of reduced nausea (46–53). Three studies show placebo effects on nausea experienced during a nausea-inducing activity after verbal suggestions (47, 48, 51), although the effect was limited to women in one study (51) and to men in another (48). A possible reason for the non-significant findings in the other studies (46, 52, 53) is that in these studies, participants were not previously made familiar with the nausea-inducing task, possibly resulting in a low expectation of nausea that cannot be reduced further with placebo. Other studies have shown that suggestions of reduced nausea can reduce the disgust experienced when viewing disgusting stimuli (49, 50). With respect to behavioral outcomes, participants did not tolerate the nauseating stimulus for longer after a verbal suggestion of a ginger treatment, regardless of whether there was an effect on reported symptoms (51, 52). Similarly, no differences between the placebo and control groups were detected with an electrogastrogram in any study (46, 51, 52), except for one (53), where participants who received a suggestion of reduced nausea actually showed more abnormal gastric activity. The two functional magnetic resonance imaging (fMRI) studies (49, 50) indicate an effect of a placebo with the suggestion of nausea reduction, showing decreased activity in the insula (particularly the left) and increased connectivity between the dorsomedial prefrontal cortex and the amygdala. The latter finding is consistent with processes of cognitive reappraisal of aversive stimuli, while the insula is a region associated with disgust and pain perception as well as pain analgesia (54–56). The overall pattern indicates that a placebo effect on nausea after verbal suggestion is found only on self-reported measures in some subgroups and under specific conditions.

Itch. Six recent studies have examined the effect of suggestions on itch (11, 34, 57–60). In most studies experienced itch was not successfully reduced (11, 34, 57, 59, 60), although it was in one study (58). All but one of the studies that did not find an effect gave only the suggestion, without a separate placebo (11, 59) or used a nonspecific suggestion (34, 60). Regardless of self-reported itch, none of the studies reported an effect on a physiological measure, be it weal size (58, 59), flare (59), skin temperature (59), heart rate (34), or skin conductance (34). Taken together, producing a placebo effect on itch seems to require more than just a verbal suggestion, with effects appearing only with very convincing suggestions or under specific circumstances.

Overall, placebo effects from a verbal suggestion do not seem to be as generally effective in other symptoms as they are in pain. The many studies showing clear effects on self-reported fatigue that extend to performance measures echo results on placebo analgesia, where verbal suggestion alone seems to be effective at reducing pain (3, 19). However, dyspnea, nausea, and itch were not reduced after a verbal suggestion in many studies, and seem to require certain conditions (such as specific phrasing of the suggestion) to be effective. Physiological correlates such as heart rate, lung function, or weal size show little evidence of being affected for any symptom.

PLACEBO EFFECTS EVOKED THROUGH CONDITIONING

In a conditioning procedure in a placebo study, participants can personally experience the beneficial effect of the placebo. This is generally done by modifying the intensity of the presented noxious stimulus, such as lowering the heat of a heat pain stimulus when a placebo cream is applied. While conditioning and suggestion were in the past sometimes seen as competing explanations of placebo effects, more recent perspectives (61, 62) generally consider them complementary, both contributing to the expectations that then influence the experience of noxious sensations. Note that when a study involves conditioning, this is almost always classical conditioning; while some studies into operant conditioning in the context of placebo and nocebo effects exist (63, 64), they are as of yet too rare too draw any general conclusions.

Fatigue. The combination of verbal suggestion and conditioning to produce a placebo effect on fatigue has been much less studied than the effect of verbal suggestion alone. Only two studies have adopted the method (31, 36). Both studies also include a group where only verbal suggestion was applied, allowing conclusions about the added effect of combining the methods. No effects on fatigue or perceived exhaustion were found in one study (31), while in the other (36), the self-report measure was only affected in the combined verbal suggestion and conditioning group, with no effect of suggestion alone. In both studies, participants in the combination condition showed larger effects on physical performance than those who only received a placebo and the suggestion. The study by Fiorio et al. (31), using transcranial magnetic stimulation, supports the idea that a placebo procedure influences a central mechanism (35), and extends these findings by suggesting that this results in rapid increases in excitability in the corticospinal system for the specific muscle involved. While low in number, these studies suggest greater placebo effects on fatigue and motor performance when verbal suggestion and conditioning were combined.

Dyspnea. We are not aware of studies using a design combining verbal suggestion and conditioning or using conditioning alone that investigated placebo effects on dyspnea.

Nausea. Two studies have combined verbal suggestion and conditioning to evoke a placebo effect on nausea (48, 65). Horing et al. (65) found that a combination of suggestion and conditioning was effective in reducing both self-reported nausea symptoms as well as behavioral consequences (how often participants could move their head during the nauseating task and how long they could tolerate the task). No results were found on electrogastrogram measures of digestive tract activity. The other study (48) similarly found that self-reported nausea was reduced after a procedure of suggestion and conditioning, but noted that suggestion seemed to be only effective for men, while conditioning was only effective for women. Both studies found an effect that was more elusive in studies that only used a verbal suggestion, indicating that conditioning may have some added value in reducing nausea, but further research will have to elucidate to what extent and for which groups this applies.

For nausea, there is also a line of research into using conditioning alone, without verbal suggestion, to induce placebo effects. These studies use two strategies. The first is overshadowing, where during a learning phase the nausea-inducing stimulus is associated with a very salient stimulus (e.g., a strong-tasting beverage) which is then not present at test (66–68). Because the nausea is associated with the salient stimulus, the absence of the stimulus may reduce nausea. The other is latent inhibition, where participants are exposed to the environment where the nausea is induced several times before the nausea induction (66, 69, 70). There, the fact that the environment is not just associated with nausea but also with previous neutral experiences will make it less nausea-inducing. These protocols have been used to reduce anticipatory nausea (66–69) and nocebo nausea (70). This seems to be generally effective (67–70), although the study implementing both interventions found no differences between the latent inhibition, overshadowing, combination, and control groups, and there were some indications that the latent inhibition intervention actually increased nausea (66). The one behavioral measure of rotation tolerance was not affected (69). Physiological results are mixed: some findings for heart rate correspond to self-report measures (68), but hormone measures either show no effect (67) or follow the unexpected effect of showing increased symptoms for latent inhibition (66). The results of the conditioning studies look promising in reducing self-reported anticipatory nausea and might stimulate other fields to continue to develop optimized conditioning procedures.

Itch. Only two studies specifically investigated the effect of verbal suggestion with conditioning on itch (57, 71). In both cases, the placebo consisted of an electrode, with the suggestion that it modified the intensity of the electrically-induced itch. The first study (57) found that only the combination of verbal suggestion and conditioning reduced self-reported itch, with either method individually not producing significant results. The second study (71) further indicated that this combination could also reverse nocebo effects on itch that had earlier been induced by a similar procedure. This reduced itch, however, did not result in reduced scratching behavior (72). While the evidence is limited, these studies suggest that the combination of verbal suggestion and conditioning is needed to successfully induce placebo effects on itch.

Overall, procedures that combine conditioning and verbal suggestion seem to more reliably induce a placebo effect on fatigue, nausea, and itch than those that use verbal suggestion alone. This aligns with results in pain (20, 21). It should be noted, however, that these results are based on a small number of studies, and more confirmatory work will still need to be done. One possible exception and example is the work in nausea, where a stronger tradition of studies has confirmed the utility of conditioning both with and without a verbal suggestion.

NOCEBO EFFECTS

Whereas placebo effects involve the reduction of noxious symptoms, nocebo effects consist of evoking or enhancing these symptoms. The experimental setup of a nocebo study is generally much like a placebo study, where a noxious agent is applied, and the participant learns through a verbal suggestion or conditioning to experience it differently. Nocebo research is still limited because of its relative novelty and the ethical concerns involved. In pain, studies have shown that nocebo effects require fewer learning trials than placebo effects (73) and are resistant to extinction (74). This would suggest more robust findings for nocebo studies than placebo studies. It has also been suggested that nocebo effects on pain might be more reliably evoked with just a verbal suggestion than placebo effects, making the addition of conditioning less necessary [(20); see also Ref. (2)]. We studied whether these findings also apply to fatigue, dyspnea, nausea, and itch.

NOCEBO EFFECTS EVOKED THROUGH VERBAL SUGGESTIONS

Fatigue. Three studies have investigated a nocebo effect on fatigue from verbal suggestion alone (25, 75, 76). One study (25) found that the suggestion of a fatigue-inducing drink increased participants' rate of exhaustion, but did not decrease their performance or influence cardio-respiratory, muscle, and blood lactate measures, while another found the opposite result, with no effect on rate of exhaustion but a reduction in force output (76). The final study (75) did not find increased fatigue after a nonspecific suggestion of ultrasonic noise. This suggests that nocebo effects from verbal suggestion are possible for fatigue when the suggestion is specific enough, but more evidence is needed.

Dyspnea. Five studies, all using asthmatic participants, have investigated the nocebo effect of suggestion on dyspnea (39, 40, 42, 44, 77). The results are relatively equivocal: two studies found an effect on reported symptoms (39, 77) while two others found no effect (40, 44) and another only found an effect in a subgroup of highly nervous participants (42). Similarly mixed results are found for lung measures, with two studies finding an effect (44, 77), which was not confirmed in two other studies (40, 42). One study additionally found an effect on a measure of airway inflammation (40). The evidence for nocebo effects on dyspnea and related lung function measures arising from verbal suggestion alone is thus rather tenuous. The overall results are very mixed and no clear methodological trend seems to explain them.

Nausea. There are three studies examining nocebo effects from verbal suggestion on nausea (46, 75, 78). No studies found the hypothesized results, reporting no effect on experienced nausea (75, 78), an effect only in men on motion tolerance (78), and a reversed effect (46), where reported nausea and gastric tachyarrhythmia were actually lower for the nocebo group compared to control. The suggestions used in two of these studies were not optimal however, either referring generally to effects of ultrasonic noise (75) or to a drug that would increase nausea but reduce other symptoms of motion sickness (46). These studies suggest that verbal suggestions are not effective for evoking or worsening nausea, but studies using a more specific or unilateral suggestion may prove to be more effective in the future.

Itch. Five studies have investigated nocebo effects from the suggestion of increased itch (11, 79–82). All of them indicate that self-reported itch worsened after the nocebo suggestion, although the results were not consistent for every measure in one study (82). Scratching duration was also increased in one study in the group that received a very negative compared to a more neutral suggestion (81), but this also applied to the group receiving no information, and the difference was only seen in patients. The results on self-reported measures seem to transfer to the associated skin reactions (80), although again not consistently for every measure in one study (82). Napadow and colleagues (79) also performed fMRI analyses, finding increased activity in the dorsolateral prefrontal cortex, caudate, and intraparietal sulcus associated with nocebo itch. These areas responded in similar ways to an actual allergen, suggesting this activation may be specific for itch and not applicable to nocebo effects more generally. The results of these studies indicate that nocebo suggestions can worsen experienced itch, while the evidence is more mixed for behavioral and physiological correlates.

Overall, the studies investigating the effect of only verbal suggestions to induce nocebo effects are less numerous than the corresponding placebo studies, and do not provide enough evidence for solid conclusions. Only in itch are consistent nocebo effects seen, which may be due to the unique qualities of that symptom: itch is known to arise even when it is just talked about or observed in others [contagious itch; see Ref. (83) for a review]. The results for itch seem to most resemble those in pain, where nocebo effects seem easier to evoke than placebo effects. For dyspnea and nausea, the results for placebo and nocebo studies are both mixed, and for fatigue the results for placebo are more consistent than for nocebo effects.

NOCEBO EFFECTS EVOKED THROUGH CONDITIONING

Fatigue. We are aware of only a single study that has examined nocebo effects on fatigue elicited by a combination of verbal suggestion and conditioning (76). The results indicate no effect on perceived exhaustion, though this might also be due to a training effect emerging throughout the repeated sessions of the experiment. The procedure did lead to an overall reduction in performance, although the effect was not larger in the condition combining verbal suggestion and conditioning than in the verbal suggestion alone condition.

Dyspnea. Eight studies have investigated a nocebo effect on dyspnea using conditioning. Two of them combine verbal suggestion and conditioning [Refs. (84–86); note that the latter two use the same dataset), and six rely on conditioning while offering either no suggestion or a similar suggestion in both conditions (87–92). Two studies (84, 87) offer the participant an inhaler and are thus clearly placebo studies, while the others expose participants to scented air *via* a special breathing apparatus but do not offer a physical treatment that would be universally recognized as a placebo. All studies show an increase in self-reported asthma symptoms after conditioning. However, in some studies this increase in self-reported symptoms applied only under certain conditions [i.e., when the conditioning procedure featured an unpleasant and not a pleasant scent (89, 91, 92)] or on some of the included measures [Ref. (87); only subjective airway obstruction was affected, and not feelings of dyspnea or hyperventilation]. Physiological measures of lung functioning and breathing were not affected in three studies (87, 88, 92) while five other studies found an effect on some of the included physiological outcomes (84, 85, 89–91). Many of these studies use healthy samples (84–86, 88–90, 92); the results do not differ systematically between the results of these studies and those where participants were asthmatics (84, 87) or psychosomatic patients (91). These studies together provide convincing evidence that a conditioning procedure can evoke self-reported symptoms of dyspnea, much more clearly than verbal suggestion alone, although the results remain somewhat inconsistent for physiological measures.

Nausea. Four studies have used either conditioning alone (78, 93) or the combination of verbal suggestion and conditioning (70, 94) to induce nocebo effects on nausea. In all cases, self-reported nausea was increased in participants, although one study (78) found the same gender pattern as in placebo nausea, where women responded more strongly than men to the conditioning procedure. The gender pattern also applied when considering how long participants could endure the nausea-inducing rotation. Another study using only conditioning (93) found that participants consumed less of a drink that was associated with the rotation, but no effect on tolerance of rotation and also no effect on two hormonal outcomes. The findings indicate that gender may be an important factor in placebo and nocebo nausea. The combination of verbal suggestion and conditioning seems to be quite effective at influencing nausea, and more effective than suggestion alone, although very limited evidence suggests this might not extend to physiological correlates of nausea.

Itch. The three available studies indicate that the combination of verbal suggestion and conditioning is effective for inducing nocebo effects on itch (57, 71, 95). All of the available studies find a nocebo effect on self-reported itch when using a procedure combining suggestion and conditioning, although one follow-up analysis (72) did not find consistent effects on scratching behavior. Moreover, the study by van de Sand et al. (95) used fMRI to investigate neural activity associated with nocebo itch, finding increased activity in the rolandic operculum and increased connectivity between the insula and periaqueductal grey in the nocebo condition. These results do not correspond to those found in the earlier fMRI study into nocebo itch (79), which did not use conditioning and only tested patients. Activity in the operculum is also found in fMRI nocebo hyperalgesia studies (96), but these results do not overlap with imaging studies for other symptoms. While no immediate pattern emerges from behavioral or physiological outcomes, self-reported itch is clearly influenced when conditioning and verbal suggestion are combined.

The low number of studies on nocebo effects that use conditioning makes it hard to draw a conclusion across symptoms that is not pre-emptive. The limited results available would suggest that nocebo effects on dyspnea and nausea are more robust after the combination of verbal suggestion and conditioning than they are after verbal suggestion alone. The combination procedure did not seem to lead to more robust effects in fatigue, where results are limited but appear weak, or in itch, where verbal suggestion alone already produced clear nocebo effects. In this sense, only the results for itch seems to echo those on pain, where it has also been suggested that nocebo effects can be evoked as easily with suggestion alone as with a combination of suggestion and conditioning (20).

THE MEDIATING ROLE OF EXPECTANCIES

A common theoretical view is that placebo and nocebo effects function by means of expectancies: you will feel less pain when you expect to (61, 97, 98). In pain, research has shown that the expectation of analgesia or hyperalgesia is indeed a contributing factor to placebo and nocebo effects [e.g., Refs. (99–100)]. Current theoretical perspectives generally consider verbal suggestion and conditioning complementary forces that together influence the expectations that in turn influence the experience of noxious sensations (61, 62).

Fatigue. One study (25) found a strong relation between the expectation of increased or decreased fatigue and increases and decreases in performance. Other studies found an effect of the suggestion on participants' expectations, but no relationship between expectations and fatigue (34) or performance (37).

Dyspnea. De Peuter and colleagues (84) found that participants undergoing a nocebo procedure had higher expectations for asthma symptoms as well as higher asthma symptom ratings; however, expectations were only statistically related for asthmatics and not the whole sample. From another angle, a study that specifically tried to not to instill any expectations in participants also found no effects on dyspnea (101).

Nausea. Four studies have directly investigated the role expectations in placebo and nocebo effects on nausea (47, 51, 52, 70), but only one of them (47) found the hypothesized effect, with both expectations of nausea and self-reported nausea lower in the placebo than in the control group. The other studies show discrepancies; either expectancies were affected but nausea was not (52), nausea was effected but expectancies were not (51), or there was a relationship between expectations and nausea for nocebo effects but not for placebo effects (70).

Itch. The study by van Laarhoven and colleagues (11) showed a correlation between expected itch and nocebo-induced itch ratings. Another study found increased expectations but no corresponding effect on itch (34), while a third found a relation between positive expectations and reduced symptoms only in the experimental group (59). An investigation of the mechanisms behind placebo and nocebo effects on itch (102) found that placebo responders self-generated fewer itch expectations in a separate task, although corresponding results were not found for nocebo responders.

The available evidence points to differential effects of expectations for every symptom, with stronger evidence for expectations as a mediator in itch and some evidence in dyspnea, but more evidence against a mediating relationship in fatigue and nausea. Further research is needed to elucidate what underlying mechanisms might additionally play a role in placebo and nocebo effects in these symptoms, especially for nausea and fatigue where expectations might not play an important role. Other mechanisms such as attention and fear have been suggested [e.g., Refs. (103, 104)], but have only been investigated infrequently, especially outside of pain.

IDENTIFYING THE PLACEBO RESPONDER

The question whether it is possible to recognize the placebo responder is almost as old as the study of placebo effects itself (105), but consistent findings have been elusive (106). One possible reason for the lack of consistent findings could be that predictors are different for different symptoms. We therefore review the findings from the included studies for each of the discussed symptoms.

Fatigue. The only study that investigated outcomes on fatigue as well as individual characteristics (34) found no moderating effect of neuroticism, extraversion, positive or negative affectivity, depression, anxiety, catastrophizing, or body vigilance.

Dyspnea. Based on a fear learning model (107), it has been hypothesized that participants high in negative affectivity might respond more strongly to negative suggestions of impaired breathing. This has been examined in several studies, with three finding the expected relationship (42, 87, 88) but four others no relationship (41, 89, 91) or an effect only for one of six subjective breathing measures (84). Suggestibility has also been examined as a possible predictor, with one study finding a relationship (77) that was not confirmed in three other studies (39, 41, 42). Likewise, no effect was found in one study for positivity (41). A final study (91) found no effect for information seeking and a negative effect of a blunting behavioral style.

Nausea. Two studies investigated the relationship between a placebo effect and multiple individual characteristics. One found a larger placebo effect for participants with lower scores on general self-efficacy, internal locus of control, generalized self, and mobility of nervous processes (108), while the other found no effect of the same variables as well as no effect of anxiety or optimism (51). As mentioned before, in other studies an effect is seen for gender, with men showing larger effects on placebo and nocebo nausea after suggestion and women showing larger effects after conditioning (48, 78), although one study also found suggestion effective only in women (51). There is some indication that this effect may be due to the gender of the experimenter (52).

Itch. Several studies in itch have examined many individual characteristics, but found almost no effects for any of them, regardless of whether they found actual placebo or nocebo effects (11, 34, 57, 71). The variables investigated in these studies are theorized to relate to expectations and include neuroticism, extraversion, positive and negative affectivity, depression, anxiety, catastrophizing, body vigilance, optimism, hope, worrying, impulsivity, self-efficacy, general future expectations, suggestibility, and social desirability characteristics. The only one of these studies to find effects (57) did so only in the group where conditioning and verbal suggestion were combined, which was also the only condition that showed effects. Here, a greater placebo effect was associated with less hope, while greater nocebo effects were associated with less hope and extraversion and more worrying, and negative effect. Another study investigating fewer variables (109) found a positive relationship between a placebo effect and ego resiliency but none with neuroticism. Considering the many variables investigated across these studies, the few observed associations should be interpreted with care.

Taken together, these results suggest that individual characteristics do not consistently predict placebo or nocebo effects on fatigue, dyspnea, nausea, and itch. The search for predictors is inconvenienced by the fact that different studies tend to investigate different variables and many results still need to be replicated. It should also be noted that, compared to some other symptoms, the type of variables under consideration is rather narrow, being almost entirely limited to personality factors. Other placebo and nocebo studies have, for example, found indications of genetic predispositions (110) or neurochemical indicators (9). Since placebo effects seem to be determined by a variety of different factors (social, psychological, neurobiological, genetic), future studies may need to incorporate more sophisticated statistical methods to test the combined effect of several predictors at once in order to identify the placebo responder [for some recent examples in pain, see, e.g., Refs. (111, 112)].

DISCUSSION

This review investigated to what extent findings from studies on placebo analgesia and nocebo hyperalgesia also apply to fatigue, dyspnea, nausea, and itch. Broad similarities can be observed in that placebo and nocebo effects are evoked for these symptoms in a large proportion of studies using similar methods. Some specific results also appear to be consistent: placebo effects are more likely after a procedure combining conditioning and verbal suggestion than verbal suggestion alone, and there is no clear evidence which individual characteristics predict who will respond to placebo and who will not. Other findings do not clearly confirm those in pain. We find little evidence that verbal suggestion alone can consistently evoke placebo and nocebo effects across symptoms, with the exception of placebo effects on fatigue and nocebo effects on itch. For dyspnea and nausea only, nocebo effects seem to be larger after a combination of verbal suggestion and conditioning than suggestion alone. There is some evidence for a mediating role of expectations in placebo and nocebo effects across symptoms, although to a lesser extent in nausea or fatigue. Altogether, it seems that placebo and nocebo studies on pain provide a reasonable starting point for predicting these effects in other sensations, but a number of differences caution against extrapolating every finding in pain to other symptoms.

Each of the sensations we discuss has been studied in a line of research separated from the others, each with its own strengths and opportunities for further inquiry. Studies that examine fatigue tend to come from the field of sport psychology, and therefore focus on improving athletic performance. This has led to placebo effects being investigated much more than nocebo effects. Performance is generally the primary outcome, with perceived exhaustion as just one extra variable. Participants in these studies are generally physically active individuals, sometimes even professional athletes. These factors obviously limit the generalizability of these findings to medical contexts, where fatigue is a large problem (113); it remains to be seen to what extent the findings apply to patients suffering from chronic or mental fatigue. In the context of improving performance, investigating mechanisms behind the effect is perhaps a secondary concern, and fewer studies examine the effect of conditioning or individual characteristics that predict the response. Several researchers have, however, started the work of performing tightly controlled experimental studies that offer more insight into the exact mechanisms of placebo and nocebo effects on fatigue [e.g., Refs. (31, 76)]. It would be fruitful to extend these toward the clinical domain, especially since two separate trials have already shown patients suffering from fatigue can benefit from a placebo intervention (114, 115).

In dyspnea, there is a strong clinical focus, since the background of many of these studies comes from the study and treatment of asthma and somatic symptom disorders. A large proportion of studies therefore also uses asthmatics as participants. This, in turn, also limits generalizability for some findings, albeit in another direction than in the case of fatigue. Since this field features older studies, it also shows more methodological limitations, such as low participant numbers, nonspecific suggestions, and unclear symptom induction methods that can easily be rectified in new studies. Studies that include both conditioning and verbal suggestion, allowing the effects to be compared, would also be a valuable addition. A perhaps bigger issue is that no research group seems to have focused specifically on placebo and nocebo effects in dyspnea. This has led to a lack of common methods and conceptualizations that would facilitate comparisons within the subdiscipline and to other subdisciplines, despite having one of the longest traditions of placebo research [reaching as far back as the study in Ref. (116)]. This might be helped by systematic review or meta-analysis, of the type that exists for other fields [e.g., Refs. (117, 118)].

A clear experimental tradition exists in placebo and nocebo effects on nausea. The field originated in the study of anticipatory nausea in chemotherapy (68, 119), so it has a clear clinical angle, even though later studies focus on healthy participants. The subdiscipline also sports two dedicated research groups and insightful reviews (118, 119). A strong theoretical foundation in conditioning has not only improved upon mixed initial results (46, 52) but has also led to the development of the latent inhibition and overshadowing paradigms that are, as of yet, rarely applied in the rest of the placebo literature. We echo earlier calls (120) that these results should be replicated and applied to other fields of placebo research. This subdiscipline also offers conclusions that deviate the most from findings in pain, with an increased importance of gender [(48, 51, 78); see also Ref. (121) for a recent nuanced overview] and indications of a reduced role of expectations (51, 52, 70). The latter finding is further confirmed by findings in clinical trials that report similarly inconsistent results when expectations are explicitly investigated (122, 123). Our findings do appear to fit with earlier speculation that the gustatory system may have a special capability for unconscious conditioning (124). Due to its connection with the digestive system, nausea may have more in common with symptoms like hormone levels that are more affected by unconscious conditioning than consciously accessible expectations (10). However, since pain is also affected by implicit conditioning (125), further comparisons are needed to resolve this question.

Most studies of placebo and nocebo effects on itch are comparatively recent. This has allowed the field to benefit from advances in other subdisciplines, and thus the studies cover different methods and avoid some of the limitations of earlier work. Itch studies also feature a large number of individual variables as possible moderators, although no consistent findings have emerged. This may be taken as an indication that individual predictors, at least of the kind that can be measured by questionnaires, might not provide much further insight in experimental studies of placebo and nocebo effects. Several studies in the field have also investigated effects arising from verbal suggestion without a physical placebo (11, 59, 80–82), one of which also forgoes deception (59). These are interesting explorations of alternative applications of placebo effects that can also be considered in other subdisciplines. Although the two fMRI studies of nocebo itch do not report clearly congruous results, this is an important first step in investigating whether there is a common nocebo network across symptoms.

Aside from pain, fatigue, dyspnea, nausea, and itch, many other symptoms exist that can be affected by placebo and nocebo effects. Results indicate effects on variables as varied as sleep quality (126), symptoms of Parkinson disease (10), and depression (9). The current review was limited to sensations that share several important similarities with pain, but the question of generalizability of course applies to other sensations as well. Comparisons between these other symptoms can also answer important questions about underlying mechanisms and predictors that cannot be answered for the included symptoms in this review. For example, the neurological underpinnings of placebo effects in Parkinson disease have been studied more (9) than similar mechanisms in dyspnea or nausea. Similarly, there are studies of genetic predictors of placebo effects on pain (127) and fatigue (115), but the available research does not allow a comparison of genetic predictors between the symptoms included in this review. Comparisons might also be valuable for predictors with clear implications for clinical practice, such as the perceived cost of the placebo (128, 129), the odds of receiving placebo (51, 130), the invasiveness of the placebo (131, 132), other interventions that could enhance the effect of placebos (133), or pre-existing associations that could influence symptom acquisition [e.g., the color red being associated with pain (134)].

In order to translate findings to clinical practice, a comparison must also be made between healthy and patient populations. The included studies mostly use healthy volunteers as participants, but a reasonable number focus on patients. While the number of studies that compare healthy and patient populations is too low for a meaningful analysis, there is some indication that patients show different or stronger results (79, 81, 84). A meta-analysis of placebo-like effects on pain in patients (99) tentatively indicated that effects on chronic pain are smaller than on experimentally induced or acute procedural pain, possibly because of a relatively high number of unsuccessful treatment experiences in chronic pain patients. These same experiences, however, should theoretically increase the likelihood of nocebo effects. This is especially relevant considering multiple theories that argue that certain chronic conditions may be exacerbated by or find their etiology in learning effects (107, 135, 136). These theories focus on sensitization, fear learning, conditioning, and generalization, which all likely play a role in nocebo effects. More research that compares healthy groups to those suffering chronically from the relevant symptoms or investigates the progression of these chronic complaints is sorely needed to indicate how much support there is for these theories. This would allow knowledge of placebo and nocebo effects to be utilized to prevent the development and aid the treatment of chronic conditions, such as by counterconditioning the nocebo effect (71).

Our conclusions are limited by the small number of studies available. More studies are needed for solid conclusions, especially about nocebo effects and the added value of combining verbal suggestions with conditioning. Many of the included studies include methodological limitations, such as a small sample size, the omission of a baseline measure, ineffective induction of noxious sensation, or a less convincing verbal suggestion. The included studies also show a large amount of heterogeneity in terms of the methods they use to induce noxious sensations or evoke placebo and nocebo effects. Lastly, the lack of a systematic approach means the review is not exhaustive.

In conclusion, learning mechanisms of placebo and nocebo effects show large overlap, but also important differences across pain, fatigue, dyspnea, nausea, and itch. Knowledge of these differences can be used to optimally control these effects in experimental and clinical studies and increase placebo and reduce nocebo effects in clinical practice. As the separate subdisciplines for each symptom not only provide different results, but also differ in the amount and type of studies available, this review also highlights future promising research possibilities.

AUTHOR CONTRIBUTIONS

FW drafted the manuscript, supported by AE and KP. All authors fully read the final draft and provided their approval.

Organization for Scientific Research (NWO) (Grant No. 453-16-004) and an ERC Consolidator Grant from the European Research Council (ERC) (Grant No. 617700), both granted to AE.

REFERENCES

1. Klinger R, Colloca L, Bingel U, Flor H. Placebo analgesia: clinical applications. *Pain* (2013) 155(6):1–16. doi: 10.1016/j.pain.2013.12.007
2. Petersen GL, Finnerup NB, Colloca L, Amanzio M, Price DD, Jensen TS, et al. The magnitude of nocebo effects in pain: a meta-analysis. *Pain* (2014) 155(8):1426–34. doi: 10.1016/j.pain.2014.04.016
3. Vase L, Petersen GL, Riley JL, Price DD. Factors contributing to large analgesic effects in placebo mechanism studies conducted between 2002 and 2007. *Pain* (2009) 145(1–2):36–44. doi: 10.1016/j.pain.2009.04.008
4. Evers AWM, Colloca L, Blease C, Annoni M, Atlas LY, Benedetti F, et al. Implications of placebo and nocebo effects for clinical practice: expert consensus. *Psychother Psychosom* (2018) 87(4):204–10. doi: 10.1159/000490354
5. Benedetti F, Lanotte M, Lopiano L, Colloca L. When words are painful: unraveling the mechanisms of the nocebo effect. *Neuroscience* (2007) 147(2):260–71. doi: 10.1016/j.neuroscience.2007.02.020
6. Klinger R, Blasini M, Schmitz J, Colloca L. Nocebo effects in clinical studies. *PAIN Reports* (2017) 2(2):e586. doi: 10.1097/PR9.0000000000000586
7. Kroenke K, Arrington ME, Manglesdorff A. The prevalence of symptoms in medical outpatients and the adequacy of therapy. *Arch Intern Med* (1990) 150(8):1685–9. doi: 10.1001/archinte.150.8.1685
8. Breivik H, Eisenberg E, O'Brien T. The individual and societal burden of chronic pain in Europe: the case for strategic prioritisation and action to improve knowledge and availability of appropriate care. *BMC Public Health* (2013) 13(1):1229–43. doi: 10.1186/1471-2458-13-1229
9. Benedetti F. Mechanisms of placebo and placebo-related effects across diseases and treatments. *Annu Rev Pharmacol Toxicol* (2008) 48(1):33–60. doi: 10.1146/annurev.pharmtox.48.113006.094711
10. Benedetti F, Pollo A, Lopiano L, Lanotte M, Vighetti S, Rainero I. Conscious expectation and unconscious conditioning in analgesic, motor, and hormonal placebo/nocebo responses. *J Neurosci* (2003) 23(10):4315–23. doi: 10.1523/JNEUROSCI.23-10-04315.2003
11. Van Laarhoven AIM, Vogelaar ML, Wilder-Smith OH, Van Riel PLCM, Van De Kerkhof PCM, Kraaimaat FW, et al. Induction of nocebo and placebo effects on itch and pain by verbal suggestions. *Pain* (2011) 152(7):1486–94. doi: 10.1016/j.pain.2011.01.043
12. Schmelz M. Itch and Pain Differences and Commonalities. In: Schaible H-G, editor. *Pain Control*, vol. 227. Heidelberg: Springer-Verlag Berlin Heidelberg (2015). p. 285–301. doi: 10.1007/978-3-662-46450-2_14
13. Ariel G, Saville W. Anabolic steroids: the physiological effects of placebos. *Med Sci Sports* (1972) 4(2):124–6. doi: 10.1249/00005768-197200420-00015
14. Godfrey S, Silverman M. Demonstration by placebo response in asthma by means of exercise testing. *J Psychosom Res* (1973) 17(4):293–7. doi: 10.1016/0022-3999(73)90106-2
15. Kroenke K. Patients presenting with somatic complaints: epidemiology, psychiatric co-morbidity and management. *Int J Methods Psychiatr Res* (2003) 12(1):34–43. doi: 10.1002/mpr.140
16. Matterne U, Apfelbacher C, Loerbroks A, Schwarzer T, Büttner M, Ofenloch R, et al. Prevalence, correlates and characteristics of chronic pruritus: a population-based cross-sectional study. *Acta Derm Venereol* (2011) 91(6):674–9. doi: 10.2340/00015555-1159
17. Verhoeven EWM, Kraaimaat FW, van de Kerkhof PCM, van Weel C, Duller P, van der Valk PGM, et al. Prevalence of physical symptoms of itch, pain and fatigue in patients with skin diseases in general practice. *Br J Dermatol* (2007) 156(6):1346–49. doi: 10.1111/j.1365-2133.2007.07916.x
18. Lorber W, Mazzoni G, Kirsch I. Illness by suggestion: expectancy, modeling, and gender in the production of psychosomatic symptoms. *Ann Behav Med* (2007) 33(1):112–6. doi: 10.1207/s15324796abm3301_13
19. Vase L, Riley JL, Price DD. A comparison of placebo effects in clinical analgesic trials versus studies of placebo analgesia. *Pain* (2002) 99(3):443–52. doi: 10.1016/S0304-3959(02)00205-1
20. Colloca L, Sigaudo M, Benedetti F. The role of learning in nocebo and placebo effects. *Pain* (2008) 136(1–2):211–8. doi: 10.1016/j.pain.2008.02.006
21. Klinger R, Soost S, Flor H, Worm M. Classical conditioning and expectancy in placebo hypoalgesia: a randomized controlled study in patients with atopic dermatitis and persons with healthy skin. *Pain* (2007) 128(1–2):31–9. doi: 10.1016/j.pain.2006.08.025
22. Bąbel P, Bajcar EA, Adamczyk W, Kicman P, Lisińska N, Świder K, et al. Classical conditioning without verbal suggestions elicits placebo analgesia and nocebo hyperalgesia. *PLoS One* (2017) 12(7):e0181856. doi: 10.1371/journal.pone.0181856
23. Bräscher AK, Kleinböhl D, Hölzl R, Becker S. Differential classical conditioning of the nocebo effect: increasing heat-pain perception without verbal suggestions. *Front Psychol* (2017) 8:1–12. doi: 10.3389/fpsyg.2017.02163
24. Bräscher AK, Witthöft M, Becker S. The underestimated significance of conditioning in placebo hypoalgesia and nocebo hyperalgesia. *Pain Res Manag, 2018* (2018) 2018:6841985. doi: 10.1155/2018/6841985
25. Bottoms L, Buscombe R, Nicholettos A. The placebo and nocebo effects on peak minute power during incremental arm crank ergometry. *Eur J Sports Sci* (2014) 14(4):362–7. doi: 10.1080/17461391.2013.822564
26. Brietzke C, Asano RY, De Russi de Lima F, Pinheiro FA, Franco-Alvarenga PE, Ugrinowitsch C, et al. Caffeine effects on VO2max test outcomes investigated by a placebo perceived-as-caffeine design. *Nutr Health* (2017) 23(4):231–8. doi: 10.1177/0260106017723547
27. Broelz EK, Wolf S, Schneeweiss P, Niess AM, Enck P, Weimer K. Increasing effort without noticing: a randomized controlled pilot study about the ergogenic placebo effect in endurance athletes and the role of supplement salience. *PLoS One* (2018) 13(6):1–14. doi: 10.1371/journal.pone.0198388
28. Duncan MJ. The effect of caffeine ingestion on anaerobic performance in moderately trained adults. *Serbian J Sports Sci* (2010) 3(4):99–106.
29. Duncan MJ, Lyons M, Hankey J. Placebo effects of caffeine on short-term resistance exercise to failure. *Int J Sports Physiol Perform* (2009) 4(2):244–53. doi: 10.1123/ijspp.4.2.244
30. Fanti-Oren S, Birenbaum-Carmeli D, Eliakim A, Pantanowitz M, Nemet D. The effect of placebo on endurance capacity in normal weight children – a randomized trial. *BMC Pediatr* (2019) 19(15):1–5. doi: 10.1186/s12887-019-1394-x
31. Fiorio M, Emadi Andani M, Marotta A, Classen J, Tinazzi M. Placebo-induced changes in excitatory and inhibitory corticospinal circuits during motor performance. *J Neurosci* (2014) 34(11):3993–4005. doi: 10.1523/JNEUROSCI.3931-13.2014

32. Kalasountas V, Reed J, Fitzpatrick J. The effect of placebo-induced changes in expectancies on maximal force production in college students. *J Appl Sports Psychol* (2007) 19(1):116–24. doi: 10.1080/10413200601123736
33. McClung M, Collins D. "Because i know it will!": placebo effects of an ergogenic aid on athletic performance. *J Sport Exerc Psychol* (2007) 29(3):382–94. doi: 10.1123/jsep.29.3.382
34. Peerdeman KJ, Van Laarhoven AIM, Donders ART, Hopman MTE, Peters ML, Evers AWM. Inducing expectations for health: effects of verbal suggestion and imagery on pain, itch, and fatigue as indicators of physical sensitivity. *PLoS ONE* (2015) 10(10):1–16. doi: 10.1371/journal.pone.0139563
35. Piedimonte A, Benedetti F, Carlino E. Placebo-induced decrease in fatigue: evidence for a central action on the preparatory phase of movement. *Eur J Neurosci* (2015) 41(4):492–7. doi: 10.1111/ejn.12806
36. Pollo A, Carlino E, Benedetti F. The top-down influence of ergogenic placebos on muscle work and fatigue. *Eur J Neurosci* (2008) 28(2):379–88. doi: 10.1111/j.1460-9568.2008.06344.x
37. Tallis J, Muhammad B, Islam M, Duncan MJ. Placebo effects of caffeine on maximal voluntary concentric force of the knee flexors and extensors. *Muscle Nerve* (2016) 54(3):479–86. doi: 10.1002/mus.25060
38. Tolusso DAVT, Aurent CMAL, Ullenkamp ADAMMF. Placebo effect: influence on repeated intermittent sprint performance on consecutive days. *J Strength Cond Res* (2015) 29(7):1915–24. doi: 10.1519/JSC.0000000000000844
39. Isenberg SA, Lehrer PM, Hochron S. The effects of suggestion on airways of asthmatic subjects breathing room air as a suggested bronchoconstrictor and bronchodilator. *J Psychosom Res* (1992) 36(8):769–76. doi: 10.1016/0022-3999(92)90135-O
40. Jaén C, Dalton P. Asthma and odors: the role of risk perception in asthma exacerbation. *J Psychosom Res* (2014) 77(4):302–08. doi: 10.1016/j.jpsychores.2014.07.002
41. Kemeny ME, Rosenwasser LJ, Panettieri RA, Rose RM, Berg-Smith SM, Kline JN. Placebo response in asthma: a robust and objective phenomenon. *J Allergy Clin Immunol Pract* (2007) 119(6):1375–81. doi: 10.1016/j.jaci.2007.03.016
42. Put C, Van Den Bergh O, Van Ongeval E, De Peuter S, Demedts M, Verleden G. Negative affectivity and the influence of suggestion on asthma symptoms. *J Psychosom Res* (2004) 57(3):249–55. doi: 10.1016/S0022-3999(03)00541-5
43. Wechsler ME, Kelley JM. Active albuterol or placebo, sham acupuncture, or no intervention in asthma. *N Engl J Med* (2011) 365(2):119–26. doi: 10.1056/NEJMoa1103319
44. Wigal JK, Kotses H, Rawson JC, Creer TL. The effects of suggestion on the total respiratory resistance of nonasthmatic female subjects. *J Psychosom Res* (1988) 32(4–5):409–16. doi: 10.1016/0022-3999(88)90024-4
45. Teeter JG, Bleecker ER. Relationship between airway obstruction and respiratory symptoms in adult asthmatics. *Chest* (1998) 113(2):272–7. doi: 10.1378/chest.113.2.272
46. Levine ME, Stern RM, Koch KL. The effects of manipulating expectations through placebo and nocebo administration on gastric tachyarrhythmia and motion-induced nausea. *Psychosom Med* (2006) 68(3):478–86. doi: 10.1097/01.psy.0000221377.52036.50
47. Müller V, Remus K, Hoffmann V, Tschöp MH, Meissner K. Effectiveness of a placebo intervention on visually induced nausea in women – a randomized controlled pilot study. *J Psychosom Res* (2016) 91:9–11. doi: 10.1016/j.jpsychores.2016.09.012
48. Quinn VF, Colagiuri B. Sources of placebo-induced relief from nausea: the role of instruction and conditioning. *Psychosom Med* (2016) 78(3):365–72. doi: 10.1097/PSY.0000000000000265
49. Schienle A, Übel S, Schöngaßner F, Ille R, Scharmüller W. Disgust regulation *via* placebo: an fMRI study. *Soc Cogn Affect Neurosci* (2014) 9(7):985–90. doi: 10.1093/scan/nst072
50. Schienle A, Übel S, Wabnegger A. When opposites lead to the same: a direct comparison of explicit and implicit disgust regulation via fMRI. *Soc Cogn Affect Neurosci* (2017) 12(3):445–51. doi: 10.1093/scan/nsw144
51. Weimer K, Horing B, Muth ER, Scisco JL, Klosterhalfen S, Enck P. Different disclosed probabilities to receive an antiemetic equally decrease subjective symptoms in an experimental placebo study: to be or not to be sure. *Clin Ther* (2017) 39(3):487–501. doi: 10.1016/j.clinthera.2016.11.022
52. Weimer K, Schulte J, Maichle A, Muth ER, Scisco JL, Horing B, et al. Effects of ginger and expectations on symptoms of nausea in a balanced placebo design. *PLoS ONE* (2012) 7(11):e49031. doi: 10.1371/journal.pone.0049031
53. Williamson MJ, Thomas MJ, Stern RM. The contribution of expectations to motion sickness symptoms and gastric activity. *J Psychosom Res* (2004) 56(6):721–6. doi: 10.1016/S0022-3999(03)00130-2
54. Lieberman MD, Jarcho JM, Berman S, Naliboff BD, Suyenobu BY, Mandelkern M, et al. The neural correlates of placebo effects: a disruption account. *Neuroimage* (2004) 22(1):447–55. doi: 10.1016/j.neuroimage.2004.01.037
55. Wager TD, Atlas LY, Leotti LA, Rilling JK. Predicting individual differences in placebo analgesia: contributions of brain activity during anticipation and pain experience. *J Neurosci* (2011) 31(2):439–52. doi: 10.1523/JNEUROSCI.3420-10.2011
56. Zubieta JK, Yau WY, Scott DJ, Stohler CS. Belief or need? Accounting for individual variations in the neurochemistry of the placebo effect. *Brain Behav Immun* (2006) 20(1):15–26. doi: 10.1016/j.bbi.2005.08.006
57. Bartels DJP, Van Laarhoven AIM, Haverkamp EA, Wilder-Smith OH, Donders ART, Van Middendorp H, et al. Role of conditioning and verbal suggestion in placebo and nocebo effects on itch. *PLoS One* (2014) 9(3):e91727. doi: 10.1371/journal.pone.0091727
58. Darragh M, Chang JWH, Booth RJ, Consedine NS. The placebo effect in inflammatory skin reactions: the influence of verbal suggestion on itch and weal size. *J Psychosom Res* (2015) 78(5):489–94. doi: 10.1016/j.jpsychores.2015.01.011
59. Meeuwis SH, Van Middendorp H, Veldhuijzen DS, Van Laarhoven AIM, De Houwer J, Lavrijsen APM, et al. Placebo effects of open-label verbal suggestions on itch. *Acta Derm Venereol* (2018) 98(2):268–74. doi: 10.2340/00015555-2823
60. Skvortsova A, Veldhuijzen DS, Van Middendorp H, Van Den Bergh O, Evers AWM. Enhancing placebo effects in somatic symptoms through oxytocin. *Psychosom Med* (2018) 80(4):353–60. doi: 10.1097/PSY.0000000000000571
61. Colloca L, Miller FG. How placebo responses are formed: a learning perspective. *Philos Trans R Soc B Biol Sci* (2011) 366(1572):1859–69. doi: 10.1098/rstb.2010.0398
62. Kirsch I, Lynn SJ, Vigorito M, Miller RR. The role of cognition in classical and operant conditioning. *J Clin Psychol* (2004) 60(4):369–92. doi: 10.1002/jclp.10251
63. Adamczyk WM, Wiercioch-Kuzianik K, Bajcar EA, Bąbel P. Rewarded placebo analgesia: a new mechanism of placebo effects based on operant conditioning. *Eur J Pain (United Kingdom)* (2019) 23(5):923–35. doi: 10.1002/ejp.1360
64. Lenaert B, Jansen R, van Heugten CM. You make me tired: an experimental test of the role of interpersonal operant conditioning in fatigue. *Behav Res Ther* (2018) 103:12–7. doi: 10.1016/j.brat.2018.01.006
65. Horing B, Weimer K, Schrade D, Muth ER, Scisco JL, Enck P, et al. Reduction of motion sickness with an enhanced placebo instruction. *Psychosom Med* (2013) 75(5):497–504. doi: 10.1097/PSY.0b013e3182915ee7
66. Hall G, Stockhorst U, Enck P, Klosterhalfen S. Overshadowing and latent inhibition in nausea-based context conditioning in humans: theoretical and practical implications. *Q J Exp Psychol (Hove)* (2015) 69(6):1227–38. doi: 10.1080/17470218.2015.1080739
67. Stockhorst U, Hall G, Enck P, Klosterhalfen S. Effects of overshadowing on conditioned and unconditioned nausea in a rotation paradigm with humans. *Exp Brain Res* (2014) 232(8):2651–64. doi: 10.1007/s00221-014-3998-6
68. Stockhorst U, Weiner JA, Klosterhalfen W, Aul C, Steingruber HJ. Effects of overshadowing on conditioned nausea in cancer patients: an experimental study. *Physiol Behav* (1998) 64(5):743–53. doi: 10.1016/S0031-9384(98)00135-8
69. Klosterhalfen S, Kellermann S, Stockhorst U, Wolf J, Kirschbaum C, Hall G, et al. Latent inhibition of rotation chair-induced nausea in healthy male and female volunteers. *Psychosom Med* (2005) 67(2):335–40. doi: 10.1097/01.psy.0000156930.00201.e0
70. Quinn VF, Livesey EJ, Colagiuri B. Latent inhibition reduces nocebo nausea, even without deception. *Ann Behav Med* (2017) 51(3):432–41. doi: 10.1007/s12160-016-9867-8
71. Bartels DJP, Van Laarhoven AIM, Stroo M, Hijne K, Peerdeman KJ, Donders ART, et al. Minimizing nocebo effects by conditioning with verbal

suggestion: a randomized clinical trial in healthy humans. *PLoS ONE* (2017) 12(9):1–19. doi: 10.1371/journal.pone.0182959

72. Bartels DJP, van Laarhoven AIM, de Kerkhof PCM, Evers AWM. Nocebo effects and scratching behaviour on itch. *Acta Derm Venereol* (2018) 98(10):943–50. doi: 10.2340/00015555-2979
73. Colloca L, Petrovic P, Wager TD, Ingvar M, Benedetti F. How the number of learning trials affects placebo and nocebo responses. *Pain* (2010) 151(2):430–9. doi: 10.1016/j.pain.2010.08.007
74. Colagiuri B, Quinn VF, Colloca L. Nocebo hyperalgesia, partial reinforcement, and extinction. *J Pain* (2015) 16(10):995–1004. doi: 10.1016/j.jpain.2015.06.012
75. Fletcher MD, Lloyd Jones S, White PR, Dolder CN, Leighton TG, Lineton B. Effects of very high-frequency sound and ultrasound on humans. Part II: a double-blind randomized provocation study of inaudible 20-kHz ultrasound. *J Acoust Soc Am* (2018) 144(4):2521–31. doi: 10.1121/1.5063818
76. Pollo A, Carlino E, Vase L, Benedetti F. Preventing motor training through nocebo suggestions. *Eur J Appl Physiol Occup Physiol* (2012) 112(11):3893–903. doi: 10.1007/s00421-012-2333-9
77. Leigh R, Macqueen G, Tougas G, Hargreave FE, Bienenstock J. Change in forced expiratory volume in 1 second after sham bronchoconstrictor in suggestible but not suggestion-resistant asthmatic subjects: a pilot study. *Psychosom Med* (2003) 65(5):791–5. doi: 10.1097/01.PSY.0000079454.48714.1B
78. Klosterhalfen S, Kellermann S, Braun S, Kowalski A, Schrauth M, Zipfel S, et al. Gender and the nocebo response following conditioning and expectancy. *J Psychosom Res* (2009) 66(4):323–8. doi: 10.1016/j.jpsychores.2008.09.019
79. Napadow V, Li A, Loggia ML, Kim J, Mawla I, Desbordes G, et al. The imagined itch: brain circuitry supporting nocebo-induced itch in atopic dermatitis patients. *Allergy* (2015) 70(11):1485–92. doi: 10.1111/all.12727
80. Scholtz OB, Hermanns N. Illness behavor and cognitions influence the perception of itching of patients suffering from atopic dermatitis. *Z Klin Psychol* (1994) 23(2):127–35.
81. Schut C, Rädel A, Frey L, Gieler U, Kupfer J. Role of personality and expectations for itch and scratching induced by audiovisual itch stimuli. *Eur J Pain* (2016) 20:14–18. doi: 10.1002/ejp.751
82. Stumpf A, Zerey V, Heuft G, Ständer S, Pfleiderer B, Schneider G. Itch perception and skin reactions as modulated by verbal suggestions: role of participant's and investigator's sex. *Acta Derm Venereol* (2016) 96(5):619–23. doi: 10.2340/00015555-2336
83. Schut C, Grossman S, Gieler U, Kupfer J, Yosipovitch G. Contagious itch: what we know and what we would like to know. *Front Hum Neurosci* (2015) 9:1–6. doi: 10.3389/fnhum.2015.00057
84. De Peuter S, Van Diest I, Lemaigre V, Li W, Verleden G, Demedts M, et al. Can subjective asthma symptoms be learned? *Psychosom Med* (2005) 67(3):454–61. doi: 10.1097/01.psy.0000160470.43167.e2
85. Fannes S, Van Diest I, Meulders A, De Peuter S, Vansteenwegen D, Van den Bergh O. To inhale or not to inhale: conditioned avoidance in breathing behavior in an odor-20% CO2 paradigm. *Biol Psychol* (2008) 78(1):87–92. doi: 10.1016/j.biopsycho.2008.01.003
86. Meulders A, Fannes S, Van Diest I, De Peuter S, Vansteenwegen D, Van den Bergh O. Resistance to extinction in an odor-20% CO2 inhalation paradigm: further evidence for a symptom learning account of multiple chemical sensitivity. *J Psychosom Res* (2010) 68(1):47–56. doi: 10.1016/j.jpsychores.2009.03.009
87. De Peuter S, Put C, Lemaigre V, Demedts M, Verleden G, Van Den Bergh O. Context-evoked overperception in asthma. *Psychol Health* (2007) 22(6):737–48. doi: 10.1080/14768320601151702
88. Devriese S, Winters W, Stegen K, Van Diest I, Veulemans H, Nemery B, et al. Generalization of acquired somatic symptoms in response to odors: a pavlovian perspective on multiple chemical sensitivity. *Psychosom Med* (2000) 62(6):751–9. doi: 10.1097/00006842-200011000-00003
89. Van den Bergh O, Kempynck PJ, Van de Woestijne KP, Baeyens F, Eelen P. Respiratory learning and somatic complaints: a conditioning approach using CO2-enriched air inhalation. *Behav Res Ther* (1995) 33(5):517–27. doi: 10.1016/0005-7967(94)00080-4
90. Van den Bergh O, Stegen K, Diest I. Van, Raes C. E. Al.. Acquisition and extinction of somatic symptoms in response to odours: a pavlovian paradigm relevant to multiple chemical sensitivity. *Occup Environ Med* (1999) 56(5):295–301. doi: 10.1136/oem.56.5.295
91. Van den Bergh O, Stegen K, Van De Woestijne KP. Learning to have psychosomatic complaints: conditioning of respiratory behavior and somatic complaints in psychosomatic patients. *Psychosom Med* (1997) 59(1):13–23. doi: 10.1097/00006842-199701000-00003
92. Van den Bergh O, Stegen K, Van De Woestijne KP. Memory effects on symptom reporting in a respiratory learning paradigm. *Health Psychology* (1998) 17(3):241–8. doi: 10.1037/0278-6133.17.3.241
93. Klosterhalfen S, Rüttgers A, Krumrey E, Otto B, Stockhorst U, Riepl RL, et al. Pavlovian conditioning of taste aversion using a motion sickness paradigm. *Psychosom Med* (2000) 62(5):671–7. doi: 10.1097/00006842-200009000-00011
94. Quinn VF, MacDougall HG, Colagiuri B. Galvanic vestibular stimulation: a new model of placebo-induced nausea. *J Psychosom Res* (2015) 78(5):484–8. doi: 10.1016/j.jpsychores.2014.12.011
95. van de Sand MF, Menz MM, Sprenger C, Büchel C. Nocebo-induced modulation of cerebral itch processing – an fMRI study. *Neuroimage* (2018) 166(2017):209–18. doi: 10.1016/j.neuroimage.2017.10.056
96. Amanzio M, Palermo S, Benedetti F. Nocebo and Pain. In: *The Neuroscience of Pain, Stress, and Emotion: Psychological and Clinical Implications*. Cambridge: Academic Press (2016). doi: 10.1016/B978-0-12-800538-5.00006-6
97. Kirsch I. Response expectancy as determinant of experience and behavior. *Am Psychol* (1985) 40(11):1189–202. doi: 10.1037//0003-066X.40.11.1189
98. Peerdeman KJ, van Laarhoven AIM, Peters ML, Evers AWM. An integrative review of the influence of expectancies on pain. *Front Psychol* (2016) 7:1–7. doi: 10.3389/fpsyg.2016.01270
99. Peerdeman KJ, Van Laarhoven AIM, Keij SM, Vase L, Rovers MM, Peters ML, et al. Relieving patients' pain with expectation interventions: a meta-analysis. *Pain* (2016) 157(6):1179–91. doi: 10.1097/j.pain.0000000000000540
100. Pollo A, Amanzio M, Arslanian A, Casadio C, Maggi G, Benedetti F. Response expectancies in placebo analgesia and their clinical relevance. *Pain* (2001) 93(1):77–84. doi: 10.1016/S0304-3959(01)00296-2
101. O'Donnell CR, Lansing RW, Schwartzstein RM, Banzett R. The effect of aerosol saline on laboratory-induced dyspnea. *Lung* (2017) 195(1):37–42. doi: 10.1007/s00408-016-9971-3
102. Bartels DJP, van Laarhoven AIM, Heijmans N, Hermans D, Debeer E, van de Kerkhof PCM, et al. Cognitive schemas in placebo and nocebo responding: role of autobiographical memories and expectations. *Clin Ther* (2017) 39(3):502–12.e1. doi: 10.1016/j.clinthera.2017.02.004
103. Flaten MA, Aslaksen PM, Lyby PS, Bjorkedal E. The relation of emotions to placebo responses. *Philos Trans R Soc B Biol Sci* (2011) 366(1572):1818–27. doi: 10.1098/rstb.2010.0407
104. Gibbons FX, Carver CS, Scheier MF, Hormuth SE. Self-focused attention and the placebo effect: fooling some of the people some of the time. *J Exp Soc Psychol* (1979) 15(3):263–74. doi: 10.1016/0022-1031(79)90037-4
105. Lasagna LC. Placebos. *Sci Am* (1955) 193:68–71. doi: 10.1038/scientificamerican0855-68
106. Kaptchuk TJ, Kelley JM, Deykin A, Wayne PM, Lasagna LC, Epstein IO, et al. Do "placebo responders" exist? *Contemp Clin Trials* (2008) 29(4):587–95. doi: 10.1016/j.cct.2008.02.002
107. Janssens T, Verleden G, De Peuter S, Van Diest I, Van den Bergh O. Inaccurate perception of asthma symptoms: a cognitive-affective framework and implications for asthma treatment. *Clin Psychol Rev* (2009) 29(4):317–27. doi: 10.1016/j.cpr.2009.02.006
108. Horing B, Weimer K, Muth ER, Enck P. Prediction of symptom change in placebo versus no-treatment group in experimentally induced motion sickness. *Appl Psychophysiol Biofeedback* (2015) 40(3):163–72. doi: 10.1007/s10484-015-9284-y
109. Darragh M, Booth RJ, Consedine NS. Trait predictors of placebo responses in itch. *Psychol, Health Med* (2016) 21(6):769–75. doi: 10.1080/13548506.2015.1115106
110. Colagiuri B, Schenk LA, Kessler MD, Dorsey SG, Colloca L. The placebo effect: from concepts to genes. *Neuroscience* (2015) 307:171–90. doi: 10.1016/j.neuroscience.2015.08.017
111. De Pascalis V, Scacchia P. The influence of reward sensitivity, heart rate dynamics and EEG-delta activity on placebo analgesia. *Behav Brain Res* (2019) 359:320–32. doi: 10.1016/j.bbr.2018.11.014

112. Zhou L, Wei H, Zhang H, Li X, Bo C, Wan L, et al. The influence of expectancy level and personal characteristics on placebo effects: psychological underpinnings. *Front Psychiatry* (2019) 10:1–10. doi: 10.3389/fpsyt.2019.00020
113. Rosenthal TC, Majeroni BA, Pretorius R, Malik K. Fatigue: an overview. *Am Fam Physician* (2008) 78(10):1173–9.
114. Hoenemeyer TW, Kaptchuk TJ, Mehta TS, Fontaine KR. Open-label placebo treatment for cancer-related fatigue: a randomized-controlled clinical trial. *Sci Rep* (2018) 8(1):4–11. doi: 10.1038/s41598-018-20993-y
115. Zhou ES, Hall KT, Michaud AL, Blackmon JE, Partridge AH, Recklitis CJ. Open-label placebo reduces fatigue in cancer survivors: a randomized trial. *Support Care Cancer* (2018) 27:(6):2179–87. doi: 10.1007/s00520-018-4477-6
116. Luparello T, Lyons HA, Bleecker ER, McFadden ER. Influences of suggestion on airway reactivity in asthmatic subjects. *Psychosom Med* (1968) 30(6):819–25. doi: 10.1097/00006842-196811000-00002
117. Fiorio M. Modulation of the Motor System by Placebo and Nocebo Effects. In: *International Review of Neurobiology.*, 1st ed., vol. 139. Amsterdam: Elsevier (2018). doi: 10.1016/bs.irn.2018.07.012
118. Quinn VF, Colagiuri B. Placebo interventions for nausea: a systematic review. *Ann Behav Med* (2015) 49(3):449–62. doi: 10.1007/s12160-014-9670-3
119. Stockhorst U, Steingrueber H-J, Enck P, Klosterhalfen S. Pavlovian conditioning of nausea and vomiting. *Auton Neurosci* (2006) 129(1–2):50–7. doi: 10.1016/j.autneu.2006.07.012
120. Quinn VF, Colagiuri B. Using learning strategies to inhibit the nocebo effect. In: *International Review of Neurobiology.*, 1st ed., vol. 138. Cambridge: Academic Press (2018). doi: 10.1016/bs.irn.2018.01.011
121. Enck P, Klosterhalfen S. Does sex/gender play a role in placebo and nocebo effects? conflicting evidence from clinical trials and experimental studies. *Front Neurosci* (2019) 13:160. doi: 10.3389/fnins.2019.00160
122. Roscoe JA, Ph D, Neill MO, Jean-pierre P, Ph D, Heckler E, et al. An exploratory study on the effects of an expectancy manipulation on chemotherapy-related nausea. *J Pain Symptom Manage* (2010) 40(3):379–90. doi: 10.1016/j.jpainsymman.2009.12.024
123. Shelke AR, Roscoe JA, Morrow GR, Colman LK, Banerjee TK, Kirshner JJ. Effect of a nausea expectancy manipulation on chemotherapy-induced nausea: a university of rochester cancer center community clinical oncology program study. *NIH Public Access* (2008) 35(4):381–7. doi: 10.1016/j.jpainsymman.2007.05.008
124. Lovibond PF, Shanks DR. The role of awareness in pavlovian conditioning: empirical evidence and theoretical implications. *J Exp Psychol: Anim Behav Processes* (2002) 28(1):3–26. doi: 10.1037/0097-7403.28.1.3
125. Bräscher AK, Witthöft M. Nocebo hyperalgesia induced by implicit conditioning. *J Behav Ther Exp Psychiatry* (2019) 64:106–12. doi: 10.1016/j.jbtep.2019.03.006
126. Fratello F, Curcio G, Ferrara M, Marzano C, Couyoumdjian A, Petrillo G, et al. Can an inert sleeping pill affect sleep? effects on polysomnographic, behavioral and subjective measures. *Psychopharmacology* (2005) 181(4):761–70. doi: 10.1007/s00213-005-0035-2
127. Yu R, Gollub RL, Vangel M, Kaptchuk TJ, Smoller JW, Kong J. Placebo analgesia and reward processing: integrating genetics, personality, and intrinsic brain activity. *Hum Brain Mapp* (2014) 35(9):4583–93. doi: 10.1002/hbm.22496
128. Espay AJ, Norris MM, Eliassen JC, Dwivedi A, Smith MS, Banks C, et al. Placebo effect of medication cost in parkinson disease: a randomized double-blind study. *Neurology* (2015) 85(8):742–3. doi: 10.1212/WNL.0000000000001879
129. Faasse K, Cundy T, Gamble G, Petrie KJ. The effect of an apparent change to a branded or generic medication on drug effectiveness and side effects. *Psychosom Med* (2013) 75(1):90–6. doi: 10.1097/PSY.0b013e3182738826
130. Rief W, Glombiewski JA. The hidden effects of blinded, placebo-controlled randomized trials: an experimental investigation. *Pain* (2012) 153(12):2473–7. doi: 10.1016/j.pain.2012.09.007
131. Fässler M, Meissner K, Kleijnen J, Hróbjartsson A, Linde K. A systematic review found no consistent difference in effect between more and less intensive placebo interventions. *J Clin Epidemiol* (2014) 68(4):442–51. doi: 10.1016/j.jclinepi.2014.11.018
132. Kaptchuk TJ, Goldman P, Stone DA, Stason WB. Do medical devices have enhanced placebo effects? *J Clin Epidemiol* (2000) 53(8):786–92. doi: 10.1016/S0895-4356(00)00206-7
133. Elsenbruch S, Roderigo T, Enck P, Benson S. Can a brief relaxation exercise modulate placebo or nocebo effects in a visceral pain model? *Front Psychiatry* (2019) 10:1–14. doi: 10.3389/fpsyt.2019.00144
134. Wiercioch-Kuzianik K, Bąbel P. Color hurts. the effect of color on pain perception. *Pain Med* (2019) 00(0):1–8. doi: 10.1093/pm/pny285
135. Lenaert B, Boddez Y, Vlaeyen JWS, van Heugten CM. Learning to feel tired: a learning trajectory towards chronic fatigue. *Behav Res Ther* (2018) 100:54–66. doi: 10.1016/j.brat.2017.11.004
136. Tanaka M, Watanabe Y. A new hypothesis of chronic fatigue syndrome: co-conditioning theory. *Med Hypotheses* (2010) 75(2):244–9. doi: 10.1016/j.mehy.2010.02.032

18

The Knowledge of Contextual Factors as Triggers of Placebo and Nocebo Effects in Patients with Musculoskeletal Pain: Findings from a National Survey

*Giacomo Rossettini[1], Alvisa Palese[2], Tommaso Geri[1], Mattia Mirandola[1], Fabio Tortella[1] and Marco Testa[1]**

[1] Department of Neuroscience, Rehabilitation, Ophthalmology, Genetics, Maternal and Child Health, University of Genova, Savona, Italy, [2] Department of Medical Sciences, University of Udine, Udine, Italy

***Correspondence:**
Marco Testa
marco.testa@unige.it

Backgrounds: Contextual factors (CFs) have been recently proposed as triggers of placebo and nocebo effects in musculoskeletal pain. CFs encompass the features of the clinician (e.g. uniform), patient (e.g. expectations), patient–clinician relationship (e.g. verbal communication), treatment (e.g. overt therapy), and healthcare setting (e.g. design). To date, the researchers' understanding of Italian patients' knowledge about the role of CFs in musculoskeletal pain is lacking.

Objectives: The aim of this study was to investigate attitudes and beliefs of Italian patients with musculoskeletal pain about the use of CFs in clinical practice.

Methods: A national sample of Italian patients with musculoskeletal pain was recruited from 12 outpatient private clinics in Italy. An invitation to participate in an online survey was sent to patients: a) exhibiting musculoskeletal pain; b) aged 18–75; c) with a valid e-mail account; and d) understanding Italian language. Survey Monkey software was used to deliver the survey. The questionnaire was self-reported and included 17 questions and 2 clinical vignettes on the patients' behavior, beliefs, and attitudes towards the adoption of CFs in clinical practice. Descriptive statistics and frequencies described the actual number of respondents to each question.

Results: One thousand one hundred twelve patients participated in the survey. Five hundred seventy-four participants were female (52%). The average age of patients was 41.7 ± 15.2 years. Patients defined CFs as an intervention with an unspecific effect (64.3%), but they believed in their clinical effectiveness. They identified several therapeutic effects of CFs for different health problems. Their use was considered ethically acceptable when it exerts beneficial psychological effects (60.4%), but it was banned if considered deceptive (51.1%). During clinical practice, patients wanted to be informed about the use of CFs (46.0%) that are accepted as an addition to other interventions to optimize clinical responses (39.3%). Moreover, patients explained the power of CFs through body–mind connections (37.1%).

Conclusion: Patients with musculoskeletal pain had positive attitudes towards the use and effectiveness of CFs when associated with evidence-based therapy. They mostly perceived the adoption of CFs in clinical practice as ethical.

Keywords: placebo effect, nocebo effect, pain, musculoskeletal, survey, conditioning, learning, expectation

INTRODUCTION

Placebo and nocebo effects represent an emerging area of interest in musculoskeletal treatment. In this field, for several years, researchers have considered placebo and nocebo as incidental elements to be supervised in randomized controlled trials aimed at isolating the specific effect of a treatment (1). However, in the last decades, the modern neurobiological perspective has conceptualized placebo and nocebo effects as results of the psychosocial context surrounding every healthcare intervention, capable of influencing patients' pain (2).

Placebo effects are the beneficial result of a patient's exposure to a positive context (3), while nocebo effects are adverse consequences of a patient's interaction with a negative context (4). Expectations and conditioning are the main psychological mechanisms underlying placebo and nocebo effects, although social learning and mindset theories have also been demonstrated as explanations of their existing and their functioning (5–7). From a neurobiological perspective, the release of specific neurotransmitters is associated with the exposure to specific contexts: endogenous opioids, dopamine, cannabinoids, oxytocin, and vasopressin have been observed in positive contexts, while opioid and dopamine deactivation and cholecystokinin and cyclooxygenase-prostaglandins activation were observed in negative contexts (8–11). Moreover, different contexts can modulate neural pathways involved in the descending control of pain, influencing the activity of anterior cingulate cortex, dorsolateral prefrontal cortex, periaqueductal grey, and spinal cord (12–16).

The context is composed of several therapeutic signs, symbols, metaphors, and healing rituals (17, 18), called Contextual Factors (CFs), that inform the patients on the value and the meaning of treatment delivered and can influence their healthcare experience by triggering placebo and nocebo effects (19). The therapeutic encounter is strongly characterized by CFs such as a) the clinicians' beliefs and behaviors; b) the patients' expectations and his/her previous experiences; c) the colour and the shape of the intervention; d) the verbal and non-verbal element of communication; and e) the ornaments and the colour of the healthcare setting (2). A robust body of evidence informs clinicians about the positive impact of CFs on therapeutic outcomes such as pain, disability, satisfaction, and perceived quality in different healthcare field as medicine, nursing, physiotherapy, musculoskeletal, and neurological rehabilitation (2, 20–23). As a consequence, a recent experts consensus suggested the adoption of CFs to stimulate placebo effects and to avoid nocebo effects, thus increasing the overall effectiveness of established evidence-based interventions (24).

Abbreviations: CFs, Contextual Factors; EQI, EuroQol Index; CHERRIES, Checklist for Reporting Results of Internet E-Surveys; STROBE, STrengthening the Reporting of OBservational Studies in Epidemiology.

From a clinical perspective, the patient's point of view about CFs has been proposed as a central line of investigation (25). Up to now, qualitative and quantitative researches have investigated the participants' point of view towards placebo using focus groups (26, 27), interviews (28–30), and surveys (31–39–44). Studies have been performed in different countries such as the US (28, 29, 32–33, 34, 38, 39), Asia (27, 42, 43), Australia (36), and Europe (26, 30, 31, 35, 37, 40, 41, 44), involving healthy subjects (26, 27, 32, 34, 41–43) and patients with acute/chronic health conditions (30, 36–39, 40, 44), depression (43), irritable bowel syndrome (28, 29), and rheumatic and musculoskeletal pain (31, 33, 35). Overall, findings revealed a) a heterogeneous understanding of placebo effects, ranging from limited (27, 32, 33, 35, 36, 40) to well-expressed knowledge (30, 31, 37, 39); b) a dualistic conceptualization of placebo effects, as a beneficial element to be legitimized or as ineffective (26, 28); and c) an open vision about placebos in clinical practice, revealing the deception and the lack of informed consent as major ethical issues of their use (27, 30, 32–38, 39, 44). However, the cultural differences and the various adopted definitions of "placebo treatment" threatened the development of a coherent body of evidence and require more research in the field (25, 39), particularly in Italy, where no studies have investigated the attitudes and beliefs of Italian patients towards CFs.

Moreover, among other different chronic conditions greatly affecting the quality of life of patients, musculoskeletal pain medicine represents an interesting and open field of investigation, given its high frequency and its pervasion by CFs (2). Aligned with this vision, the aims of our study were to explore: a) the clinical behaviors, b) the definition, c) the beliefs, d) the ethical concerning, e) the communication implications, f) the circumstances of application, and g) the mechanism of actions of CFs in a nationwide sample of Italian patients with musculoskeletal pain.

MATERIALS AND METHODS

Design

A quantitative web-based cross-sectional survey herein reported in accordance with the Checklist for Reporting Results of Internet E-Surveys (CHERRIES) guidelines (45) and STrengthening the Reporting of OBservational Studies in Epidemiology (STROBE) (46) was performed. The Liguria Clinical Experimental Ethics Committee (P.R.236REG2016, accepted on 19/07/2016) approved the present study.

Participants and Setting

A national sample of Italian patients with musculoskeletal pain was recruited from 12 outpatients' private clinics located in different regions of Italy (North, n = 4; Centre, n = 4; South, n = 4) between May and August 2018.

Managers of each clinic provided the list of patients recruited for this survey to the principal investigator. The patients were included/excluded in accordance with the physician's judgement based on the defined criteria. The inclusion criteria were as follows: a) age between 18 and 75 (38, 39); b) being currently affected by musculoskeletal pain due to either acute traumatic events (e.g., a fracture) or chronic complaints (e.g., overuse) (47); c) having a valid e-mail account; d) good understanding of the Italian language (33); and e) a EuroQol Index (EQI) < 1. The EQI has values ranging from 0 (worst) to 1 (best) and was calculated using the specific normative data of the Italian population (48). The EQI was calculated starting from the answers given in the EuroQol 5-dimensional scale (EQ-5D-3L), that is, a descriptive system composed of five closed three-level single answer questions, exploring mobility, self-care, usual activities, pain/discomfort, and anxiety/depression domains. Patients affected by cancer or by non-musculoskeletal cause of pain (e.g. neuropathic pain) (33) were excluded.

The number of eligible people who responded to the survey was 1,112. With this sample size, a relative standard error of 3% of the true estimate in the population with a 95% confidence level within 0.03 percentage points was expected, using a simple random sampling approach and with the population proportion set to 50% (49).

Questionnaire Development and Pre-Testing

A survey instrument which included questions and clinical vignettes was developed adapting a previous survey on CFs performed among Italian physical therapists and nursing by our research group (50, 51). Questions and clinical vignettes were linguistically adapted to facilitate patient's understanding and answers by the research group. In the whole questionnaire, the word "placebo" was avoided preferring the word "contextual factors" aimed at improving the number of responses by participants (26, 50–52).

The initial list was composed of 22 questions and 2 clinical vignettes that were critically appraised for face and content validity (53) using a panel of seven experts with a wide experience in placebo and survey design (a psychologist, a nurse, and five physical therapists). The experts checked the list independently providing feedback on content accuracy, relevance, wording clarity, and survey structure. Following the feedback received, some adjustments were made and the number of questions was reduced from 22 to 17 because there were overlapping and redundancy.

Once consensus on the final questionnaire was reached among the experts, a preliminary version of the survey, composed of 17 questions and 2 clinical vignettes, was piloted in a convenience sample of 45 patients with musculoskeletal pain and coming from different Italian regions (North, n = 15, Centre, n = 15; South, n = 15) (54).

After the pilot, a telephone debriefing session was performed (53). Experts interviewed the convenience sample of patients about the possible problems encountered during the survey (e.g. recognizing questions that needed additional explanation, wording that was hard to read or that participants found unclear). The outcome of the pilot phase offered the opportunity to reword three items (regarding ethics, communication, and mechanism of action) and to improve the readability of the entire survey.

Questionnaire Implementation

The self-administered questionnaire (**Supplementary file 1** – English version, **Supplementary file 2** – Italian version) adopted in this study was divided into three sections (A, B, C), which used both open-ended and closed multiple-choice questions (55).

Section A investigated the socio-demographic variables using six questions (age, sex, geographical region, social status, workplace, and education). Three closed multiple-choice single answer questions explored the features of musculoskeletal pain (anatomical location, time of onset, and intensity using Numeric Rating Scale 0–10) (56).

In Section B, two clinical vignettes were presented as two closed multiple-choice questions with, respectively, single and multiple answers:

1) the first vignette was about the use of massage in a patient with low back pain and high expectations towards this treatment based on previous positive experience. Participant were asked to choose what they considered the best action in this situation in which the clinician knew that massage was not indicated and that the low back pain would have spontaneously disappeared in a short time;
2) the second vignette described a clinical case of patient with shoulder pain who responded positively when a sham laser (with power-off) replaced the active laser therapy. In this scenario, participants were asked to draw a conclusion about the efficacy and effectiveness of the sham laser.

Section C comprised eight closed questions. Three closed multiple-choice single answer questions investigated the definition of CFs ("How would you define the therapeutic role of CFs?"), the participants' CFs belief (Likert from 0 "not at all" to 4 "a lot of"), and the potential beneficial effects of CFs ("What are the potential effects of CFs in the following health problems?"). Moreover, five closed multiple-choice multiple answers explored the ethical implications perceived in adopting CFs (e.g. "The use of CFs for therapeutic purposes can be considered ethically acceptable when…."), communication implications about CFs ("How do you communicate to the patient the use of CFs at the end of treatment?'), the circumstances under which they are applied ("Under what circumstances would you use CFs?"), and the possible mechanisms of action ("What mechanism of action can explain the effect of CFs?").

Data Collection Procedure

Survey Monkey (Survey-Monkey, Palo Alto, California, www.surveymonkey.com) online survey tool was adopted to administer the questionnaire. The survey was disseminated over a 12-week period between 18th May 2018 and 18th August 2018. Participants were contacted using the mailing list of the 12-outpatient private clinics (55). An email including the survey link (https://it.surveymonkey.com/r/contestopazientiitalianimsk) and a brief note outlining a) the aim of the study, b) data handling (anonymity), c) the informed consent statement, and d) the invitation to complete the survey was distributed. More specifically, the statement in the email informed the recipient that, by clicking on the survey link, the respondents were providing their consent to participate in the study (55). Moreover, an operational definition of CFs was provided to introduce participants to the topic, thus avoiding misinterpretation (30, 35–39): "CFs represent a series of relational or environmental situations capable of influencing the perception of your healthcare condition. Examples of CFs are: the words and posture used by the clinician, the smells, the sounds, and the furnishing of the therapeutic setting" (2).

Three email reminders were sent 4 and 8 and 12 weeks after the initial contact to encourage those who did not take part in the survey to complete it. The time required to complete the survey was 10–15 min (12 min on average), as per the optimal time required to increase response rates in online surveys (57). Participation was voluntary, and no incentives were offered to participants (55). Due to forced response validation, participants were required to answer all questions to prevent missing data (58). Participants were able to review or change responses using a back button before getting to the end of the questionnaire. At the end of the survey, a summary of the answers was provided to the participants (55). Data were copied and deposited in an encrypted computer, and only the project leader could access information achieved in all stages of the study (55). Participants' identities remained concealed to researchers; all data were anonymized (names and mail addresses) to ensure confidentiality and data protection and to avoid psychological harm (55).

Data Analysis

Survey data were downloaded from SurveyMonkey into .xls format and reviewed for data quality.

For descriptive statistics, continuous variables were reported using mean and standard deviation (SD). The five response options for the domain beliefs about CFs were also analyzed with mean and SD in order to have an average distribution of each single belief. Dichotomous, nominal, and ordinal variables, coming from single answer questions, were described using absolute and relative frequencies. Intervals of the observed estimates were calculated with a 95% confidence level (95%CI). For the questions with multiple answers, the absolute and relative frequencies were calculated for each combination of responses given by each participant. For example, considering that the fields (n) asked in the domain "Non-ethic" were three with dichotomous responses (r), we did not calculate the absolute frequency of the three possible fields, but of their eight combinations, given by the formula r^n, to better describe the groups of participants giving multiple answers present in the population.

The association between the individual characteristics (section A of the survey) and the single choice responses given in sections B and C of the survey was investigated with Cramer's V, which is a measure of strength and direction of association derived from chi-square statistics, which was not considered for the analysis of the differences because its significance depends on the size of the sample. For this purpose, age was transformed into ordinal variables considering a decade as variable levels for the analysis of correlations, as described below. Only correlation values above the threshold of acceptance set at 0.60 were reported.

Data analysis was handled using R software (59) and the psych (60) and ggplot2 (61) packages.

RESULTS

Participants' Characteristics

The majority of patients (n = 574; 51.6%; 95%CI 48.6–54.6) were female; their average age was 41.7 ± 15.2 years. 43.9% of participants (n = 488; 95%CI 40.9–46.9) were living in the North of Italy at the time of the survey.

Fifty point three percent of participants were high school graduate (n = 559; 95%CI 47.3–53.2); a large part of them were employed (n = 755; 67.9%; 95%CI 65.0–70.6) in intellectual, scientific, and highly specialized professions (n = 164; 14.7%; 95%CI 12.7–17.0).

Participants reported musculoskeletal pain principally located in the cervical spine and head region (n = 258; 23.2%; 95%CI 20.8–25.8). They had been suffering from pain for >6 months (n = 563; 50.6%; 95%CI 47.6–53.6) with a mean level of severity of 4.9 out of 10 (95%CI 4.8–5.0). The EQI presented a mean of 0.85 out of 1 ± 0.12.

The respondents' demographics are described in **Table 1**.

Clinical Vignette 1

The most frequently chosen solution to the first vignette was "to suggest the possibility of delivering massage if the clinical condition fails to improve" (n = 525; 47.2%; 95%CI 44.2–50.2). The least frequent answer instead was to "try to convince the patient of the uselessness of massage" (n = 79; 7.1%; 95%CI 5.7–8.8). The overall overview of data is reported in **Figure 1**.

Clinical Vignette 2

The most frequent answer to the second vignette was "pain is not organic but psychological" (n = 496; 44.6%; 95%CI 41.7–47.6), while the least frequent one was "supporting patient determined improvements after treatment with sham laser (power-off)" (n = 99; 8.9%; 95%CI 7.3–10.8). The single items and their combinations are presented in **Figure 2**.

Definition of CFs

The majority of patients defined CFs as "an intervention without a specific effect for the condition being treated, but with a

TABLE 1 | Participant characteristics (n = 1,112).

Demographic	Values	95%CI
Gender, *n* (%)		
Female	574 (51.6)	48.6–54.6
Male	538 (48.4)	45.4–51.4
Years, mean (SD)	41.7 (15.2)	40.8–42.6
Italian region, *n* (%)		
North	488 (43.9)	40.9–46.9
Centre	323 (29)	26.4–31.8
South	301 (27.1)	24.5–29.8
Social status, *n* (%)		
Employed	755 (67.9)	65.0–70.6
Student	149 (13.4)	11.5–15.6
Retired	119 (10.7)	9.0–12.7
Housewife	59 (5.3)	4.1–6.8
Unemployed	30 (2.7)	1.9–3.9
Type of job*, *n* (%)		
Nothing	357 (32.1)	29.4–34.9
Intellectual, scientific, highly specialized profession	164 (14.7)	12.7–17.0
Trade, service	162 (14.6)	12.6–16.8
Office workers	139 (12.5)	10.6–14.6
Technician	96 (8.6)	7.1–10.5
Laborer, farmer, artisan	94 (8.5)	6.9–10.3
Unqualified profession	36 (3.2)	2.3–4.5
Legislator, businessman, manager	25 (2.2)	1.5–3.3
Drivers	24 (2.2)	1.4–3.2
Military profession	15 (1.3)	0.8–2.3
Education, *n* (%)		
High school	559 (50.3)	47.3–53.2
Bachelor's degree	328 (29.5)	26.8–32.3
Secondary school	133 (12.0)	10.1–14.0
Master's degree	56 (5.0)	3.9–6.5
Primary school	22 (1.9)	1.3–3.0
PhD	14 (1.3)	0.7–2.2
Anatomical region of pain, *n* (%)		
Cervical spine–head	258 (23.2)	20.8–25.8
Lumbar spine–pelvis	252 (22.7)	20.2–25.3
Shoulder–arm	193 (17.4)	15.2–19.7
Knee–leg	155 (13.9)	12.0–16.1
Ankle–foot	70 (6.3)	5.0–7.9
Hip–thigh	55 (4.9)	3.8–6.4
Thoracic spine–ribs	47 (4.2)	3.1–5.6
Wrist–hand	44 (4.0)	2.9–5.3
Elbow–forearm	25 (2.2)	1.5–3.3
Jaw	13 (1.2)	0.6–2.0
Duration of pain, *n* (%)		
Over 6 months	563 (50.6)	47.6–53.6
Less than 3 months	355 (31.9)	29.2–34.8
From 3 to 6 months	194 (17.4)	15.3–19.8
Intensity of pain, mean (SD)	4.9 (2.1)	4.8–5.0
EQI, mean (SD)	0.85 (0.12)	0.85–0.86

n, number of participants; %, percentage; SD, standard deviation; 95%CI, 95% confidence interval; >, more; visual analog scale, visual; EQI, EuroQol Index.
**According to "Nomenclature and classification of work" provided by ISTAT http://professioni.istat.it/sistemainformativoprofessioni/cp2011/*

possible unspecific effect" (n = 715; 64.3%; 95%CI 61.4–67.1). Instead, the minority of patients identified CFs as "a sham treatment used as control tests for safety and efficacy of active treatment" (n = 109; 9.8%; 95%CI 8.1–11.7). The remaining considered CFs as "a harmless or inert intervention" (n = 167; 15.0%; 95%CI 13.0–17.3) or "an intervention that has a special effect through known physiological mechanisms" (n = 121; 10.9%; 95%CI 9.1–12.9).

Beliefs

The mean score of beliefs was 2.6 out of 5 (95%CI 2.5–2.6), thus denoting a substantial level of belief towards CFs among patients. In detail, the most believed CFs were (in descending order): "overt therapy" (mean = 3.4; 95%CI 3.3–3.4), "empathetic therapeutic alliance with the patient" (mean = 3.3; 95%CI 3.2–3.3), "verbal communication" (mean = 3.1; 95%CI 3.0–3.1), and "patient-centered approach" (mean = 3.1; 95%CI 3.0–3.1). The least believed CFs were (in descending order): "adequate design" (mean = 1.8; 95%CI 1.8–1.9), "uniform" (mean = 1.8; 95%CI 1.8–1.9), and "physical contact with the patient" (mean = 1.5; 95%CI 1.4–1.5). An overall description of beliefs towards CFs is presented in **Table 2**.

Therapeutic Effect

Patients mainly chose "physiological and psychological" therapeutic effects for health problems such as acute pain (n = 640; 57.5%; 95%CI 54.6–60.5), chronic pain (n = 629; 56.6%; 95%CI 53.6–59.5), and insomnia (n = 562; 50.5%; 95%CI 47.6–53.5). The "psychological" effect was predominantly reported for emotional (n = 689; 62.0%; 95%CI 59.0–64.8) and cognitive disorders (n = 616; 55.4%; 95%CI 52.4–58.3) and oncological problems (n = 513; 46.1%; 95%CI 43.2–49.1). Patients identified the therapeutic effects behind several health conditions such as gastrointestinal (n = 451; 40.6%; 95%CI 37.7–43.5) and cardiovascular problems (n = 405; 36.4%; 95%CI 33.6–39.3) as "physiological." Infectious (n = 629; 56.6%; 95%CI 53.6–59.5), immune/allergic (n = 566; 50.9%; 95%CI 47.9–53.9), drug, and medication addictions (n = 531; 47.8%; 95%CI 44.8–50.7) were selected as having "no benefit." An overall report of therapeutic effects is presented in **Table 3**.

Ethical Implications

The adoption of CFs was considered ethical when "it exerts beneficial psychological effects" (n = 672; 60.4%; 95%CI 57.5–63.3). In this field, the least selected answer was "the patient wants or expects this treatment" (n = 51; 4.6%; 95%CI 3.5–6.0). The detailed responses are presented in **Figure 3**.

The adoption of CFs was instead considered non-ethical when "it is based on deception" (n = 568; 51.1%; 95%CI 48.1–54.0). Differently, the least frequent selected answer was when "the evidence available is insufficient" (n = 164; 14.7%; 95%CI 12.7–17.0). The overall responses are presented in **Figure 4**.

Communication

Participants desired to be informed about the use of CFs, thus selecting with a higher frequency the communication "it is a treatment without a specific effect for your problem, but capable of improving your condition" (n = 512; 46.0%; 95%CI 43.1–49.0). The least frequent chosen item was "it can help but you are not sure about its effect" (n = 26; 2.3%; 95%CI 1.6–3.5). The full combinations of responses are reported in **Figure 5**.

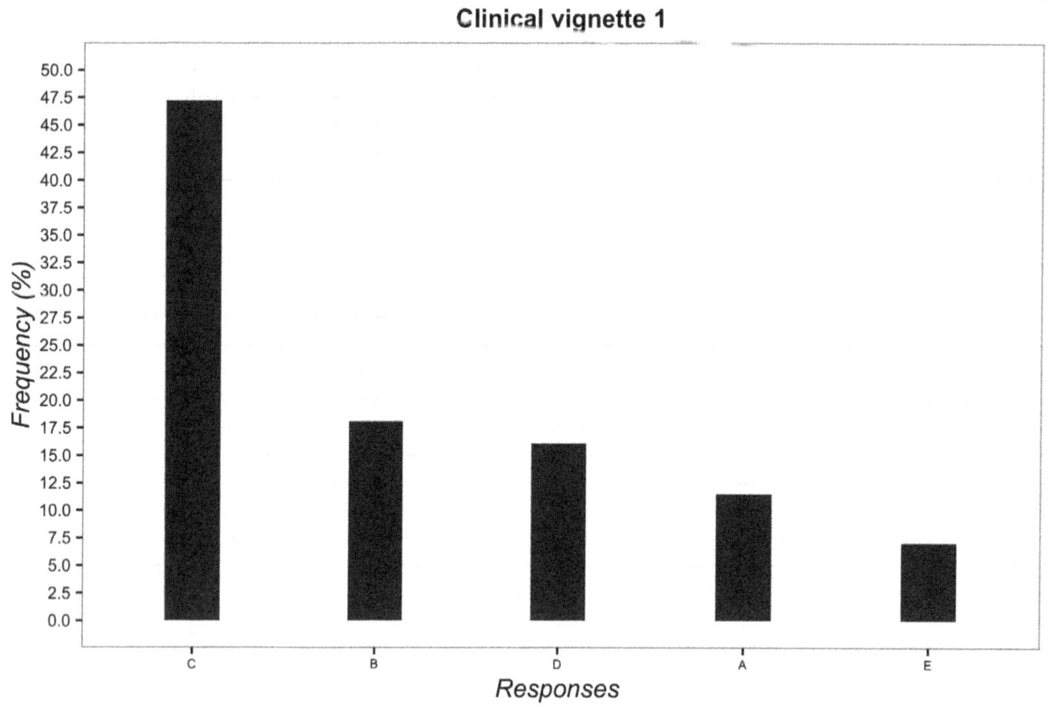

FIGURE 1 | Percentages of responses for clinical vignette 1. **(A)** deliver massage; **(B)** tell the patient that low back pain would resolve itself in a few days; **(C)** suggest the possibility of delivering massage if the clinical condition fails to improve; **(D)** advise a different treatment commonly used for low back pain; **(E)** try to convince the patient of the futility of the massage.

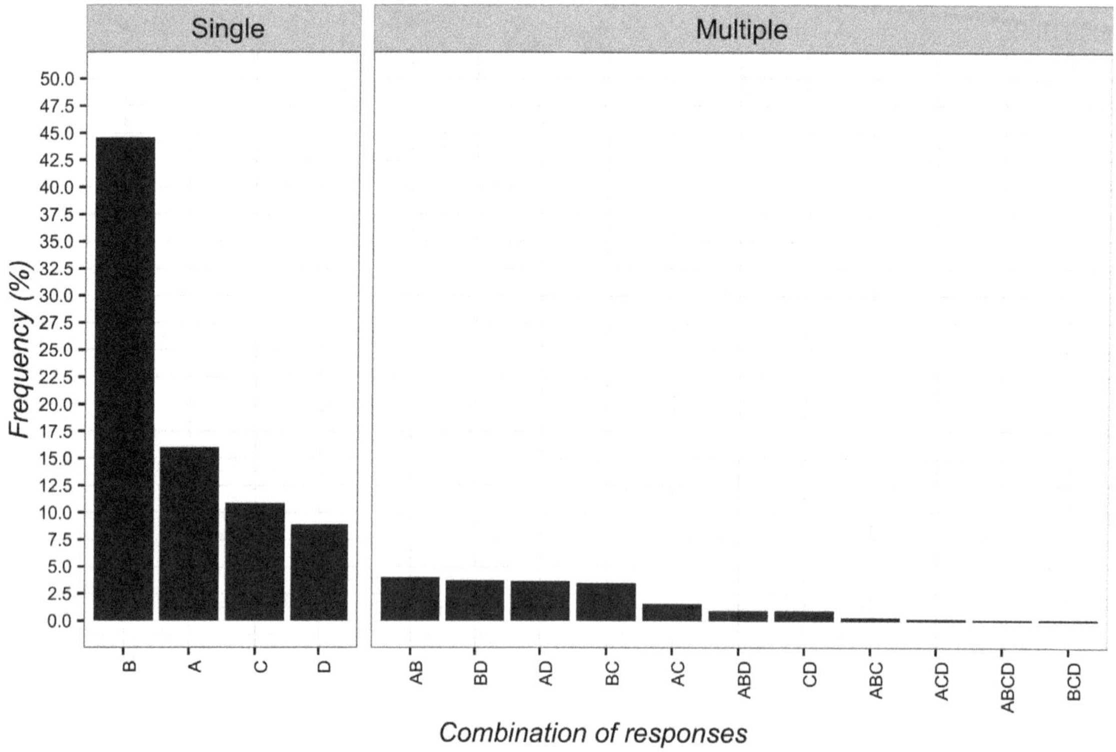

FIGURE 2 | Percentages of responses for clinical vignette 2. **(A)** the positive attention of the healthcare team leads to decreased pain; **(B)** pain is not organic but psychological; **(C)** the patient is very suggestible; **(D)** the supporting patient saw an improvement after treatment with laser switched off.

TABLE 2 | Beliefs regarding contextual factors (*n* = 1,112).

Contextual factor items[a]	Likert score mean (95%CI)	4 *n* (%); 95%CI	3 *n* (%); 95%CI	2 *n* (%); 95%CI	1 *n* (%); 95%CI	0 *n* (%); 95%CI
A: Professional reputation (e.g. qualification, expertise)	2.1 (2.0–2.1)	70 (6.3); 5.0–7.9	266 (23.9); 21.5–26.6	513 (46.1); 43.2–49.1	192 (17.3); 15.1–19.6	71 (6.4); 5.0–8.0
A: Uniform (e.g. white coat)	1.8 (1.8–1.9)	65 (5.8); 4.6–7.4	229 (20.6) 18.3–23.1	431 (38.8); 35.9–41.7	241 (21.7); 19.3–24.2	146 (13.1); 11.2–15.3
A: Positive attitudes and behavior (e.g. towards a patient's dysfunctions)	2.7 (2.6–2.7)	156 (14.0) 12.1–16.2	577 (51.9) 48.9–54.9	276 (24.8); 22.3–27.5	78 (7.0); 5.6–8.7	25 (2.2); 1.5–3.4
B: Patient's expectation and preference (e.g. towards a treatment)	2.2 (2.2–2.3)	97 (8.7); 7.2–10.6	408 (36.7); 33.9–39.6	326 (29.3); 26.7–32.1	210 (18.9); 16.7–21.3	71 (6.4); 5.1–8.0
B: Patient's previous experience (e.g. towards a treatment)	2.7 (2.7–2.8)	168 (15.1); 13.1–17.4	586 (52.7); 49.7–55.7	272 (24.5); 22.0–27.1	64 (5.8); 4.5–7.3	22 (2.0); 1.3–3.0
C: Verbal communication (e.g. positive messages associated with the treatment)	3.1 (3.0–3.1)	334 (30.0); 27.4–32.8	582 (52.3); 49.3–55.3	151 (13.6); 11.6–15.8	29 (2.6); 1.8–3.8	16 (1.4); 0.9–2.4
C: Non-verbal communication (e.g. posture, gestures, eye contact, facial expressions)	2.9 (2.8–2.9)	251 (22.6); 20.2–25.2	572 (51.4); 48.5–54.4	205 (18.4); 16.2–20.9	62 (5.6); 4.3–7.1	22 (2.0); 1.3–3.0
C: Empathetic therapeutic alliance with the patient (e.g. active listening)	3.3 (3.2–3.3)	545 (49.0); 46.0–52.0	384 (34.6); 31.8–37.4	136 (12.2); 10.4–14.3	40 (3.6); 2.6–4.9	7 (0.6); 0.3–1.4
D: Overt therapy (e.g. possibility for the patient to see the treatment using a mirror)	3.4 (3.3–3.4)	578 (52.0); 49.0–54.9	398 (35.8); 33.0–38.7	99 (8.9); 7.3–10.8	29 (2.6); 1.8–3.8	8 (0.7); 0.3–1.5
D: Patient-centered approach (e.g. shared-decision of treatment)	3.1 (3.0–3.1)	346 (31.1); 28.4–33.9	578 (52.0); 49.0–54.9	150 (13.5); 11.6–15.7	26 (2.3); 1.6–3.5	12 (1.1); 0.6–1.9
D: Professional approach to patient (e.g. privacy, punctuality)	3.0 (3.0–3.1)	380 (34.2) 31.4–37.1	496 (44.6); 41.6–47.6	154 (13.8); 11.9–16.1	56 (5.0); 3.9–6.5	26 (2.3); 1.6–3.5
D: Physical contact with the patient (e.g. touch to inform, assist, prepare, take care)	1.5 (1.4–1.5)	63 (5.7); 4.4–7.2	168 (5.7); 13.1–17.4	200 (18.0); 15.8–20.4	491 (44.2); 41.2–47.1	190 (17.1); 14.9–19.5
E: Comfortable setting (e.g. little noise, music, fragrances, temperature)	2.7 (2.6–2.7)	174 (15.6); 13.6–17.9	562 (50.5); 47.6–53.5	259 (23.3); 20.9–25.9	86 (7.7); 6.3–9.5	31 (2.8); 1.9–4.0
E: Adequate environmental architecture (e.g. windows and skylights, supportive indicators)	2.3 (2.2–2.4)	120 (10.8); 9.1–12.8	338 (30.4); 27.7–33.2	456 (41.0); 38.1–44.0	151 (13.6); 11.6–15.8	47 (4.2); 3.2–5.6
E: Adequate design (e.g. decorations, ornaments and colors)	1.8 (1.8–1.9)	63 (5.7); 4.4–7.2	189 (17.0); 14.9–19.4	478 (43.0); 40.1–46.0	286 (25.7); 23.2–28.4	96 (8.6); 7.1–10.5

%, percentage; n, number of participants; 95%CI, 95% confidence interval; 0, not at all; 1, few; 2, enough; 3, much; 4, a lot of; A, physical therapist domain; B, patient domain; C, physical therapist–patient relationship domain; D, therapy domain; E, healthcare setting domain.

[a]The items were reported from: Testa M, Rossettini G. Enhance placebo, avoid nocebo: How contextual factors affect physiotherapy outcomes. Man Ther. 2016;24:65–74.

TABLE 3 | Therapeutic effect(s) of contextual factors (*n* = 1,112).

Clinical conditions	Psychological and physiological *n* (%); 95%CI	Psychological *n* (%); 95%CI	Physiological *n* (%); 95%CI	No benefit *n* (%); 95%CI
Acute pain	640 (57.5); 54.6–60.5	210 (18.9); 16.6–21.3	132 (11.9); 10.1–13.9	130 (11.7); 9.9–13.8
Chronic pain	629 (56.6); 53.6–59.5	244 (21.9); 19.6–24.5	123 (11.1); 9.3–13.1	116 (10.4); 8.7–12.4
Cognitive disorder	227 (20.4); 18.1–22.9	616 (55.4); 52.4–58.3	65 (5.8); 4.6–7.4	204 (18.3); 16.1–20.8
Emotional disorder	336 (30.2); 27.5–33.0	689 (62.0); 59.0–64.8	50 (4.5); 3.4–5.9	37 (3.3); 2.4–4.6
Gastrointestinal problem	367 (33.0); 30.3–35.9	134 (12.0); 10.2–14.1	451 (40.6); 37.7–43.5	160 (14.4); 12.4–16.6
Sexual problem	505 (45.4); 42.5–48.4	336 (30.2); 27.5–33.0	99 (8.9); 7.3–10.8	172 (15.5); 13.4–17.8
Drug and medication addiction	283 (25.4); 22.9–28.1	258 (23.2); 20.8–25.8	40 (3.6); 2.6–4.9	531 (47.8); 44.8–50.7
Neurological problem	471 (42.4); 39.4–45.3	244 (21.9); 19.6–24.5	198 (17.8); 15.6–20.2	199 (17.9); 15.7–20.3
Rheumatologic problem	452 (40.6); 37.7–43.6	251 (22.6); 20.2–25.2	257 (23.1); 20.7–25.7	152 (13.7); 11.7–15.9
Immune/allergic problem	227 (20.4); 18.1–22.9	150 (13.5); 11.6–15.7	169 (15.2); 13.2–17.5	566 (50.9); 47.9–53.9
Oncological problem	310 (27.9); 25.3–30.6	513 (46.1); 43.2–49.1	74 (6.6); 5.3–8.3	215 (19.3); 17.1–21.8
Cardiovascular problem	297 (26.7); 24.1–29.4	185 (16.6); 14.5–19.0	405 (36.4); 33.6–39.3	225 (20.2); 17.9–22.7
Infectious problem	191 (17.2); 15.0–19.5	125 (11.2); 9.5–13.3	167 (15.0); 13.0–17.3	629 (56.6); 53.6–59.5
Insomnia	562 (50.5); 47.6–53.5	413 (37.1); 34.3–40.1	50 (4.5); 3.4–5.9	87 (7.8); 6.3–9.6

%, percentage; n, number of participants; 95%CI, 95% confidence interval.

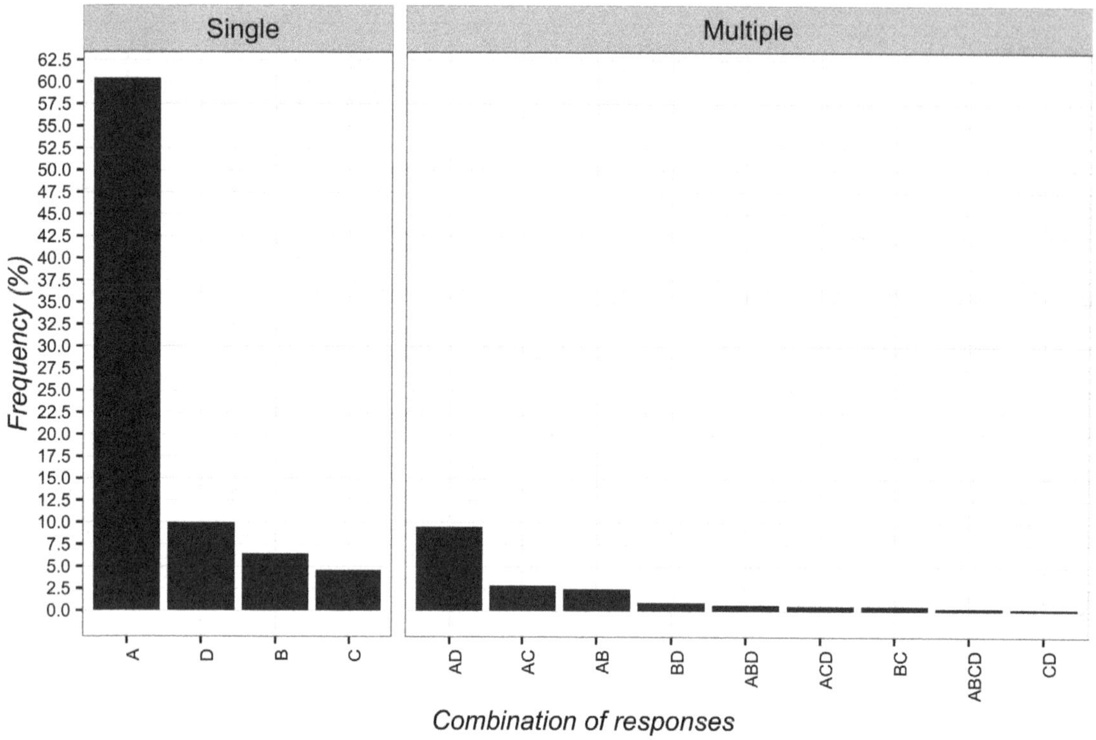

FIGURE 3 | Percentages of responses for the ethical use of Contextual Factors. **(A)** it exerts beneficial psychological effects; **(B)** the other therapies are over; **(C)** the patient wants or expects this treatment; **(D)** effectiveness shown by clinical experience.

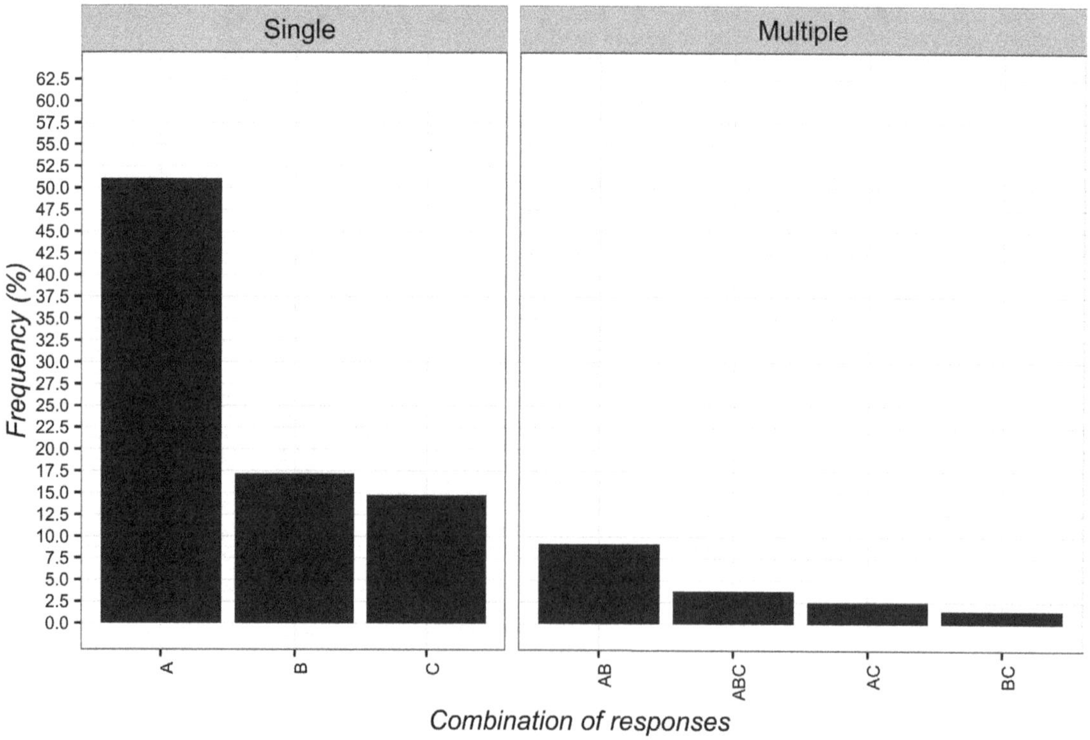

FIGURE 4 | Percentages of responses for not-ethical use of Contextual Factors. **(A)** it is based on deception; **(B)** it undermines trust between patient and clinician; **(C)** the evidence is insufficient.

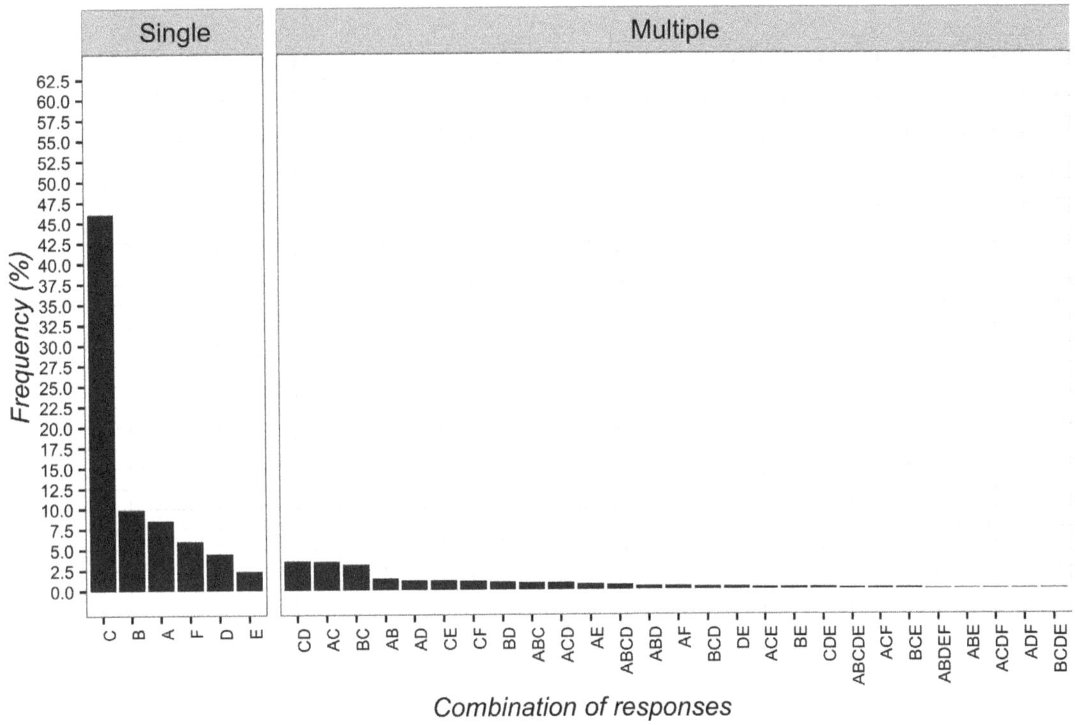

FIGURE 5 | Percentages of responses for communicating to patients the implications of Contextual Factors. **(A)** it is a treatment that can help and will not hurt; **(B)** it is an effective treatment; **(C)** it is a treatment without a specific effect for your problem, but capable of improving your condition; **(D)** it is a treatment that induces a psychological change; **(E)** it can help but you are not sure about its effect; **(F)** you do not receive any information.

Circumstances of CF Application and Mechanism of Action

As for the circumstances of CF application, the most frequent item was "as an adjunct to other interventions to optimize clinical responses" (n = 437; 39.3%; 95%CI 36.4–42.2). The least frequent answers were two items: "for non-specific problems" (n = 15; 1.3%; 95%CI 0.8–2.3) and "to control pain" (n = 13; 1.2%; 95%CI 0.6–2.0). Globally, the combinations of responses are presented in **Figure 6**.

In terms of mechanism of action, patients selected "mind–body connections" as most frequent option (n = 413; 37.1%; 95%CI 34.3–40.1). The least frequent answers were instead "natural history of disease" (n = 14; 1.3%; 95%CI 0.7–2.2) and "spiritual energies" (n = 10; 0.9%; 95%CI 0.5–1.7) as reported in **Figure 7**.

Correlation between Variables

The strength of association was considered weak with a Cramer's V lower than the established threshold (Cramer's V < 0.60) for all the correlations, such as between the characteristics reported in **Table 1** (gender, age, Italian region, social status, type of job, education, anatomical region of pain, duration of pain, intensity of pain, EQI) and the responses given in sections B and C of the survey.

DISCUSSION

To the best of our knowledge, this is the first research investigating the awareness of Italian patients about the therapeutic effect of CFs on musculoskeletal pain. The main findings of our study suggest that patients: a) conceptualized CFs as an intervention with an unspecific effect; b) believed in the clinical effectiveness of CFs; c) identified several possible therapeutic effects of CFs for various health problems; d) considered the use of CFs to stimulate beneficial psychological effects as ethically correct; e) saw as non-ethical the deceptive adoption of CFs; f) desired transparent information about CFs; g) recognized the application CFs as an adjunct to other interventions to optimize clinical responses; and h) proposed mind–body connection as a principal mechanism of action of CFs.

Therefore, according to our and former findings, it is recommended to extend the consideration of CFs in clinical policies and research designs, as they are also a patients' perspective expression, and not only a significant contribution to the therapeutic outcome from clinicians' point of view (18, 21, 25, 26, 29, 34). Namely, if patients present an adequate knowledge of CFs, their implementation can be ethically acceptable by clinicians and researchers. On the contrary, if patients report a misconception about CFs, clinicians and researchers should adequately reconceptualise their point of view before adopting CFs.

Responding to clinical vignette 1, about 50% of our participants suggested the possibility of delivering the expected intervention (massage) if clinical condition did not improve. As reported in previous qualitative researches (62, 63), patients with low back pain considered the fulfilment of expectation as a milestone of the decision-making process capable of improving clinical outcome(s) and adherence to treatment; therefore, clinicians should adopt it

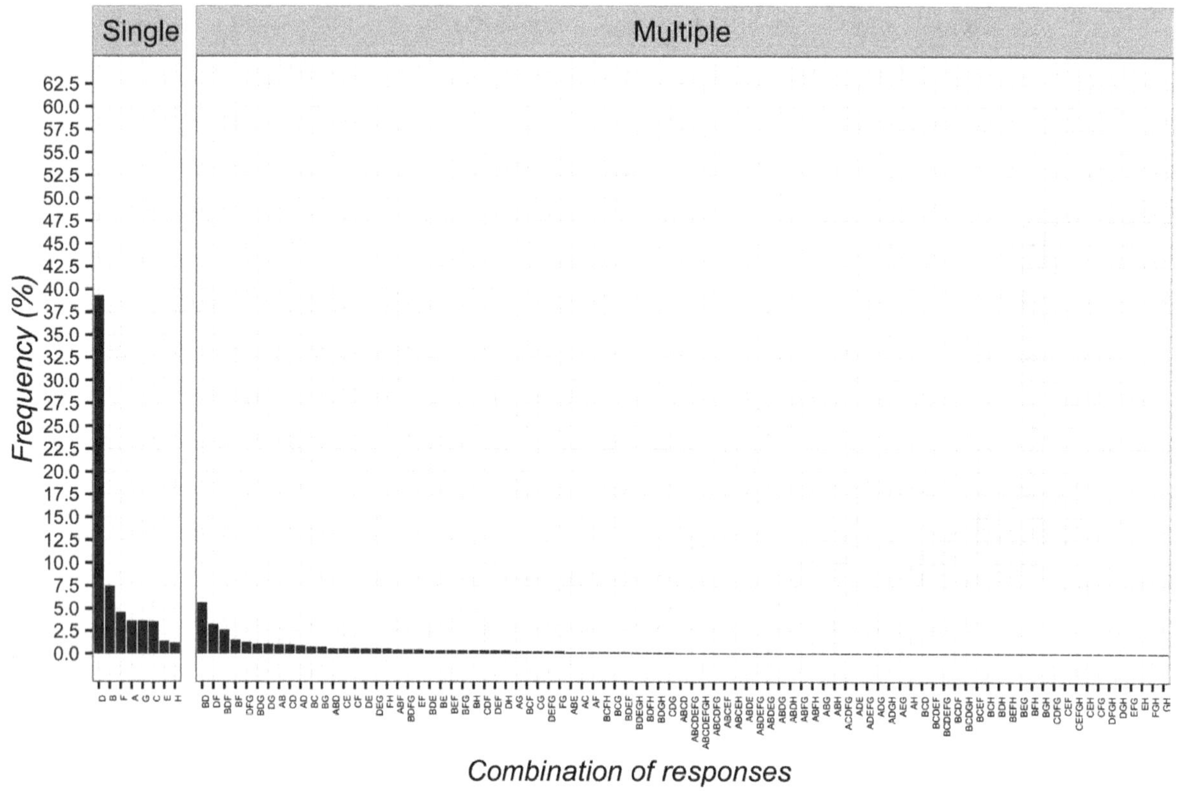

FIGURE 6 | Percentages of responses for circumstances of Contextual Factors application. **(A)** as a result of unjustified and constant demands for healthcare interventions; **(B)** to calm down the patient; **(C)** when all other therapies are over; **(D)** in addition to other interventions to optimize clinical responses; **(E)** for non-specific problems; **(F)** to gain time; **(G)** as a diagnostic tool to differentiate between psychological and physiological problems; **(H)** to control pain.

aimed at enhancing therapeutic responses (2). However former studies did not explore the ethical implications we proposed to patients in our survey. Our observations made clinicians aware that satisfying patients' expectations cannot exceed ethical boundaries of professional deontology not only for their personal moral values but also for specific willingness of the patients. In other words, they desire that clinician avoids the administration of the expected intervention when it is detrimental or simply useless.

As resulted in clinical vignette 2, the majority of Italian patients considered the recovery of shoulder pain with laser switched off as explained by symptoms of psychological origin. In accordance with previous international surveys on placebo (30, 35, 36), participants recognized the patients' psychological profile as an important predictor of placebo effects, able to explain the reduction in complaints (64). Therefore, clinicians should remember that patients are aware that their psychological condition affects their health status, so healthcare providers may have to weight this component in each healthcare interaction they have.

Our results made us consider CFs as an intervention lacking specificity capable of influencing patients' clinical condition through an unspecific effect. This confirms the patients' vision of placebo as an inert (32, 39), sham (37), fake (28) substance without any pharmacological active ingredient (30) rather than an active contextual process (25). This old conceptualization of placebos among patients can be the result of the patients' socio-cultural context (education, friends and family) (29) and of the external information received (books, newspapers, social media, and the internet) (26, 52). Routinely, clinicians should assess their patients' knowledge on placebo effects and try to correct misconceptions and inconsistencies with the current scientific thinking (65), for example, by encouraging the acquisition of information from evidence-based websites (66).

In line with previous surveys on placebos (30, 31, 35–39), Italian patients believed that CFs can influence therapeutic outcome(s). Namely, the most believed CFs are related to the therapeutic encounter (e.g. empathetic therapeutic alliance, communication, and overt therapy); the least believed CFs concerned healthcare design, the clinician's uniform and the touch. Previous surveys focused on evaluating patients' given value only on a part of possible CFs in each study, never trying to draft an importance ranking (26, 28, 31, 35, 37, 39). In our study, we aimed to draw up a classification, but this result suggests that patients assign the therapeutic value of CFs on a case-by-case basis. From a translational perspective, this finding pushes clinicians to assess patients' beliefs about specific CFs in order to adopt and reinforce the CFs most believed to trigger placebo and to reduce nocebo effects.

Italian patients identified several therapeutic effects of CFs for various health problems ranging from physiological and psychological issues to no benefit. While in previous surveys the expected therapeutic effect was limited to diseases in which psychological influence plays an important role (pain) (30, 31, 35, 36, 39), our participants' responses seem to be more articulated

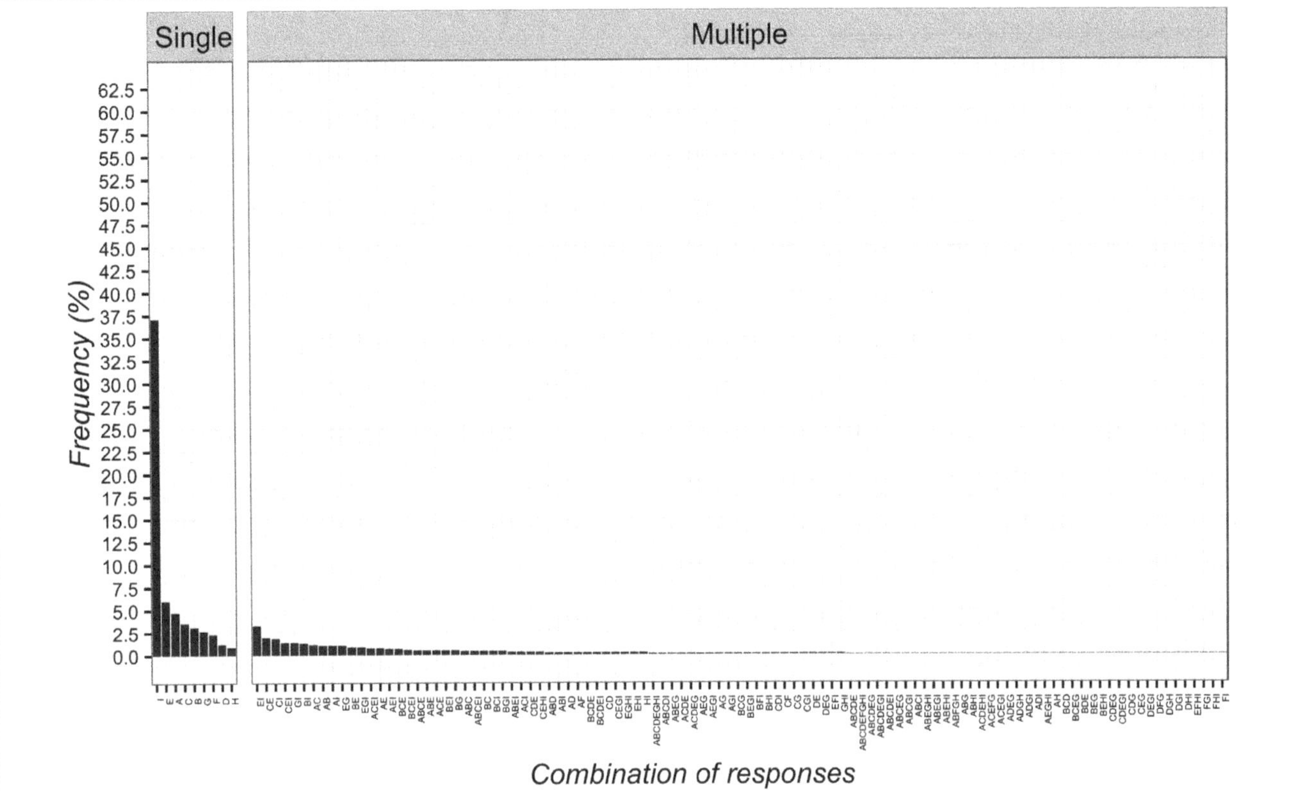

FIGURE 7 | Percentages of responses for Contextual Factors mechanism of action. **(A)** patient's expectation; **(B)** conditioning; **(C)** suggestibility; **(D)** natural history of disease; **(E)** psychological factors; **(F)** unexplained; **(G)** physiological/biological factors; **(H)** spiritual energies; **(I)** mind–body connections.

and support the idea that: a) CFs do not work in all diseases; b) CFs can act with different therapeutic effects (e.g. physiological and psychological); and c) the therapeutic effect of CFs depends on the specific nature and the severity of the disease. This heterogeneity could be related to the ethno cultural background that differ between patients from Northern (e.g. United Kingdom) and Southern Europe (e.g. Italy), and between European patients compared to other populations from different continents, as reported in former surveys on placebo (67). However, our findings are not conclusive, requiring further studies aimed at identifying patients' perspective on the therapeutic effects of CFs in different health problems.

In accordance with the position of a recent expert consensus on placebo and nocebo for clinical practice (24), the majority of Italian patients considered as ethical and acceptable the use of CFs as therapy enhancers when they stimulate beneficial psychological effects and improve patients' symptoms. The pursuit of patients' benefit, the lack of harm, the absence of other effective treatments, and the presence of pain or other conditions of suffering are other main reasons for the ethical implementation of placebo treatments reported in literature (26, 30, 32–33, 34, 36–40). On the contrary, among surveys, the use of placebo is considered as non-ethical when: a) it conflicts with available scientific evidence; b) it provides advantages to clinicians; c) it determines dysfunctional attachment behavior between clinicians and patients; d) it is harmful; or e) it worsens clinical outcomes (26, 32–33, 34, 36, 38, 40).

Our participants considered as non-ethical the deceptive use of CFs. In accordance with previous surveys on placebo (26, 33, 34, 38, 44), deception was considered negatively as it determines a violation of the patients' autonomy and right to be informed about the treatment delivered. Indeed, it can compromise the trust towards clinicians particularly when deceptive treatment resulted in negative outcomes (37, 39). Surprisingly, in other surveys, participants expressed a more tolerant opinion and considered deception acceptable when it helps patients to improve without damaging patient–clinician relationship (36, 41–43). The heterogeneity of these data highlights the complexity behind the ethical domain of CFs, thus the need for further research on the topic across countries.

As for communication, the majority of Italian patients desired transparent information about CFs. In line with previous surveys (26, 30, 37–38, 39, 44), our result confirms the need to notify patients without lying when they receive a non-specific treatment. Communication is a central aspect of the patient–clinician relationship and constitutes one of the most important CFs capable of triggering placebo or nocebo response with a relevant effect on clinical outcomes (2). Two strategies to inform patients have been reported in literature: 1) a direct message ("this is a placebo pill") (37–39) or 2) an indirect general message ("this pill has helped others in the past") that avoids the "placebo" word to limit misunderstanding related to the term (26, 30). Nevertheless, some results of previous surveys supported the non-transparent use of placebo treatments (35, 38–40): some respondents claimed that a clinician should not tell patients that the treatment was a placebo to avoid a potential lack of benefit. Currently, this vision appears dated and incompatible with the evidence available on several health conditions such as irritable bowel syndrome, depression, allergic rhinitis, back pain, and attention deficit hyperactivity disorder (68) that report positive clinical effects also to open-label placebo administration.

According to a previous survey among patients with musculoskeletal complaints (33), in our investigation, CFs are mainly seen by Italian patients as additional interventions that can optimize clinical responses. Overall, our finding suggests a patient's positive attitude towards CFs, thus stimulating their adoption among clinicians to boost the result of evidence-based interventions (2, 22).

Mind–body connection has been proposed as the main mechanism of action of CFs by participants, in accordance with previous surveys on placebo (26, 28, 30, 38). Within a Cartesian dualistic perspective, the power of mind is able to activate patients' inner resources and capacity of self-healing, thus directly influencing symptoms from body (28), relegating to a less relevant role other mechanisms such as expectation, conditioning, hope, psychological (e.g. attitudes, beliefs, and desire), and physiological factors (e.g. real change in the brain) (26, 28, 29, 31, 69, 70). The future analysis about the mechanisms behind the clinical effectiveness of CFs represents a research agenda capable to enrich the knowledge of patients' perspective involved in the creation of placebo/nocebo effects.

STRENGTHS AND LIMITATIONS

We have investigated for the first time the knowledge of CFs among Italian patients with musculoskeletal pain, thus expanding, also by involving a wider sample, findings of research in this field previously conducted in other countries (31, 33). Furthermore, the patients' health status as measured with the EQI was similar to that of the general population (48). Compared to focus group methodology, the use of a questionnaire-based survey has contributed to expand the focus of our analysis and revealed the complexity behind CF construct (71). Moreover, the adoption of clinical vignettes helped to gradually introduce a potentially unfamiliar topic such as CFs to patients (26).

Despite the novelty of this study, we recognize several limitations that could affect our findings. First, we have recruited only participants from outpatient clinics, thus limiting the generalization of findings in different contexts (e.g. inpatient services). Second, although not correlated to CF knowledge in our sample, participants had a generally high education and work position, introducing a possible source of bias (38). Third, social desirability and recall bias could have occurred due to self-reported and retrospective nature of data (36, 37). Finally, the distribution of response in question with multiple choice (either with single or multiple answers) revealed the presence of different strata. Therefore, the confidence level of the estimate varies when the proportion of responses is different from the estimated 50% that occurred in non-dichotomic questions. We suggest using our result in future research to estimate the required sample size more precisely using stratified random sampling.

CONCLUSION

Italian outpatient with musculoskeletal pain reported positive attitudes and beliefs towards the implementation of CFs in clinical practice, and this may have an impact at different levels.

According to the patients' opinion, it is ethically welcome for clinicians to adopt CFs as an additional treatment integrated with the evidence-based intervention aimed at enhancing therapeutic outcomes.

To support a mindful clinical use of CFs, educational courses should be implemented in academic curricula to expand the knowledge among healthcare providers.

Moreover, following the patients' vision, policymakers and managers should create the conditions and the normative frame to ease the appropriate integration of CFs in clinical practice.

Future surveys are needed to explore how patients conceptualise mechanisms of actions and the role of CFs in different health conditions and across countries.

ETHICS STATEMENT

The present study consists in a web-based survey of which protocol was approved by the Liguria Clinical Experimental Ethics Committee (P.R.236REG2016, accepted on 19/07/2016). Participants were contacted by an email including the survey link (https://it.surveymonkey.com/r/contestopazientiitalianimsk) and a brief note outlining a) the aim of the study, b) data handling (anonymity), c) the informed consent statement, and d) the invitation to complete the survey. Moreover, the email specifically informed the recipient that by clicking on the survey link he would have provided his consent to participate in the study. Participants' identities remained concealed to researchers; all data were anonymized (name and email address) to ensure confidentiality and data protection.

AUTHOR CONTRIBUTIONS

Conceptualization: GR, MT. Data curation: GR, TG. Formal analysis: TG. Investigation: GR, MT. Methodology: GR, AP, TG, MM, FT, MT. Project administration: GR, MT. Resources: GR, MT. Software: GR, TG. Supervision: AP, MM, FT. Validation: GR, AP, TG, MM, FT, MT. Visualization: GR, AP, TG, MM, FT, MT. Writing – original draft: GR, AP, TG, MM, FT, MT. Writing – review & editing: GR, AP, TG, MM, FT, MT.

ACKNOWLEDGMENTS

The authors would like to thank all the Italian patients who took part in the survey.

REFERENCES

1. Paterson C, Dieppe P. Characteristic and incidental (placebo) effects in complex interventions such as acupuncture. *BMJ* (2005) 330:1202–5. doi: 10.1136/bmj.330.7501.1202
2. Rossettini G, Carlino E, Testa M. Clinical relevance of contextual factors as triggers of placebo and nocebo effects in musculoskeletal pain. *BMC Musculoskelet Disord* (2018) 19:27. doi: 10.1186/s12891-018-1943-8
3. Benedetti F. Placebo and the new physiology of the doctor-patient relationship. *Physiol Rev* (2013) 93:1207–46. doi: 10.1152/physrev.00043.2012
4. Blasini M, Corsi N, Klinger R, Colloca L. Nocebo and pain: an overview of the psychoneurobiological mechanisms. *Pain Rep* (2017) 2, e585. doi: 10.1097/PR9.0000000000000585
5. Enck P, Bingel U, Schedlowski M, Rief W. The placebo response in medicine: minimize, maximize or personalize? *Nat Rev Drug Discov* (2013) 12:191–204. doi: 10.1038/nrd3923
6. Crum AJ, Leibowitz KA, Verghese A. Making mindset matter. *BMJ* (2017) 356:j674. doi: 10.1136/bmj.j674
7. Colloca L, Benedetti F. Placebo analgesia induced by social observational learning. *Pain* (2009) 144:28–34. doi: 10.1016/j.pain.2009.01.033
8. Carlino E, Benedetti F. Different contexts, different pains, different experiences. *Neuroscience* (2016) 338:19–26. doi: 10.1016/j.neuroscience.2016.01.053
9. Levine JD, Gordon NC, Fields HL. The mechanism of placebo analgesia. *Lancet* (1978) 2:654–7. doi: 10.1016/S0140-6736(78)92762-9
10. Colloca L, Pine DS, Ernst M, Miller FG, Grillon C. Vasopressin boosts placebo analgesic effects in women: a randomized trial. *Biol Psychiatry* (2016) 79:794–802. doi: 10.1016/j.biopsych.2015.07.019
11. Amanzio M, Benedetti F. Neuropharmacological dissection of placebo analgesia: expectation-activated opioid systems versus conditioning-activated specific subsystems. *J Neurosci* (1999) 19:484–94. doi: 10.1523/JNEUROSCI.19-01-00484.1999
12. Atlas LY. Wager TD. A meta-analysis of brain mechanisms of placebo analgesia: consistent findings and unanswered questions. *Handb Exp Pharmacol* (2014) 225:37–69. doi: 10.1007/978-3-662-44519-8_3
13. Bingel U, Lorenz J, Schoell E, Weiller C, Büchel C. Mechanisms of placebo analgesia: rACC recruitment of a subcortical antinociceptive network. *Pain* (2006) 120:8–15. doi: 10.1016/j.pain.2005.08.027
14. Eippert F, Finsterbusch J, Bingel U, Büchel C. Direct evidence for spinal cord involvement in placebo analgesia. *Science* (2009) 326:404. doi: 10.1126/science.1180142
15. Wager TD, Rilling JK, Smith EE, Sokolik A, Casey KL, Davidson RJ, et al. Placebo-induced changes in FMRI in the anticipation and experience of pain. *Science* (2004) 303:1162–7. doi: 10.1126/science.1093065
16. Lui F, Colloca L, Duzzi D, Anchisi D, Benedetti F, Porro CA. Neural bases of conditioned placebo analgesia. *Pain* (2010) 151:816–24. doi: 10.1016/j.pain.2010.09.021
17. Wager TD, Atlas LY. The neuroscience of placebo effects: connecting context, learning and health. *Nat Rev Neurosci* (2015) 16:403–18. doi: 10.1038/nrn3976
18. Geuter S, Koban L, Wager TD. The cognitive neuroscience of placebo effects: concepts, predictions, and physiology. *Annu Rev Neurosci* (2017) 40:167–88. doi: 10.1146/annurev-neuro-072116-031132
19. Carlino E, Frisaldi E, Benedetti F. Pain and the context. *Nat Rev Rheumatol* (2014) 10:348–55. doi: 10.1038/nrrheum.2014.17
20. Di Blasi Z, Harkness E, Ernst E, Georgiou A, Kleijnen J. Influence of context effects on health outcomes: a systematic review. *Lancet* (2001) 357:757–62. doi: 10.1016/S0140-6736(00)04169-6
21. Castelnuovo G, Giusti EM, Manzoni GM, Saviola D, Gabrielli S, Lacerenza M, et al. What is the role of the placebo effect for pain relief in neurorehabilitation? Clinical implications from the Italian Consensus Conference on Pain in Neurorehabilitation. *Front Neurol* (2018) 9:310. doi: 10.3389/fneur.2018.00310
22. Testa M, Rossettini G. Enhance placebo, avoid nocebo: how contextual factors affect physiotherapy outcomes. *Man Ther* (2016) 24:65–74. doi: 10.1016/j.math.2016.04.006
23. Palese A, Rossettini G, Colloca L, Testa M. The impact of contextual factors on nursing outcomes and the role of placebo/nocebo effects: a discussion paper. *PAIN Rep* (2019) 4:e716. doi: 10.1097/PR9.0000000000000716
24. Evers AWM, Colloca L, Blease C, Annoni M, Atlas LY, Benedetti F, et al. Implications of placebo and nocebo effects for clinical practice: expert consensus. *Psychother Psychosom* (2018) 87:204–10. doi: 10.1159/000490354
25. Hardman DI, Geraghty AW, Lewith G, Lown M, Viecelli C, Bishop FL. From substance to process: a meta-ethnographic review of how healthcare professionals and patients understand placebos and their effects in primary care. *Health (London)* (2018), 1363459318800169. doi: 10.1177/1363459318800169
26. Bishop FL, Aizlewood L, Adams AEM. When and why placebo-prescribing is acceptable and unacceptable: a focus group study of patients' views. *PLoS One* (2014) 9:e101822. doi: 10.1371/journal.pone.0101822
27. Asai A, Ohnishi M, Nishigaki E, Sekimoto M, Fukuhara S, Fukui T. Focus group interviews examining attitudes toward medical research among the Japanese: a qualitative study. *Bioethics* (2004) 18:448–70. doi: 10.1111/j.1467-8519.2004.00409.x
28. Bishop FL, Jacobson EE, Shaw JR, Kaptchuk TJ. Scientific tools, fake treatments, or triggers for psychological healing: how clinical trial participants conceptualise placebos. *Soc Sci Med* (2012) 74:767–74. doi: 10.1016/j.socscimed.2011.11.020
29. Kaptchuk TJ, Shaw J, Kerr CE, Conboy LA, Kelley JM, Csordas TJ, et al. "Maybe I made up the whole thing": placebos and patients' experiences in a randomized controlled trial. *Cult Med Psychiatry* (2009) 33:382–411. doi: 10.1007/s11013-009-9141-7
30. Tandjung R, Tang H, Fässler M, Huber CA, Rosemann T, Fent R, et al. The patient's perspective of placebo use in daily practice: a qualitative study. *Swiss Med Wkly* (2014) 144:w13899. doi: 10.4414/smw.2014.13899
31. Hughes J, Greville-Harris M, Graham CA, Lewith G, White P, Bishop FL. What trial participants need to be told about placebo effects to give informed consent: a survey to establish existing knowledge among patients with back pain. *J Med Ethics* (2017) 43:867–70. doi: 10.1136/medethics-2016-103964
32. Kisaalita NR, Robinson ME. Analgesic placebo treatment perceptions: acceptability, efficacy, and knowledge. *J Pain* (2012) 13:891–900. doi: 10.1016/j.jpain.2012.06.003
33. Kisaalita N, Staud R, Hurley R, Robinson M. Placebo use in pain management: the role of medical context, treatment efficacy, and deception in determining placebo acceptability. *Pain* (2014) 155:2638–45. doi: 10.1016/j.pain.2014.09.029
34. Kisaalita NR, Roditi D, Robinson ME. Factors affecting placebo acceptability: deception, outcome, and disease severity. *J Pain* (2011) 12:920–8. doi: 10.1016/j.jpain.2011.02.353
35. Berthelot JM, Maugars Y, Abgrall M, Prost A. Interindividual variations in beliefs about the placebo effect: a study in 300 rheumatology inpatients and 100 nurses. *Joint Bone Spine* (2001) 68:65–70. doi: 10.1016/S1297-319X(00)00225-6
36. Chen G-F, Johnson MH. Patients' attitudes to the use of placebos: results from a New Zealand survey. *N Z Med J* (2009) 122:35–46.
37. Fässler M, Gnädinger M, Rosemann T, Biller-Andorno N. Placebo interventions in practice: a questionnaire survey on the attitudes of patients and physicians. *Br J Gen Pract* (2011) 61:101–7. doi: 10.3399/bjgp11X556209
38. Ortiz R, Chandros Hull S, Colloca L. Patient attitudes about the clinical use of placebo: qualitative perspectives from a telephone survey. *BMJ Open* (2016) 6:e011012. doi: 10.1136/bmjopen-2015-011012
39. Hull SC, Colloca L, Avins A, Gordon NP, Somkin CP, Kaptchuk TJ, et al. Patients' attitudes about the use of placebo treatments: telephone survey. *BMJ* (2013) 347:f3757. doi: 10.1136/bmj.f3757
40. Lynöe N, Mattsson B, Sandlund M. The attitudes of patients and physicians towards placebo treatment—A comparative study. *Soc Sci Med* (1993) 36:767–74. doi: 10.1016/0277-9536(93)90037-5
41. Köteles F, Ferentzi E. Ethical aspects of clinical placebo use: what do laypeople think? *Eval Health Prof* (2012) 35:462–76. doi: 10.1177/0163278712453993
42. Nitzan U, Feffer K, Bloch Y, Lichtenberg P, Lev-Ran S, Becker G, et al. Consenting not to be informed: a survey on the acceptability of placebo use in the treatment of depression. *J Nerv Ment Dis* (2013) 201:345–7. doi: 10.1097/NMD.0b013e318288e2e7
43. Feffer K, Lichtenberg P, Becker G, Bloch Y, Netzer R, Nitzan U. A comparative study with depressed patients on the acceptability of placebo use. *Gen Hosp Psychiatry* (2016) 41:53–6. doi: 10.1016/j.genhosppsych.2016.05.004
44. Wolter T, Kleinmann B. Placebo acceptability in chronic pain patients: more dependent on application mode and resulting condition than on individual factors. *PLoS One* (2018) 13:e0206968. doi: 10.1371/journal.pone.0206968

45. Eysenbach G. Improving the quality of web surveys: the checklist for reporting results of internet e-surveys (CHERRIES). *J Med Internet Res* (2004) 6:e34. doi: 10.2196/jmir.6.3.e34
46. von Elm E, Altman DG, Egger M, Pocock SJ, Gøtzsche PC, Vandenbroucke JP, et al. Strengthening the Reporting of Observational Studies in Epidemiology (STROBE) statement: guidelines for reporting observational studies. *BMJ* (2007) 335:806–808. doi: 10.1136/bmj.39335.541782.AD
47. Dieppe P. Chronic musculoskeletal pain. *BMJ* (2013) 346:f3146. doi: 10.1136/bmj.f3146
48. Scalone L, Cortesi PA, Ciampichini R, Belisari A, D'Angiolella LS, Cesana G, et al. Italian population-based values of EQ-5D health states. *Value Health* (2013) 16:814–22. doi: 10.1016/j.jval.2013.04.008
49. National Statistical Service. Sample size calculator. (2017) Available at: http://www.abs.gov.au/websitedbs/D3310114.nsf/home/Sample+Size+Calculator.
50. Rossettini G, Palese A, Geri T, Fiorio M, Colloca L, Testa M. Physical therapists' perspectives on using contextual factors in clinical practice: findings from an Italian national survey. *PLoS One* (2018) 13:e0208159. doi: 10.1371/journal.pone.0208159
51. Palese A, Cadorin L, Testa M, Geri T, Colloca L, Rossettini G. Contextual factors triggering placebo and nocebo effects in nursing practice: findings from a national cross-sectional study. *J Clin Nurs* (2019) 28:1966–78. doi: 10.1111/jocn.14809
52. Bennett GJ. Does the word "placebo" evoke a placebo response? *Pain* (2018) 159:1928–31. doi: 10.1097/j.pain.0000000000001269
53. de Leeuw D, Hox J, Dillman D. *International handbook of survey methodology (European Association of Methodology Series). first.* New York (USA): Taylor and Francis group (2008).
54. Beaton DE, Bombardier C, Guillemin F, Ferraz MB. Guidelines for the process of cross-cultural adaptation of self-report measures. *Spine* (2000) 25:3186–91. doi: 10.1097/00007632-200012150-00014
55. Eysenbach G, Wyatt J. Using the Internet for surveys and health research. *J Med Internet Res* (2002) 4:E13. doi: 10.2196/jmir.4.2.e13
56. Haefeli M, Elfering A. Pain assessment. *Eur Spine J* (2006) 15:S17–24. doi: 10.1007/s00586-005-1044-x
57. Fan W, Yan Z. Factors affecting response rates of the web survey: a systematic review. *Comput Human Behav* (2010) 26:132–9. doi: 10.1016/j.chb.2009.10.015
58. Peerdeman KJ, Tekampe J, van Laarhoven AIM, van Middendorp H, Rippe RCA, Peters ML, et al. Expectations about the effectiveness of pain and itch relieving medication administered via different routes. *Eur J Pain* (2018) 22:774–83. doi: 10.1002/ejp.1163
59. R Development Core Team: *A Language and Environment for Statistical Computing.* Vienna, Austria: R Foundation for Statistical Computing (2015).
60. Revelle W. *psych: Procedures for Psychological, Psychometric, and Personality Research.* Evanston, Illinios: Northwestern University (2016).
61. Wickham H. *ggplot2: elegant graphics for data analysis.* New York: Springer-Verlag (2009). doi: 10.1007/978-0-387-98141-3
62. Stenner R, Swinkels A, Mitchell T, Palmer S. Exercise prescription for non-specific chronic low back pain (NSCLBP): a qualitative study of patients' experiences of involvement in decision making. *Physiotherapy* (2016) 102:339–44. doi: 10.1016/j.physio.2015.08.005
63. Darlow B, Perry M, Dean S, Mathieson F, Baxter GD, Dowell A. Putting physical activity while experiencing low back pain in context: balancing the risks and benefits. *Arch Phys Med Rehabil* (2016) 97:245–51.e7. doi: 10.1016/j.apmr.2015.09.020
64. Horing B, Weimer K, Muth ER, Enck P. Prediction of placebo responses: a systematic review of the literature. *Front Psychol* (2014) 5:1079. doi: 10.3389/fpsyg.2014.01079
65. Kisaalita NR, Hurley RW, Staud R, Robinson ME. Placebo use in pain management: a mechanism-based educational intervention enhances placebo treatment acceptability. *J Pain* (2016) 17:257–69. doi: 10.1016/j.jpain.2015.10.017
66. Greville-Harris M, Bostock J, Din A, Graham CA, Lewith G, Liossi C, et al. Informing patients about placebo effects: using evidence, theory, and qualitative methods to develop a new website. *JMIR Res Protoc* (2016) 5:e106. doi: 10.2196/resprot.5627
67. Bachiocco V, Credico C, Tiengo M. The pain locus of control orientation in a healthy sample of the Italian population: sociodemographic modulating factors. *J Cult Divers* (2002) 9:55–62.
68. Charlesworth JEG, Petkovic G, Kelley JM, Hunter M, Onakpoya I, Roberts N, et al. Effects of placebos without deception compared with no treatment: a systematic review and meta-analysis. *J Evid Based Med* (2017) 10:97–107. doi: 10.1111/jebm.12251
69. Stone DA, Kerr CE, Jacobson E, Conboy LA, Kaptchuk TJ. Patient expectations in placebo-controlled randomized clinical trials. *J Eval Clin Pract* (2005) 11:77–84. doi: 10.1111/j.1365-2753.2004.00512.x
70. Di Blasi Z, Crawford F, Bradley C, Kleijnen J. Reactions to treatment debriefing among the participants of a placebo controlled trial. *BMC Health Serv Res* (2005) 5:30. doi: 10.1186/1472-6963-5-30
71. Schmidt WC. World-Wide Web survey research: benefits, potential problems, and solutions. *Behav Res Methods Instrum Comput* (1997) 29:274–9. doi: 10.3758/BF03204826

19

Effects of Open- and Closed-Label Nocebo and Placebo Suggestions on Itch and Itch Expectations

Stefanie H. Meeuwis[1,2], Henriët van Middendorp[1,2], Antoinette I.M. van Laarhoven[1,2,3], Dieuwke S. Veldhuijzen[1,2], Adriana P.M. Lavrijsen[4] and Andrea W.M. Evers[1,2,3]*

[1] Health, Medical and Neuropsychology Unit, Faculty of Social and Behavioural Sciences, Institute of Psychology, Leiden University, Leiden, Netherlands, [2] Leiden Institute for Brain and Cognition, Leiden University Medical Center, Leiden, Netherlands, [3] Department of Psychiatry, Leiden University Medical Center, Leiden, Netherlands, [4] Department of Dermatology, Leiden University Medical Center, Leiden, Netherlands

***Correspondence:**
Stefanie H. Meeuwis
s.h.meeuwis@fsw.leidenuniv.nl

Placebo and nocebo effects have been shown to influence subjective symptoms such as itch. These effects can be induced by influencing outcome expectations through, for example, combining the application of an inert substance (e.g., a cream) with verbal suggestions on the anticipated effects of this substance. Interestingly, placebo effects also occur when it is known that a treatment is inert (i.e., open-label placebo). However, no study to date has examined the efficacy of negative and positive verbal suggestions under similar open-label and closed-label (i.e., concealed placebo/nocebo) conditions in itch. A randomized controlled between-subjects study design was applied in which healthy volunteers ($n = 92$) were randomized to 1) an open-label positive verbal suggestion group, 2) a closed-label positive verbal suggestion group, 3) an open-label negative verbal suggestion group, or 4) a closed-label negative verbal suggestion group. Verbal suggestions were made regarding the topical application of an inert substance. Itch was evoked experimentally by histamine iontophoresis at baseline and again following suggestions. Itch expectations, self-reported itch during and following iontophoresis, and skin response parameters were measured. Positive suggestions were found to result in significantly lower expected itch than were negative suggestions in both open- and closed-label conditions. No effects of the suggestions on itch during iontophoresis were found, but significantly lower itch was reported in the 4 min following iontophoresis in the (combined open- and closed-label) positive compared with negative verbal suggestion groups. In addition, a smaller increase in skin temperature was found in the positive compared with negative suggestion groups. The findings illustrate a potential role of (open- and closed-label) placebo for optimizing expectations and treatment effects for itch in clinical practice.

Clinical Trial Registration: Netherlands Trial Register, trial number: NTR6530.

Keywords: placebo, nocebo, itch, suggestion, pruritus

INTRODUCTION

Itch is the most common somatosensory symptom in dermatological conditions. It is a hallmark symptom of atopic eczema (1), and its prevalence in psoriasis is high (2). Moreover, itch is a common symptom of various other disorders, including kidney failure, liver disease, cancer, allergy, and diabetes mellitus (3–5). Due to its high prevalence—approximately 8% of the general population and over 50% of dermatological patients—the burden of itch and its impact on society are high (6, 7). Often, patients report significantly lowered quality of life, increased depressive and anxious symptoms, and sleep disturbances due to chronic itch (8). While current treatments aim to suppress itch through pharmacological interventions, oftentimes, limited effects and significant side effects are reported (3, 9). As such, it is important to identify factors that contribute to treatment efficacy.

One of the factors that may be especially relevant for treatment outcomes is the placebo effect. Placebo effects are defined as beneficial effects of otherwise pharmacologically inert substances (10, 11) and have been studied in a variety of medical conditions and symptoms, including itch and pain (12–14). Multiple pathways through which these effects can be elicited have been identified, including associative learning processes, social learning, or instructional learning (12, 15–17). Within these pathways, expectancy is a key component. To illustrate, a positive expectation may be elicited through past experiences with the beneficial effects of a certain type of medication (associative learning), through observation of treatment efficacy in others (social learning), or through receiving positive (verbal) information about a treatment (instructional learning) (17). In turn, this positive expectation can then result in psychoneurobiological changes and symptom reduction (18, 19). On the other hand, when expectations regarding a treatment outcome are low or negative outcomes are expected, symptoms may worsen or the occurrence of treatment side effects may increase, known as the nocebo effect (12, 20).

The current literature indicates that at least 30% of itch reduction in clinical practice might be attributable to placebo effects (21). Placebo and nocebo effects can be experimentally induced for itch by changing expectations through verbal suggestions regarding inert treatments or through the use of associative learning mechanisms (22–28). However, not all studies confirm these findings (28, 29). In addition, there is some evidence that it may be necessary to combine multiple placebo induction methods (e.g., associative learning and positive suggestions) and that a single induction method may not be sufficient to elicit significant placebo effects (22). Hence, further study of the circumstances under which placebo effects may be elicited for itch is relevant.

Most studies on placebo effects take on a traditional approach, in which patients or healthy individuals are told that a pharmacologically effective substance (e.g., a pill or cream) is given, whereas in reality, the substance is pharmacologically inert (30, 31). While this concealing or deceptive approach is useful for studying the underlying mechanisms of placebo effects in general, it may become problematic when it comes to utilizing these effects in clinical practice, where concealment or deception regarding the treatment provided brings along ethical issues. For a long time, it was believed that this would prevent strategic use of the placebo effect in clinical practice (30). In the past years, however, studies have demonstrated that placebo effects can also occur when it is explicitly told that, although a given substance is inert, placebo effects may still help in alleviating symptoms. These so-called open-label placebo effects have been found to significantly reduce symptoms of irritable bowel syndrome, depression, attention deficit hyperactivity disorder, chronic low back pain, and allergic rhinitis (31–39). Most of these studies induce open-label placebo effects through a combination of an attribute (e.g., an inert pill) that may trigger previously learned associations between medicine and symptom reduction in general, and a scripted briefing in which the positive effects of placebo pills are emphasized (a suggestive framework) (31–34, 36–38). Findings on whether these effects can be attributed to the provided pill or the provided explanation alone are contradictory (35, 39, 40).

In view of the previous findings, further research is needed to demonstrate the efficacy of both open-label and closed-label (i.e., concealed) placebo effects for itch. It is not yet known whether effect sizes of open-label and closed-label placebo effects are comparable. Moreover, no study to date has investigated whether nocebo effects can be induced under both closed-label and open-label conditions for itch. To this end, we investigated in the current study whether negative or positive outcome expectations, induced by a suggestive framework (negative and positive verbal suggestions, provided in an open-label and closed-label context) combined with an attribute (an inert tonic), can influence self-reported itch during an experimental itch induction by histamine in healthy volunteers. We primarily tested the effects of the positive and negative suggestions on itch by combining open- and closed-label groups. Secondarily, we tested these effects for open-label and closed-label contexts separately to see whether these effects were comparable, and we investigated the effects of suggestions on other markers of the response to this test, for example, the physical skin response to histamine. We expected a decrease in itch following positive verbal suggestions compared with an increase in itch following negative verbal suggestions for both the open-label and closed-label conditions.

MATERIALS AND METHODS

The study was approved by the Medical Ethical Committee at the Leiden University Medical Center, the Netherlands (NL58792.058.16), and registered in the Dutch Trial Register (NTR6530). The study was performed in accordance with the Declaration of Helsinki (41). All participants provided written informed consent.

Participants

Healthy male and female participants were recruited through advertisements at Leiden University and through social media (e.g., Facebook). Inclusion criteria consisted of an age between 18 and 35 years and a good understanding of the Dutch written and spoken language. Interested volunteers were excluded in case of self-reported severe somatic or psychological morbidity that could interfere with the participant's safety or study protocol [e.g., heart or lung diseases, histamine intolerance, or Diagnostic and Statistical Manual of Mental Disorders - Fourth Edition Text Revised (DSM-IV-TR) psychiatric diagnoses]; current chronic itch or pain complaints; current use of analgesics, anti-inflammatory medication, antihistamines, or antibiotics; and (suspected) pregnancy. Participants were asked to refrain from the consumption of heavy meals, caffeine, and smoking 2 h, exercise 12 h, and alcohol as well as drugs 24 h prior to the sessions to prevent potential influences on study outcomes. Adherence to these lifestyle guidelines, as well as the exclusion criteria, was verified at the start of each session by means of interviewing.

Study Design

A between-subjects, single-blinded, randomized controlled experimental trial design was applied. Eligible participants were randomized to (I) an open-label positive verbal suggestion (VS) group, (II) a closed-label positive VS group, (III) an open-label negative VS group, or (IV) a closed-label negative VS group. Randomization sequence was acquired using an online random number generator (www.random.org, Dublin, Ireland). Allocation was not concealed for experimenters. Participants were invited for a baseline and an experimental session, which were timed 1 week apart. An overview of the study design and measurement schedule is provided in **Figure 1**.

Measures and Materials

Verbal Suggestions

Before the study, participants were informed that the study aimed to investigate individual differences in the sensitivity to itch and the role of psychological factors in explaining these differences. They were informed that the itch induction method would elicit a response similar to a mosquito bite (e.g., that their skin may become red and swollen). During the experimental session, participants were told that, prior to itch induction, a tonic would be applied that influences sensitivity to itch. In reality, this tonic was a pink-colored skin disinfectant (Orphi Pharma B.V., Dordrecht, the Netherlands). The itch induction during the baseline session was used as a reference point for the suggestions. In the positive VS groups (I and II), the following suggestion was given: "This tonic has an itch-reducing effect and will make the skin less sensitive to itch. From previous research we know that the application of this tonic will reduce itch for most people, meaning around 95 percent of the studied people. As such, we expect that you will experience less itch, compared to the previous test." Participants in the negative VS groups (III and IV) were given the same information, but negative words were used instead of positive words (e.g., "itch-increasing" rather than "itch-reducing").

When participants were allocated to one of the two open-label groups, additional instructions were given. For the positive VS

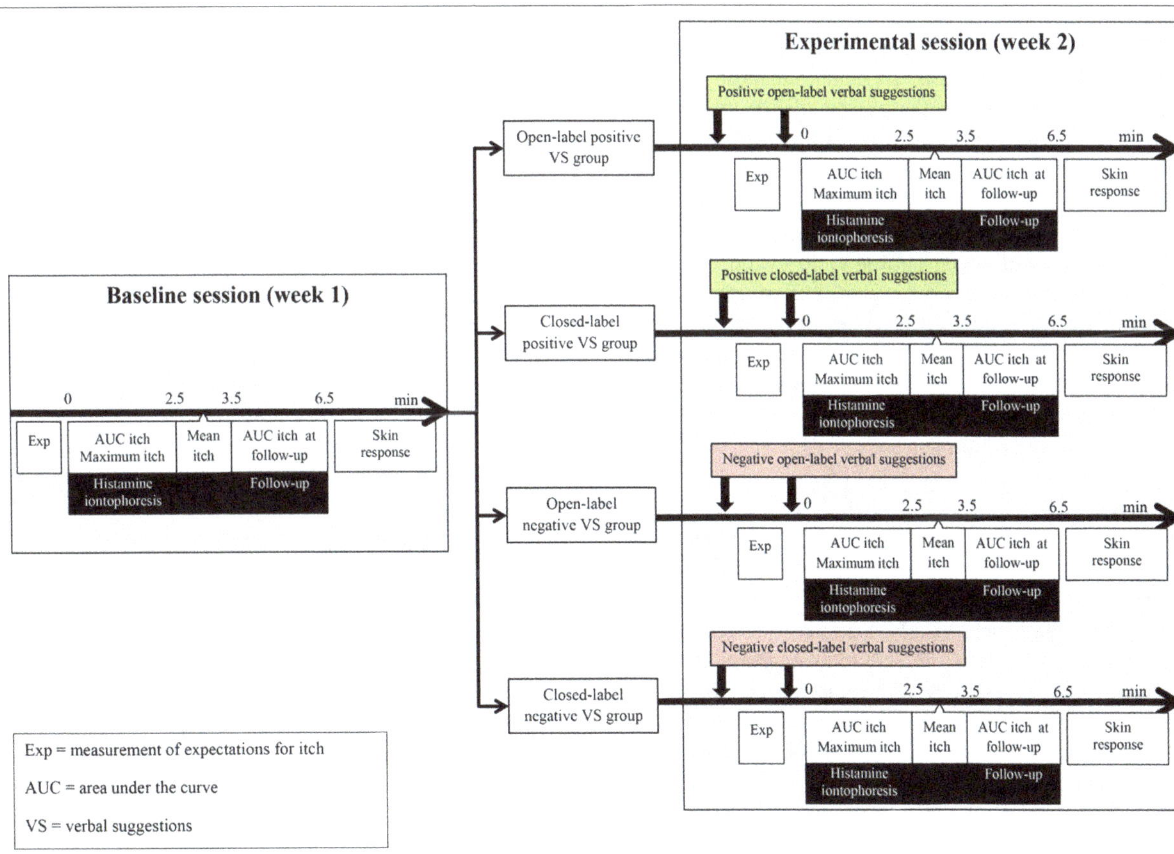

FIGURE 1 | Overview of the design of the study and the measurement schedule for the different verbal suggestions (VS) groups.

group, these were: "I just told you that the tonic reduces itch. In fact, the tonic is a placebo. From research we know that the expectation that a remedy reduces itch will really cause people to experience less itch. This is caused by different processes, for example itch-reducing substances that are released in the brain. These substances are also released when people know that they receive a placebo. So, even though I told you this, you will likely experience less itch during the test." For the open-label negative VS groups, negative words were again used in the instructions instead of positive words. During application of the tonic, the provided suggestions and, if applicable, open-label instructions were briefly repeated in a single sentence.

Expected Itch

Expected itch in response to histamine iontophoresis was assessed on a Numeric Rating Scale (NRS) ranging from 0 ("no itch") to 10 ("worst itch imaginable"). Participants rated the amount of itch they expected to experience during iontophoresis twice: once at the start of the baseline session and once during the experimental session, following the verbal suggestions but prior to histamine iontophoresis.

Histamine Iontophoresis

Histamine was applied to the skin by transdermal iontophoresis (Chattanooga Group, Hixson, TN, USA). This method has been previously validated and reliably induces itch in healthy populations (22, 28, 29, 35). A 0.6% diphosphate (equivalent to 1% histamine dihydrochloride) histamine solution was prepared in distilled water with propylene glycol and hypromellose 4,000 mPa by the local pharmacy. In preparation of iontophoresis, the skin was cleaned with either a transparent disinfectant (alcohol 70%; baseline session) or a pink-colored disinfectant (0.5% chlorhexidine in alcohol 70%, with rhodamine; experimental session) suggested to be itch-reducing or itch-increasing, depending on placebo or nocebo condition. A 2.5-cc electrode (Iogel, Iomed, DJO Global, Hannover, Germany; active surface: 11.7 cm^2) was treated with the histamine solution and applied to the volar side of the non-dominant forearm. A reference electrode was placed on the volar side of the upper arm. The electrode nodes were spaced approximately 10 cm apart. Histamine was applied to the skin by iontophoresis with a current level set at 0.4 mA for 2.5 min, following which the electrodes and any residual histamine were removed from the skin.

Self-Reported Itch

Self-reported itch in response to histamine iontophoresis was assessed using the same 0–10 NRS as described under Expected Itch. During iontophoresis, participants continuously rated itch using a vertical bar slide depicting the NRS. Scores were sampled at a 10-Hz rate using E-Prime 2.0 (42). Directly following iontophoresis, mean itch was verbally assessed by asking participants how much itch (on a 0–10 scale) they experienced in general during the test. From 1 to 4 min after iontophoresis, participants were asked to rate self-reported itch every 30 s on the bar slide as a follow-up period. The primary study outcome was the area under the curve (AUC) of itch during the 2.5 min of iontophoresis. Secondary outcomes were maximum itch reported during the 2.5 min of iontophoresis, verbally assessed mean itch, and AUC itch during the 4-min follow-up. AUC of itch and maximum itch during iontophoresis were computed using MATLAB Release 2012b (The MathWorks, Inc., Natick, MA, USA).

Subjective Skin Response

Participants filled in the Sensitive Scale-10 (SS-10) (43) to measure their subjective skin response. The SS-10 contains 10 items, of which 9 items assessed specific skin symptoms (e.g., itch, pain, general discomfort, and heat sensations). Participants were asked to rate in what intensity they had experienced these symptoms over the past 3 days as a baseline measurement, as well as during histamine iontophoresis. Symptoms were rated on NRS ranging from 0 ("zero intensity") to 10 ("intolerable intensity"). An additional symptom ("redness of the skin") was assessed on a 0–10 NRS (43). Total scores were calculated by summing all items and ranged from 0 to 100. Cronbach's alpha ranged from .83 to .87 in the current study for baseline and post-iontophoresis assessments of the SS-10.

Physical Skin Response

Wheal size and flare areas following histamine application were measured after the 4-min follow-up period after the iontophoresis test. The size of the skin response was measured by drawing the outline of the redness and thickening of the skin onto a 1-cm^2 gridded transparent sheet with a 0.4-mm black permanent marker (Staedtler, Germany). The sheets were scanned and then retraced using ImageJ software (44), after which the wheal and flare area (in cm^2) were calculated. In addition, skin temperature was measured following iontophoresis, using a handheld infrared digital thermometer (accuracy ± 2.0 °C, resolution 0.1 °C; BaseTech, Conrad Electronic Benelux B.V.). Measurements were taken with the thermometer held vertically and approximately 1 cm above the center of the histamine application area. To control for individual differences in skin temperature, a baseline measurement was taken prior to iontophoresis, with change from baseline temperature being used as the outcome measure.

Procedures

Prior to participation, written information regarding the study was provided, and volunteers were asked to fill in an online questionnaire assessing the study's inclusion and exclusion criteria. When volunteers were considered eligible for participation, they were invited to the lab for a 30-min baseline session and a 45-min experimental session, which were timed 1 week apart. At the start of the baseline session, the study procedures were explained, and written informed consent was provided. Next, personality questionnaires were administered, which are not further described here as they are unrelated to the aim of the current study. Baseline measurements of itch expectation and subjective skin responses in the past 3 days were taken. Next, the skin of the non-dominant forearm was disinfected, and electrodes were placed on the arm, after which the histamine test was conducted. Measurements of itch and physical skin responses were taken, followed by an assessment of subjective skin responses. After 1 week, the experimental session took place. First, the general procedure of the second session was explained, and verbal suggestions were given (the content of which depended on group allocation). Measurements of post-VS expected itch and of subjective skin responses in the past 3 days were taken. Next, the skin was cleaned using the pink disinfectant, during which the verbal suggestions were briefly repeated. Histamine iontophoresis was conducted; and measurements of itch, physical skin response, and subjective skin response were taken. At the end of the session, participants were asked to fill in a final questionnaire assessing the general amount of itch experienced during both baseline and post-VS iontophoresis and, for the open-label groups only, how believable and convincing participants thought the open-label rationale was (on a 0–10 NRS). Upon completion, they were debriefed on the true purpose of the study. For each session, participants received a compensation of €7.50.

Statistical Analyses

As input for the power calculation, we used the effect size of Cohen's $d = 1.10$, that was found by Napadow et al. (25), who investigated nocebo effects induced by an inert substance (i.e., a sham allergen solution) on itch. As the current study investigated not only nocebo effects following application of an inert substance but also placebo effects, and both were investigated under closed-label and open-label conditions, a more conservative effect size of $d = 0.90$ was used for computation of sample sizes for the separate open-label and closed-label analyses. A power calculation for an analysis of covariance (ANCOVA) using G*Power 3.1 (45) indicated that 21 participants per group would be needed at a power of $\beta = .80$ and a significance level of $\alpha = .05$ for the primary outcome of AUC itch during iontophoresis in the experimental session between the (separate closed-label or open-label) positive verbal suggestion group and the negative verbal suggestion group while controlling for AUC itch at baseline. A missing data rate of 10% was taken into account, resulting in a sample size of 23 participants in each group.

Analyses were performed using SPSS 21.0 for Windows (IBM SPSS Inc., Chicago, IL, USA). Normal distribution of the variables and the assumptions of each analysis were checked prior to analysis. To test for group differences in demographics and baseline variables, chi-square tests and one-way analyses of variance (ANOVAs) were conducted. As *a priori* determined primary analysis, differences between the combined negative VS groups and positive VS groups in AUC itch during iontophoresis were assessed by a general linear model (GLM) ANCOVA, controlled for AUC itch during baseline iontophoresis. Similar analyses were conducted for the secondary outcome parameters, maximum itch during iontophoresis, mean itch (assessed verbally following iontophoresis), AUC itch during the 4-min follow-up, subjective skin response, and the physical skin response parameters.

Due to technical difficulties with the NRS bar slide and E-Prime, data of some participants ($n = 6$) were missing for the analyses of AUC itch and maximum itch during iontophoresis. Data of one participant were missing for the skin temperature measurements. For those variables that were non-normally distributed (i.e., AUC itch during follow-up), a change score was calculated by subtracting baseline scores from those measured post-VS (with zero indicating no change, negative scores indicating a decrease, and positive scores indicating an increase from baseline to post-VS). A GLM ANOVA was then performed to detect differences in change scores between groups. For expected itch following suggestions, an ANOVA was also conducted. For each AN(C)OVA, Cohen's d was calculated, and the following interpretations were used: small effect size 0.20, medium effect size 0.50, and large effect size 0.80 (46). When appropriate, covariate-adjusted means were used for calculation of Cohen's d. In addition, paired sample t-tests were conducted within each group to assess changes in each outcome parameter from the baseline to post-VS measurements. In order to examine whether the effects of verbal suggestions were similar regardless of participants knowing about the expectation induction, all analyses were repeated for the separate open-label and closed-label conditions. As the effects of suggestions were expected to be similar under open-label and closed-label contexts, differences between open- and closed-label groups were not tested statistically. Rather, effect sizes generated by the separate open-label and closed-label analyses were used for indirect comparisons.

To explore potential group differences in the strength of associations between the process measure of post-VS itch expectation and the outcome measures of itch and skin response, Pearson's r correlations were calculated within each group, and Cohen's q was computed as an effect size for the difference in strength of association, with the following categories of interpretation: no effect < 0.10, small effect size 0.10 < 0.30, medium effect size 0.30 < 0.50, and large effect size ≥ 0.50 (46). For AUC itch during follow-up, Spearman's rho was calculated. The open-label groups were compared on how believable and convincing participants thought the open-label rationale was by independent-samples t-tests. All analyses were conducted two sided with $\alpha = .05$. For the secondary analyses (i.e., AN(C)OVAs and paired-sample t-tests for separate open-label and closed-label analyses), Bonferroni's correction for multiple comparisons was used, thus resulting in a significance level of $\alpha/2 = .025$. To correct for alpha inflation due to multiple itch outcomes, an additional Bonferroni's correction was applied for the secondary itch outcomes, resulting in a significance level of $\alpha/3 = .017$ for the combined-group analyses and $(\alpha/3)/2 = .008$ for the separate-group analyses of the secondary itch outcomes. All values described in the Results section represent mean ± SD, unless stated otherwise.

RESULTS

Participants

A total of 138 potential participants expressed interest in the study, of whom 44 were not included (18 had somatic or psychological morbidity, 4 were non-proficient in the Dutch language, and 22 gave no response following screening). Two participants dropped out after the baseline session and were replaced. This resulted in the intended sample size of 92 participants (16 males, 17.4%; 76 females, 82.6%), whose age ranged from 18 to 30 ($M = 21.8 \pm 2.7$). Participants were randomized into 1) the open-label positive VS group ($n = 22$), 2) the closed-label positive VS group ($n = 23$), 3) the open-label negative VS group ($n = 23$), or 4) the closed-label negative VS group ($n = 24$). The groups did not differ in demographic factors (all $p \geq .42$), baseline itch expectation prior to iontophoresis ($p = .13$), baseline self-reported itch parameters (all $p \geq .58$), and baseline subjective and physical skin condition (all $p \geq .12$). An overview of the means and standard deviations of the baseline and outcome measures is presented in **Table 1** (combined open-label and closed-label groups) and in **Supplementary Table S1** (separate open-label and closed-label groups).

Expected Itch

A large-sized effect of verbal suggestions on expected itch was found; $F(1,90) = 20.94, p < .001$, Cohen's $d = 0.96$. As illustrated in **Figure 2**, expected itch following suggestions was significantly lower in the combined positive VS groups ($M = 2.62 \pm 1.82$) compared with the combined negative VS groups ($M = 4.41 \pm 1.93$).

A secondary analysis showed a large-sized effect of suggestions in the open-label groups [$F(1,43) = 15.84, p < .001$, Cohen's $d = 1.21$] and a medium-sized effect in the closed-label groups [$F(1,45) = 6.15, p = .017$, Cohen's $d = 0.74$], both indicating significantly lower expected itch in the positive VS group (open label: $M = 2.35 \pm 1.88$; closed label: $M = 2.88 \pm 1.77$) than in the negative VS group (open label: $M = 4.59 \pm 1.91$; closed label: $M = 4.24 \pm 1.99$).

Primary Itch Measure: Area Under the Curve (AUC) of Itch during Histamine Iontophoresis

For the primary outcome AUC itch, a small-sized non-significant difference between the combined positive VS groups and the combined negative VS groups was found; $F(1,83) = 1.75, p = .19$, Cohen's $d = 0.29$. Secondary analyses for the separate open- and closed-label groups revealed similar findings (both $p \geq .31$; see **Figure 3**). Within-group analyses of baseline to post-VS changes indicated that AUC itch decreased marginally in the combined positive VS groups [$t(39) = 1.98, p = .055$] but did not change in the combined negative VS groups [$t(45) = -0.19, p = .85$]. No within-group changes in AUC itch from baseline to post-VS were detected for the separate open- and closed-label groups (all $p \geq .12$). An overview of within-group comparisons for AUC itch and other outcome measures is presented in **Table 2** (combined

TABLE 1 | Means ± standard deviations for the combined open- and closed-label positive and the combined open- and closed-label negative verbal suggestion groups.

		Combined open- and -closed-label			
	n	Positive VS (*n* = 45)	Negative VS (*n* = 47)	AN(C)OVA	
				p-value	Cohen's *d*
Process measure					
Pre-iontophoresis itch expectation	92	5.15 ± 1.95	4.82 ± 1.75	.40	
Post-VS itch expectation[A]	92	2.62 ± 1.82	4.41 ± 1.93	<.001	0.96
Baseline histamine iontophoresis					
AUC itch[B]	88	369.79 ± 241.69	361.35 ± 230.24	.87	
Maximum itch	88	3.95 ± 2.44	3.78 ± 2.26	.73	
Mean itch[C]	92	3.10 ± 1.90	2.93 ± 1.75	.66	
Post-VS histamine iontophoresis					
AUC itch[B,D]	86	314.61 ± 237.34	367.54 ± 266.63	.19	0.29
Maximum itch[D]	86	3.44 ± 2.54	3.81 ± 2.45	.24	0.26
Mean itch[C,D]	92	2.83 ± 1.93	3.19 ± 2.09	.076	0.38
Change from baseline to post-VS scores					
AUC itch during follow-up[B,E]	90	−3.38 ± 6.37	0.02 ± 6.88	.017	0.52
Baseline skin response to iontophoresis					
Subjective skin response[F]	92	24.37 ± 11.77	22.78 ± 12.25	.53	
Wheal area (cm^2)	92	10.52 ± 3.47	11.09 ± 3.00	.40	
Flare area (cm^2)	92	47.74 ± 11.05	48.16 ± 12.45	.86	
Change in skin temperature (°C)[G]	91	1.70 ± 1.01	1.58 ± 1.22	.61	
Post-VS skin response to iontophoresis					
Subjective skin response[D,F]	91	21.08 ± 12.31	20.79 ± 12.21	.58	0.12
Wheal area (cm^2)[D]	92	10.12 ± 3.80	10.68 ± 3.69	.78	0.06
Flare area (cm^2)[D]	92	45.54 ± 13.11	47.17 ± 11.75	.54	0.13
Change in skin temperature (°C)[D,G]	90	1.83 ± 1.15	2.34 ± 1.62	.018	0.52

[A]VS, verbal suggestions. [B]AUC, area under the curve. [C]Assessed verbally on a Numeric Rating Scale ranging from 0 to 10. [D]Group differences assessed by ANCOVA, controlled for baseline. Cohen's d was calculated with the estimated marginal means (controlled for baseline). [E]Calculated as post-VS measure–baseline measure (session 2–session 1) and corrected for significant outliers. [F]As measured by an adjusted version of the Sensitive Scale-10 (43). [G]Calculated as post-iontophoresis temperature–pre-iontophoresis temperature.

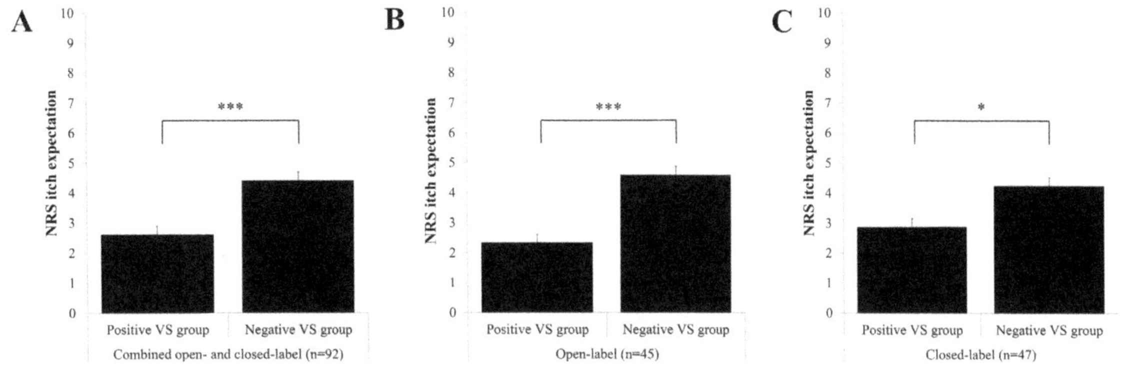

FIGURE 2 | Mean Numeric Rating Scale (NRS) score for post-verbal suggestions (VS) itch expectation with the standard error of the mean (SEM) for **(A)** the combined open- and closed-label positive VS group (n = 45) and negative VS group (n = 47); **(B)** the open-label positive VS group (n = 22) and open-label negative VS group (n = 23); and **(C)** the closed-label positive VS group (n = 23) and closed-label negative VS group (n = 24). $^{***}p < .001$, $^{*}p < .05$.

open-label and closed-label groups) and **Supplementary Table S2** (separate open-label and closed-label groups).

Secondary Itch Measures during and Following Histamine Iontophoresis

Maximum Itch and Mean Itch during Iontophoresis

Findings for maximum itch during iontophoresis were similar to those of AUC itch, with no effects of suggestions for the combined as well as separate groups (all $p \geq .24$) and a marginal decrease from baseline to post-VS exclusively for the combined positive VS groups [$t(39) = 2.00$, $p = .053$]. The combined positive VS groups showed a small-sized tendency to report lower (post-iontophoresis-assessed) mean itch ($M = 2.83 \pm 1.93$) than did the combined negative VS groups ($M = 3.19 \pm 2.09$); $F(1,89) = 3.22$, $p = .076$, Cohen's $d = 0.38$. No effects of verbal suggestions were found when open- and closed-label groups were separated, nor were changes from baseline to post-VS scores detected for any of the groups (all $p \geq .19$).

AUC of Itch during Follow-Up Following Iontophoresis

A significant and medium-sized difference in the change scores of AUC for itch during the 4-min follow-up was found when open- and closed-label groups were combined [$F(1,88) = 6.09$, $p = .016$, Cohen's $d = 0.52$], with AUC itch during follow-up decreasing significantly in the combined positive VS groups ($M = -3.73 \pm 7.55$) compared with the combined negative VS groups ($M = 0.02 \pm 6.88$). A small-sized non-significant effect of verbal suggestions was found in the open-label groups; $F(1,43) = 2.11$, $p = .15$, Cohen's $d = 0.43$, and a marginal and medium-sized effect in the closed-label groups, in the same direction as for the combined groups; $F(1,43) = 4.94$, $p = .032$, Cohen's $d = 0.67$. A significant change from baseline to post-VS in AUC itch during follow-up was demonstrated for the combined positive VS groups [$t(42) = 3.24$, $p = .002$]. In the combined negative VS groups, however, no change was detected [$t(46) = -0.02$, $p = .98$]. Separating open- and closed-label groups revealed a non-significant change within the open-label positive VS group [$t(21) = 1.87$, $p = .075$] and a significant change within the closed-label positive VS group [$t(20) = 3.14$, $p = .005$].

Skin Response

Subjective Skin Response (SS-10)

For subjective skin response following the histamine test, no significant difference was found between the combined positive and negative VS groups, nor between the separate open- and closed-label positive and negative VS groups (all $p \geq .12$). A significant decrease in subjective skin response from baseline to post-VS was demonstrated in the combined positive VS groups [$t(43) = 2.59$, $p = .013$], but not in the negative VS groups [$t(46) = 1.61$, $p = .12$]. When analyses were conducted for separate open- and closed-label groups, a significant decrease was demonstrated only for the closed-label positive VS group; $t(22) = 3.75$, $p < .001$.

Physical Skin Response

No effects of verbal suggestions on wheal or flare areas were found for either the combined or separate open- and closed-label groups (all $p \geq .23$). Regarding skin temperature, the combined positive VS groups showed a medium-sized lower increase in skin temperature from before to after iontophoresis ($M = 1.83 \pm 1.15$) than did the combined negative VS groups ($M = 2.34 \pm 1.62$); $F(1,87) = 5.84$, $p = .018$, Cohen's $d = 0.52$. In the same direction, marginally significant medium-sized effects of verbal suggestions on skin temperature increase were found in the open-label [$F(1,41) = 3.01$, $p = .090$, Cohen's $d = 0.54$] and closed-label groups [$F(1,43) = 2.93$, $p = .094$, Cohen's $d = 0.52$], respectively. Within-group comparisons for both combined and separate open- and closed-label positive and negative VS groups showed that skin temperature increased significantly from baseline to post-VS for the negative VS groups (all $p \leq .048$), but not for the positive VS groups (all $p \geq .12$).

Associations between Expected Itch and the Outcome Measures of Itch

In the combined open- and closed-label groups, expected itch following suggestions was significantly and positively associated

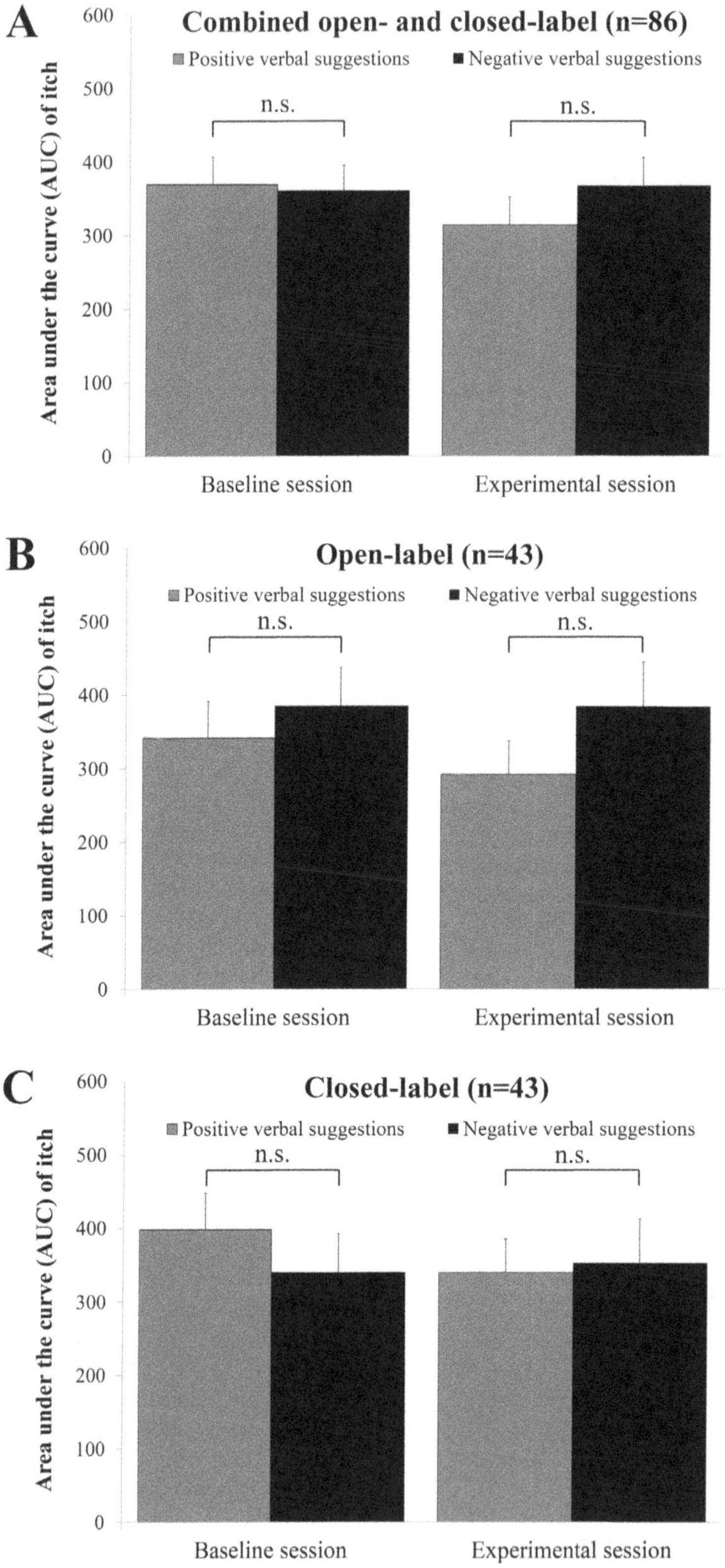

FIGURE 3 | Mean area under the curve (AUC) of self-rated itch during histamine iontophoresis in the baseline and experimental session, with the standard error of the mean (SEM) for **(A)** the combined open- and closed-label positive VS group (n = 40) and negative VS group (n = 46); **(B)** the open-label positive VS group (n = 21) and open-label negative VS group (n = 22); and **(C)** the closed-label positive VS group (n = 19) and closed-label negative VS group (n = 24). n.s. = not significant ($p > .05$).

TABLE 2 | Within-group mean changes from baseline and separate paired sample *t*-test results for the combined open- and closed-label positive verbal suggestion groups and combined negative verbal suggestion groups.

	Combined open- and closed-label positive VS groups (n = 45)				Combined open- and closed-label negative VS groups (n = 47)			
	n	Mean change	t	p	n	Mean change	t	p
Histamine iontophoresis								
AUC itch[A]	40	−46.91	1.98	.055	46	6.19	−0.19	.85
Maximum itch	40	−0.44	2.00	.053	46	0.02	−0.07	.94
Mean itch[B]	45	−0.26	1.34	.19	47	0.26	−1.30	.20
Post-iontophoresis follow-up								
AUC itch[A]	43	−3.73	3.24	.002	47	0.02	−0.02	.98
Skin response to iontophoresis								
Subjective skin response[C]	44	−3.30	2.59	.013	47	−2.00	1.61	.12
Wheal area (cm^2)	45	−0.40	0.79	.43	47	−0.41	0.87	.39
Flare area (cm^2)	45	−2.20	1.31	.20	47	−0.99	0.50	.62
Change in skin temperature (°C)[D]	44	0.14	−0.88	.38	46	0.76	−3.88	<.001

Mean change was calculated as post-verbal suggestions score–baseline score, with negative values indicating a decrease from baseline and positive scores indicating an increase from baseline. [A]AUC, area under the curve. [B]Assessed verbally on a Numeric Rating Scale ranging from 0 to 10. [C]As measured by an adjusted version of the Sensitive Scale-10 (43). [D]Calculated as post-iontophoresis temperature–pre-iontophoresis temperature.

with all itch measures during and following iontophoresis (all $r \geq .43$, all $p \leq .01$). Comparisons of the strength of the association between expected itch and the itch outcome measures showed small-sized to no differences in associative strength between the combined positive and combined negative VS groups (all Cohen's $q \leq 0.15$). In the separate open-label and closed-label groups, findings were similar, with one exception: in the open-label positive VS group exclusively, itch expectations were not associated with mean itch and AUC of itch during follow-up (both $p \geq .11$). An overview of Pearson's r and Spearman's ρ correlation coefficients can be found in **Table 3** (combined open- and closed-label groups) and **Supplementary Table S3** (separate open- and closed-label groups).

Open-Label Instruction Believability

Overall, participants in the open-label conditions rated the instructions as very clear (M = 7.90 ± 2.32). Ratings on how convincing the instructions had been were more ambiguous (M = 5.37 ± 2.46). In general, participants in the open-label groups believed that expectations are able to influence itch (M = 6.49 ± 1.97) but rated the extent in which their own itch experience was influenced by the application of the tonic as low (M = 3.81 ± 2.43). Groups did not differ in their ratings of the instructions (all $p \geq .21$).

TABLE 3 | Within-group Pearson's *r* and Spearman's rho correlations for the process measure of post-VS itch expectation and outcome measures of self-reported itch and skin response for the combined open- and closed-label group comparisons, with Cohen's *q* as estimate of the difference in effect size between groups.

	Combined open- and closed-label groups		
	Positive VS (n = 45)	Negative VS (n = 47)	Cohen's q
Post-VS histamine iontophoresis			
AUC itch[A]	.67***	.58***	0.15
Maximum itch	.63***	.59***	0.06
Mean itch[B]	.52***	.60***	0.12
Post-VS follow-up on iontophoresis			
AUC itch during follow-up[A,C]	.43**	.49***	0.08
Post-VS skin response to iontophoresis			
Subjective skin response[D]	.50***	.59***	0.13
Wheal area (cm^2)	−.09	−.01	0.08
Flare area (cm^2)	.03	−.23	0.26
Change in skin temperature (°C)[E]	.04	−.19	0.23

*[A]AUC, area under the curve. [B]Assessed verbally on a Numeric Rating Scale ranging from 0 to 10. [C]Calculated using the non-parametric Spearman's rho. [D]As measured by an adjusted version of the Sensitive Scale-10 (43). [E]Calculated as post-iontophoresis temperature–pre-iontophoresis temperature. **p < .01; ***p < .001.*

DISCUSSION

The current study investigated whether positive and negative outcome expectations, induced by open-label and closed-label positive and negative verbal suggestions regarding an inert tonic, could influence self-reported itch in response to a histamine test. For the first time, open- and closed-label placebo effects for itch were investigated within a single study, including a comparison with open- and closed-label nocebo effects. It was demonstrated that both open-label and closed-label verbal suggestions were able to influence itch expectations. For the primary outcome of area under the curve for itch during histamine iontophoresis, a small-sized but non-significant effect of verbal suggestions was found. Participants in the combined open- and closed-label positive VS groups reported lower itch during an immediate follow-up period after iontophoresis compared to the negative VS groups. *Post hoc* tests indicated that this was mostly due to differences between positive and negative VS groups under closed-label conditions. In addition, a significantly smaller increase in skin temperature was observed in the combined positive VS groups compared with the negative VS groups, but no effects on other markers of the physical skin response to histamine were found. Overall, the current study shows that verbal suggestions regarding a topical application of a substance can influence expectations for itch, regardless of whether or not participants know about receiving suggestions, and provides limited evidence that these suggestions may influence itch and skin response in response to histamine.

The findings that verbal suggestions were able to influence itch in the follow-up period after histamine iontophoresis are in line with a previous study that found medium-to-large-sized effects of positive suggestions on histamine-induced itch (24). While that particular study made use of a cream to help induce placebo effects, the current study used a pink-colored tonic. Potentially, the use of this particular attribute may have led towards smaller effects in the current study, since a cream could be perceived as a common treatment for itch by some participants, could trigger previously learned associations, and could thus potentially elicit stronger effects overall (47). Moreover, negative verbal suggestions did not elicit negative expectations for itch in the current study and did not increase itch either during or following the histamine test, which is not in line with previous evidence for verbal suggestion-induced nocebo effects in itch (25, 26, 28). It should be noted though that these previous studies have induced nocebo effects through negative suggestions regarding the experimental itch induction method that was used, whereas the current study provided suggestions regarding the topical application of an attribute prior to itch induction. While this did allow for a direct comparison of positive and negative expectation induction, potentially, it may have influenced the credibility of the negative verbal suggestions as well. Topical application of, for example, a cream or tonic in a laboratory setting might be associated more easily with symptom reduction rather than worsening of symptoms. In comparison, information regarding an experimental itch induction method, though less clinically relevant, may provide a more neutral basis for induction of nocebo effects through suggestions. Alternatively, although the baseline histamine application was valuable for participants as a comparison point for the second application, nocebo effects induced through negative verbal suggestions could have been influenced by participants being less anxious about the second histamine test, in comparison with the first test (since participants were generally unfamiliar with histamine iontophoresis prior to participating in the study). Future research may utilize a counterbalanced design to examine this more in detail. Likewise, more research is needed to investigate under which circumstances and through which attributes placebo and nocebo effects may be elicited for itch.

An effect of negative verbal suggestions on change in skin temperature due to histamine application was demonstrated. This finding is similar to previous work on placebo effects in autonomically controlled parameters and wheal responses (26, 48), a meta-analysis of clinical trials demonstrating placebo effects on physical outcome parameters controlled by the autonomic nervous system (49), and early studies on suggestions and hypnosis (50–52). Considering that either the outcome measure differed from these previous studies (i.e., skin temperature change rather than wheal size) or the expectation induction method was different (i.e., verbal suggestions given without hypnosis), caution is needed in interpreting these results. Moreover, the verbal suggestions in the current study did not influence wheal and flare areas to histamine, which is in line with most recent studies (24, 29, 35, 53, 54).

Our design allowed for the first time comparisons of effect sizes of positive and negative verbal suggestions under open- and closed-label conditions for itch. The findings demonstrate that positive verbal suggestions are able to significantly reduce expectations of itch under both open-label and closed-label conditions, with open-label verbal suggestions seemingly inducing larger expectancy effects. Overall, the effects of positive and negative verbal suggestions on itch were approximately similar sized under open-label and closed-label conditions. However, some differences between the conditions could be seen when examining the within-group changes from baseline. Closed-label suggestions appeared slightly more effective for itch, as illustrated by the significant within-group changes in itch during follow-up from baseline to post-suggestions under closed-label conditions. That open-label placebo treatment can significantly influence expectations and, potentially, symptoms of itch is in line with previous findings on other outcome parameters (31, 32, 34–39). It also provides further preliminary support for the notion that concealment of treatment is not necessary to elicit placebo responses, and that placebo mechanisms can potentially be utilized in clinical practice. Small differences between the open-label instructions of the current study and previous work need to be noted. Previous studies [e.g., Refs. 31–34, 40] began their open-label placebo instructions by indicating that the pill that was used was a placebo, prior to indicating the efficacy and mechanisms of these effects. The current study on the other hand began by introducing the tonic as an effective tool for itch reduction and explaining that it was a placebo afterwards, together with a rationale on why it would still be effective. Differences in the order in which this type of information is presented may impact the strength of open-label placebo and nocebo effects. In addition, previous work has incorporated the concept of learning in the open-label instructions (i.e., by giving the example of Pavlov's dog). This aspect has been omitted here, as the current study investigates placebo responses evoked by conscious expectancy (i.e., verbal information) rather than associative learning mechanisms. Potentially, this may have influenced the efficacy of the open-label rationale. Some caution needs to be taken in interpreting the effects of negative verbal suggestions under the separate open-label and closed-label conditions, since neither type of negative verbal suggestions was able to increase expectations of itch.

Some strengths and limitations need to be taken into account. This is the first study that compares open- and closed-label positive and negative verbal suggestions to elicit placebo and nocebo effects in itch and other responses to histamine.

Since the study was conducted single blinded, a reporting bias cannot be ruled out, as participants may have adjusted their answers to the experimenters' expectations. To minimize influences of response bias on assessments of expectations and itch, participants used a (computerized) bar slide to indicate these parameters. Future research might, however, consider using a double-blinded approach. The effect sizes found in the current study are considerably small, which may be due to the itch stimulus being perceived as low by participants. As such, the study may have been underpowered to find small effects, which seems to be supported by finding more significant effects of the combined open- and closed-label groups than for the separate groups. Moreover, the design of the current study did not include a no-treatment group. This prevents an estimation of a true placebo or nocebo response, as itch may reduce from the first to second histamine test regardless of group allocation. Though habituation to the itch stimulus cannot be ruled out, its role is likely small, since the itch stimuli were relatively short and presented with 1 week in between. Alternatively, anxiety may have resulted in higher itch ratings during baseline. Including a no-treatment group to control for these reductions or utilizing a counterbalanced design could provide better estimates of a true placebo and nocebo response. Lastly, verbal suggestions were given regarding an inert tonic. While this approach may have worked for placebo induction, potentially, it may have been harder to elicit nocebo effects in this manner, as negative consequences regarding such a treatment method may be counterintuitive. To compare open-label and closed-label nocebo effects for itch, a different approach could be needed. For example, future research could investigate whether nocebo effects can be induced when the effects of an inert substance on itch are introduced as side effects of this substance, as changing to such an introduction of negative effects may be more closely related to how negative effects would be experienced in clinical practice.

In conclusion, this study provides evidence for the first time that positive verbal suggestions can induce expectations for itch reduction under both open-label and closed-label conditions. Suggestions are able to reduce the amount of itch experienced after histamine iontophoresis under both open-label and closed-label conditions, with closed-label suggestions appearing more effective in reducing itch during follow-up. However, experienced itch during histamine iontophoresis was not influenced by suggestions. Future research may aim to investigate under which circumstances and with which type of attribute these suggestions could elicit effects for itch. Further demonstrating the efficacy of open-label placebo effects may help facilitate the application of these effects in clinical practice.

AUTHOR CONTRIBUTIONS

SM, HvM, and AE designed the study and wrote the protocol. AvL and DV commented on the protocol. SM and AvL undertook the statistical analysis. SM and HvM wrote the first draft of the manuscript. AvL, DV, AL and AE commented on the manuscript.

FUNDING

This study was funded by a European Research Council Consolidator Grant 2013 (ID: ERC-2013-CoG-617700_EXPECT HEAL-TH, granted to AE). The funders had no role in study design, data collection or analysis, decision to publish, or writing this manuscript.

ACKNOWLEDGMENTS

The authors would like to thank Ir. Elio E. Sjak-Shie for his help with developing the NRS bar slide used for histamine iontophoresis and would like to thank Dr. Victor L. Knoop for his help with analyzing the bar slide data generated by E-Prime.

REFERENCES

1. Yew YW, Thyssen JP, Silverberg JI. A systematic review and meta-analysis of the regional and age-related differences of atopic dermatitis clinical characteristics. *J Am Acad Dermatol* (2018) 80(2):390–401. doi: 10.1016/j.jaad.2018.09.035
2. Shahwan KT, Kimball AB. Itch intensity in moderate-to-severe plaque psoriasis versus atopic dermatitis: a meta-analysis. *J Am Acad Dermatol* (2017) 76(6):1198–200.e1191. doi: 10.1016/j.jaad.2017.02.002
3. Grundmann S, Ständer S. Chronic pruritus: clinics and treatment. *Ann Dermatol* (2011) 23(1):1–11. doi: 10.5021/ad.2011.23.1.1
4. Krajnik M, Zylicz Z. Understanding pruritus in systemic disease. *J Pain Symptom Manage* (2001) 21(2):151–68. doi: 10.1016/S0885-3924(00)00256-6
5. Pereira MP, Ständer S. Assessment of severity and burden of pruritus. *Allergol Int* (2017) 66(1):3–7. doi: 10.1016/j.alit.2016.08.009
6. Matterne U, Apfelbacher CJ, Loerbroks A, Schwarzer T, Buttner M, Ofenloch R, et al. Prevalence, correlates and characteristics of chronic pruritus: a population-based cross-sectional study. *Acta Derm Venereol* (2011) 91(6):674–9. doi: 10.2340/00015555-1159
7. Schut C, Dalgard FJ, Halvorsen JA, Gieler U, Lien L, Tomas Aragones LR, et al. Occurrence, chronicity and intensity of itch in a clinical consecutive sample of patients with skin diseases: a multi-centre study in 13 European countries. *Acta Derm Venereol* (2019) 99(2):146–51. doi: 10.2340/00015555-3040
8. Fostini AC, Girolomoni G. Experimental elicitation of itch: evoking and evaluation techniques. *J Dermatol Sci* (2015) 80(1):13–7. doi: 10.1016/j.jdermsci.2015.06.004
9. Leslie TA. Itch. *Medicine* (2013) 41(7):367–71. doi: 10.1016/j.mpmed.2013.04.004
10. Benedetti F, Benedetti E, Carlino A. How placebos change the patient's brain. *Neuropsychopharmacology* (2011) 36(1):339–54. doi: 10.1038/npp.2010.81
11. Colloca L, Miller FG. How placebo responses are formed: a learning perspective. *Philos Trans R Soc Lond B Biol Sc* (2011a) 366(1572):1859–69. doi: 10.1098/rstb.2010.0398

12. Bartels DJP, van Laarhoven AIM, van de Kerkhof PCM, Evers AWM. Placebo and nocebo effects on itch: effects, mechanisms, and predictors. *Eur J Pain* (2016) 20(1):8–13. doi: 10.1002/ejp.750
13. Vase L, Petersen GL, Riley JL, 3rd, Price DD. Factors contributing to large analgesic effects in placebo mechanism studies conducted between 2002 and 2007. *Pain* (2009) 145(1–2):36–44. doi: 10.1016/j.pain.2009.04.008
14. Vase L, Riley JL, III, Price DD. A comparison of placebo effects in clinical analgesic trials versus studies of placebo analgesia. *Pain* (2002) 99(3):443–52. doi: 10.1016/S0304-3959(02)00205-1
15. Benedetti F, Mayberg HS, Wager TD, Stohler CS, Zubieta J-K. Neurobiological mechanisms of the placebo effect. *J Neurosci* (2005) 25(45):10390. doi: 10.1523/JNEUROSCI.3458-05.2005
16. Pacheco-López G, Engler H, Niemi M-B, Schedlowski M. Expectations and associations that heal: immunomodulatory placebo effects and its neurobiology. *Brain Behav Immun* (2006) 20(5):430–46. doi: 10.1016/j.bbi.2006.05.003
17. Peerdeman KJ, van Laarhoven AI, Peters ML, Evers AW. An integrative review of the influence of expectancies on pain. *Front Psychol* (2016) 7:1270. doi: 10.3389/fpsyg.2016.01270
18. Geuter S, Koban L, Wager TD. The cognitive neuroscience of placebo effects: concepts, predictions, and physiology. *Ann Rev Neurosci* (2017) 40:167–88. doi: 10.1146/annurev-neuro-072116-031132
19. Tekampe J, van Middendorp H, Meeuwis SH, van Leusden JW, Pacheco-Lopez G, Hermus AR, et al. Conditioning immune and endocrine parameters in humans: a systematic review. *Psychother Psychosom* (2017) 86(2):99–107. doi: 10.1159/000449470
20. Colloca L, Miller FG. The nocebo effect and its relevance for clinical practice. *Psychosom Med* (2011b) 73(7):598–603. doi: 10.1097/PSY.0b013e3182294a50
21. van Laarhoven AIM, van der Sman-Mauriks IM, Donders AR, Pronk MC, van de Kerkhof PC, Evers AWM. Placebo effects on itch: a meta-analysis of clinical trials of patients with dermatological conditions. *J Invest Dermatol* (2015) 135(5):1234–43. doi: 10.1038/jid.2014.522
22. Bartels DJP, Van Laarhoven AIM, Haverkamp EA, Wilder-Smith OH, Donders ART, Van Middendorp H, et al. Role of conditioning and verbal suggestion in placebo and nocebo effects on itch. *PLoS ONE* (2014) 9(3):e91727. doi: 10.1371/journal.pone.0091727
23. Bartels DJP, Van Laarhoven AIM, Stroo M, Hijne K, Peerdeman KJ, Donders ART, et al. Minimizing nocebo effects by conditioning with verbal suggestion: a randomized clinical trial in healthy humans. *PLoS ONE* (2017) 12(9):e0182959. doi: 10.1371/journal.pone.0182959
24. Darragh M, Chang JWH, Booth RJ, Consedine NS. The placebo effect in inflammatory skin reactions: the influence of verbal suggestion on itch and weal size. *J Psychosom Res* (2015) 78(5):489–94. doi: 10.1016/j.jpsychores.2015.01.011
25. Napadow V, Li A, Loggia ML, Kim J, Mawla I, Desbordes G, et al. The imagined itch: brain circuitry supporting nocebo-induced itch in atopic dermatitis patients. *Allergy Eur J Allergy Clin Immunol* (2015) 70(11):1485–92. doi: 10.1111/all.12727
26. Stumpf A, Zerey V, Heuft G, Stander S, Pfleiderer B, Schneider G. Itch perception and skin reactions as modulated by verbal suggestions: role of participant's and investigator's sex. *Acta Derm Venereol* (2016) 96(5):619–23. doi: 10.2340/00015555-2336
27. van de Sand MF, Menz MM, Sprenger C, Büchel C. Nocebo-induced modulation of cerebral itch processing—an fMRI study. *NeuroImage* (2018) (166):209–18. doi: 10.1016/j.neuroimage.2017.10.056
28. van Laarhoven AIM, Vogelaar ML, Wilder-Smith OH, van Riel PLCM, van de Kerkhof PCM, Kraaimaat FW, et al. Induction of nocebo and placebo effects on itch and pain by verbal suggestions. *Pain* (2011) 152(7):1486–94. doi: 10.1016/j.pain.2011.01.043
29. Skvortsova A, Veldhuijzen DS, Van Middendorp H, Van den Bergh O, Evers AWM. Enhancing placebo effects in somatic symptoms through oxytocin. *Psychosom Med* (2018) 80(4):353–60. doi: 10.1097/PSY.0000000000000571
30. Blease C, Colloca L, Kaptchuk TJ. Are open-label placebos ethical? Informed consent and ethical equivocations. *Bioethics* (2016) 30(6):407–14. doi: 10.1111/bioe.12245
31. Kaptchuk TJ, Friedlander E, Kelley JM, Sanchez MN, Kokkotou E, Singer JP, et al. Placebos without deception: a randomized controlled trial in irritable bowel syndrome. *PLoS ONE* (2010) 5(12):e15591. doi: 10.1371/journal.pone.0015591
32. Carvalho C, Caetano JM, Cunha L, Rebouta P, Kaptchuk TJ, Kirsch I. Open-label placebo treatment in chronic low back pain: a randomized controlled trial. *Pain* (2016) 157(12):2766–72. doi: 10.1097/j.pain.0000000000000700
33. Hoenemeyer TW, Kaptchuk TJ, Mehta TS, Fontaine KR. Open-label placebo treatment for cancer-related fatigue: a randomized-controlled clinical trial. *Sci Rep* (2018) 8(1):2784. doi: 10.1038/s41598-018-20993-y
34. Kelley JM, Kaptchuk TJ, Cusin C, Lipkin S, Fava M. Open-label placebo for major depressive disorder: a pilot randomized controlled trial. *Psychother Psychosom* (2012) 81(5):312–4. doi: 10.1159/000337053
35. Meeuwis SH, Van Middendorp H, Veldhuijzen DS, Van Laarhoven AIM, De Houwer J, Lavrijsen APM, et al. Placebo effects of open-label verbal suggestions on itch. *Acta Derm Venereol* (2018) 98(2):268–74. doi: 10.2340/00015555-2823
36. Sandler AD, Bodfish JW. Open-label use of placebos in the treatment of ADHD: a pilot study. *Child Care Health Dev* (2008) 34(1):104–10. doi: 10.1111/j.1365-2214.2007.00797.x
37. Sandler AD, Glesne C, Bodfish JW. Conditioned placebo dose reduction: a new treatment in attention-deficit hyperactivity disorder? *J Dev Behav Pediatr* (2010) 31(5):369–75. doi: 10.1097/DBP.0b013e3181e121ed
38. Schaefer M, Harke R, Denke C. Open-label placebos improve symptoms in allergic rhinitis: a randomized controlled trial. *Psychother Psychosom* (2016) 85(6):373–4. doi: 10.1159/000447242
39. Schaefer M, Sahin T, Berstecher B. Why do open-label placebos work? A randomized controlled trial of an open-label placebo induction with and without extended information about the placebo effect in allergic rhinitis. *PLoS ONE* (2018) 13(3):e0192758. doi: 10.1371/journal.pone.0192758
40. Locher C, Frey Nascimento A, Kirsch I, Kossowsky J, Meyer A, Gaab J. Is the rationale more important than deception? A randomized controlled trial of open-label placebo analgesia. *Pain* (2017) 158(12):2320–8. doi: 10.1097/j.pain.0000000000001012
41. World Medical Association. World Medical Association Declaration of Helsinki: ethical principles for medical research involving human subjects. *Jama* (2013) 310(20):2191–4. doi: 10.1001/jama.2013.281053
42. Schneider W, Eschman A, Zuccolotto A. *E-Prime reference guide*. Pittsburgh: Psychology Software Tools, Inc. (2012).
43. Misery L, Jean-Decoster C, Mery S, Georgescu V, Sibaud V. A new ten-item questionnaire for assessing sensitive skin: the Sensitive Scale-10. *Acta Derm Venereol* (2014) 94(6):635–9. doi: 10.2340/00015555-1870
44. Schneider CA, Rasband WS, Eliceiri KW. NIH Image to ImageJ: 25 years of image analysis. *Nat Methods* (2012) 9(7):671–5. doi: 10.1038/nmeth.2089
45. Faul F, Erdfelder E, Lang A-G, Buchner A. G*Power 3: a flexible statistical power analysis program for the social, behavioral, and biomedical sciences. *Behav Res Methods* (2007) 39(2):175–91. doi: 10.3758/BF03193146
46. Cohen J. *Statistical power analysis for the behavioral sciences. 2nd ed.* In. Hillsdale, NJ: Erlbaum (1988).
47. Peerdeman KJ, Tekampe J, van Laarhoven AIM, van Middendorp H, Rippe RCA, Peters ML, et al. Expectations about the effectiveness of pain- and itch-relieving medication administered via different routes. *Eur J Pain* (2018) 22(4):774–83. doi: 10.1002/ejp.1163
48. Meissner K. Placebo responses on cardiovascular, gastrointestinal, and respiratory organ functions. In: Benedetti F, Enck P, Frisaldi E, Schedlowski M, editors. *Placebo. Handbook of experimental pharmacology.*, vol. 225. Berlin, Heidelberg: Springer (2014). doi: 10.1007/978-3-662-44519-8_11
49. Meissner K, Distel H, Mitzdorf U. Evidence for placebo effects on physical but not on biochemical outcome parameters: a review of clinical trials. *BMC Med* (2007) 5:3. doi: 10.1186/1741-7015-5-3
50. Grabert JC, Bregman NJ, McAllister HA. Skin temperature regulation: the effects of suggestions and feedback. *Int J Neurosci* (1980) 10(4):217–21. doi: 10.3109/00207458009162047

51. Hájek P, Jakoubek B, Kýhos K, Radil T. Increase in cutaneous temperature induced by hypnotic suggestion of pain. *Percept Mot Skills* (1992) 74(3, Pt 1):737–8. doi: 10.2466/PMS.74.3.737-738
52. Kistler A, Mariauzouls C, Wyler F, Bircher AJ, Wyler-Harper J. Autonomic responses to suggestions for cold and warmth in hypnosis. *Forsch Komplementmed* (1999) 6(1):10–4. doi: 10.1159/000021188
53. Booth RJ, Petrie KJ, Brook RJ. Conditioning allergic skin responses in humans: a controlled trial. *Psychosom Med* (1995) 57(5):492–5. doi: 10.1097/00006842-199509000-00012
54. Darragh M, Booth RJ, Koschwanez HE, Sollers J, Broadbent E. Expectation and the placebo effect in inflammatory skin reactions. A randomised-controlled trial. *J Psychosom Res* (2013) 74(5):439–43. doi: 10.1016/j.jpsychores.2012.12.010

20

Classical Conditioning as a Distinct Mechanism of Placebo Effects

Przemysław Bąbel*

Pain Research Group, Institute of Psychology, Jagiellonian University, Kraków, Poland

***Correspondence:**
Przemysław Bąbel
przemyslaw.babel@uj.edu.pl

Classical conditioning was suggested as a mechanism of placebo effects in the 1950s. It was then challenged by response expectancy theory, which proposed that classical conditioning is just one of the means by which expectancies are acquired and changed. According to that account, placebo effects induced by classical conditioning are mediated by expectancies. However, in most of the previous studies, either expectancies were not measured or classical conditioning was combined with verbal suggestions. Thus, on the basis of those studies, it is not possible to conclude whether expectancies are involved in placebo effects induced by pure classical conditioning. Two lines of recent studies have challenged the idea that placebo effects induced by classical conditioning are always mediated by expectancies. First, some recent studies have shown that a hidden conditioning procedure elicits both placebo analgesia and nocebo hyperalgesia, neither of which is predicted by expectancy. Second, there are studies showing that visual cues paired with pain stimuli of high or low intensity induce both placebo analgesia and nocebo hyperalgesia when they are presented subliminally without participants' awareness. The results of both lines of studies suggest that expectancy may not always be involved in placebo effects induced by classical conditioning and that conditioning may be a distinct mechanism of placebo effects. Thus, these results support the idea that placebo effects can be learned by classical conditioning either consciously or unconsciously. However, the existing body of evidence is limited to classically conditioned placebo effects in pain, that is, placebo analgesia and nocebo hyperalgesia.

Keywords: classical conditioning, nocebo effect, Pavlovian conditioning, placebo effect, response expectancy

THE ORIGINS OF THE CLASSICAL CONDITIONING ACCOUNT OF PLACEBO EFFECTS

Classical conditioning was independently suggested as a mechanism of placebo effects for the first time in 1957 by Gliedman, Gantt, and Teitelbaum (1) and Kurland (2). It is interesting that just 2 years earlier, Beecher (3) had published his seminal paper that is now considered the starting point of scientific interest in placebo effects. Thus, classical conditioning has been regarded as a mechanism of placebo effects since the very beginning of research on placebo. However, Wickramasekera (4, 5) was the first to propose a broad and coherent theoretical account of placebo effects as conditional reflexes.

According to the classical conditioning approach, placebo is a conditioned stimulus and placebo effects are conditioned responses. The first studies in which classical conditioning with an active drug as an unconditioned stimulus was used to induce placebo effects were conducted in animals (6–8). However, in fact, Pavlov (9) was the first to describe the effects of repeated applications of active drugs that his collaborators had found. Dr. Podkopaev associated the sound of a definite pitch with the effects of a dose of apomorphine in dogs. In effect, the sound of the note alone produced all the symptoms of the drug. Similarly, when Dr. Krylov repeatedly injected morphine into dogs, he observed that the preliminaries of the injection were sufficient to produce all the symptoms of the drug. Nevertheless, these early studies started two very important lines of research, that is, studies on conditioned immunopharmacological effects (10) derived from Ader and Cohen's (6) experiment and studies on conditioned drug tolerance (11) derived from Sigel's (8) experiment. In both lines of research, responses to stimuli that accompany the application of pharmacologically active drugs are classically conditioned. However, these studies do not aim to explore the mechanisms of placebo effects, and they focus on conditioning of physiological responses.

Voudouris, Peck, and Coleman (12–14) developed the classical conditioning paradigm to induce placebo effects in humans. By surreptitiously pairing an inactive cream with decreasing nociceptive stimulation, they strengthened the placebo effect induced by verbal suggestion of the analgesic action of the cream (12, 13). Moreover, in spite of the fact that they had previously induced the placebo effect by verbal suggestion of the analgesic action of an inactive cream, they were subsequently able to induce the nocebo effect by pairing the same cream with increasing nociceptive stimulation (12, 13). Most importantly, they also found that placebo analgesia can be induced by classical conditioning alone (without verbal suggestions); that is, the placebo effect was found in a group that was informed that they had received an inactive cream, which was then surreptitiously paired with decreasing nociceptive stimulation (14). However, it should be noted that the cream used in these studies might have raised expectancy based on previous experiences with active treatment creams and that expectancy might have biased the results. These studies started a new line of research on placebo effects induced by classical conditioning. The aim of the paper is to briefly summarize recent findings and, based on them, draw conclusions on the differential roles of classical conditioning and expectancy in placebo effects. It should be noted that subjective responses, that is, pain, are subject to conditioning in this new line of research. Thus, this paper focuses on classical conditioning of placebo effects in pain, including placebo analgesia and nocebo hyperalgesia.

THE CLASSICAL CONDITIONING ACCOUNT IS CHALLENGED BY RESPONSE EXPECTANCY THEORY

In the same year as the first study on classical conditioning of placebo effects in humans was published (12), Kirsch (15) published his seminal paper on response expectancy in which he proposed another account of placebo effects. His theory assumes that placebo effects result from expectancies concerning placebo intervention. Kirsch (15) highlighted that, among other processes, classical conditioning is involved in the acquisition and modification of expectancy. According to this viewpoint, classical conditioning is one of the means by which expectancies are acquired and modified; that is, the effects of conditioning are mediated by expectancy (15). In other words, there is only one mechanism of placebo effects—expectancy; classical conditioning is only a method that is used to acquire or change expectancy.

This view is reflected in the popular learning model of placebo effects proposed by Colloca and Miller (16). In this model, placebo effects result from expectancies acquired by decoding information from the psychosocial context, including conditioned stimuli, among others. Thus, according to the model, classical conditioning is a mean by which placebo effects may be induced and expectancies play a central role in the formation of placebo effects induced by classical conditioning.

It should be noted that expectancies are by definition consciously accessible (17–19). According to a recent definition, expectation is understood to mean a "conscious, conceptual belief about the future occurrence of an event" (20).

Kirsch's (15) account of the role of expectancy in the formation of placebo effects induced by classical conditioning is based on a current view on classical conditioning, which is best summarized by Rescorla (21). This modern view differs substantially from Pavlov's (9) account, as is well reflected in the title of Rescorla's (21) seminal paper: "Pavlovian conditioning: It's not what you think it is." According to this current view, classical conditioning is not a mechanical process in which one stimulus passes control over a response from another stimulus; instead, conditioning is now seen as the learning of relations among events, which allows the organism to represent its environment. As a consequence, cognitive involvement is assumed for classical conditioning. From this perspective, conditioning produces the expectancy that certain stimuli will be followed by other stimuli, and it is this expectancy that produces the response. In other words, expectancies mediate the effects of conditioning (18).

THE CHALLENGE CONTINUES IN STUDIES CONTRASTING CLASSICAL CONDITIONING AND EXPECTANCY

Kirsch (15) not only challenged the classical conditioning account of placebo effects on theoretical grounds but also conducted an empirical test of his theory. Montgomery and Kirsch (22) showed that the effects of classical conditioning on placebo analgesia induced by verbal suggestions are completely mediated by expectancies and that when participants were informed that they were undergoing the conditioning procedure (i.e., pairing placebo cream with decreasing nociceptive stimulation), the conditioning did not have an effect on placebo analgesia induced by verbal suggestions.

Montgomery and Kirsch's (22) study together with Voudouris and collaborators' (12–14) investigations started the conditioning versus expectancy debate, which has still not been fully resolved. The essence of this debate is whether classical conditioning is a distinct mechanism of placebo effects or the effects of conditioning are mediated by expectancy. The early stage of this debate was reviewed by Stewart-Williams and Podd (19). However, during 15 years since their seminal paper was published, new research findings have been collected that shed light on the debate.

So far, few studies have been conducted in which both classical conditioning was applied and expectancy was measured. Although most of these studies suggest that the effects of conditioning are correlated with expectancy (23–26), predicted by expectancy (27), or mediated by expectancy (22, 28–30), their results are limited to participants in whom both verbal suggestions of analgesia or hyperalgesia and classical conditioning were applied. Thus, based on these findings, one cannot draw any conclusions on the role of expectancy in placebo effects induced by pure classical conditioning. Instead, it can be concluded that expectancy is involved in the effects of conditioning on placebo effects induced by verbal suggestions.

Moreover, the sparse studies in which pure classical conditioning was applied (without verbal suggestions) and expectancy was measured usually failed to induce placebo effects (25, 31, 32), probably due to limited conditioning trials (from 12 to 30, including 6–15 in which placebo was paired with changes in nociceptive stimulation). Even if it succeeded in one study (i.e., placebo analgesia was found in the group subjected to pure conditioning), the results of regression analysis revealing the prediction of the placebo effect by expectancies were based on the results from all the study groups, including those in which verbal suggestions of analgesia were provided (33). Thus, it is not possible to conclude whether expectancies predicted placebo analgesia found in the group subjected to pure classical conditioning. Interestingly, in that study, classical conditioning produced the placebo effect, regardless of whether or not participants were informed that they were undergoing the conditioning procedure (i.e., pairing placebo cream with decreasing nociceptive stimulation) and regardless of whether they were informed that active or inactive intervention was used (in fact placebo) (33). These results contradict Montgomery and Kirsch's (22) findings.

CHALLENGE ACCEPTED: PLACEBO EFFECTS INDUCED BY PURE CLASSICAL CONDITIONING

Unfortunately, most of the few studies in which pure classical conditioning without verbal suggestions succeeded in inducing placebo effects did not involve the measurement of expectancy (34–36). For many years, the only study in which pure classical conditioning effectively induced the placebo effect and expectancy was measured was the one conducted by Voudouris and collaborators (14). In one of the groups, participants were informed that they were in a control group and they would receive a neutral cream. They were then subjected to conditioning procedure in which the cream was paired with decreased nociceptive stimulation without participants' knowledge. However, in that study, expectancy was measured only once (before the pre-test), so it is impossible to determine whether the conditioning that was performed after the pre-test changed expectancies.

Recently, two lines of studies have challenged the idea that placebo effects induced by classical conditioning are always mediated by expectancies. In the first line, hidden conditioning without verbal suggestions is conducted, and expectancies are measured on a trial-by-trial basis. Conditioning procedure may be conducted in two ways: by informing or not informing participants that there is a relationship between the placebo (i.e., a conditioned stimulus) and the active drug or procedure (i.e., an unconditioned stimulus). When participants are aware of the relationship, this is referred to as open conditioning; when they are not aware of it, this is called hidden conditioning. Thus, the role of consciousness is the main difference between hidden and open conditioning.

In three recent studies, hidden conditioning was used to induce placebo analgesia (37, 38) and nocebo hyperalgesia (38, 39), and expectancies were measured on a trial-by-trial basis. These studies found that not only hidden conditioning was effective in producing placebo effects but also, primarily, expectancies predicted or mediated neither placebo analgesia nor nocebo hyperalgesia (37–39), even though conditioning had an effect on expectancies (37). Moreover, when participants were asked at the end of the study whether they had noticed the contingency between placebo stimuli and differences in pain intensity, most of them denied (37). Thus, based on these results, it seems that it is possible to induce placebo effects without the awareness of the participants.

The second line of research that sheds light on the role of expectancy in placebo effects induced by pure classical conditioning involves placebo stimuli presented subliminally without participants' awareness. In this paradigm, clearly recognizable visual stimuli are first paired with pain stimuli of high or low intensity. After a conditioning phase is completed, the same conditioned visual cues are presented subliminally in a testing phase. It has been found that pain stimuli preceded by subliminally presented conditioned visual stimuli are rated as less or more painful depending on whether they have previously been paired with high or low pain stimuli, indicating that placebo analgesia and nocebo hyperalgesia are induced without awareness (40–44). Moreover, it has also been found that both placebo analgesia and nocebo hyperalgesia can be induced not only by conditioning of supraliminal stimuli but also by conditioning of subliminally presented stimuli (44). Placebo effects induced by conditioned stimuli presented subliminally without participants' awareness suggest that expectancy may not have been involved in their production, which is consistent with the results from the first line of studies. Although expectancy is not measured in those studies, participants are not aware of the presented stimuli. Thus, their expectancy should not have affected the results.

It may be argued that the studies from both lines of research did not include any placebo interventions in the form of a sugar pill, fake cream, or sham electrodes. In fact, in all of those studies, visual stimuli were paired with decreasing or/and increasing pain stimulation. However, according to Miller and Kaptchuk (45), the placebo effect is not the result of a specific intervention, but it is rather produced and enhanced by the context surrounding the treatment. Thus, even if no inert treatment is administered, the so-called placebo-related effect may still be found (46).

CONCLUSIONS

The results of both lines of studies suggest that expectancy may not be always involved in placebo effects induced by classical conditioning and that conditioning may be a distinct mechanism of placebo effects.

These findings are in line with the fact that, in some cases, classical conditioning represents an automatic process that is not mediated by cognitive expectancy (18). In fact, many phenomena could be explained by classical conditioning without cognitive mediation. They include evaluative conditioning, second-order conditioning, conditioned taste aversions and flavor preferences, conditioning with subliminally presented conditioned stimuli, conditioned immunosuppression, and conditioning in simple organisms among others (see (18) for review). Thus, only some placebo effects could be explained by classical conditioning without expectancy involvement.

However, the findings under discussion do not exclude the role of expectancy in inducing placebo effects. Expectancy ratings may not always predict placebo effects. However, pre-cognitive associations, that is, "links between events and/or objects that exist outside conscious awareness" (20), may be acquired through hidden conditioning procedures or be responsible for responses to subliminally presented conditioned stimuli. In fact, when classical conditioning is used to enhance or reduce placebo effects induced by verbal suggestions, expectancies are involved in their formation (22–30). In that case, classical conditioning is just a mean by which expectancies are acquired and modified. Moreover, expectancies might not always be easily self-reported; that is, although expectancies do exist, one might not be able to report them. However, the idea of conscious expectancies that are not self-reported should be dealt with caution as it may lead to circular reasoning (17).

These conclusions are in line with recent review (47) and previously proposed models postulating that the classical conditioning and response expectancy accounts do not exclude each other, but the range of phenomena they explain is not completely the same (19, 48). Conditioning involves either conscious learning (acquisition and modifications of expectancies) or unconscious learning (conditioning not mediated by expectancy). Expectancies can be acquired and modified by conditioning and other procedures, including verbal suggestions and observational learning. In other words, either conscious learning (expectancy and conditioning) or unconscious learning (conditioning) can be mechanisms of placebo effects. Thus, both accounts seem to be compatible rather than mutually exclusive (19, 48). From this perspective, classical conditioning is in some cases a distinct mechanism of placebo effects, and sometimes, it is just a method used to acquire or change expectancy.

Thus, the current conclusions contradict Colloca and Miller's (16) learning model of the formation of placebo effects. They suggest that conditioned placebo and nocebo responses may not always be mediated by expectancy. It seems that Colloca and Miller's (16) model does not explain the mechanism of all instances of placebo effects. However, future studies should answer the question under which circumstances placebo effects induced by classical conditioning are mediated by expectancy and when they are not mediated by expectancy. Previous studies in which expectancies were not involved in the induction of placebo effects by classical conditioning used visual stimuli as placebos together with a large number of conditioning trails. Thus, these two factors may be necessary to induce conditioned placebo effects that are not mediated by expectancy. So far, it seems only clear that placebo effects induced by both conditioning and verbal suggestions are mediated by expectancy. Further research is also needed to investigate the differential role of classical conditioning and expectancy in placebo effects outside pain. It would also be of interest to investigate whether all principles of classical conditioning found in studies outside the placebo research field (e.g., generalization and extinction) can be directly applied to placebo effects.

The finding that expectancy may not always be involved in placebo effects induced by classical conditioning has implications that have been discussed above, not only for placebo theory. It also has important implications for the methodology of placebo studies, that is, that expectancies should be measured in research on placebo effects when the role of expectancy is under study. Regardless of whether placebo effects were induced by classical conditioning, verbal suggestions, or both, the involvement or absence of expectancy might be postulated only when expectancy was measured. Most importantly, this fact also has implications for clinical practice. Pain can decrease or increase after negative or positive experiences that are associated with environmental stimuli. In effect, these environmental stimuli may increase or reduce pain symptoms, not only without any provided verbal suggestions, but—most importantly—without patients' conscious awareness. Thus, pain changes can occur even when patients do not anticipate them. The decrease or increase of pain may result from uncontrollable contextual factors. Identifying the elements, that is, the conditioned stimuli that change pain experiences, could be an essential part of pain management programs. However, as significant differences between experimental and clinical settings exist, further studies are needed before translating laboratory research results into clinical practice.

AUTHOR CONTRIBUTIONS

The author confirms being the sole contributor of this work.

FUNDING

This manuscript was prepared under grant number 2014/14/E/HS6/00415 from the National Science Centre, Poland.

REFERENCES

1. Gliedman LH, Gantt WH, Teitelbaum HA. Some implications of conditional reflex studies for placebo research. *Am J Psychiatry* (1957) 113:1103–7. doi: 10.1176/ajp.113.12.1103
2. Kurland AA. The drug placebo—its psychodynamic and conditional reflex action. *Behav Sci* (1957) 2(2):101–10. doi: 10.1002/bs.3830020203
3. Beecher HK. The powerful placebo. *J Am Med Assoc* (1955) 159(17):1602–6. doi: 10.1001/jama.1955.02960340022006
4. Wickramasekera I. A conditioned response model of the placebo effect predictions from the model. *Biofeedback Self Regul* (1980) 5(1):5–18. doi: 10.1007/BF00999060
5. Wickramasekera I. A conditioned response model of the placebo effect: predictions from the model. In: White L, Tursky B, Schwartz GE, editors. *Placebo: theory, research, and mechanisms.* The Guilford Press (1985). p. 255–87.
6. Ader R, Cohen N. Behaviorally conditioned immunosuppression. *Psychosom Med* (1975) 37(4):333–40. doi: 10.1097/00006842-197507000-00007
7. Herrnstein RJ. Placebo effect in the rat. *Science* (1962) 138(3541):677–8. doi: 10.1126/science.138.3541.677
8. Siegel S. Evidence from rats that morphine tolerance is a learned response. *J Comp Physiol Psychol* (1975) 89(5):498–506. doi: 10.1037/h0077058
9. Pavlov IP. *Conditioned reflexes: an investigation of the physiological activity of the cerebral cortex.* Oxford, England: Oxford Univ. Press (1927). p. xv, 430.
10. Lückemann L, Unteroberdörster M, Kirchhof J, Schedlowski M, Hadamitzky M. Applications and limitations of behaviorally conditioned immunopharmacological responses. *Neurobiol Learn Mem* (2017) 142 (Pt A):91–8. doi: 10.1016/j.nlm.2017.02.012
11. Siegel S, Baptista MA, Kim JA, McDonald RV, Weise-Kelly L. Pavlovian psychopharmacology: the associative basis of tolerance. *Exp Clin Psychopharmacol* (2000) 8(3):276–93. doi: 10.1037//1064-1297.8.3.276
12. Voudouris NJ, Peck CL, Coleman G. Conditioned placebo responses. *J Pers Soc Psychol* (1985) 48(1):47. doi: 10.1037//0022-3514.48.1.47
13. Voudouris NJ, Peck CL, Coleman G. Conditioned response models of placebo phenomena: further support. *Pain* (1989) 38(1):109–16. doi: 10.1016/0304-3959(89)90080-8
14. Voudouris NJ, Peck CL, Coleman G. The role of conditioning and verbal expectancy in the placebo response. *Pain* (1990) 43(1):121–8. doi: 10.1016/0304-3959(90)90057-K
15. Kirsch I. Response expectancy as a determinant of experience and behavior. *Am Psychol* (1985) 40(11):1189–202. doi: 10.1037/0003-066X.40.11.1189
16. Colloca L, Miller FG. How placebo responses are formed: a learning perspective. *Philos Trans R Soc Lond B Biol Sci* (2011) 366(1572):1859–69. doi: 10.1098/rstb.2010.0398
17. Kirsch I. Conditioning, expectancy, and the placebo effect: comment on Stewart-Williams and Podd (2004). *Psychol Bull* (2004) 130(2):341–3; discussion 344-345. doi: 10.1037/0033-2909.130.2.341
18. Kirsch I, Lynn SJ, Vigorito M, Miller RR. The role of cognition in classical and operant conditioning. *J Clin Psychol* (2004) 60(4):369–92. doi: 10.1002/jclp.10251
19. Stewart-Williams S, Podd J. The placebo effect: dissolving the expectancy versus conditioning debate. *Psychol Bull* (2004) 130(2):324. doi: 10.1037/0033-2909.130.2.324
20. Wager TD, Atlas LY. The neuroscience of placebo effects: connecting context, learning and health. *Nat Rev Neurosci* (2015) 16(7):403–18. doi: 10.1038/nrn3976
21. Rescorla RA. Pavlovian conditioning. It's not what you think it is. *Am Psychol* (1988) 43(3):151–60. doi: 10.1037//0003-066X.43.3.151
22. Montgomery GH, Kirsch I. Classical conditioning and the placebo effect. *Pain* (1997) 72(1):107–13. doi: 10.1016/S0304-3959(97)00016-X
23. Corsi N, Colloca L. Placebo and nocebo effects: the advantage of measuring expectations and psychological factors. *Front Psychol* (2017) 8:308. doi: 10.3389/fpsyg.2017.00308
24. Price DD, Milling LS, Kirsch I, Duff A, Montgomery GH, Nicholls SS. An analysis of factors that contribute to the magnitude of placebo analgesia in an experimental paradigm. *Pain* (1999) 83(2):147–56. doi: 10.1016/S0304-3959(99)00081-0
25. Reicherts P, Gerdes ABM, Pauli P, Wieser MJ. Psychological placebo and nocebo effects on pain rely on expectation and previous experience. *J Pain* (2016) 17(2):203–14. doi: 10.1016/j.jpain.2015.10.010
26. Schafer SM, Colloca L, Wager TD. Conditioned placebo analgesia persists when subjects know they are receiving a placebo. *J Pain* (2015) 16(5):412–20. doi: 10.1016/j.jpain.2014.12.008
27. Colagiuri B, Quinn VF, Colloca L. Nocebo hyperalgesia, partial reinforcement, and extinction. *J Pain* (2015) 16(10):995–1004. doi: 10.1016/j.jpain.2015.06.012
28. Colagiuri B, Quinn VF. Autonomic arousal as a mechanism of the persistence of nocebo hyperalgesia. *J Pain* (2018) 19(5):476–86. doi: 10.1016/j.jpain.2017.12.006
29. Jepma M, Wager TD. Conceptual conditioning: mechanisms mediating conditioning effects on pain. *Psychol Sci* (2015) 26(11):1728–39. doi: 10.1177/0956797615597658
30. Kirsch I, Kong J, Sadler P, Spaeth R, Cook A, Kaptchuk TJ, et al. Expectancy and conditioning in placebo analgesia: separate or connected processes? *Psychol Conscious* (2014) 1(1):51. doi: 10.1037/cns0000007
31. Bąbel P. Psychologiczne mechanizmy negatywnego działania placebo. Analiza empiryczna [Psychological mechanisms of negative placebo action. An empirical analysis]. *Stud Psychol Psychol Stud* (2008) 46(1):13–24.
32. Rhudy JL, Güereca YM, Kuhn BL, Palit S, Flaten MA. The influence of placebo analgesia manipulations on pain report, the nociceptive flexion reflex, and autonomic responses to pain. *J Pain* (2018) 19(11):1257–74. doi: 10.1016/j.jpain.2018.04.012
33. de Jong PJ, van Baast R, Arntz A, Merckelbach H. The placebo effect in pain reduction: the influence of conditioning experiences and response expectancies. *Int J Behav Med* (1996) 3(1):14–29. doi: 10.1207/s15327558ijbm0301_2
34. Amanzio M, Benedetti F. Neuropharmacological dissection of placebo analgesia: expectation-activated opioid systems versus conditioning-activated specific subsystems. *J Neurosci* (1999) 19(1):484–94. doi: 10.1523/JNEUROSCI.19-01-00484.1999
35. Bräscher A-K, Kleinböhl D, Hölzl R, Becker S. Differential classical conditioning of the nocebo effect: increasing heat–pain perception without verbal suggestions. *Front Psychol* (2017) 8:2163. doi: 10.3389/fpsyg.2017.02163
36. Klinger R, Soost S, Flor H, Worm M. Classical conditioning and expectancy in placebo hypoalgesia: a randomized controlled study in patients with atopic dermatitis and persons with healthy skin. *Pain* (2007) 128(1):31–9. doi: 10.1016/j.pain.2006.08.025
37. Bąbel P, Adamczyk W, Świder K, Bajcar EA, Kicman P, Lisińska N. How classical conditioning shapes placebo analgesia: hidden versus open conditioning. *Pain Med* (2018) 19(6):1156–69. doi: 10.1093/pm/pnx177
38. Bąbel P, Bajcar EA, Adamczyk W, Kicman P, Lisińska N, Świder K, et al. Classical conditioning without verbal suggestions elicits placebo analgesia and nocebo hyperalgesia. *PLoS ONE* (2017) 12(7):e0181856. doi: 10.1371/journal.pone.0181856
39. Bajcar EA, Wiercioch-Kuzianik K, Adamczyk WM, Bąbel P. To experience or to be informed? Classical conditioning induces nocebo hyperalgesia even when placebo analgesia is verbally suggested—results of a preliminary study. *Pain Med* (2019). doi: 10.1093/pm/pnz123
40. Egorova N, Park J, Kong J. In the face of pain: the choice of visual cues in pain conditioning matters. *Eur J Pain* (2017) 21(7):1243–51. doi: 10.1002/ejp.1024
41. Egorova N, Park J, Orr SP, Kirsch I, Gollub RL, Kong J. Not seeing or feeling is still believing: conscious and non-conscious pain modulation after direct and observational learning. *Sci Rep* (2015) 5:16809. doi: 10.1038/srep16809
42. Jensen KB, Kaptchuk TJ, Chen X, Kirsch I, Ingvar M, Gollub RL, et al. A neural mechanism for nonconscious activation of conditioned placebo and nocebo responses. *Cereb Cortex N Y N* (1991) 201525(10):3903–10. doi: 10.1093/cercor/bhu275
43. Jensen KB, Kaptchuk TJ, Kirsch I, Raicek J, Lindstrom KM, Berna C, et al. Nonconscious activation of placebo and nocebo pain responses. *Proc Natl Acad Sci* (2012) 109(39):15959–64. doi: 10.1073/pnas.1202056109
44. Jensen K, Kirsch I, Odmalm S, Kaptchuk TJ, Ingvar M. Classical conditioning of analgesic and hyperalgesic pain responses without conscious awareness. *Proc Natl Acad Sci* (2015) 112(25):7863–7. doi: 10.1073/pnas.1504567112

45. Miller FG, Kaptchuk TJ. The power of context: reconceptualizing the placebo effect. *J R Soc Med* (2008) 101(5):222–5. doi: 10.1258/jrsm.2008.070466
46. Benedetti F. *Placebo effects*. New York: Oxford University Press (2014). 427 p. doi: 10.1093/acprof:oso/9780198705086.001.0001
47. Bräscher A-K, Witthöft M, Becker S. The underestimated significance of conditioning in placebo hypoalgesia and nocebo hyperalgesia. *Pan Res Manag* (2018) 6841985. doi: 10.1155/2018/6841985
48. Bąbel P. Psychologiczne mechanizmy działania placebo: warunkowanie klasyczne a oczekiwania [Psychological mechanisms of placebo action: classical conditioning and expectancy]. *Stud Psychol [Psychol Stud]* (2006) 44(3):5–15.

21

A Direct Comparison of Placebo and Nocebo Effects on Visuospatial Attention: An Eye-Tracking Experiment

Carina Höfler, Jonas Potthoff and Anne Schienle*

Department of Clinical Psychology, University of Graz, Graz, Austria

Correspondence:
Carina Höfler
carina.hoefler@uni-graz.at

Background: Placebo and nocebo effects on visual attention are still poorly understood. This eye-tracking study directly compared effects of sham transcranial magnetic stimulation (sTMS) that was administered along with the verbal suggestion that the treatment would either increase (placebo) or decrease (nocebo) left-sided visual attention.

Method: Twenty women who had reported decreased attention (nocebo responders) and 20 women who had reported increased attention (placebo responders) following sTMS completed a visual search task with three visual load levels. The task was conducted once with and once without the placebo or the nocebo (sTMS). Left-sided fixations and reaction times for left-sided targets (in comparison with right-sided targets) were analyzed.

Results: Contrary to the verbal suggestion, the nocebo responders showed more left-sided fixations in the nocebo condition (compared with the control condition) and responded faster to left-sided targets in the high-load condition. The placebo had no effect on fixations and reaction times.

Conclusion: These results indicate a more beneficial effect of a nocebo compared with a placebo for the first time. Limits and possibilities of placebo and nocebo interventions are discussed.

Keywords: placebo, nocebo, eye-tracking, visuospatial attention, sham transcranial magnetic stimulation

INTRODUCTION

Placebos and nocebos are physically or pharmacologically inert drugs, devices, or other types of sham interventions that are able to influence various clinical and physiological outcomes related to health (1). Whereas placebos have beneficial effects on specific conditions, nocebos are associated with the occurrence of negative symptoms, the worsening of symptoms, or the prevention of improvement. Both effects are considered to be 'context effects' because they are mediated by diverse mechanisms, such as learning, expectations, and social cognition (1).

It has been repeatedly shown that placebos and nocebos are able to change somatic and emotional processes. The most studied phenomena, "placebo analgesia" and "nocebo hyperalgesia," refer to the experience of either decreased or increased levels of pain after sham treatment. Other placebo/nocebo phenomena, for example, those related to perceptual processes, have been investigated less frequently and are therefore still poorly understood. A few studies have shown that placebos and nocebos are able to alter visual attention [e.g., Refs. (2–7)]. In those studies, the placebo treatments reduced visual avoidance of negative affective stimuli (4, 5, 8) and enhanced the performance on a visual search task (3). In contrast, the nocebos reduced the performance on a visual search task (3) and increased visual cortex activation during negative affective picture processing (6). Thus, there is converging evidence indicating that nocebo- or placebo-related expectations are able to influence the processing of visual inputs.

In one nocebo study on attention, a surprising effect was observed (7). Healthy individuals received sham transcranial magnetic stimulation (sTMS) along with the verbal suggestion that the treatment would elicit temporary neglect-like attention deficits in the left visual field (transitory "pseudo-neglect"). Contrary to this suggestion, in those participants who had reported experiencing attention deficits, the nocebo actually enhanced the number of left-sided fixations and facilitated target detection. These results point to a paradoxical yet positive aspect of nocebo treatment, where the suggestion of unilateral attention deficits actually provokes unilateral attention improvements (7).

This unexpected finding raises questions relating to an analogous situation: what would be the effects of a placebo sTMS combined with the verbal suggestion of a unilateral improvement in attention? In general, placebo/nocebo mechanisms are still poorly understood and controversial topics of discussion. While some findings indicate that placebos and nocebos are "evil twins" that produce effects that are counterparts of one common phenomenon [e.g., Refs. (9, 10)], others argue that placebo/nocebo responses are distinct phenomena with distinct neurobiological representations [e.g., Refs. (11, 12)].

In order to better understand both mechanisms, comparative studies, which include both placebo and nocebo conditions, are needed. In the present study, the effects of equivalent placebo and nocebo suggestions on visual-spatial attention were directly compared with each other. The study design was based on a previous nocebo study (7), which was extended by adding a placebo group. Participants completed a visual search task after being treated with a placebo or nocebo device: this device was an sTMS system, which was administered with the verbal instruction that the stimulation would either induce temporary left-sided attention improvements (placebo) or deficits (nocebo). Differences in left-sided fixation frequency, as well as reaction times for left-sided targets (in comparison with right-sided targets) during sham treatment, were compared between the placebo and the nocebo groups. Based on previous placebo studies on general visual attention [e.g., Ref. (3)], it was expected that the placebo would enhance left-sided attention as reflected by an increase in left-sided fixations and faster reactions to left-sided targets (in comparison with right-sided targets). This placebo-related improvement should be more pronounced than the previously observed increase in left-sided attention during nocebo treatment (7).

METHOD

Sample

A total of 40 right-handed healthy university students with a mean age of 21.06 years (SD = 2.58) were included in the study sample. Exclusion criteria were the presence of mental/neurological disorders, medication intake (except contraceptives), participation in a previous study with a real TMS system and attention deficits as assessed by a clinical interview, and an attention test (d2) (13). All participants had normal or corrected-to-normal vision. They were recruited *via* announcements at the university campus and gave written informed consent. The study was conducted in accordance with the Declaration of Helsinki and approved by the ethics committee of the university.

Design and Procedure

The subjects either participated in the placebo arm of the study (n = 20) or in the nocebo arm (n = 20). The placebo arm consisted of two counterbalanced conditions (with placebo vs. without placebo). The same was true for the nocebo arm (two counterbalanced conditions: with nocebo vs. without nocebo). The two conditions were separated by approximately 1 week. The design of the study is displayed in the **Supplementary Table S1**.

The placebo/nocebo device was an sTMS system, which was administered with the verbal suggestion that the stimulation would either induce temporary left-sided attention improvements (placebo) or deficits (nocebo). In fact, the sTMS system was a head massage tool, which induced symmetrical vibrations across the head (**Figure 1**) associated with a whirring sound. The system was presented as an innovative portable low-intensity repetitive TMS system for neurological rehabilitation. Given the increasing relevance of TMS in this field [especially in the treatment of visual neglect symptoms, e.g., Ref. (14)], this type of treatment was chosen. In order to increase the credibility of the cover story, the participants were provided with technical illustrations and a fictitious scientific article about the TMS system and its possible applications.

The sTMS system was administered for 4 min with verbal instructions either suggesting temporary left-sided attention improvements (placebo) or deficits (nocebo).

Placebo: "TMS can induce left-sided attention improvements … The visual exploration on the left side will be perceived as significantly easier and can be done faster…"

Nocebo: "TMS can induce left-sided [neglect-like] attention deficits…. The visual exploration on the left side will be perceived as significantly more challenging and exhausting…"

After the sTMS, the system was removed and the eye-tracking experiment with the visual search task started. Before and after the experiment, the affective state of the participants was assessed *via* the self-assessment manikin (1–9, 9 = happy, aroused, dominant) (15). At the end of the placebo/nocebo condition, the efficacy of the sTMS system was rated (0–100%), and the participants were asked to report experienced symptoms induced by the sTMS. At the end of the study, all participants were debriefed.

The participants of the nocebo arm were 20 "nocebo responders" [subsample of a previous study by Höfler et al. (7)], who had rated the sTMS stimulation as most effective. Effectiveness was defined as perceived change in visual attention (in the suggested direction) in percent (100% = very effective). For the placebo arm of the study, 20 women were selected from a bigger sample of 50 women ("placebo responders"). These responders did not differ from the nocebo responders in their effectiveness ratings for the sTMS (nocebo = 49.50%, SE = 3.18; placebo = 54.35%, SE = 4.03; $p > .28$). The two

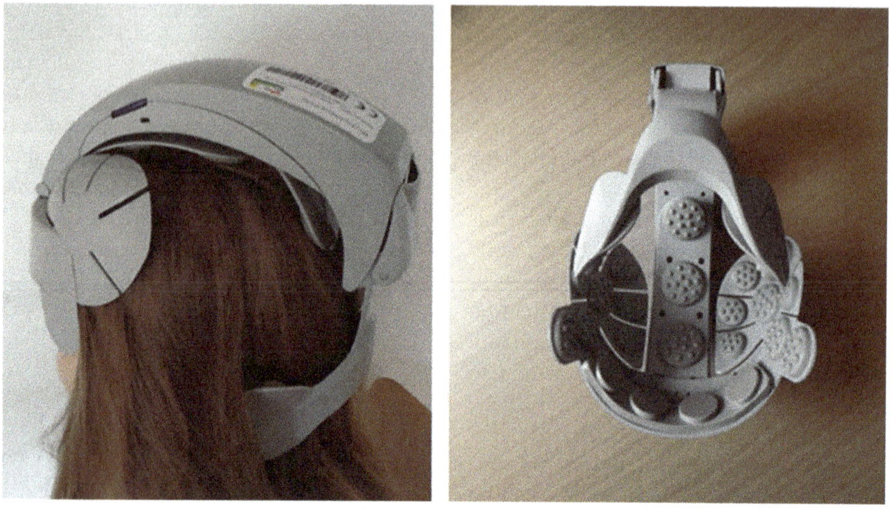

FIGURE 1 | Sham device for transcranial magnetic stimulation (sTMS).

groups (placebo, nocebo) did not differ in mean age (nocebo = 21.00 years, SD = 2.41; placebo = 22.20 years, SD = 2.67; $p > .14$), average value of d2-attention (nocebo = 107.55, SE = 2.19; placebo = 109.65, SE = 1.48; $p = .43$), mean reaction time (nocebo = 11,209.73 ms, SE = 660.02; placebo = 10,535.56 ms, SE = 470.31; $p = .41$), and hit rate of targets in the visual search task (nocebo = 98.82%, SE = .29; placebo = 98.89%, SE = .28; $p = .86$).

We only selected "responders" for the present investigation because previous studies showed that the effects of placebos/nocebos are associated with the expected and experienced efficacy of the sham treatment [e.g., Refs. (7, 16, 17)]. Placebo/nocebo effects are mediated by diverse processes, including expectations, beliefs, and social cognition (1). In this sense, a positive/negative belief is a prerequisite for the placebo/nocebo effect to occur.

Visual Search Task

Participants performed a visual search task, the adapted version of the balloons test (18). The balloons task had three visual load conditions with either 50, 100, or 200 schematic black balloons depicted on a white background (**Figure 2**). Each balloon was represented by a black circle with an adjoining black vertical line originating from the bottom of the circle. The diameter of each circle was 11 mm; the line had a length of 7 mm. The balloons functioned as distractors, and one black circle without a line was the target. Participants were instructed to localize the target as fast as possible on the computer screen and confirm the detection *via* mouse click (the cursor was not visible during the search task). The mouse click was used to determine the reaction time. Subsequently, the participants were asked to point to the target to verify the correct localization. Prior to each visual load condition, a blank white screen was shown for 30 s. The sequence of the conditions was counterbalanced. Each condition comprised 12 trials; each trial had a maximum duration of 90 s. In each trial, the target had a different position oriented on a balanced 4:3 grid (six targets at each side per condition). The sequence of target location was randomized. Prior to the task, the participants performed two example tasks (target on the left/right) to get familiar with the procedure.

During the search task, two-dimensional eye movements were recorded with an SMI RED250mobile (sampling rate: 250 Hz, nine-point calibration). We calibrated both eyes and analyzed data from the eye, which produced a better spatial resolution (>0.35° visual angle). The data were only analyzed if the spatial resolution was above 0.5°. The experiment was controlled with the SMI Experiment Suite. The data were exported with SMI Begaze and customized Python scripts. For event detection, standard

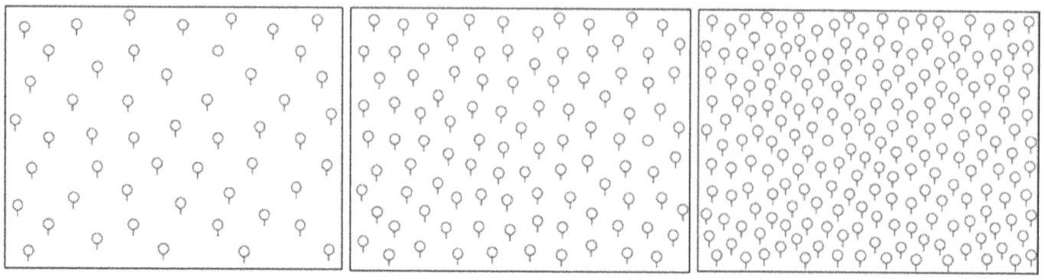

FIGURE 2 | Balloon task with three visual load levels.

thresholds of the SMI BeGaze Software (Version 3.6.52) for high-speed eye-tracking data (sampling rate >200 Hz) were used: The velocity threshold for saccade detection was 40°/s. Fixations were defined by an absence of saccades and blinks (defined as moments without registered gaze positions) that lasted at least 50 ms. Participants sat about 60 cm away from the computer monitor. To minimize head movements and standardize the head position, we additionally used a chin rest. Prior to the recording, a nine-point calibration procedure was used. The paradigm was presented on a 24-in. widescreen TFT monitor with a resolution of 1,920 × 1,080 pixels.

Data Analyses

For the analysis of the data from the balloons test, the computer screen was divided into the left and right sides (area of interest). To identify changes in directed attention due to the placebo/nocebo treatment, the percentage of left-sided (relative to right-sided) fixations was calculated (mean percent of total fixations per trial, which was within the left area of interest: values above 50% indicate a left-sided bias, values below 50% indicate a right-sided bias). Further, the lateralization index (LI) (19) of the mean reaction time for targets on the left vs. right side was determined (positive values indicate slower reactions to left-sided targets; negative values indicate faster reactions to left-sided targets).

Separate repeated-measures 3 × 2 ANOVAs were performed for the percent of the left-sided fixations and the LI of the reaction time with the within-subject factors visual load (50, 100, 200 balloons) and treatment (nocebo OR placebo, control) for the placebo and nocebo groups.

In order to compare the attention bias between the placebo and the nocebo treatments, two separate ANOVAs for the difference scores for the percent of left-sided fixations [treatment (placebo OR nocebo) minus control] and LI reaction time [treatment (placebo OR nocebo) minus control] were computed with visual load (50, 100, 200 balloons) as within-subjects factor and group (placebo, nocebo) as between-subjects factor.

To assess possible group differences in affective states, separate ANOVAs including the within-subjects factor time of measurement (before, after search task) and the between-subjects factor group were computed for the difference score of valence, arousal, and dominance [treatment (placebo OR nocebo) minus control]. We report Bonferroni adjusted p-values and partial eta squared ($\eta 2p$) as effect size measure.

RESULTS

Eye-Tracking

Descriptive statistics for the left-sided bias (fixations and reaction times) in the placebo and nocebo groups are displayed in **Table 1**.

Placebo: The conducted ANOVA for the percentages of left-sided fixations and LI reaction time in the placebo group revealed no significant main effects or interactions for the factor treatment (all $p > .06$).

Nocebo: In the nocebo group, the ANOVAs for fixation count [$F(1, 19) = 18.65, p < 0.001, \eta 2p = .495$] and LI reaction time [$F(1, 19) = 13.01, p = .002, \eta 2p = .406$] showed a significant main effect treatment. More left-sided fixations were observed, and reaction time for left-sided targets (in relation to right-sided targets) was lower in the nocebo condition compared with the control condition. The interactions treatment × visual load revealed no significant results ($p > .18$).

Placebo vs. Nocebo: The conducted ANOVA for left-sided fixations in the sTMS condition relative to the control condition showed a significant main effect group [$F(1, 38) = 4.426, p = 0.042, \eta 2p = .104$]. The nocebo group displayed more left-sided fixations due to the treatment than the placebo group. Other effects were not significant (all $p > .09$). Means and standard errors for left-sided fixations (treatment minus control) are displayed in **Figure 3**.

The ANOVA for the differences in LI reaction time (treatment minus control) revealed a significant main effect group [$F(1, 38) = 7.12, p = 0.011, \eta 2p = .158$] and a significant interaction group × visual load [$F(2, 76) = 4.41, p = 0.015, \eta 2p = .104$]. The conducted *post hoc t*-tests showed that sTMS decreased response times for left-sided targets in the nocebo group in comparison with the placebo group in the high-load condition ($p = .001$) but not in the low- and medium-load conditions (both $p > .15$). The main effect visual load was not significant ($p > .70$). Means and standard errors for LI scores are shown in **Figure 4**.

TABLE 1 | Percentages of left-sided fixations and LI reaction time (means and standard errors) in the placebo and nocebo groups (treatment minus control) for the different visual load levels.

	Placebo group						Nocebo group					
	Placebo treatment			Control			Nocebo treatment			Control		
	Low	Medium	High	Low	Medium	High	Low	Medium	High	Low	Medium	High
Left-sided fixations (%)	51.08 (1.89)	51.91 (1.81)	52.44 (2.09)	49.11 (2.07)	50.76 (2.46)	53.73 (2.08)	55.26 (2.54)	53.08 (2.70)	55.75 (2.01)	50.16 (2.81)	46.23 (2.09)	53.49 (1.89)
Reaction time (LI)	–.005 (.031)	.013 (.043)	–.110 (.053)	.110 (.049)	–.002 (.0538)	–.217 (.056)	–.048 (.036)	–.110 (.045)	–.246 (.035)	.013 (.053)	–.009 (.046)	–.048 (.051)

Visual load conditions (low: 50, medium: 100, high: 200 distractors); left-sided fixations (above 50% = more left-sided fixations); reaction time LI (lateralization index): negative values indicate faster reactions to left-sided targets.

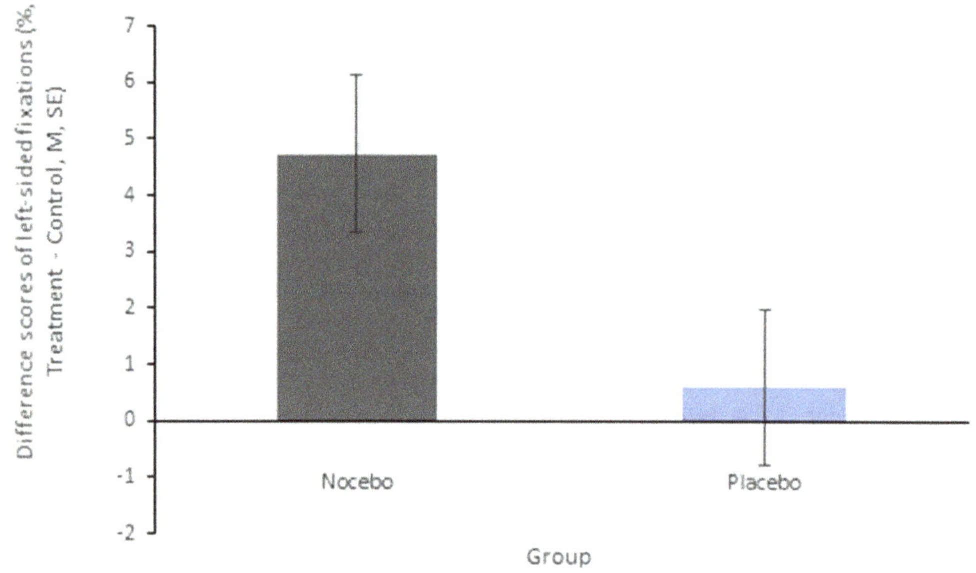

FIGURE 3 | Mean difference scores and standard errors for percentages of left-sided fixations for the main effect group. Positive values indicate a higher percentage of left-sided fixations in the treatment condition (placebo or nocebo) compared with the control condition.

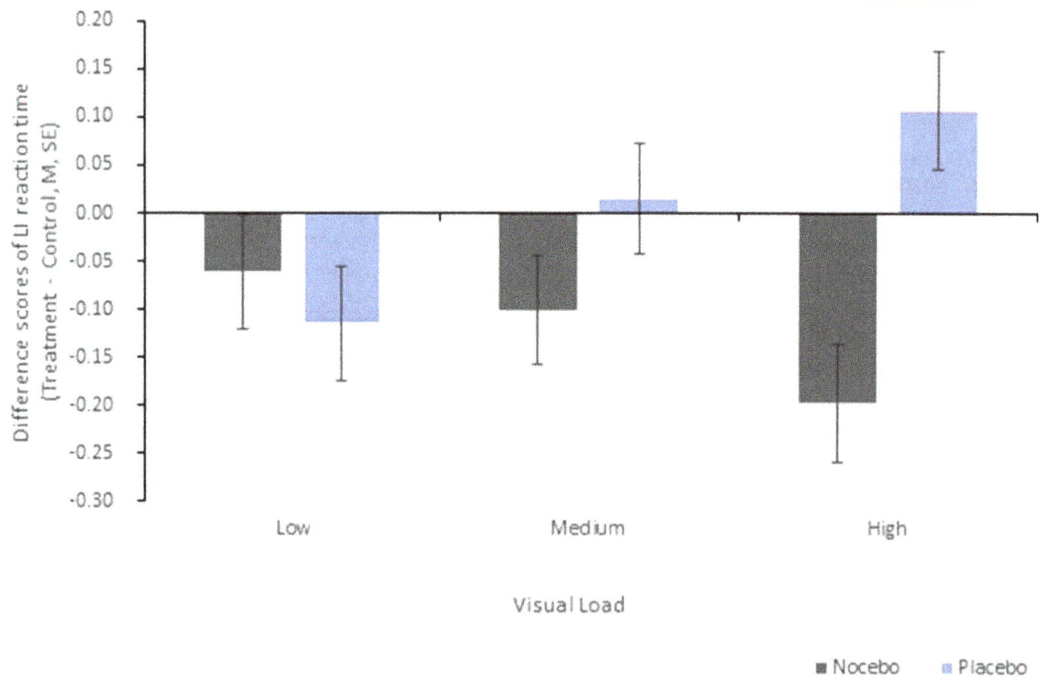

FIGURE 4 | Mean difference scores and standard errors for the lateralization index reaction time for the interaction group × visual load. Negative values indicate faster reactions for left-sided targets in the treatment condition compared with the control condition.

Self-Report

Affective ratings: The ANOVAs for the difference scores of arousal and dominance revealed a significant main effect group. The nocebo group reported higher arousal [$F(1, 38) = 4.43$, $p = 0.042$, $\eta 2p = .104$] and lower dominance [$F(1, 38) = 9.08$, $p = 0.005$, $\eta 2p = .193$] in the treatment relative to the control condition. The conducted ANOVA for the difference scores of valence (treatment minus control) produced no significant results (all $p > .17$). Means and standard errors for the affective ratings can be found in the **Supplementary Table S2.**

Reported symptoms: The following nocebo-induced symptoms were reported by the nocebo group: slower search behavior

(40%), heavy eye-lid (30%), blurred vision (20%), reduced concentration (45%), and other nonspecific symptoms (60%, e.g., numbness in the left side of the body). The placebo group reported: enhanced concentration (70%), faster search behavior (45%), twitching of the eyelids (5%), perceptual changes (10%, e.g., left-sided targets appeared bigger), and other nonspecific symptoms (15%, e.g., increased sensitivity in the left side of the body) in the treatment condition.

An exploratory correlation analysis indicated that the treatment-related affective changes [treatment (placebo or nocebo) minus control] in arousal, dominance, and valence (before, as well as after the search task) were not associated with the placebo/nocebo responsiveness (percentages of left-sided fixations and LI reaction time during sTMS; all $p > .11$).

DISCUSSION

This eye-tracking study directly compared the effects of a placebo and a nocebo on visuospatial attention in healthy individuals. The participants reported experiencing improved attention in the placebo condition, although no changes in gaze behavior and reaction time occurred. Contrary to this, the nocebo significantly increased the number of left-sided fixations and decreased reaction time for left-sided compared with right-sided targets, especially in the condition with the highest visual load. Thus, the placebo had no effects on attention, whereas the nocebo exerted effects in the opposite direction of the verbal suggestion.

These results indicate a more beneficial effect of a nocebo, relative to a placebo, for the first time. The suggestion of a deficit in the nocebo group seemed to have prompted a need for compensation, and thus elicited a paradoxical effect. In other words, the suggestion of negative symptoms actually led to improvement. To the best of our knowledge, this is the first report on positive nocebo effects. In contrast, paradoxical placebo effects have been described before. Here, a sham treatment introduced as an agent to reduce symptoms actually made a condition worse or elicited negative side effects [for a review see (20)].

According to the present results, paradoxical interventions could be more effective than a common goal-directed placebo intervention, at least in some cases. In psychotherapy, the usefulness of paradoxical interventions has long been recognized. Particularly, when the commitment to change or therapy motivation is low, paradoxical interventions can be helpful for achieving therapy goals [e.g., Ref. (21)]. This especially applies to neuropsychological therapy where lack of compliance is a common problem in patients with disorders such as anosognosia (e.g., hemiplegia, aphasia; visual neglect). These patients are not aware of their deficit and therefore do not use, or pursue learning, compensatory strategies (22). In this specific case, nocebo interventions could open new doors in neuropsychological therapy, perhaps helping achieve positive therapy outcomes when goal-directed suggestions do not work.

The placebo group also found the treatment to be effective and experienced a subjective increase in left-sided attention. Objectively, however, this was not present. To explain this, it is very likely that the participants reduced their individual effort during the search task because of the assumed support by the sTMS treatment. This might even be considered a negative placebo effect because the participants overestimated their own attention abilities. Partly in line with this effect, when sTMS was applied, participants in the placebo group described themselves as generally more relaxed and self-confident (i.e., lower arousal and increased dominance) than those in the nocebo group. In any case, these effects portray an interesting dissociation between subjective and objective placebo/nocebo effects.

The findings of the present investigation raise basic questions regarding the possibilities and limits of placebo and nocebo treatments. It is known that placebos show differential effectiveness depending on the particular condition being treated. For example, substantial placebo effects have been found in the treatment of some disorders (e.g., depression, irritable bowel syndrome) but not in others (e.g., bacterial infections, the common cold) (23). In healthy individuals, pronounced effects have also been observed, such as when attempting to change emotional responses *via* placebo. Schienle et al. (5) administered a disgust placebo to their participants (labeled as an anti-nausea drug), while they were presented with stimuli commonly perceived as repulsive (e.g., spoiled food, excrements). The placebo reduced the intensity of experienced disgust by more than half of its original value.

In the present study, a neglect-like reaction was suggested to participants. Inducing "pseudo-neglect" (or "pseudo-unilateral attention focusing") may be more difficult because healthy individuals have no experience with this specific phenomenon. It has been argued that direct experience (conditioning) is the most powerful way of inducing placebo-related expectancies and associated placebo responses (24); in other words, more commonly experienced reactions may be more susceptible to placebo effects. In the present investigation, a left-sided improvement/reduction of attention was suggested. This is a very specific symptom. Healthy individuals are very likely more familiar with feelings of generally reduced or increased attention and alertness. When such general changes in attention have been suggested, visual search performance was able to be altered *via* placebo/nocebo treatment (3).

It is important to acknowledge the following limitations of the present study. We only investigated women due to sex-related differences in placebo/nocebo responses [e.g., Refs. (25, 26)]. Therefore, the results cannot be generalized to men. Moreover, we did not assess or control the intake of nicotine and caffeine prior to the investigation, which might have introduced unspecific effects on general visual attention. Further, since only placebo and nocebo responders were included in the analyses, the sample size was relatively small and only allows for conclusions regarding individuals who subjectively experienced left-sided attention improvements/deficits. Finally, the nocebo group reported higher arousal and lower dominance, which may reflect a higher subjective value of the suggested left-sided deficits (as compared with left-sided improvements). However, the affective ratings were not correlated with the responsiveness to the sTMS (e.g., percentages of left-sided fixations). Therefore, it seems unlikely that the nocebo effects were mediated *via* enhanced arousal.

In summary, the present results indicate an interesting dissociation between subjectively experienced effects of placebos/nocebos and the resulting behavioral changes.

AUTHOR CONTRIBUTIONS

CH and AS designed the study and wrote the manuscript. CH and JP recruited participants for the study, collected the data, and conducted the statistical analysis of the data.

ACKNOWLEDGMENTS

The authors acknowledge the financial support by the University of Graz.

REFERENCES

1. Wager TD, Atlas LY. The neuroscience of placebo effects: connecting context, learning and health. *Nat Rev Neurosci* (2015) 16:403. doi: 10.1038/nrn3976
2. Sterzer P, Frith C, Petrovic P. Believing is seeing: expectations alter visual awareness. *Curr Biol* (2008) 18:R697–R698. doi: 10.1016/j.cub.2008.06.021
3. Colagiuri B, Livesey EJ, Harris JA. Can expectancies produce placebo effects for implicit learning? *Psychon Bull Rev* (2011) 18:399–405. doi: 10.3758/s13423-010-0041-1
4. Schienle A, Übel S, Scharmüller W. Placebo treatment can alter primary visual cortex activity and connectivity. *Neuroscience* (2014) 263:125–9. doi: 10.1016/j.neuroscience.2014.01.016
5. Schienle A, Gremsl A, Übel S, Körner C. Testing the effects of a disgust placebo with eye tracking. *Int J Psychophysiol* (2016) 101:69–75. doi: 10.1016/j.ijpsycho.2016.01.001
6. Höfler C, Wabnegger A, Schienle A. Investigating visual effects of a disgust nocebo with fMRI. *J Integr Neurosci* (2018a) 17:83–91. doi: 10.3233/JIN-170041
7. Höfler C, Gremsl A, Schienle A. Nocebo and pseudo-neglect: paradoxical effects detected with eye-tracking. *Int J Psychophysiol* (2018b) 125:29–34. doi: 10.1016/j.ijpsycho.2018.01.014
8. Gremsl A, Schwab D, Höfler C, Schienle A. Placebo effects in spider phobia: an eye-tracking experiment. *Cogn Emot* (2018) 32(8):1571–7. doi: 10.1080/02699931.2017.1422698
9. Schmid J, Theysohn N, Gaß F, Benson S, Gramsch C, Forsting M, et al. Neural mechanisms mediating positive and negative treatment expectations in visceral pain: a functional magnetic resonance imaging study on placebo and nocebo effects in healthy volunteers. *Pain* (2013) 154(11):2372–80. doi: 10.1016/j.pain.2013.07.013
10. Schmid J, Bingel U, Ritter C, Benson S, Schedlowski M, Gramsch C, et al. Neural underpinnings of nocebo hyperalgesia in visceral pain: a fMRI study in healthy volunteers. *NeuroImage* (2015) 120:114–22. doi: 10.1016/j.neuroimage.2015.06.060
11. Kong J, Gollub RL, Polich G, Kirsch I, Laviolette P, Vangel M, et al. A functional magnetic resonance imaging study on the neural mechanisms of hyperalgesic nocebo effect. *J Neurosci* (2008) 28(49):13354–62. doi: 10.1523/JNEUROSCI.2944-08.2008
12. Freeman S, Yu R, Egorova N, Chen X, Kirsch I, Claggett B, et al. Distinct neural representations of placebo and nocebo effects. *NeuroImage* (2015) 112:197–207. doi: 10.1016/j.neuroimage.2015.03.015
13. Brickenkamp R, Schmidt-Atzert L, Liepmann D. Test d2-Revision: Aufmerksamkeits-und Konzentrationstest: Hogrefe Göttingen. (2010).
14. Cazzoli D, Rosenthal CR, Kennard C, Zito GA, Hopfner S, Müri RM, et al. Theta burst stimulation improves overt visual search in spatial neglect independently of attentional load. *Cortex* (2015) 73:317–29. doi: 10.1016/j.cortex.2015.09.009
15. Bradley MM, Lang PJ. Measuring emotion: the self-assessment manikin and the semantic differential. *J Behav Ther Exp Psychiatry* (1994) 25:49–59. doi: 10.1016/0005-7916(94)90063-9
16. Wager TD, Fields HL. Placebo analgesia. In: McMahon S, Koltzenburg M, Tracey I, Turk DC, editors. *Wall & Melzack's Textbook of Pain*. Philadelphia: Elsevier Health Sciences (2013).
17. Corsi N, Colloca L. Placebo and nocebo effects: the advantage of measuring expectations and psychological factors. *Front Psychol* (2017) 8. doi: 10.3389/fpsyg.2017.00308
18. Edgeworth JA, Robertson IH, McMillan TM. The Balloons Test: a test for visual inattention: Harcourt Assessment. (1998).
19. Wilke M, Lidzba K. LI-tool: a new toolbox to assess lateralization in functional MR-data. *J Neurosci Methods* (2007) 163(1):128–36. doi: 10.1016/j.jneumeth.2007.01.026
20. Rosenzweig P, Brohier S, Zipfel A. The placebo effect in healthy volunteers: influence of experimental conditions on the adverse events profile during phase I studies. *Clin Pharmacol Therapeutics* (1993) 54:578–83. doi: 10.1038/clpt.1993.190
21. Beutler LE, Moleiro C, Talebi H. Resistance in psychotherapy: what conclusions are supported by research. *J Clin Psychol* (2002) 58(2):207–17. doi: 10.1002/jclp.1144
22. Kerkhoff G, Schenk T. Rehabilitation of neglect: an update. *Neuropsychologia* (2012) 50:1072–9. doi: 10.1016/j.neuropsychologia.2012.01.024
23. Hróbjartsson A, Gøtzsche PC. Is the placebo powerless? An analysis of clinical trials comparing placebo with no treatment. *N Engl J Med* (2001) 344(21):1594–602. doi: 10.1056/NEJM200105243442106
24. Kirsch I. The placebo effect revisited: lessons learned to date. *Complement Ther Med* (2013) 21(2):102–4. doi: 10.1016/j.ctim.2012.12.003
25. Ondo WG, Hossain MM, Gordon MF, Reess J. Predictors of placebo response in restless legs syndrome studies. *Neurology* (2013) 81:193–4. doi: 10.1212/WNL.0b013e31829a33bd
26. Casper RC, Tollefson GD, Nilsson ME. No gender differences in placebo responses of patients with major depressive disorder. *Biol Psychiatry* (2001) 49(2):158–60. doi: 10.1016/S0006-3223(00)00966-5

Permissions

All chapters in this book were first published by Frontiers; hereby published with permission under the Creative Commons Attribution License or equivalent. Every chapter published in this book has been scrutinized by our experts. Their significance has been extensively debated. The topics covered herein carry significant findings which will fuel the growth of the discipline. They may even be implemented as practical applications or may be referred to as a beginning point for another development.

The contributors of this book come from diverse backgrounds, making this book a truly international effort. This book will bring forth new frontiers with its revolutionizing research information and detailed analysis of the nascent developments around the world.

We would like to thank all the contributing authors for lending their expertise to make the book truly unique. They have played a crucial role in the development of this book. Without their invaluable contributions this book wouldn't have been possible. They have made vital efforts to compile up to date information on the varied aspects of this subject to make this book a valuable addition to the collection of many professionals and students.

This book was conceptualized with the vision of imparting up-to-date information and advanced data in this field. To ensure the same, a matchless editorial board was set up. Every individual on the board went through rigorous rounds of assessment to prove their worth. After which they invested a large part of their time researching and compiling the most relevant data for our readers.

The editorial board has been involved in producing this book since its inception. They have spent rigorous hours researching and exploring the diverse topics which have resulted in the successful publishing of this book. They have passed on their knowledge of decades through this book. To expedite this challenging task, the publisher supported the team at every step. A small team of assistant editors was also appointed to further simplify the editing procedure and attain best results for the readers.

Apart from the editorial board, the designing team has also invested a significant amount of their time in understanding the subject and creating the most relevant covers. They scrutinized every image to scout for the most suitable representation of the subject and create an appropriate cover for the book.

The publishing team has been an ardent support to the editorial, designing and production team. Their endless efforts to recruit the best for this project, has resulted in the accomplishment of this book. They are a veteran in the field of academics and their pool of knowledge is as vast as their experience in printing. Their expertise and guidance has proved useful at every step. Their uncompromising quality standards have made this book an exceptional effort. Their encouragement from time to time has been an inspiration for everyone.

The publisher and the editorial board hope that this book will prove to be a valuable piece of knowledge for researchers, students, practitioners and scholars across the globe.

List of Contributors

Verena Hoffmann, Marina Lanz and Jennifer Mackert
Institute of Medical Psychology, Faculty of Medicine, LMU Munich, Munich, Germany

Timo Müller and Matthias Tschöp
Helmholtz Diabetes Center, Helmholtz Zentrum München, German Research Center for Environmental Health (GmbH), Munich, Germany
German Center for Diabetes Research (DZD), Garching bei München, Germany

Karin Meissner
Institute of Medical Psychology, Faculty of Medicine, LMU Munich, Munich, Germany
Division of Health Promotion, Coburg University of Applied Sciences, Coburg, Germany

Younbyoung Chae
Acupuncture and Meridian Science Research Center, College of Korean Medicine, Kyung Hee University, Seoul, South Korea

Ye-Seul Lee
Acupuncture and Meridian Science Research Center, College of Korean Medicine, Kyung Hee University, Seoul, South Korea
Department of Anatomy and Meridians, College of Korean Medicine, Gachon University, Seongnam, South Korea

Paul Enck
Department of Internal Medicine, Psychosomatic Medicine and Psychotherapy, University of Tübingen, Tübingen, Germany

Kristina Fuhr and Dustin Werle
Clinical Psychology and Psychotherapy, Department of Psychology, University of Tuebingen, Tuebingen, Germany

Lili Zhou, Huijuan Zhang and Xuejing Lu
CAS Key Laboratory of Mental Health, Institute of Psychology, Chinese Academy of Sciences, Beijing, China
Department of Psychology, University of Chinese Academy of Sciences, Beijing, China

Lawrence H. Price, Linda L. Carpenter and Audrey R. Tyrka
Mood Disorders Research Program, Laboratory for Clinical and Translational Neuroscience, Butler Hospital, Department of Psychiatry and Human Behavior, Alpert Medical School, Brown University, Providence, RI, United States

Xiaoyun Li, Cunju Bo and Li Wan
Key Laboratory of Cognition and Personality, Ministry of Education, Faculty of Psychology, Southwest University, Chongqing, China

Li Hu
CAS Key Laboratory of Mental Health, Institute of Psychology, Chinese Academy of Sciences, Beijing, China
Department of Psychology, University of Chinese Academy of Sciences, Beijing, China
Key Laboratory of Cognition and Personality, Ministry of Education, Faculty of Psychology, Southwest University, Chongqing, China
Department of Pain Management, The State Key Clinical Specialty in Pain Medicine, The Second Affiliated Hospital of Guangzhou Medical University, Guangzhou, China

Johannes A. C. Laferton
Department of Psychiatry, Brigham and Women's Hospital, Harvard Medical School, Harvard University, Boston, MA, United States
Department of Clinical Psychology and Psychotherapy, Friedrich-Alexander-Universität Erlangen-Nürnberg, Erlangen, Germany
Department of Clinical Psychology and Psychotherapy, Psychologische Hochschule Berlin, Berlin, Germany

Sagar Vijapura, Lee Baer, Alisabet J. Clain, Abigail Cooper, George Papakostas, Maurizio Fava and David Mischoulon
Depression Clinical and Research Program, Department of Psychiatry, Massachusetts General Hospital, Harvard Medical School, Boston, MA, United States

Rebecca K. Webster
Department of Psychological Medicine, Institute of Psychiatry, Psychology & Neuroscience, King's College London, London, United Kingdom
The National Institute for Health Research Health Protection Research Unit in Emergency Preparedness and Response, King's College London, London, United Kingdom

Lauren C. Howe
Department of Business Administration, University of Zurich, Zurich, Switzerland

Kate Faasse
School of Psychology, University of New South Wales, Sydney, NSW, Australia

G. James Rubin
Department of Psychological Medicine, Institute of Psychiatry, Psychology & Neuroscience, King's College London, London, United Kingdom
The National Institute for Health Research Health Protection Research Unit in Emergency Preparedness and Response, King's College London, London, United Kingdom

Charlotte R. Blease
Program in Placebo Studies, Beth Israel Deaconess Medical Center, Harvard Medical School, Boston, MA, United States
School of Psychology, University College Dublin, Dublin, Ireland

Kari A. Leibowitz and Alia J. Crum
Department of Psychology, Stanford University, Stanford, CA, United States

Hojjat Daniali
Department of Humanity Sciences, Shahed University, Tehran, Iran

Arve Flaten
Department of Psychology, Norwegian University of Science and Technology, Trondheim, Norway

Marko Curkovic
Department for Diagnostics and Intensive Care, University Psychiatric Hospital Vrapce, Zagreb, Croatia

Andro Kosec
Department of Otorhinolaryngology and Head and Neck Surgery, University Hospital Center Sestre Milosrdnice, Zagreb, Croatia

Aleksandar Savic
Department for Diagnostics and Intensive Care, University Psychiatric Hospital Vrapce, Zagreb, Croatia
Department of Psychiatry, University of Zagreb School of Medicine, Zagreb, Croatia

Piotr Gruszka
Mental Health Research and Treatment Center, Faculty of Psychology, Ruhr-Universität Bochum, Bochum, Germany

W.M. Evers
Health, Medical and Neuropsychology Unit, Institute of Psychology, Faculty of Social and Behavioral Sciences, Leiden University, Leiden, Netherlands
Leiden Institute for Brain and Cognition, Leiden University, Leiden, Netherlands
Department of Psychiatry, Leiden University Medical Center, Leiden, Netherlands

Paul Enck and Stephan Zipfel
Psychosomatic Medicine and Psychotherapy, Department of Internal Medicine VI, University Hospital Tübingen, Tübingen, Germany

Sigrid Elsenbruch, Till Roderigo and Sven Benson
Institute of Medical Psychology and Behavioral Immunobiology, University Hospital Essen, Essen, Germany

Christoph Burger
Department of Basic Psychological Research and Research Methods, Faculty of Psychology, University of Vienna, Vienna, Austria
Department of Applied Psychology: Work, Education and Economy, Faculty of Psychology, University of Vienna, Vienna, Austria

Mark P. Jensen
Department of Rehabilitation Medicine, University of Washington, Seattle, WA, United States

Suzanne G. Helfer
Department of Psychology, Adrian College, Adrian, MI, United States

Kirsten Barnes and Ben Colagiuri
School of Psychology, University of Sydney, Sydney, NSW, Australia

Andrew L. Geers
Department of Psychology, University of Toledo, Toledo, OH, United States

Alexander Winkler and Christiane Hermann
Department of Clinical Psychology and Psychotherapy, Justus-Liebig-University, Giessen, Germany

Irving Kirsch
Harvard Medical School, Boston, MA, United States

Fabian Wolters and Kaya J. Peerdeman
Health, Medical and Neuropsychology Unit, Institute of Psychology, Faculty of Social and Behavioral Sciences, Leiden University, Leiden, Netherlands
Leiden Institute for Brain and Cognition, Leiden University, Leiden, Netherlands

Alvisa Palese
Department of Medical Sciences, University of Udine, Udine, Italy

Przemysław Bąbel
Pain Research Group, Institute of Psychology, Jagiellonian University, Kraków, Poland

Giacomo Rossettini, Tommaso Geri, Mattia Mirandola, Fabio Tortella and Marco Testa
Department of Neuroscience, Rehabilitation, Ophthalmology, Genetics, Maternal and Child Health, University of Genova, Savona, Italy

Stefanie H. Meeuwis, Henriët van Middendorp and Dieuwke S. Veldhuijzen
Health, Medical and Neuropsychology Unit, Faculty of Social and Behavioural Sciences, Institute of Psychology, Leiden University, Leiden, Netherlands
Leiden Institute for Brain and Cognition, Leiden University Medical Center, Leiden, Netherlands

Antoinette I. M. van Laarhoven and Andrea W. M. Evers
Health, Medical and Neuropsychology Unit, Faculty of Social and Behavioural Sciences, Institute of Psychology, Leiden University, Leiden, Netherlands
Leiden Institute for Brain and Cognition, Leiden University Medical Center, Leiden, Netherlands
Department of Psychiatry, Leiden University Medical Center, Leiden, Netherlands

Adriana P.M. Lavrijsen
Department of Dermatology, Leiden University Medical Center, Leiden, Netherlands

Carina Höfler, Jonas Potthoff and Anne Schienle
Department of Clinical Psychology, University of Graz, Graz, Austria

Index

R

S

T

V

W